Outdoor Emergency Care

*Comprehensive First Aid
for Nonurban Settings*

Outdoor Emergency Care

Comprehensive First Aid for Nonurban Settings

Second Edition

Warren D. Bowman, M.D.

The material in this text and in the National Ski Patrol System, Inc. Winter Emergency Care program is consistent with universally accepted standards of emergency and medical care that have been endorsed by many respected medical groups and authorities. The National Ski Patrol cannot and does not accept any responsibility for liability claims that may develop as the result of specialized applications of the text material of this outdoor emergency care publication in situations other than the purposes for which this course was created, as discussed in the Introduction and Appendix C.

Credits

Education Director: Judy Over
Editor: Rebecca W. Ayers
Graphic Designer/Illustrator:
   Reata Bitter, Bitter-Sweet Studio
Typography: About Faces
Printer: American Web

Cover Photos: Background photo by Bob Winsett for Ski the Summit, Colorado. Inset photos (top row, left to right) by Jack Affleck for Vail, Colorado; and Deer Valley Resort; (middle row) Bob Winsett for Ski the Summit; and Larry Pierce for Steamboat Springs, Colorado; (bottom row) Ben Blankenburg for Ski the Summit; and Lori Adamski-Peek for Park City Ski Area, Utah.

ISBN 0-929752-01-5

Library of Congress
Card Catalog Number 93-84167

Printed in the United States of America

Table of Contents

Acknowledgements   vii

About the Author   ix

Part I

	Introduction	2
Chapter 1	Adapting to the Outdoor Environment	8
Chapter 2	Overview of Human Anatomy and Physiology	32
Chapter 3	Surface Anatomy and Vital Signs	64
Chapter 4	Basic Patient Assessment and Life Support Techniques	82
Chapter 5	Oxygen and Other Types of Respiratory System Support	112
Chapter 6	Bleeding and Shock	124
Chapter 7	Skin and Soft-tissue Injuries, Burns, and Bandaging	136
Chapter 8	Emergency Care of Bone and Joint Injuries: General Principles	152
Chapter 9	Mechanisms and Patterns of Injury	178
Chapter 10	Specific Injuries to the Upper Extremity	186
Chapter 11	Specific Injuries to the Lower Extremity and Pelvis	196
Chapter 12	Injuries to the Head, Eye, Face, and Throat	210
Chapter 13	Injuries to the Neck and Back	226
Chapter 14	Chest Injuries	244
Chapter 15	Injuries to the Abdomen, Pelvis, and Genitalia	256
Chapter 16	Common Medical Complaints	266
Chapter 17	Medical Emergencies	286
Chapter 18	Environmental Emergencies	306
Chapter 19	Advanced Assessment	328
Chapter 20	Extrication and Transport	354
Chapter 21	Ski Injuries	382
Chapter 22	Triage	392
Chapter 23	Poisoning	406
Chapter 24	Hazardous Plants and Animals	412
Chapter 25	Water Emergencies	426
Chapter 26	Emergency Childbirth	438

Part II

Appendix A	**Legal Aspects of Emergency Care**	448
Appendix B	**Basic Life Support**	454
Appendix C	**Principles of Wilderness Emergency Care**	474
Appendix D	**Emergency Care Kits**	496
Appendix E	**Examples of Useful Forms**	502
Appendix F	**Guidelines for Prevention of AIDS, Hepatitis, and other Bloodborne Infections**	508
Appendix G	**Useful Knots**	512

	Glossary	516
	Index	534

Acknowledgements

Producing a textbook of this magnitude would have been impossible without many useful suggestions and contributions from members of the National Ski Patrol and others interested in outdoor emergency care. The entire manuscript has been reviewed in depth by members of the National Ski Patrol's Winter Emergency Care Program Administration Committee (WECPAC), the National Medical Advisory Committee, the Winter Emergency Care Supervisors, and a special Expert Medical Review Committee composed of nationally known experts in prehospital emergency care.

The author is particularly indebted to Executive Director Steve Over and to the National Ski Patrol Board of Directors for their strong support, to Education Director Judy Over for compiling and reviewing the text and illustrations, to Communications Director Rebecca W. Ayers for editing the manuscript and overseeing production, to Reata Bitter for her excellent graphic design and illustrations, and to my secretary, Luann Pfeiffer, for her timely and uncomplaining help.

The following persons reviewed the early drafts of the textbook:

National Ski Patrol Winter Emergency Care Program Administration Committee

Jack Mason
Jeff Olsen
Warren Bowman, M.D.
John Clair
Mary Davis
Daven Decker
Kathy Ferrigan
Dick Pearson
*Marlen Guell
*John Chandler, M.D.
*Carol Smith
*Doug Carlberg

National Medical Advisory Committee

Kevin Park, M.D.
    Alaska Division
Nancy Brooke, M.D.
    Central Division
Fred Spannaus, M.D.
    Eastern Division
Les Folio, D.O.
    European Division
David Chittenden, M.D.
    Far West Division
William Fogarty, M.D.
    Intermountain Division
*T. W. McCowin, M.D.
    Intermountain Division
Jon Anderson, M.D.
    Northern Division
David Herfindahl, M.D.
    Pacific Northwest Division
*Roger Sherman, M.D.
    Professional Division
John (Chip) Woodland, M.D.
    Professional Division
Mark Frank, M.D.
    Rocky Mountain Division
Kermit Lowry, Jr., M.D.
    Southern Division

Division Winter Emergency Care Supervisors

Paul Brooks
    Alaska Division
*Ray Clouatre
    Alaska Division
Kotaro (Jim) Hori
    USSP-Asia Division
Janet Bell
    Central Division
Kathy Ferrigan
    Central Division
Carl Roloff
    Central Division
Kenneth LaPlante, Jr.
    Eastern Division
James Miller
    Eastern Division
Mary Murrett
    Eastern Division
Howard Wyandt
    Eastern Division
*Adam Cohen
    European Division
James DeWitt
    European Division
*Timothy Jankowski, O.D.
    Far West Division
RoseAnn Jankowski
    Far West Division
Tim O'Brien
    Far West Division
*Jack Wright
    Intermountain Division
Frank Ziebert
    Intermountain Division
*Douglas Follick
    Northern Division
Russell Sigman
    Northern Division
Robert Hendricks
    Pacific Northwest Division
*Dolores LaLiberte
    Pacific Northwest Division
Luann Dodge
    Rocky Mountain Division
Michael Schene
    Rocky Mountain Division
Mary Lou Argow
    Southern Division
*former committee members

Expert Medical Review Committee

Paul Auerbach, M.D.
Alex Butman, REMT-P
Peter Hackett, M.D.
Norman McSwain, M.D.
Joseph B. Serra, M.D.
Richard Withington, M.D.

The following persons contributed significantly to or reviewed specific sections of the text:

R. Morgan Armstrong
Cherry Blondell, BSN, RNC
Marc Bond, J.D.
David Calhoun, M.D.
Sandy Henry Call
James Dodge, M.D.
R. J. Frascone, M.D.
Harry Friedman
Walter Gregg, J.D.
James Harris, M.D.
Peter Hutchinson
John McGrath
Edward J. Otten, M.D.
Scott D. Phillips, M.D.
Thomas J. Puskas, D.O.
Richard Rech, Ph.D.
Peter Reitz, J.D.
Joseph Rich, M.D.
Robert E. Riddle
Bruce Ries, J.D.
Mike Shellito
Bernie Smith
Ronald M. Sturtz, J.D.
John B. Sullivan, M.D.
Robert Waddell II
Frances Walker

Special thanks are owed to the following people for their comprehensive review and constructive criticism:

Patricia Beagle
Marc Bond, J.D.
Alex Butman, REMT-P
John Clair
Mark Frank, M.D.
Jack Mason
Norman McSwain, M.D.
Mary Murrett
Carl Roloff
Richard Withington, M.D.

About the Author

Warren D. Bowman, M.D. specializes in internal medicine and hematology and has special interests in wilderness and mountain medicine.

Dr. Bowman has been a member of the Department of Internal Medicine, Billings Clinic, Billings, Montana, since 1960.

He is a clinical associate professor of medicine at the University of Washington Medical School. Dr. Bowman has been a member of the Beartooth Ski Patrol at Red Lodge Mountain, Montana, since 1964 and has served the National Ski Patrol as its national medical advisor since 1970.

He is a fellow of the American College of Physicians and a former governor of the Montana Chapter of the ACP. Dr. Bowman also belongs to the International Society for Ski Safety, the International Society for Mountain Medicine, and the medical commission of the Union International des Associations d'Alpinisme (UIAA). He is a member of the medical committee of the American Alpine Club and is a founding member, board member, and president-elect of the Wilderness Medical Society. He is former chairman of the medical committee for the National Association for Search and Rescue (NASAR) and a former board chairman of the Midland Empire Chapter of the American Red Cross.

As a ski patroller, Dr. Bowman also has served as Northern Division ski mountaineering advisor, has twice received the national award as outstanding administrative patroller, and was given the Minot Dole Award in 1990. He is a nationally registered avalanche and ski mountaineering instructor and holds National Appointment #3537.

Dr. Bowman is a member of the editorial board of the *Journal of Wilderness Medicine.* He has written many journal articles on medical subjects, textbook chapters on cold injury and wilderness survival, and first aid manuals, including the National Ski Patrol's *Winter First Aid Manual.*

This textbook is dedicated to the thousands of ski patrollers past and present who have spent untold hours in the wind and cold ministering to the injured and ill in the snowy mountains.

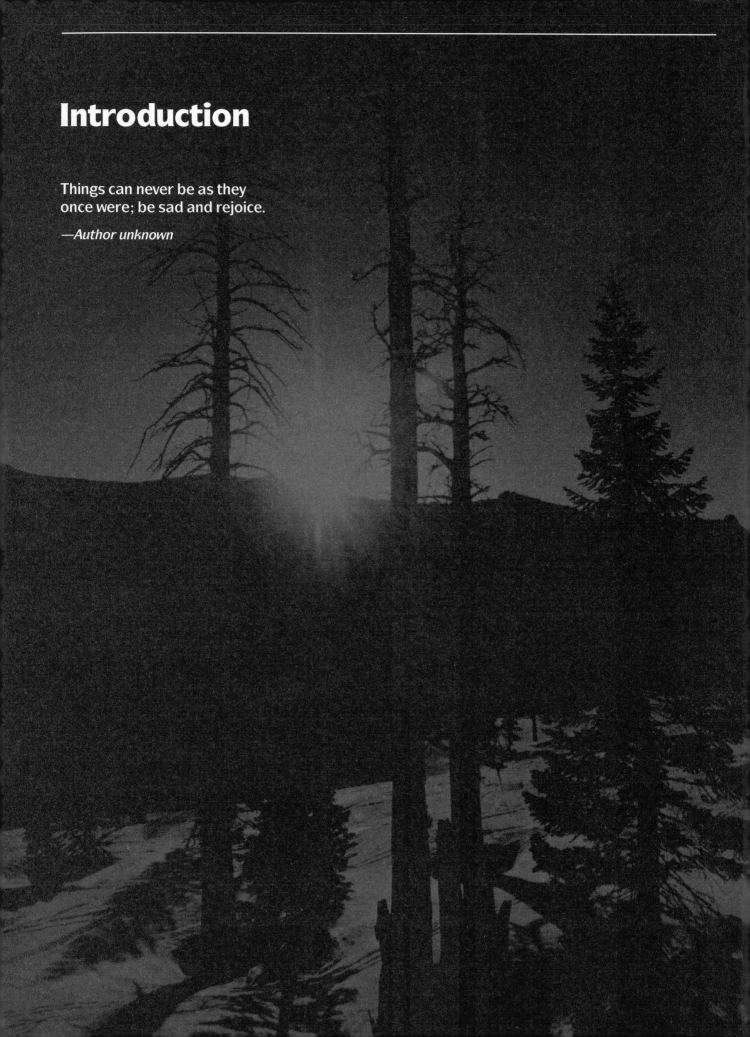

Introduction

Things can never be as they
once were; be sad and rejoice.

—*Author unknown*

First Edition

The discovery of sulfa drugs and antibiotics during the 1930s was the beginning of a revolution in medical care. As ancient scourges such as syphilis, tuberculosis, leprosy, smallpox, and malaria were controlled or eliminated, infection—once the greatest killer of mankind—was superseded by trauma and degenerative diseases. Hospital care also improved dramatically as new techniques of diagnosis and treatment were introduced and breakthroughs in technology led to the marvels of open-heart surgery, organ transplantation, and the artificial kidney. The care of the critically ill improved markedly with the development of the intensive care unit. (However, it remains to be seen whether the latest epidemic, acquired immunodeficiency syndrome [AIDS], will yield as easily to our efforts.)

Despite these advances, by the 1960s it was obvious that *care of the patient prior to reaching the hospital* had not kept pace with improvements in in-hospital care. Injuries were the leading cause of death and disability in children and young people, and the poor quality of prehospital care was a national disgrace.

In 1966, the National Research Council produced a landmark report, *Accidental Death and Disability: The Neglected Disease of Modern Society,* that stimulated a national effort to create the Emergency Medical Services (EMS) system, a closely-linked, interdependent network of emergency departments and emergency vehicles manned by trained emergency medical technicians (EMTs), prepared to reach patients rapidly, provide modern emergency care, and transport them to the hospital.

During this time, the American Academy of Orthopaedic Surgeons produced the EMT "bible," *Emergency Care and Transportation of the Sick and Injured*, based on the National EMS Standard Curriculum developed by the National Highway Traffic Safety Administration, United States Department of Transportation (DOT).

The EMS system has dramatically improved prehospital care, but, as noted by the National Research Council in 1985, every year one in every three Americans is injured and more than 140,000 die from trauma. There still is much to be done.

Before 1985, the National Ski Patrol (NSP) required its members to be trained in basic first aid by taking the American Red Cross Advanced First Aid and Emergency Care Course. Patrollers also had to complete a special course in winter first aid that emphasized training in high-altitude and cold-weather illnesses and injuries, ski injuries, and the special equipment and techniques used by patrollers.

The National Ski Patrol has always been in a unique position compared to other providers of prehospital care. In addition to caring for seldom-seen illnesses and injuries such as deep frostbite and acute mountain sickness, its members often serve in locations far from hospitals and frequently must provide care for an hour or more before patients can be turned over to the EMS system. Nordic ski patrollers and ski mountaineers can be many hours or even days from a doctor or hospital.

In the fall of 1985, the National Ski Patrol reexamined available first aid training courses. The American Red Cross Advanced First Aid and Emergency Care Course was designed primarily for urban laypersons with quick access to the EMS system. EMT training, primarily oriented toward heart attacks and auto accidents in an urban setting, was designed for ambulance attendants and, in some cases, was dependent upon radio support from emergency room physicians. Without extensive modification, neither of these two major training systems was suited to the needs of ski patrollers. These findings motivated the National Ski Patrol to develop its Winter Emergency Care (WEC) program, a new program in emergency care that reflects the NSP's primary concern with the winter environment.

Outdoor Emergency Care is designed as a textbook for the NSP Winter Emergency Care program. The knowledge and skills presented here are fundamental; they differ only as appropriate to the outdoor environment and closely follow the DOT's National EMS Standard Curriculum, 1984 revision. The WEC program's main purpose is to prepare ski patrol candidates without previous first aid or EMT training to handle the prehospital emergency care problems seen at an alpine or nordic ski area. However, because patient care in nonurban settings generally has lagged behind aid available in urban settings, this textbook is designed to be useful to *any* person who may need to provide first aid outdoors. The contents are not limited to cold-weather emergency situations. This textbook covers all types of outdoor problems, including patient care when definitive medical help may be hours or days away because of distance, adverse travel conditions, or communication difficulties.

Outdoor Emergency Care uses a carefully selected, minimal number of medical terms. The terms are defined when first used and are listed in the glossary. They are a form of shorthand: each one replaces several words or a sentence of nontechnical English, and all are commonly used in the EMS system. Serious rescuers who coordinate with the EMS system will find them useful and time-saving.

Other terms used in this textbook also need to be explained. First, the word "rescuer" is used to designate a ski patroller, backcountry search and rescue group member, leader of a backcountry recreational party, or any other person who provides care in an emergency. The word "patient" applies to the ill or injured person who requires such care. The author believes that this word—which in the past has referred only to persons cared for by physicians and nurses—is better than the alternatives. "Patient" has replaced "victim" in the EMS literature and is defined by *Webster's New Collegiate Dictionary* as "the recipient of any of various personal services." The term "victim" has unattractive implications of causation, the term "subject" is nonspecific, and the term "casualty"—commonly used in British Commonwealth countries—connotes trauma alone.

"Definitive medical care" refers to care given in a hospital or physician's office. An "emergency medical technician," or "EMT," is a person who has passed a basic or advanced EMT course sanctioned by his or her state and the U.S. Department of Transportation. "EMS system" refers to the interconnected network of hospitals, emergency departments, ambulances, helicopters, physicians, nurses, and EMTs that provides most prehospital emergency care. The terms "first aid" and "emergency care" will be used somewhat interchangeably, but the author prefers to use "first aid" for simpler techniques that do not require much equipment and that rely on speedy coordination with the EMS system, and to use "emergency care" for more sophisticated, EMT-level techniques where EMS interaction may be delayed.

In-depth material on anatomy and physiology is included to stimulate interest in understanding human body function and the location of important body parts, although some of this information may not be immediately applicable in emergency care.

Although specific descriptions of emergency care techniques are provided in this textbook, the student should understand that there is never only one "correct" way of managing a specific problem. Any technique that is consistent with well-recognized principles of anatomy, physiology and emergency care, does the job well, and does not injure the patient is acceptable.

The student will not become an expert care provider simply by studying this textbook or by successfully completing the National Ski Patrol Winter Emergency Care Course or other similar course. However, this course will furnish the groundwork for the continuing study, practice, and review necessary to be "worthy to serve the suffering." One aim of this textbook is to prepare the student to analyze and devise rational emergency care for unusual situations not specifically covered in training. To this end, special emphasis will be given to a solid foundation in anatomy, physiology, in-depth patient assessment for both injuries and medical illnesses, and improvisation of first aid equipment and techniques.

Warren D. Bowman, M.D., F.A.C.P.
National Medical Advisor
National Ski Patrol System, Inc.

The Billings Clinic
Billings, Montana
January 1988

Second Edition

Over four years have passed since the first edition of *Outdoor Emergency Care* was published. Since then it has been tested and critiqued, and it appears to have been accepted both by ski patrollers and others in the outdoor community to fill an empty space between orthodox emergency care textbooks and books on wilderness medicine.

Based on this experience, the second edition has been prepared with continued emphasis on the student. The goal has been to present information in a systematic and logical format so that the student can use this textbook as a tool for understanding and attaining knowledge about important and sometimes complicated concepts. All chapters have been brought up to date and in some cases expanded in line with changes in emergency care. Errors have been sought diligently and corrected where found. In areas where controversy exists—such as the care of accidental poisoning, snakebite, and spinal injuries—I have tried to present a consensus based on recommendations from the more experienced and credible authorities in the field.

I have had invaluable assistance from the scores of experts in prehospital emergency care who have read the first drafts of this second edition. They include experienced ski patrollers, physicians, nurses, paramedics, and EMTs. I owe each a great debt and have tried to give each credit elsewhere in the book. The ultimate decision on what to include in the book and what advice to follow has been mine, however. I accept the blame for any errors of omission or commission, and any suggestions or criticisms of its contents should be directed to me.

Basic anatomy and physiology, both normal and abnormal, are emphasized so that the student, when confronted with a situation not covered in his or her training, will have the tools to improvise the correct solution to the emergency care problem at hand. Both similarities and differences between injuries and illnesses are presented to help the student care correctly for patients with such commonly seen signs and symptoms as shortness of breath, abdominal pain, or shock—without the necessity for a precise diagnosis.

The nonurban aspects of illnesses and injuries continue to form the basis of this text, especially in the areas of prevention, the analysis of mechanisms and patterns of injury, and the improvisation of splints and other emergency care equipment. Medical illnesses— even minor ones such as nosebleeds and colds—are covered as well as injuries to familiarize the student with the management of common medical problems seen at home and in the outdoor environment.

Mechanisms of injury continue to be emphasized so the student will develop the habit of always thinking of how laws of physics and peculiarities of human anatomy and physiology can be used to predict the locations and types of injuries, particularly internal injuries.

In preparing this edition, I have tried to follow widely accepted principles taught in national training programs in prehospital trauma life support (PHTLS) and advanced trauma life support (ATLS), modifying these principles only as appropriate to the outdoor, nonurban environment. Although the knowledge and skills presented in this text frequently go far beyond those included in standard "First Responder" texts, I have tried to include all the components of the existing curricula developed by the U.S. Department of Transportation (DOT) and the American Society for Testing and Materials (ASTM).

The beginning student of emergency care may feel overcome and even prematurely defeated by the number of facts to be learned and new concepts to be mastered. Emergency care textbook authors and course instructors face with varying degrees of success the difficult job of organizing facts and techniques into easily grasped and remembered groups and trying to make the principles of anatomy, physiology, injury, disease, and emergency care understandable, clear, and retainable. These tasks are made easier if the following principles are understood beforehand by both student and instructor.

1. To some extent, the student already is familiar with his or her own body functions and structure, and has had some personal contact with illness and injury. The instructor can build on this knowledge and experience.
2. Unlike automobiles and other complicated machines, the human body is not reissued each year or two in a changed model.
3. The body has a finite number of ways to respond to the many injuries and illnesses that may affect it.
4. The number of emergency care procedures to be learned is limited. These support the body systems that have been adversely affected, no matter what the type of injury or illness.
5. The specific emergency care procedures required are fairly obvious if the student has a sound knowledge of basic anatomy and physiology. This knowledge allows the student to *adapt* to the challenge of each new problem and to *improvise* equipment and techniques if necessary.
6. Emergency care for many injuries and illnesses is temporary and/or unsatisfactory, and frequently the most important part of emergency care is to *transport* the patient as rapidly and safely as possible to *definitive medical care.*

Important basic changes from the first edition include the following:

1. Assessment is simplified so that the assessment of the *unresponsive* patient is identical to that taught in classes on basic life support or cardiopulmonary resuscitation. This means that the student has to learn only two types of primary survey rather than three: standard assessment and triage assessment. Among other things, this change is intended to improve the student's retention of basic life support knowledge and skills. Whenever a new system or body area is introduced, the assessment of that system or area is repeated in detail.

   A chapter on advanced assessment (Chapter 19) has been added. As the student progresses through the book, he or she is exposed to increasingly more complicated injuries and illnesses requiring more and more sophisticated assessment. Chapter 19 presents an overall view of assessment where the many possible findings are listed, and their possible meanings are recounted and discussed in detail.
2. New sections on Prevention of AIDS, Hepatitis, and Other Blood-borne Infections (Appendix F), Useful Forms (Appendix E), and Useful Knots (Appendix G) have been added. Since the core of basic life support is covered in Chapter 4, the first edition chapter on basic life support has become Appendix B.
3. Extensive use is made of scenarios. At least one scenario has been included in every chapter in which a scenario is appropriate; some have several. These are not brief para-

graphs where the student is given a short summary of the situation and asked what he or she would do. They are written in the form of a script, are quite detailed, and are intended to be realistic. It is hoped that, as the student concentrates on the scenario, it will be possible to imagine him- or herself a part of the action, getting a feel for how an experienced patroller or outdoorsperson handles increasingly complicated injuries and illnesses as the book progresses.

Other important changes include the following:

1. Chapter 4 (Basic Patient Assessment and Life Support Techniques) and Appendix B (Basic Life Support) have been revised based on the February 1992 National Conference on Cardiopulmonary Resuscitation (CPR) and Emergency Cardiac Care (ECC) as reported in "Guidelines for Cardiopulmonary Resuscitation and Emergency Cardiac Care," *Journal of the American Medical Association,* 268:16, October 28, 1992. It is not my intention to make recommendations that conflict with those of the organizations that will be responsible for developing the instructors' and students' guidelines for nationally taught courses in basic life support and CPR; however, publication deadlines have required me to make some assumptions about what these new guidelines are likely to be.

2. Vital signs have been moved into Chapter 3 (Surface Anatomy), where they logically belong.

3. Starting with Chapter 4, the term "rigid collar" is introduced to replace other terms such as "extrication collar" and "C-collar."

4. In Chapter 13 (Injuries to the Neck and Back), where practical, the logroll is de-emphasized in favor of the direct ground lift. The straddle slide has been dropped because it involves dangerous rescuer body mechanics. The use of short spine boards, vest-type devices, and scoop stretchers is deemphasized in favor of the direct ground lift both in Chapter 13 and Chapter 20 (Extrication and Transport).

5. In Chapter 25 (Water Emergencies), the "head splint" technique taught in the American Red Cross Lifeguard Course has replaced earlier methods of logrolling an immersion victim with a possible neck injury.

Important additions include the following:

1. The concept of increased intra-cranial pressure.

2. The neurosurgical emergency triad of decreasing responsiveness, increasing enlargement of one pupil, and increasing weakness on the opposite side.

3. Ineffective breathing and its care.

4. The need to pause during the primary survey to assess and provide care for causes of abnormal respirations and/or an abnormal pulse.

5. Critical Incident Stress Debriefing.

6. An adaptation of the "jams-and-pretzels" approach to extrication of a patient from a difficult location, as taught in the National Association of Search and Rescue (NASAR) Wilderness EMT course and other courses.

7. Snowboard and mono-ski injuries.

8. Childbirth complications such as breech presentation, twinning, hemorrhage, fetal death, abruption of the placenta, placenta previa, and toxemia of pregnancy.

Warren D. Bowman, M.D., F.A.C.P.
National Medical Advisor
National Ski Patrol System, Inc.

The Billings Clinic
Billings, Montana
January 1993

Chapter 1

Adapting to the Outdoor Environment

If the external air is of a high temperature, it does not take up the superfluous heat of the body fast enough, and we complain of too much heat: if it is very cold, it absorbs the heat too fast and produces the sensation of cold. To remedy this, we interpose a covering, which acting as a strainer, lets less air come into contact with the body, and checks the escape of the vital heat. As the atmospheric air becomes colder, more heat is conducted from the body. As it would be inconvenient in the day to be burthened with a mass of clothing entirely equivalent to great degrees of cold, we have to resort to fire and warm rooms to correct the state of the atmosphere, as a supplement to our clothing.

—Thomas Jefferson
  Notes on the State of Virginia

Most inhabitants of the Western world spend a large part of their lives in artificial cocoons, where indoor temperatures can be regulated; food, water, and clothing are easy to obtain; and shelter is always available. As a result, our ancestors' hard-won knowledge of how to survive in the wilderness is unlearned or forgotten. The underpinnings of technology that support modern living are fragile, as can be seen when a natural or manmade disaster occurs: the amenities of civilization collapse, and basics such as food, water, and shelter are difficult or impossible to obtain. Even a temporary power outage illustrates the thinness of civilization's veneer. Modern man is at a loss when electric stoves, refrigerators, furnace thermostats, and air conditioners cease to function.

Because of increased leisure time and a growing interest in outdoor activities, more and more people are spending their spare hours in non-urban environments—at times in actual wilderness. Some of these bring their "cocoons" with them, as can be seen any weekend in the recreational vehicle areas of Forest Service campgrounds. Others pride themselves on making do with a minimum of equipment. In either case, equipment failure, becoming lost, or a natural calamity such as a severe storm may suddenly require complete dependence on whatever mental and physical resources are immediately at hand.

The outdoor environment, particularly the wilderness, often is called "hostile" when, in fact, it is merely indifferent and impartial. Proper training and equipment, experience, good judgment, and the possession of at least a rudimentary amount of backcountry common sense can prepare anyone to enjoy the out-of-doors safely.

For basic survival, the human body needs a constant supply of oxygen; a stable core temperature; water; food; and a certain amount of self-confidence, faith, and the will to live. For comfort and optimum performance, the body also must be in top physical condition and free from disease and injury. Each of these requirements will be examined in turn, but they are obviously interrelated. For example, since most deaths in the outdoors in cold weather are due to injury, hypothermia, or both, maintenance of body temperature and physical integrity (through accident prevention) are probably the most important requirements for cold weather survival. However, dehydration, starvation, and exhaustion make temperature maintenance difficult and interfere with the rational thought and agility required to prevent accidents. Insufficient oxygen

Fig. 1.1 *The partial pressure of oxygen varies as air is taken into the body.*

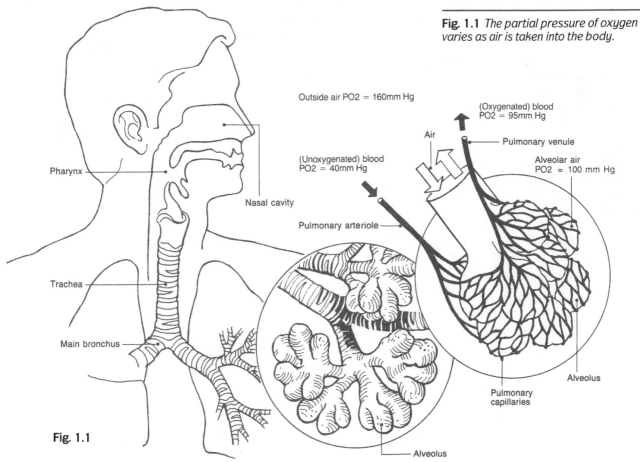

Fig. 1.1

Outside air PO2 = 160mm Hg

(Oxygenated) blood PO2 = 95mm Hg

Air

Pulmonary venule

(Unoxygenated) blood PO2 = 40mm Hg

Alveolar air PO2 = 100 mm Hg

Pharynx

Nasal cavity

Pulmonary arteriole

Trachea

Main bronchus

Alveolus

Pulmonary capillaries

Alveolus

becomes a contributing factor at extreme altitude or in the case of misfortunes such as suffocation due to avalanche burial or carbon monoxide poisoning due to cooking in an unventilated shelter. While abundant food and water will be of little value to the hypothermic person dying from insufficient clothing and shelter, lack of food and water will eventually be disastrous in an otherwise healthy and comfortable person.

During a survival experience, lack of self-confidence, faith, and the will to live may foster an attitude of panic and defeatism that tends to prevent one from taking timely survival actions such as preparing a shelter or lighting a fire. Poor physical conditioning or the presence of illness or injury will interfere with the body's ability to produce heat by shivering or other muscular activity, and will hamper wood gathering, shelter building, and other actions necessary for survival.

In a hot environment, the most important factors in survival are protection from the heat through proper clothing and shelter, and maintenance of the body's ability to cool itself by losing heat through radiation and evaporation of perspiration. Physical conditioning, hydration, and bodily integrity must be adequate to support a circulatory system that can accommodate increased skin circulation and sweat gland activity. Enough water must be available to maintain blood volume and produce perspiration.

Table 1.1

Survival Requirements

Oxygen
Stable body temperature
Water
Food
Faith and the will to live
Physical integrity

Oxygen

Air at sea level has a barometric pressure of 760 millimeters of mercury (mm Hg) and is composed of 21 percent oxygen and 78 percent nitrogen. The remaining 1 percent is made up of a small amount of carbon dioxide and trace amounts of rare gases such as argon and neon. From the standpoint of human survival and well-being, the most important physical property of oxygen is its **partial pressure,** i.e., the percentage of total air pressure accounted for by oxygen. At sea level, this is 160 mm Hg (0.21 x 760 mm Hg). When air is drawn into the lungs, it travels to the most distant parts of the respiratory tract, the **alveoli** (smallest air sacs of the lungs), where it is diluted by the carbon dioxide and water vapor found there. This dilution lowers the partial pressure of oxygen (PO_2) in the alveolar air to 100 mm Hg (Fig. 1.1).

The blood must provide the body cells with a constant supply of oxygen and must constantly remove carbon dioxide, a major waste product of metabolism. (This topic will be discussed further in Chapter 2.) The exchange of oxygen and carbon dioxide between the air and the blood occurs in the alveoli. The blood in the tiny alveolar vessels (capillaries) is separated from the alveolar air by two thin membranes: the walls of the capillaries and the walls of the alveoli, which together have a thickness of only a few microns (one micron = .000039 inches or .001 millimeter). An important law of the behavior of gases states that any gas tends to diffuse from an area of higher pressure into an area of lower pressure. Thus, the higher PO_2 in the alveolar air drives oxygen across the thin intervening membranes into the unoxygenated capillary blood, increasing its PO_2 from 40 mm Hg to 95 mm Hg, or just slightly below the 100 mm Hg PO_2 of alveolar air. (Similarly, the higher partial pressure of carbon

dioxide [PCO_2] in the capillary blood drives the carbon dioxide [CO_2] from the blood into the alveolar air where it can be excreted through the lungs). As the now oxygenated (arterial) blood circulates through the body, cells extract 58 percent of its oxygen (55 mm Hg), so that deoxygenated (venous) blood has a PO_2 of 40 mm Hg.

If the circulatory and respiratory systems are normal, a sea level atmospheric PO_2 of 160 mm Hg is more than adequate for normal body function. However, at high altitude or in the case of accident, injury, or illness, oxygen in the air is insufficient or normal transport pathways may be interrupted. Common examples of these circumstances are listed in Table 1.2. Each will be discussed in detail in following chapters.

Emergency care in each of these situations includes administering **medical oxygen,** which is described in detail in later sections of this textbook.

As one ascends from sea level, the barometric pressure drops by 20 mm Hg for each 1,000 feet (305 meters) of elevation (Fig. 1.2). At 10,000 feet (3,048 meters), the barometric pressure is two-thirds that at sea level; at 18,000 feet (5,486 meters), it is only half. The percent of oxygen in the air remains constant at 21 percent, but the partial pressure drops along with the barometric pressure.

If a person adjusted to low altitudes is taken suddenly to high altitude without supplemental oxygen, the lowest alveolar PO_2 at which that person can survive without immediately losing consciousness is 37 to 40 mm Hg, equivalent to an altitude of about 18,000 feet. At altitudes of 25,000 feet (7,700 meters) or above, death soon follows unconsciousness unless descent is rapid or supplemental oxygen is available.

Table 1.2

Causes of Interrupted Oxygen Supply

1. Insufficient Oxygen in the Outside Air
   a. High altitude
   b. Burial in a snow or dirt avalanche
   c. Poorly ventilated snow cave or other structure
   d. Malfunction of underwater breathing apparatus
   e. Near-drowning
2. Obstruction of the Upper Airway
   a. Relaxation of the tongue or pharyngeal tissues in an unconscious person
   b. Aspirated food, vomitus, dentures, or other foreign material
   c. Injury to the face or neck
3. Obstruction of the Lower Airway
   a. Inhaled foreign body
   b. Inability to cough up blood, pus, or mucus
4. Interference with Lung Function
   a. Acute
      (1) Filling of the alveoli with pus, blood, or fluid, as in pneumonia, lung hemorrhage, or pulmonary edema
      (2) Partial or total collapse of the lung because of blood, fluid, or air pressing on the outside of the lung
      (3) Spasm and thickening of bronchial walls and plugging of small bronchi with mucous, as in an attack of asthma
   b. Chronic
      (1) Thickening of the alveoli walls, as in pulmonary fibrosis
      (2) Loss of some alveoli, enlargement of others, and narrowing of the bronchi, as in emphysema
      (3) Replacement of lung tissue by tumor (benign or malignant)
5. Interference with Chest Integrity or Function
   a. Paralysis of the nerve supply to the diaphragm and/or chest muscles, as in spinal cord injury
   b. Crushing injury to the chest, as in flail chest caused by multiple rib fractures
   c. Open chest wound
6. Interference with the Brain's Control of Breathing
   a. Head injury
   b. Meningitis
   c. Stroke
7. Abnormal Function of the Circulatory System
   a. Illness
      (1) Heart attack
      (2) Chronic heart failure
      (3) Fluid in the sac around the heart
      (4) Blood clot in the lung blocking blood flow through its vessels (pulmonary embolus)
   b. Injury
      (1) Shock
      (2) Direct injury to the heart or blood vessels
8. Interference with the Blood's Oxygen-carrying Capacity
   a. Anemia
   b. Carbon monoxide poisoning

Despite these limitations, humans have walked to the summit of Mt. Everest (29,028 feet or 8,848 meters) without supplemental oxygen. Measurements on the summit of Everest have recorded a barometric pressure of 253 mm Hg, PO_2 of the inhaled air 53 mm Hg and alveolar PO_2 about 35 mm Hg. There also are permanent human habitations at altitudes close to 18,000 feet in the Chilean Andes and in Tibet. This is possible because the body is able to adjust to high altitudes by **acclimatization,** a process that is partly accomplished within several days but takes several weeks or longer to complete. The first stage of acclimatization is an increase in the rate and depth of breathing, or **hyperventilation,** which removes carbon dioxide and adds oxygen rapidly enough to raise the alveolar PO_2. The blood becomes more alkaline, which increases the ability of hemoglobin to take up oxygen. Later, the rate and depth of breathing are reset at a permanently higher level, the body produces more red cells to deliver more oxygen to the tissues, and the action of the heart and skeletal muscles becomes more efficient. People who live at high altitude develop larger chests and lungs, have higher pulmonary artery pressures, and have thicker blood because of the increased numbers of red blood cells.

Table 1.3

Summary of Acclimatization

Hyperventilation occurs.
Improvement occurs in the blood's oxygen-uptake capacity.
Improvement occurs in the blood's oxygen-carrying capacity.
The heart and skeletal muscle action becomes more efficient.

Figure 1.3 shows what happens to alveolar PO_2 and PCO_2 as travelers ascend to altitude. At about 8,000 feet (2,438 meters), the PO_2 has dropped enough to cause hyperventilation. The PO_2 drops more slowly after that, but the CO_2 drops faster as the hyperventilation washes it out of the lungs. This corresponds with the common observation that one "starts to feel the altitude" at about 8,000 feet. Serious diseases of high altitude (see Chapter 18) usually begin to occur at 7,500 to 8,000 feet (2,286 to 2,438 meters) and should be suspected in those who become ill within a day or two after arriving at these altitudes or above. This includes those who become ill after flying from their home at sea level to ski at 9,000 to 12,000 feet (2,743 to 3,658 meters) and sleep in base lodges at 8,000 to 9,000 feet.

Although **hypoxia** (lack of oxygen) is an important stress factor at high altitude, its effects are often hard to separate from those of cold, high winds, dehydration, exhaustion, hypothermia, and other stress factors commonly seen in the mountains. Climbers and ski mountaineers should have good equipment and be in good physical condition, well nourished, well rested, and free from illness and injury.

To encourage acclimatization, allow enough time for a slow ascent to altitude. Provide a rest day after ascending from sea level to 10,000 feet (3,048 meters), and limit altitude gains above 10,000 feet to 1,000 to 1,500 feet (305 to 457 meters) per day. Expeditionary mountaineers should "carry high and sleep low," i.e., ferry loads of supplies to a high cache and return to a lower camp for the night. Dehydration and hypothermia should be anticipated and prevented if possible. Time should be taken to melt enough snow for adequate water; meals and snacks should be frequent and nourishing.

During acute exposure to high altitude, the decrease in PO_2 can cause fatigue; weakness; headache; loss of appetite; nausea and vomiting; insomnia; shortness of breath on exertion; and Cheyne-Stokes respirations (waxing and waning of the depth of breathing with regular periods during which breathing ceases). These symptoms, which are discussed at greater length in Chapter 18, probably occur to some extent in everyone who goes rapidly from sea level to 8,000 feet (2,438 meters) or above.

Regulation of Body Temperature

Humans are called **homeotherms** because their metabolism is fast enough to produce heat as well as energy, and through effective mechanisms of heat production and heat loss they are able to maintain a relatively constant internal body temperature. A major benefit of homeothermy is that the body's enzyme systems, whose activity is affected by body temperature, are

---

Fig. 1.2 *Relationship Between Barometric Pressure and Altitude*

Fig. 1.3 *Changes in Alveolar Gases at Altitude*

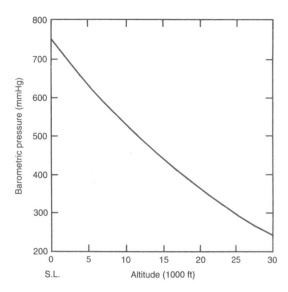

Pugh, L.G.C.E., *Journal of Physiology,* London 135, 590-610, 1957.

Fig. 1.2

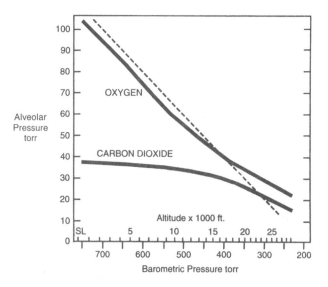

Houston, C.S., *Going Higher,* Little, Brown, 80, 1987.

Fig. 1.3

able to function efficiently all the time despite changes in the temperature of the environment. Humans and other warm-blooded creatures, unlike frogs, snakes, and other **poikilotherms** (cold-blooded creatures), do not have to lie in the sun to warm up enough to move.

The human body can be thought of as a heat-generating and heat-dissipating machine whose internal temperature is the net result of opposing mechanisms that tend to increase or decrease **body heat production, body heat loss,** and

Fig. 1.4 *Core and Shell Concept in Body Temperature Regulation*

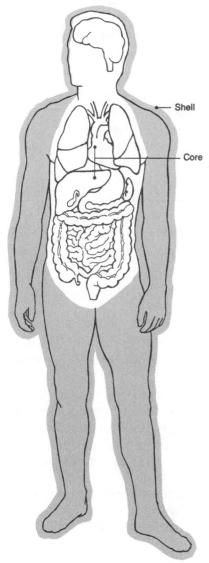

Fig. 1.4

Table 1.4

Methods of Increasing Body Heat Gain Above Basal

Involuntary	*Voluntary*
Shivering	Muscular activity
Foot stamping and other semiconscious activity	Eating
Non-shivering heat production, associated with the hormones:	Heat from hot food and drink
Thyroxin	Heat from the digestive process
Epinephrine	Heat from food metabolism
Norepinephrine	Stove, fire, sun

Table 1.5

Physical Mechanisms of Heat Loss and Gain

Conduction
Convection
Evaporation
Radiation
Respiration

the **addition of heat from the outside.** Through these mechanisms, internal body temperature can almost always be regulated successfully despite outside temperatures that can range from sub-zero temperatures to well over 100° F (47° C), depending on the season. Physiologic mechanisms that protect against excessive heat are better developed than those that protect against excessive cold.

When studying body temperature regulation, it is convenient to think of the body as being composed of a **core,** which includes the central nervous system, heart, lungs, liver, and other important internal organs, and a **shell,** composed of the skin, muscles, and extremities (Fig. 1.4).

Basal heat production, which averages 50 kilocalories per square meter of body surface per hour, is the result of never-ceasing internal metabolic processes. Additional heat can be produced by muscular activity such as shivering and exercise, by eating, by fever, and by exposure to

cold, which increases hunger and the release of hormones that stimulate heat production. Shivering can increase heat production four to five times above the basal rate; vigorous exercise up to 10 times. The body also can draw heat from external sources such as the sun, fire, and hot food and drink.

Heat is lost to or gained from the external environment in five ways: **conduction, convection, evaporation, radiation,** and **respiration.**

Conduction is the direct transfer of heat by contact, either from the warm body to a cooler object or from the cool body to a warmer object. The amount of heat transferred depends on the temperature difference and the speed with which the heat is conducted. Contact with metal or other materials that conduct heat rapidly may cause frostbite at low temperatures or burns at high temperatures. The speed of heat conduction from the body can be decreased by adding insulating clothing and increased by removing it.

Convection refers to the transfer of heat when air of a different temperature from that of the body moves across the body's surface. The amount of heat transferred depends on the speed and temperature of the air. When the air temperature is low and there is no shelter, exposure to high winds can cause dangerous heat loss. The speed of heat transfer by convection can be decreased by adding insulating clothing, especially if it is windproof, and increased by removing it.

Evaporation is the loss of heat when water or another volatile liquid on the body's surface is converted into vapor. Because of the high heat of vaporization of water (540 calories of heat are consumed during the evaporation of 1 gram of water), considerable heat can be lost through evaporation of sweat from skin or water from wet clothing. Evaporation is increased in the presence of wind and low humidity and is decreased in high humidity. This is a major source of beneficial heat loss in hot, dry climates. Frostbite caused by conduction and evaporation can occur when cold gasoline or other volatile organic liquids with freezing points below 32°F (0°C) are spilled on the skin.

Radiation refers to the transfer of heat to or from the body through infrared waves. Major amounts of heat can be lost by radiation from uncovered skin. This may be beneficial in hot climates, but people exposed to cold temperatures require adequate clothing to prevent dangerous loss of body heat by radiation. Warm head gear is especially important since considerable heat can be lost from an uncovered head because of its large surface-area-to-volume ratio and large blood supply. In hot climates, considerable heat can be gained by radiation unless the body is protected from the sun by clothing or shelter.

Body heat is lost through **respiration** as cool inhaled air is warmed to body temperature before being exhaled. The amount of heat lost depends on the outside air temperature and the rate and depth of breathing. Heat also can be gained by inhaling hot air.

To illustrate the relative importance of these mechanisms in losing heat, a resting body in still air of average humidity and a temperature of 70°F (21°C) loses 70 percent of its heat by radiation, conduction, and convection; 27 percent by evaporation; and only 3 percent through urine, feces, and the lungs. However, during hard exercise, evaporation can account for up to 85 percent of heat loss, while conduction, convection, radiation, and respiration together account for only about 15 percent.

carries otherwise would by lost by radiation, conduction, and convection. There is also some compulsion to decrease the body surface by curling up into a ball. A person can *decrease* heat loss *voluntarily* by putting on additional clothing for insulation and wind protection and by seeking shelter from the cold and wind. The body can *increase* heat loss *involuntarily* by increasing perspiration and by shunting hot blood to the shell. A person can *increase* heat loss *voluntarily* by taking off clothing and seeking shelter in a cool, breezy place. Conversely, heat gain can be increased *voluntarily* by increasing exposure to a heat source such as the hot sun or a fire, so that heat is gained by radiation, conduction, and convection.

The **human brain** is the most important organ for regulating body

Table 1.6

Methods of Decreasing Body Heat Loss

Involuntary	*Voluntary*
Decrease perspiration	Add clothing
Shunt blood away from the shell	Seek shelter from
Decrease body surface area (curl into a ball)	chilling mechanisms

Table 1.7

Methods of Increasing Body Heat Loss

Involuntary	*Voluntary*
Increase perspiration	Subtract clothing
Shunt blood to the shell	Seek shelter from
	warming mechanisms
	Expose more skin surface

The body has both **voluntary** and **involuntary** ways of decreasing or increasing heat loss or gain to stabilize its temperature. For example, the body can *decrease* heat loss *involuntarily* by decreasing perspiration and by shunting the hot blood away from the body shell, where the heat it

temperature. Conscious activities such as adding or removing clothing, seeking shelter from the environment, lighting a fire, eating and drinking, and regulating the amount of heat produced by muscular activity are more important than the body's automatic adjustments to excessive heat or cold.

Stabilization of Body Temperature

At moderate, comfortable temperatures, the body's core temperature is kept stable by constant, small adjustments in metabolic rate, muscular activity, perspiration, and skin circulation. When the body is chilled, **heat production** is augmented by a slight increase in the metabolic rate, by shivering, and by semiconscious activities such as foot stamping. At the same time, the body reduces **heat loss** by limiting perspiration and restricting blood circulation to the skin and extremities. As body temperature falls, the individual is compelled to curl up into a ball so that a smaller surface area is exposed to the environment. The brain tells the body to decrease heat loss by putting on more clothing for insulation and wind protection, and by stopping and seeking shelter. At the same time, the brain tells the body to increase heat gain by building a fire and having something to eat. Many of the body's automatic adjustments to reduce heat loss may preserve the core temperature at the expense of the shell temperature.

When the body overheats, there is a tendency to reverse these mechanisms. The body increases heat loss by increasing circulation to the skin and extremities and increasing perspiration. The body decreases heat production by resisting physical activity. A person will feel sluggish and languid, thus decreasing the amount of heat produced by muscular activity. The brain tells the body to decrease heat gain by seeking shelter from the sun, removing clothing, and fanning oneself.

The mechanisms of body temperature regulation work best if the body is well fed and hydrated, properly rested, and in good physical condition through regular exercise.

Table 1.8

Practical Ways of Decreasing Body Heat Loss

Use optimal insulation made of proper fabrics and proper lofting materials: wool, polypropylene, down, Dacron, polyester pile, foam, etc. Avoid cotton.
Use the layering principle so that clothing either can be added to prevent chilling or removed to prevent overheating and excessive perspiring.
Protect yourself from the wind to prevent windchill effect.
Use adequate coverings for body parts with a large surface-area-to-volume ratio (nose, ears, fingers, toes).
Avoid getting wet.
Avoid contact with cold substances.
Avoid excessive respiratory heat loss.
Avoid alcohol and nicotine.
Use a personal flotation device in water-related sports.

If these mechanisms fail to maintain body heat within the optimum range, injury can occur because of frostbite and hypothermia at one extreme or heat stroke at the other.

In summary, the body has three methods for avoiding dangerous degrees of cooling: it can increase internal heat production, add heat from the environment, or decrease heat loss (Table 1.8). The body also has three methods for avoiding dangerous degrees of overheating: decrease internal heat production, decrease heat intake from the outside, and increase heat loss (Table 1.11).

Adjusting to Cold Weather

Insulating garments can prevent heat loss caused by conduction, convection, and radiation. Because air conducts heat very poorly, the best garments for cold climates are those made of materials that trap a layer of still, warm air around the body and maintain this microclimate despite extremes of wind and cold. Some insulating ability is lost when garments are wet or when air spaces are reduced because the garment has become compressed or matted.

Suitable materials fall into two general groups: fibers woven into a fabric and non-woven fibers. In some cases a fiber, such as polyester, either can be made into a fabric or used as a filler. Some non-woven fibers can be incorporated into a fabric, as with polyester pile; others, such as down, are used only as a filler in quilted garments to provide loft.

Traditionally, the best and most practical insulating fabrics for cold-weather clothing have been made of wool, polyester, and acrylic; the best non-woven fibers have been down and Dacron. Wool has a special property: it remains warm even when wet because of its low wicking action and ability to suspend water droplets between its fibers without seriously affecting insulating ability. Polyester, Orlon, and related acrylic fabrics were developed to mimic the properties of wool at a lower cost. These fabrics are almost as warm as wool and are lighter, easier to dry, and less itchy. Cotton garments, particularly denim and corduroy, should not be worn in cold weather because they insulate poorly and become wet easily, which reduces their insulating value even further.

Down is unsurpassed for dry, very cold climates but is inferior to

Dacron in damp, moderately cold climates because wet down balls up and is harder to dry than wet Dacron. Foam, a lightweight plastic material containing multiple small air bubbles, is used to insulate boots, mittens, gloves, and sleeping pads.

There are a number of new fabrics woven from fibers that have lower thermal conductance, higher insulating ability, and better wicking action than conventional fibers. Examples include polypropylene, treated polyester such as Capilene, and hollow polyester such as Thermax. These new fabrics are popular choices for thermal underwear and shirts in particular.

Newer non-woven fibers include Hollofil II and Quallofil, which are hollow, synthetic fibers patterned after reindeer hair, and Thermoloft, a blend of solid and hollow fibers that trap air and block radiant heat loss. Thinsulate and Thermolite are microfibers that provide good insulating ability with lesser loft, allowing garments to be less bulky. Thermolite is claimed to block radiant heat well because its fiber diameter is the same (10u) as the wavelength of radiant heat. Polyester pile jackets are superior to wool sweaters because, in addition to being just as

warm, they are lighter, dry more easily, and do not shrink when washed.

Clothing should be **layered** to prevent both chilling and overheating. Layering allows flexibility because one or more layers may be added or subtracted as necessary. Three or four thinner layers are better than one or two thick layers. Overheating is undesirable because it increases perspiration, which can saturate clothing and increase heat loss

Fig. 1.5 *Windchill Chart*

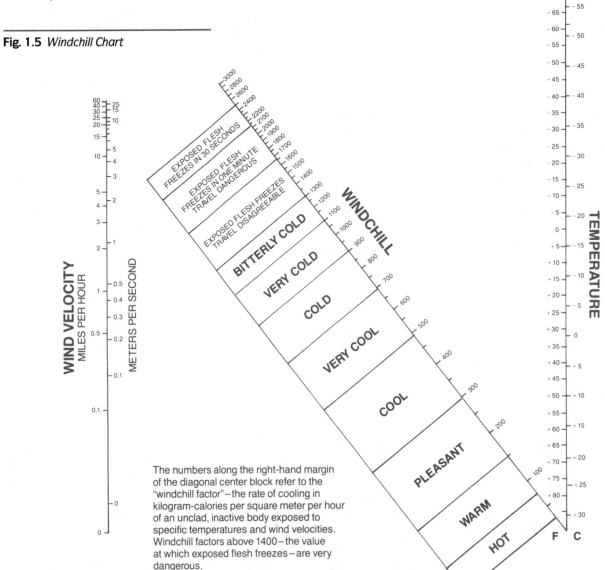

The numbers along the right-hand margin of the diagonal center block refer to the "windchill factor"—the rate of cooling in kilogram-calories per square meter per hour of an unclad, inactive body exposed to specific temperatures and wind velocities. Windchill factors above 1400—the value at which exposed flesh freezes—are very dangerous.

Fig. 1.5

Consolazio et al, *Metabolic Methods*, St. Louis, 1951, The C.V. Mosby Co.

through conduction and evaporation. Because water conducts heat away from the body 32 times faster than does air at the same temperature, wet clothing can cause rapid heat loss in cold weather. Wetting also interferes with the insulating ability of all fabrics to some extent, partly because it causes matting of the fibers with reduction of the air spaces.

Clothing should be selected with both climate and activity in mind. For example, an alpine skier who spends considerable time riding chairlifts and whose downhill speed generates significant windchill will need more layers of clothing than a nordic skier who generates more heat from muscular activity. Clothing should be easily adjustable. Sweaters, shells, and jackets should have high necks and full-length zippers that open from both top and bottom, and shells should have ventilation zippers at the armpits and upper arms. Zipper pulls should have tabs so they can be worked with mittened fingers. Outer layers should be sized generously so that inner layers can expand to their full thicknesses.

Windproof and water-resistant outer garments of nylon, nylon-cotton blends, or Gore-Tex will prevent heat loss from convection, conduction, and evaporation. These garments should include a ski or mountain parka and wind pants or warm-up pants.

As the wind velocity rises, the "effective" temperature drops (**windchill effect**). This concept refers to the *rate* of heat loss rather than the actual temperature reached as long as evaporation is not a factor. Figure 1.5 illustrates the relationship between actual temperature, wind velocity, and effective temperature at the skin surface—and underscores the necessity for windproof outer clothing and for seeking shelter during periods of cold and high wind.

Because a body in motion tends to create its own wind, a skier or snowmobiler is more susceptible to frostbite when moving than when stationary (Fig. 1.6). There is a marked danger of frostbite when the windchill factor is 1,400 or above (see Fig. 1.5), a range easily attained by a moving skier or snowmobiler when the temperature is -10°F (-23°C).

However, many skiers have suffered frostbite just by riding a chairlift while wearing insufficient clothing to protect from the wind and cold.

When the weather is cold, windy, and wet, such as during a blizzard at 32°F (0°C), evaporation, convection, radiation, and conduction combine to produce rapid heat loss. This can be a very dangerous situation for those caught unprepared (Fig. 1.7). To reduce heat loss from **infrared radiation,** wear a hat. At 5°F (-15°C), up to 70 percent of the heat produced by the body can be lost from an uncovered head. This occurs partly because there is no reduction in blood flow to the head in response to cold. The adage "if your feet are cold, put on your hat" is true (Fig. 1.8).

Prevent loss of heat from the respiratory tract by avoiding over-exertion and excessive heavy breathing. When temperatures are extremely cold, inhaled air can be warmed by protecting the mouth and nose with a hood, scarf, or neck gaiter (Fig. 1.9).

Fig. 1.6 *A moving person may be more susceptible to cold injury than a person at rest.*

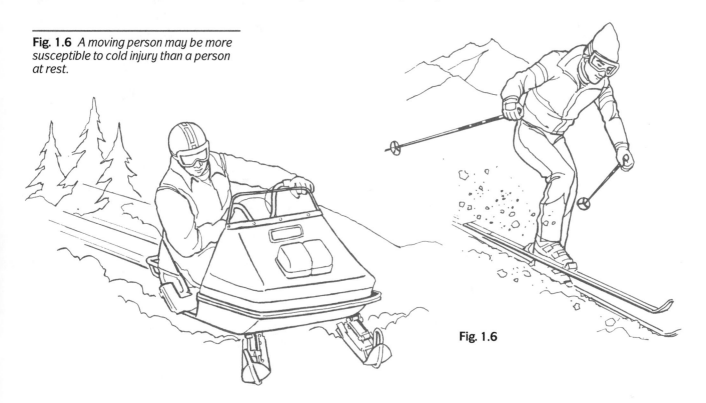

Fig. 1.6

Avoid heat loss from conduction by sitting on a toboggan, pack or log, rather than in the snow or on a cold rock or metal object (Fig. 1.10). Because bare fingers can freeze to ski bindings, crampons, and other metal objects, thin gloves (glove liners) should be worn. Avoid skin contact with gasoline or other volatile liquids with freezing points lower than water, because they will cause instant frostbite through conduction and evaporation (Fig. 1.11).

Heat loss from conduction and evaporation can be lessened by staying dry or drying off quickly when getting wet in cold weather. Ideally, outer clothing should be windproof, should not collect snow, and should shed water. However, outer clothing should not be completely waterproof because this will prevent evaporation of perspiration and cause inner garments to become wet. Designers who strive to create the ideal outer garment have a difficult task: to develop a fabric that will allow water to pass from the inside out but not from the outside in. At this time, Gore-Tex appears to do this best

although other good fabrics such as Thintech, Vapex, and Tactel are available. These garments are highly windproof, also.

Be sure to adequately cover the head, ears, hands, and feet. This counteracts the tendency of body parts with a high surface-area-to-volume ratio to lose heat rapidly by conduction, convection, and radiation. Coverings should not be so tight that they restrict blood circulation. If socks and mittens get wet, dry them or replace them with dry spares.

Heat production can be increased by increasing the level of muscular activity. If possible, walk

around, stamp your feet, swing your arms, and wiggle your fingers and toes (Fig. 1.12). If such activities combined with adding more layers of clothing do not work, it may be time to seek shelter.

Another way to keep warm is to eat. Food fuels metabolism, and the process of digestion creates heat as well. In cold weather, meals should be regular and snacks frequent. Alcohol should be avoided because it lowers blood sugar levels, increases heat loss by dilating small blood vessels in the skin, and interferes with judgment. Nicotine also should be avoided because it constricts small blood vessels in the hands and feet, predisposing them to frostbite.

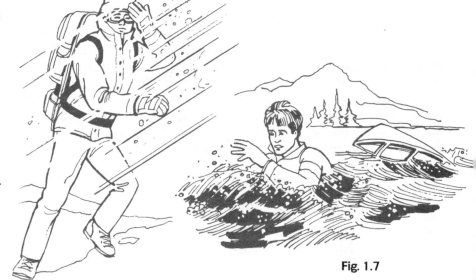

Fig. 1.7

Fig. 1.7 *The cold, windy, wet outdoor environment can be dangerous to those caught unprepared.*

Fig. 1.8 *Wear a hat in cold weather.*

Fig. 1.9 *A frost tunnel will warm inhaled air.*

Fig. 1.10 *Avoid unnecessary contact with cold objects.*

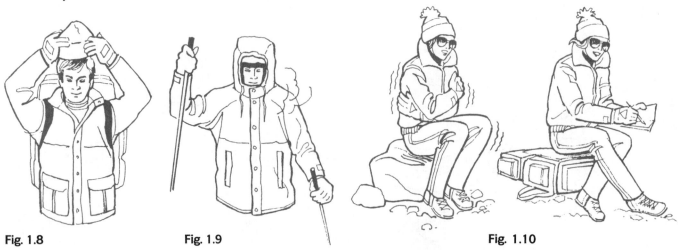

Fig. 1.8   Fig. 1.9   Fig. 1.10

Know when to quit and seek shelter. The rescuer should know how to build a fire under adverse conditions and know the basics of emergency shelter construction (Fig. 1.13). Emergency survival equipment always should be carried in the wilderness.

Sample Cold-Weather Clothing

A Four-layer System

The selection of cold-weather clothing (Fig. 1.14) depends upon the activity, expected temperature ranges, predicted amount and type of precipitation, and the expected altitude. For example, in the Coastal Alpine Zone (Cascades, Sierras, Appalachians), where temperatures are moderate and rain is common even in the winter, the rescuer should choose clothing made of materials that function well when wet, are easy to dry, and repel water (wool, polyester pile, polypropylene, Thermax,

Table 1.9

Sample Cold-Weather Survival Kit

Shelter-building equipment
Plastic or nylon tarp
Snow shovel
50 feet of 1/8-inch nylon cord
Folding saw

Fire-building equipment
Waterproof matches
Firestarter
Candle
Sturdy hunting knife

Signaling equipment
Whistle
Signal mirror
Card with ground-to-air signals
Flashlight
Two quarters for pay phone

Other
Compass
Map

Metal pot with bale
First aid kit
Toilet paper
Sunglasses
Sunburn cream
Lip salve
Spare mittens and socks
Canteen (full)
Emergency food
Extra layer of clothing, e.g., pile jacket, pants
Avalanche probe ski poles

Optional
Therm-A-Rest or piece of ensolite
Small ax (e.g., Hudson's Bay)
Stove and fuel
Snow saw
Sleeping bag

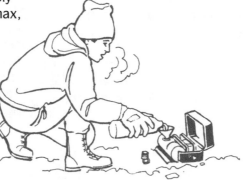

Fig. 1.11 *Avoid contact with cold liquids.*

Fig. 1.12 *Muscular activity increases heat production.*

Fig. 1.13 *Know when to quit and seek shelter.*

Fig. 1.11

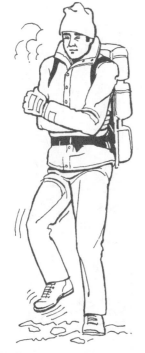

Fig. 1.12

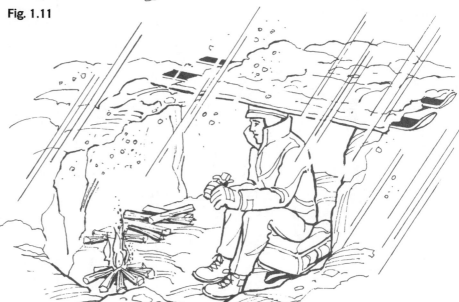

Fig. 1.13

Dacron, Quallofil, Gore-Tex). In the High Alpine Zone (Rocky Mountains and other inland ranges), where temperatures are lower and the rescuer is less apt to get wet, insulating value and windproofing are more of a concern, and down might be chosen over Dacron; nylon or nylon-cotton blends over Gore-Tex.

First Layer

Underwear: One-hundred-percent wool or 85-percent wool/15-percent nylon is a good choice, but is getting harder and harder to obtain. Thermax, Capilene, polypropylene, and blends of these are probably the new standard. Net underwear is satisfactory if it is made of wool. Synthetic combinations such as Thermolactyl and Duofold are adequate for alpine skiers; however, waffle-weaves and other types of cotton underwear are inadequate and should be avoided.

Socks: Wool and polypropylene socks are best. It is preferable to wear a pair of thin, polypropylene socks

---

Fig. 1.14 *Alpine skiers and mountaineers should apply the layering principle when selecting cold weather clothing.*

next to the skin topped with one or more pairs of heavy, wool socks.

Second Layer

Shirt: Wool, Capilene, polypropylene, and similar materials generally are the best choice; they should open completely in front or at least have a half-zipper. Turtlenecks protect the neck, as do mufflers and neck gaiters; either can be pulled up to protect the face. Orlon, nylon, or polyester blends are suitable fabrics for shirts and turtlenecks worn by alpine skiers.

Pants: Wool pants or knickers are preferable. The hard-finish wool pants found in military surplus stores are durable and reasonably priced. Downhill skiers should select pants or bibs of wool, part-wool stretch material, or quilted material. Cotton, particularly denim and corduroy, should be avoided.

Boots: Boot choice will depend on both the form of activity and the expected temperature. Boots should be roomy enough to accommodate a pair of polypropylene socks plus one or two pairs of heavy wool socks. The boots must be large enough so that the toes are neither cramped nor

likely to strike the end of the boot during downhill travel. To avoid cold feet and blisters, boots should be laced firmly enough so that the heel does not move but not so tightly that the toes cannot wiggle easily. Use gaiters in snow country to keep snow out of the tops of the boots; they should be high enough to reach the knee and are easier to get off and on if they open in front.

For moderate temperatures, lightweight fabric/leather boots are ideal for light-duty trail hiking and scrambling, but for rugged off-trail work, use sturdy full-thickness leather climbing boots 6 to 8 inches in height with rubber lug soles. Double mountaineering boots work well for the colder temperatures of winter mountaineering. These boots consist of outer boots made of leather, plastic, or nylon, and inner boots insulated with felt or foam. Boots used for ice climbing and high-angle cramponing need to be especially stiff. Boots with a removable felt inner liner such as the Sorel work well for snowshoeing and other types of nontechnical activities. For ski touring, telemarking, and ski mountaineering, special single and double ski boots

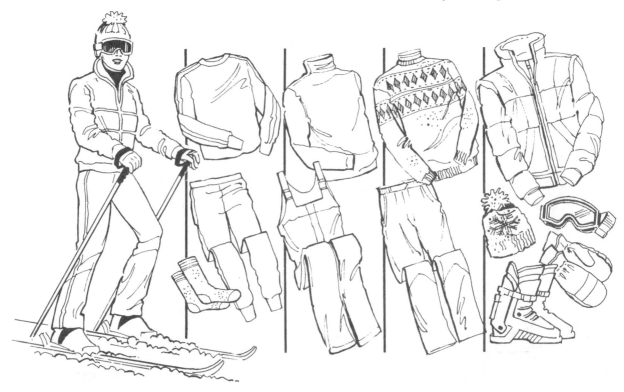

are available to fit either three-pin or mountaineering ski bindings.

Hat: The best hat choice is a wool, polypropylene, or acrylic stocking type that can be pulled down to cover the ears. Unless a neck gaiter is worn also, choose a hat with a face mask or balaclava feature, or wear a partial face mask plus ski goggles to protect the face from wind. A bill feature, light eyeshade, or tennis visor is useful for high-glare conditions. "Bomber" caps with bills and pull-down earflaps are also popular.

Glove Liners: Light polypropylene gloves are useful for moderately cold conditions, when adjusting ski bindings, or when applying a splint.

Third Layer

Parka: This garment can be a standard ski or mountain parka filled with down, Dacron, Quallofil, Thinsulate, or other lofting material. A pile or filled jacket or vest plus a shell is a more versatile combination. The parka or shell should be made of windproof and water-resistant material and have a hood with a drawstring closure. Unless bibs are worn, this garment should be fingertip

length or longer to keep the hips and waist warm and to avoid exposing bare skin when bending over. It should have multiple pockets closed with zippers, Velcro, or snaps. Metal zipper pulls and metal snaps should be shielded or situated so they do not touch bare skin; zippers should have a weather-flap. Zippered openings at the armpits make the shell more versatile. Handwarmer pockets should be included and the openings of the main cargo pockets should be accessible while wearing a first aid belt or backpack with the waist belt fastened.

Wind Pants or Warm-up Pants: These are a must for cold, windy weather, for digging a snow cave, and for working on a patient in wet or deep snow. They should be made of windproof and water-resistant material.

Mittens or Gloves: Mittens tend to be warmer than gloves but are less useful when delicate finger movements are required. A number of manufacturers are making excellent three-layer mitten sets that include windproof shells with leather palms and two sets of removable pile mittens, at least one of which attaches in place with Velcro. Similar three-layer glove systems also are

available. Another good system includes a thin polypropylene glove liner inside a heavy wool, wool/ polypropylene, or pile mitten with a windproof shell of Gore-Tex. An option that enables more finger dexterity in the cold is a polypropylene glove liner inside a fingerless wool glove inside a windproof shell. Depending on temperature, wind, and type of activity, any combination of these three-layer systems can be worn at one time. Shells should have "nose-warmers" of pile attached where they can be reached handily. They also should be long enough to cover the wrists and have palms of soft leather or sticky fabric so that ice axes or ski poles can be held securely.

Alpine skiers may prefer leather mittens or gloves lined with foam, down, or Thinsulate.

Fourth Layer

In addition to the above three layers (that are usually worn on the body), a fourth layer should be easily available in the pack or the ski patrol locker room. This should include a quilted vest or jacket filled with down or synthetic lofting material and a

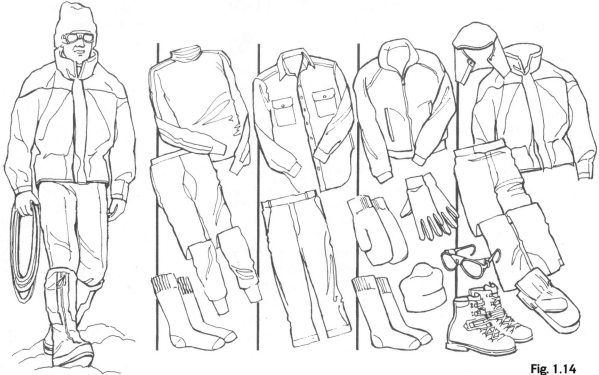

Fig. 1.14

pair of pile or quilted pants. For high-altitude mountaineering in cold weather, special insulated overboots or lined gaiters should be available.

Other Considerations

Rain Gear: In moderate climates or very wet conditions where rain or wet snow may be encountered, a set of windproof outer garments plus a set of waterproof outer garments should be carried. Ponchos do not provide as much protection as a waterproof parka and pair of rain pants, although their effectiveness may be increased by belting them at the waist.

Vapor Barrier Garments: Vapor barrier socks, long underwear, and sleeping bag liners are becoming popular. The vapor barrier system consists of a waterproof garment worn either next to the skin or over a thin garment of polypropylene or similar material. This traps a warm film of moisture next to the skin, theoretically decreases water requirements by reducing perspiration, and maintains the insulating properties of outer garments by keeping perspiration out of them.

Despite the theoretical advantages of vapor barrier systems, some people dislike the clammy feel of these garments. They should be tried out for the first time in non-survival conditions. Vapor barrier garments seem to work better in very cold weather than at moderate temperatures and probably should be avoided by those who perspire excessively. Sufficient spares should be carried to provide a dry set each day.

Adjusting to Hot Weather

Conditions that predispose humans to serious heat stress occur throughout most of the temperate zone during the summer months and in the tropics year-round. Because heat stress is related to both temperature and humidity, a moderately warm tropical environment with high humidity can be just as dangerous and uncomfortable as a hotter, drier desert environment. Death can occur if the body's core temperature rises above 104° to 105°F (4° to 40.6°C) for a significant period of time. In North America, serious heat stress can occur during marathon races run in hot weather, during long climbs on sun-exposed mountain faces, and during desert and deep canyon hikes. Vehicle breakdowns in isolated desert locations can be very hazardous to unprepared passengers.

The body adapts better to heat and altitude than to cold. It acclimatizes to heat by increasing the blood volume, dilating skin blood vessels, and improving heart efficiency so as to carry more heat from the body core to the surface. The acclimatized person starts to perspire at a lower temperature, and the volume of perspiration increases and contains less salt. After a week to 10 days, exposure to heat is noticeably less debilitating. On return to a cooler climate, these processes reverse—the most obvious sign being a temporary increase in urine volume as the blood volume contracts and the excess liquid is excreted by the kidneys.

Here are some ways to prevent problems from excessive heat:

  A. Maximize Heat Loss

    1. Increase heat loss through conduction, convection, and radiation by exposing the maximum amount of bare skin to circulating air. When in the shade, remove as much clothing as possible. When in the sun, protect the skin from sunburn. Because heat loss and perspiration may be impaired by sunscreens, a good compromise is to cover the face and hands with a sunscreen that has a high SPF (sun protection factor) number (see Chapter 18) and wear a long-sleeved shirt and long pants of thin, loose-fitting, light-colored (preferably white) cotton. Hal Brody, an expert desert hiker, recommends providing additional ventilation by cutting 3-inch triangular holes in clothing at the groin and armpits (Tierney, Gloria, "Body Heat." *Backpacker.* July 1987, p. 26). Wear a hat with a wide brim or a Foreign-Legion-style cap with a neck protector and ventilation holes in the crown.

  2. Maintain hydration by drinking adequate fluids (Fig. 1.15), some of which can contain electrolyte supplements. Among other things, this provides water to keep you perspiring freely. Enough water must be carried or be readily available in the field. Water bottles should be wrapped in clothing or other insulation and buried in a backpack to keep the water cool.

  3. Use the layering principle of clothing so that layers can be taken off during the heat of the day and added at night when the dry desert air cools rapidly. A wind shell and wind pants should be included.

4. Because of its high thermal conductivity, poor insulating ability, and good wicking ability, cotton—which should be avoided in cold weather—is the fabric of choice for hot-weather clothing. Clothing should be loose to improve air circulation.

5. Allow time to acclimatize to the heat before being exposed to prolonged or strenuous exertion in hot weather.

B. Minimize Heat Gain

1. Use coverings to protect the head and body from the direct rays of the sun.

2. Seek shade during the hottest part of the day. Make a sun shelter by suspending a tarp from cacti or by laying the tarp on a framework of poles. Because desert air is much cooler a foot above or a few inches below the ground surface, the desert traveler should lie on a platform or in a scooped-out depression rather than directly on the ground.

3. Avoid direct contact with the hot ground and other hot objects, particularly hot metal. Sturdy hiking or climbing boots should be worn, not only to protect the feet from the hot ground, but also from sharp rocks and the spines of cacti. Protect the hands with gloves. Use high-quality sunglasses to protect the eyes from glare and to block out the damaging ultraviolet and infrared rays (Fig. 1.16).

Table 1.10

Acclimatization to Hot Weather

Blood volume increases.
Heart efficiency improves.
Perspiration starts sooner and increases in volume.
Perspiration contains less salt.

Table 1.11

Avoiding Excess Body Heat

Increasing Body Heat Loss
Expose as much skin to the air as possible.
Wear loose, light-colored, cotton clothing.
Maintain hydration to promote perspiration.
Acclimatize.

Reducing Heat Gain from the Environment
Wear protective clothing.
Seek shade during the heat of the day.
Avoid touching hot objects.
Do not lie directly on the ground.

Decreasing Body Heat Production
Decrease muscular activity.

4. During rest periods, seek shade rather than resting in the direct sun.

C. Minimize Body Heat Production

1. Since active muscles produce large amounts of heat, avoid muscular exertion during periods of high heat and high humidity. Do your traveling at night or early and late in the day.

Fig. 1.15 *Drink plenty of fluids in a hot environment.*

Fig. 1.16 *Proper protective clothing is important in hot weather.*

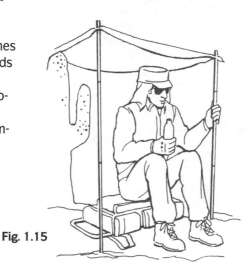

Fig. 1.15

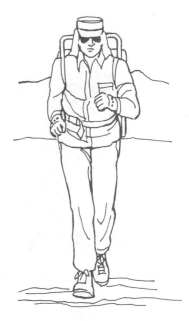

Fig. 1.16

Table 1.12

Sample Desert Survival Kit for Vehicles

Shelter-building Equipment
Plastic or nylon tarp
50 feet of 1/8-inch nylon cord
Folding saw
Short-handled folding shovel
with steel blade
Sturdy knife

Fire-building Equipment
Waterproof matches
Fire starter
Candle

Signaling Equipment
Plastic whistle
Flashlight
Signal mirror
Two quarters for pay phone
Card with ground-to-air signals
CB radio

Other
5-gallon water jug, full
Toilet paper
Spare sunglasses
Sunscreen and lip salve
Map
Compass
Spare hat
Metal pot with bale
First aid kit
Heavy gloves

Solar Still Equipment (four stills)
Four sheets of clear plastic, 6 feet
x 6 feet, reinforced in the center
by an X of duct tape
Four pieces of surgical tubing,
6 to 8 feet long
Four 1-quart plastic bowls
(Fig. 1.17).

Fig. 1.17 *Solar Still*

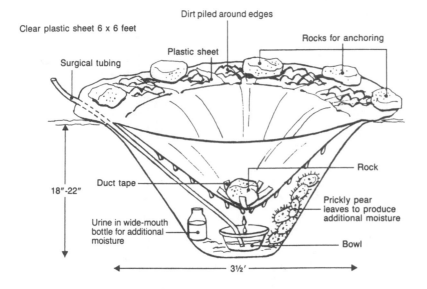

Solar Still

Clear plastic sheet 6 x 6 feet
Dirt piled around edges
Plastic sheet
Rocks for anchoring
Surgical tubing
18"-22"
Duct tape
Rock
Prickly pear leaves to produce additional moisture
Urine in wide-mouth bottle for additional moisture
Bowl
3½'

Fig. 1.17

Food and Water

Good nutrition, which includes hydration, must be a concern to outdoor travelers, especially members of rescue groups who may engage in unplanned, heavy physical activity for long periods in severe weather without adequate food or rest. Nutrition and physical fitness are the bedrock of physical performance. Performance can be enhanced if the principles of good nutrition are applied *before, during,* and *after* an outdoor experience.

Poor nutrition and dehydration, which frequently go together, have similar effects: fatigue, decreased work capacity, lack of endurance, poor recovery from exercise, lack of cold or heat tolerance (with increased susceptibility to hypothermia or heat illness), weight loss, depression, apathy, and discouragement. Coordination also may suffer, because there may not be enough glycogen in the fast-twitch muscle fibers to perform rapid corrective movements efficiently. (See **Physical Conditioning** below.)

The six groups of nutrients are **carbohydrates, fats, proteins, vitamins, minerals,** and **water.**

Table 1.13

The Six Groups of Nutrients

Carbohydrates
Fats
Proteins
Vitamins
Minerals
Water

Carbohydrates: These organic compounds are composed of carbon, hydrogen, and oxygen. When oxidized in the body, they produce energy, heat, carbon dioxide, and water. They are present in food mainly as sugars and starches, and are broken down during digestion into simple sugars that are converted into **glucose.** Glucose molecules are joined to form the complex carbohydrate **glycogen,** which is stored in the liver and muscles and can be broken down quickly into glucose to provide a rapid source of energy. However, these glycogen stores are not large and are markedly depleted by a fast as short as 24 hours. Eating a high-carbohydrate diet for several days will double the glycogen stores and can increase endurance by as much as three times that of an ordinary diet. Conversely, a low-carbohydrate diet can decrease glycogen stores and reduce endurance by as much as 50 percent. The main dietary sources of carbohydrate are fruits, vegetables, cereals, and sugar (Fig. 1.18).

Table 1.14

Food Sources of Carbohydrate

    Fruits
    Vegetables
    Cereals
    Sugar

Fats: Fats are also made up of carbon, oxygen, and hydrogen and, when metabolized, they also produce heat, energy, water, and carbon

---

Fig. 1.18 *Sources of Carbohydrate*

Fig. 1.19 *Sources of Fat*

Fig. 1.20 *Sources of Protein*

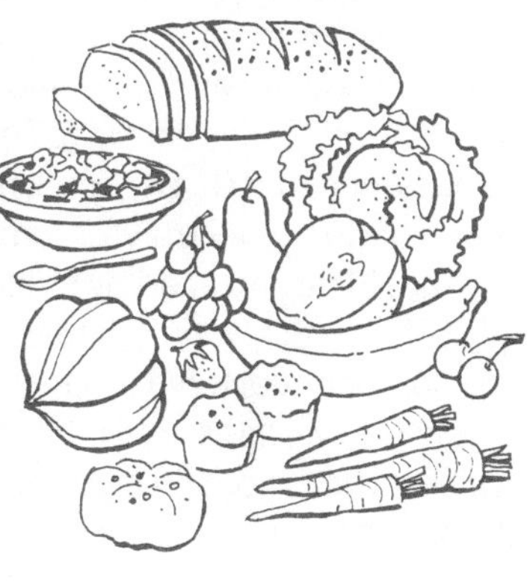

dioxide. In cases of starvation, body fat tends to be broken down into acidic compounds that are metabolized to produce heat and energy. If these compounds accumulate in the blood faster than they can be used, they cause the body tissues and blood to become excessively acidic **(acidosis).** One type of fat, **cholesterol,** has been implicated as a cause of **arteriosclerosis,** a disease characterized by thickening and loss of elasticity of arterial walls. In general, vegetable (polyunsaturated) fats are less likely to cause arteriosclerosis than animal (saturated) fats. However, some vegetable fats, such as coconut oil, are highly saturated.

Common food sources of fat are butter, lard, cooking oil, mayonnaise, chocolate, fried foods, and ice cream. Fat is also found in lesser amounts in dairy products, meat, eggs, nuts, vegetables, and cereals (Fig. 1.19).

Table 1.15

Food Sources of Fat

Butter	Dairy products
Lard	Meat
Cooking oil	Eggs
Mayonnaise	Nuts
Chocolate	Vegetables
Fried foods	Cereals
Ice cream	

In the body, fat serves as the main storage form of energy. One gram of fat when burned produces nine calories of heat or energy; a gram of

protein or carbohydrate only four. Fat in the subcutaneous tissues insulates against cold but interferes with heat loss in hot weather. During brief exercise, energy is derived equally from fat and carbohydrate. As the duration of the exercise lengthens, the percent of energy supplied by fat increases up to 80 percent. However, with strenuous exercise the body switches back to burning carbohydrate; for example, during a marathon a runner will burn about 70 percent carbohydrate and 30 percent fat.

Proteins: Proteins contain nitrogen, sulfur, and phosphorus in addition to carbon, hydrogen, and oxygen. They are complicated molecules composed of chains of **amino acids.** The body is able to synthesize all but eight of the amino acids it requires for normal growth and function. These eight amino acids, called "essential amino acids," must be obtained from food, or growth will cease and the body will sicken.

Common sources of protein are eggs, dairy products, meat, poultry, fish, legumes (peas and beans), nuts, and cereals (Fig. 1.20).

Table 1.16

Food Sources of Protein

Eggs	Peas
Dairy products	Beans
Meat	Nuts
Poultry	Cereals
Fish	

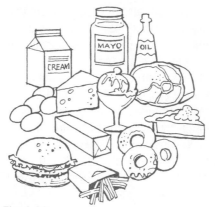

Fig. 1.18

Fig. 1.19

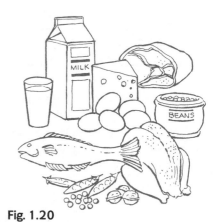

Fig. 1.20

Some proteins are called "complete proteins" because they contain all of the essential amino acids in adequate amounts to allow for tissue growth and repair. Animal products, especially eggs, are better sources of complete proteins than vegetable products. Vegetarians should include eggs and dairy products in their diets or consume a wide variety of grains and legumes to obtain all essential amino acids as well as adequate calcium, phosphorus and vitamin B_{12}. There is no benefit from eating excessive amounts of protein, since the excess will be converted into energy or stored as fat.

Vitamins: Trace amounts of these subsances are essential to the metabolic functioning of the body, where they serve mainly as cofactors and coenzymes for vital chemical reactions and as components of important substances. Because vitamins cannot be made by the body, they must be supplied in food. Fortunately, a balanced diet will supply sufficient quantities of essential vitamins. Fourteen vitamins have been identified to date: the water-soluble vitamins B_1, B_2, B_6, niacin, pantothenic acid, biotin, choline, folic acid, B_{12}, and C; and the fat-soluble vitamins A, D, E, and K.

Table 1.17

The Fourteen Vitamins

Water Soluble	*Fat Soluble*
B_1, B_2, B_6, Niacin, Pantothenic acid, Biotin, Choline, Folic acid, B_{12}, C	A, D, E, K

Water-soluble vitamins are not stored in the body and need to be consumed daily. Fat-soluble vitamins can be stored in the body. When too much vitamin A or D is ingested, a toxic condition called "hypervitaminosis" can develop. For example, eating seal or polar bear liver, which are extremely rich in vitamin A, can cause acute vitamin A toxicity.

Since a well-balanced diet already contains enough vitamins, vitamin supplements usually are unnecessary. A daily vitamin tablet does no harm, but megadoses of vitamins (more than 10 times the recommended daily allowance) may be harmful. For example, too much vitamin C can cause gout, gastritis and diarrhea; too much vitamin B_6, nerve damage; too much niacin, heart abnormalities; and too much vitamin E, headaches and weakness. In our society, vitamin supplements are overproduced, overpromoted, and overconsumed, making American sewers the world's most vitamin enriched.

Minerals: Four percent of body weight is made up of inorganic elements and simple inorganic compounds collectively called "minerals." The most common of these are calcium, phosphorus, magnesium, iron, sodium, potassium, chlorine, and sulfur, all of which are present in large amounts. Some are found in the form of electrically charged particles called "ions" and are referred to as "electrolytes." The most important of these are sodium, potassium, and chlorine. In addition, there are many essential elements present in minute amounts: chromium, cobalt, copper, fluorine, iodine, manganese, molybdenum, nickel, selenium, silicon, tin, vanadium, and zinc.

Calcium and phosphorus are the major components of bones and teeth. Iron is an essential part of the oxygen-carrying molecule hemoglobin. The electrolytes—sodium, potassium, chlorine, magnesium, and sulfur (mostly as sulfate)—are integral parts of all body fluids, both inside and outside the cells. Iodine is necessary for the metabolism-regulating hormone thyroxine. Most of the trace minerals are found in

Table 1.18

Essential Minerals

Major	*Trace*
Calcium	Chromium
Phosphorus	Cobalt
Magnesium	Copper
Iron	Fluorine
Sodium	Iodine
Potassium	Manganese
Chlorine	Molybdenum
Sulfur	Nickel
	Selenium
	Silicon
	Tin
	Vanadium
	Zinc

essential enzymes, hormones, and vitamins, such as cobalt in Vitamin B_{12} and iodine in thyroxin.

There is little need to supplement a well-balanced diet with minerals, since they are abundant in drinking water and in common foods. However, since many foods are low in iron and iron is poorly absorbed from the digestive tract, growing children and women of childbearing age may require iron supplements. People who do not get adequate calcium because of low consumption of dairy products and other good calcium sources should take calcium supplements to help prevent osteoporosis later in life. In certain parts of the United States there is little iodine in the soil so that additional iodine (usually as iodized salt) should be consumed.

During prolonged exertion in hot weather, perspiration may deplete the body of sodium and to a small extent potassium, leading to fatigue, weakness, and muscle cramps. Under these conditions, electrolytes and water should be replaced by drinking lightly salted, cold water (⅓ teaspoon salt per quart) or commercial electrolyte beverages. Even though these beverages contain electrolytes in slightly different amounts than

Table 1.19

Components of a Proper Diet

Protein:	65 grams (2.3 ounces), two-thirds from animal sources, one-third from cereals, vegetables
Carbohydrate:	150 grams (5.4 ounces), from fruits, vegetables, cereals
Fat:	45 grams (1.5 ounces), preferably polyunsaturated, from meat, fish, poultry, dairy products, vegetables, nuts, cereals
Calories:	The above contains less than 1,300 calories and needs to be supplemented to reach 2,000 to 5,000 calories.
Avoid:	Candy and other sweets, animal fat, lard, butter, cream, ice cream, coconut oil, egg yolk, shellfish, organ meats

needed, healthy individuals usually can excrete any excess in their urine. A normal diet contains so much potassium that potassium depletion is almost never a problem except when a potassium-depleting diuretic medication is taken for high blood pressure or heart disease.

In summary, the best diet is one that supplies adequate nutrients for heat and energy production, and for tissue maintenance, repair, and growth. A person of average size should eat about 65 grams (2.3 ounces) of protein daily, with two-thirds of that amount supplied by meat and dairy products and one-third by vegetables, fruits, and whole grains, including bread. About 150 grams (5.4 ounces) of carbohydrate should be eaten daily, mostly as fruits, vegetables, and whole-grain cereals. About 45 grams (1.5 ounces) of fat, preferably polyunsaturated, should be eaten daily, mainly as poultry, fish, meat and dairy products, plus the small amount found in vegetables, fruit, nuts, and whole grains. These components will provide for the basic needs of the body but will total less than 1,300 calories. The additional 2,000 to 3,000 calories that an active person needs may be obtained from a variety of foods, depending on individual choice. Foods that contain large amounts of refined sugar and/or saturated fat should be kept to a minimum (candy and other sweets, animal fat, lard, butter, cream, ice cream, coconut oil, egg yolks, shellfish, and organ meats).

Those who expect to engage in strenuous physical activity should increase the percentage of carbohydrate in their diet to 70 to 80 percent for several days *before* as well as *during* the activity by eating large amounts of potatoes, rice, pasta, and other high-carbohydrate foods. This diet also should be continued for several days *after* the activity to replenish muscle glycogen stores.

The number and size of servings can be increased to provide the calories necessary to support a given level of activity. This may be as high as 4,000 to 5,000 calories a day during a prolonged rescue effort or mountaineering expedition. Most additional calories should come from complex carbohydrates such as fruits, vegetables (especially potatoes and rice), and whole grains.

Here is an example of a back-packing menu that requires only the addition of hot or cold water.

Breakfast: Hot citrus beverage such as Tang; instant hot cereal or granola with raisins, powdered milk, brown sugar, and spices such as nutmeg or cinnamon to taste; breakfast bars; hot tea or freeze-dried coffee.

Lunch: Bread, preferably a type that will not crumble in the pack, such as hard rolls, pita bread or soft tortillas; sandwich fillers such as cheese, sausage, freeze-dried tuna or chicken salad; candy bars; powdered tea, Koolaid, or similar fruit drink.

Snacks: (to be eaten every two hours on the trail): Dried fruit, candy bars, nuts, and "gorp" (good old raisins and peanuts).

Supper: Hot jello; instant soup; commercial freeze-dried dinner; instant pudding; hot cocoa, or hot tea.

Food carried for emergency purposes or as part of a search and rescue 72-hour pack should be tasty, light in weight, high in energy, resistant to spoilage, and should not require cooking or complicated preparation. Examples include cheese, sausage, candy bars, gorp, bread, nuts, cocoa, instant breakfast drink, fruitcake, and dried fruit. Food that is unpalatable or spoiled will not be eaten, no matter how nourishing. Living off the land is a romantic notion and may be possible for experienced persons in survival situations, but (except possibly on tropical seashores), an untrained

Table 1.20

Suggested Minimum Daily Servings for Adequate Nutrition

Food Group	Servings (average size)
Milk and milk products	2
Meat and/or other high-protein food sources	2
Vegetables and fruits	4
Cereals and whole grains	4

person will not be able to find enough wild food to replace the energy expended searching for it.

Water: Water makes up about 60 percent of the body weight of an average young adult male. In females, the percentage of water is somewhat lower and the percentage of fat somewhat higher. The average sedentary person loses about 2,500 milliliters (2.7 quarts) of water each day. Of this total, 1,200 milliliters (1.3 quarts) is lost in the urine, 1,000 milliliters (1.1 quarts) through the skin and lungs, and 300 milliliters (10 ounces) in the stool. Therefore, to prevent dehydration, at least 2,500 milliliters (2.7 quarts) of water must be added daily. While about 700 milliliters (1.5 pints) of water is created daily during the metabolism of the protein, fat, and carbohydrate in food (or from body tissues if no food is available), the remaining 1,800 milliliters (2 quarts) must come from liquids and the fluids contained in such foods as meat, vegetables, and fruits.

Table 1.21

Water Balance

Gain		Loss	
Metabolism =	700 ml	Urine =	1,200 ml
Liquids and water-containing foods =	1,800 ml	Skin and lungs =	1,000 ml
		Feces =	300 ml
Total =	2,500 ml	Total =	2,500 ml

At high altitude, in hot weather, and during strenuous exercise, the amount of water lost through skin and lungs increases greatly. These losses can total 1,000 milliliters (1.1 quarts) per hour during nordic ski racing and up to 1,600 milliliters (1.8 quarts) per hour during strenuous exercise in hot weather.

Active efforts must be made to prevent dehydration in the outdoors, especially in very cold and very hot weather, and at high altitude. Cold weather decreases the sense of thirst, which may lead to a state of chronic, mild dehydration. At temperatures below freezing and at elevations above the snow line, the lack of liquid water and the time and effort required to melt snow compound the problem. In desert areas, water may be almost impossible to find.

Almost all surface water should be considered contaminated by human or animal wastes, with the possible exception of small streams and springs coming down from untracked snowfields or high, uninhabited areas at right angles to the main valley drainage. If there is any doubt about water's purity, avoid or purify it. *Giardia lamblia,* an organism found in animal and human feces that causes diarrhea and abdominal discomfort, may contaminate the most pristine wilderness water source. Purify water by boiling it, filtering it, or disinfecting it with chemicals. Remove obvious dirt by straining the water through a clean cloth. Several excellent brands of filters are available. They should have pores small enough to remove bacteria and *Giardia* cysts; most will not remove viruses. At altitudes lower than 18,000 feet (5,486 meters), simply bringing water to a boil will kill *Giardia* cysts and most harmful bacteria and viruses.

A number of products for chemical disinfection of water are available, some iodine-based and some chlorine-based. One satisfactory, widely available product is tetraglycine hydroperiodide (Potable Aqua). Persons interested in learning about other available products should consult standard mountaineering and backpacking texts. The time required to kill infectious organisms varies depending on the amount of sediment in the water, the water temperature, and the type and dose of chemical disinfectant, so the manufacturer's directions should be followed carefully and the water allowed to stand the specified amount of time before use.

Whenever open water is encountered on the trail in winter, fill all empty canteens with properly purified water. Take time in the morning to melt enough snow to provide each party member with enough to drink plus a canteenful for the day. At night, drink enough water to satisfy thirst, and sleep with a full canteen to prevent it from freezing. It is more efficient to melt ice or hard snow than to melt light, powdery snow. On warm, sunny days, snow can be spread on a dark poncho to melt.

During hot weather, especially in desert areas, carry large amounts of water since natural water sources cannot be relied on. A desert survival kit should contain the materials to make several solar stills (see Fig. 1.17), and desert travelers should be familiar with the fundamentals of desert and hot-weather survival.

At high altitude and when working hard, drink at least 3 to 4 liters (3.2 to 4.2 quarts) of water daily; in deserts, as much as a liter per hour may be needed. Urine output is a good indicator of the state of hydration. Daily urine production should equal 1 to 1.5 liters (1.1 to 1.6 quarts), and the color should be light yellow. Strenuous exercise may cause urine to be orange-brown, while vitamin supplements containing riboflavin (vitamin B_2) will turn it bright yellow. Make water more palatable, if necessary, by adding fruit flavors or making hot drinks to encourage consumption. However, when working hard and perspiring heavily, it is better to drink small amounts of plain, cold water frequently. Adding sugar to water and overfilling the stomach by drinking large amounts of liquid at one time are counterproductive because they delay gastric emptying.

If water supplies are limited, sweat should be "rationed" by avoiding over-exertion, and dietary protein should be limited since the kidney requires more water to excrete the breakdown products of protein than those of fat and carbohydrate. In desert areas, the traveler should rest in the shade during the heat of the day and travel in the early morning or at night.

Physical Conditioning

Physical fitness and conditioning are important to members of any outdoor recreational or rescue group because outdoor travel imposes unusual physical demands and presents the possibility of severe, prolonged physical stress. Therefore, rescuers should achieve and maintain a superior level of physical

fitness. Most rescuers participate in sports related to their rescue interests, such as climbing, recreational skiing, caving, and kayaking. These activities require strong, supple, durable bodies for full enjoyment. Although the best training for any sport is to practice that sport, people with demanding urban jobs may have to substitute a carefully selected set of exercises that can be performed regularly in their spare time and close to home.

Proper physical conditioning improves the strength of muscles and tendons, enhances coordination, flexibility and endurance, and reduces the chance of injury. Conditioning allows people to exert harder and longer without tiring and to recover more rapidly after rest. Conditioning also increases the margin of safety in a survival situation.

Proper conditioning slows aging and helps maintain normal weight. The drop in U.S. mortality from cardiovascular disease in the past 20 years probably is due in part to increased participation in active sports by people of all ages. The fit rescuer performs better because the fit body functions better, is better able to avoid injury, and recovers faster if injured.

Fitness can be divided into two parts: **cardiovascular** or **aerobic** (oxygen-requiring) **fitness,** which develops the heart and circulatory system to meet the body's changing needs for blood; and **motor fitness,** which develops and enhances strength, power, endurance, balance, agility, and flexibility. Suitable conditioning programs should develop both types of fitness.

Studies of skeletal muscle structure (histology) and function (physiology) indicate that there are two types of voluntary muscle fibers: Type I or "slow twitch" fibers, which are designed for sustained, slow contractions and rely mainly on aerobic metabolic processes; and Type II or "fast-twitch" fibers, which are capable of rapid contractions, tend to rely on anaerobic (non-oxygen-requiring) metabolism, and form lactic acid readily.

Successful endurance athletes such as nordic ski racers, bicycle racers, marathon runners, and long-distance swimmers tend to have more slow-twitch than fast-twitch fibers (Fig. 1.21). Athletes who engage in

Fig. 1.21 *Three Types of Endurance Athletes*

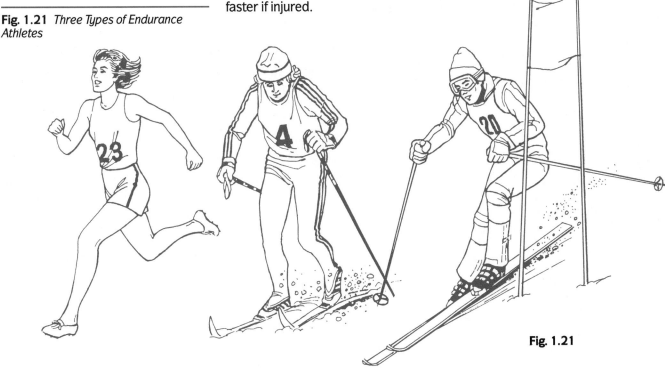

Fig. 1.21

short, intense bursts of effort, such as sprinters, jumpers, and weight lifters, do better if they have a predominance of fast-twitch fibers.

Although the proportion of fast- and slow-twitch fibers is determined at birth, selective development of one type over the other is possible to some extent. It is interesting that top alpine ski racers show wide individual variations in the relative numbers of fast- and slow-twitch fibers. This suggests that alpine skiers and ski racers employ both fiber types and that their training should emphasize aerobic techniques as well as strength, agility, and the other components of motor fitness. Training for backpacking and nordic skiing should emphasize both upper- and lower-body endurance.

The training goal for any endurance sport is to *maximize the body's ability to take up and use oxygen.* This ability can be measured by pulmonary function tests. It has been found that the greatest ability to absorb and use oxygen ($\dot{V}O_2$max) is developed through training that uses the upper and lower extremities *at the same time,* such as roller skiing and speed hiking with poles on dry land, nordic skiing on snow, and using a nordic skiing simulator.

A good fitness program should start off moderately but aim for an eventual minimum workout of at least 45 minutes four times a week (Fig. 1.22). The program should include:

A. A proper warm-up period with stretching exercises.
B. Selected calisthenics designed to develop the upper and lower extremities, back, and trunk (sit-ups, pull-ups, leg raises, push-ups, dips between parallel bars, barbell exercises, toe raises, hops over a box, etc.). Handball, racquetball, climbing boulders and artificial climbing walls, gymnastics, wrestling, and other vigorous sports and games can be substituted for calisthenics.
C. A period of aerobic exercise to build cardiovascular fitness and endurance—rhythmical, nonstop training such as swimming, jogging, bicycling, roller skiing, rollerblading, or using a rowing machine, treadmill, exercise bicycle, or nordic skiing simulator. For

minimal effectiveness, these exercises must be vigorous enough to develop and maintain a heart rate of 75 percent of the person's maximum age-related heart rate for at least 15 minutes. This maximum rate is calculated by subtracting one's age from 220 and multiplying by 0.75.
D. A cooling-down period— usually slow to moderate walking with warm-up clothes on to avoid chilling.

Table 1.22

Components of a Good Training Program

Warmup
Calisthenics or sports to develop motor fitness
Endurance training to develop cardiovascular fitness
Cooling-down period

People with chronic impairments or who have not been exercising regularly should get a thorough checkup by a physician before embarking on a fitness program. Anyone with an

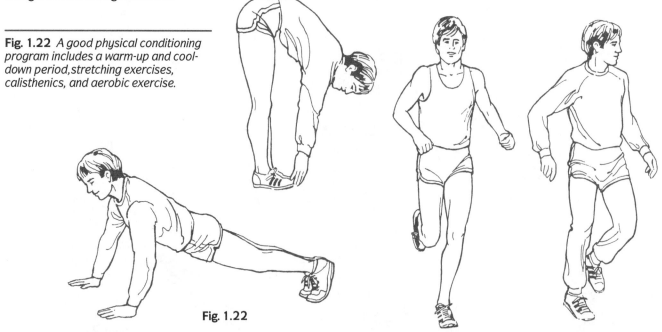

Fig. 1.22 *A good physical conditioning program includes a warm-up and cool-down period, stretching exercises, calisthenics, and aerobic exercise.*

Fig. 1.22

acute illness such as a head cold or gastrointestinal upset should abstain from exercising until recovered. Exercise should be progressive so that optimum fitness can be achieved by steadily increasing the demands made on the body. Excessive fatigue, inability to sleep the following night, a prolonged fast pulse, and persistent muscle and joint tenderness are signs that the workout has been too hard. Soon, however, the benefits of fitness become evident. The fit person feels less tired at the end of the day despite having expended more energy. Sleep is more restful, the body is less tense, and weight is maintained more easily. Individuals who follow a fitness program may not be transformed into Olympic athletes, but they will be better athletes than unfit individuals of equal natural ability and will be better able to enjoy the outdoors safely.

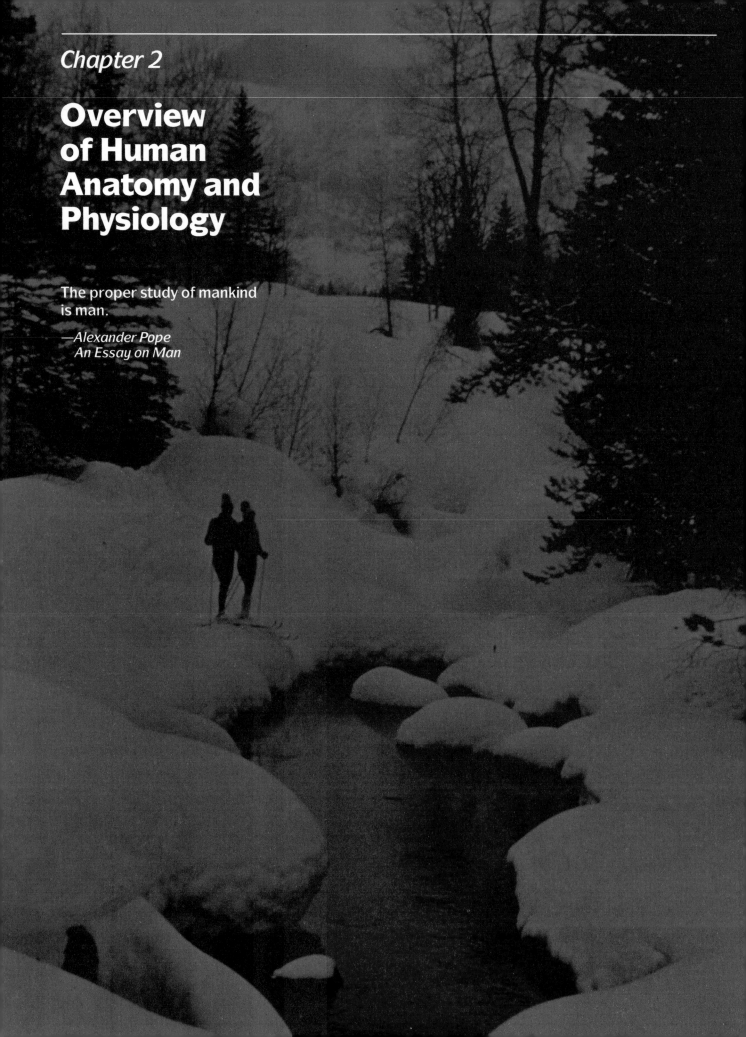

Chapter 2

Overview of Human Anatomy and Physiology

The proper study of mankind
is man.

—*Alexander Pope*
  An Essay on Man

The basic unit of all living matter is the **cell** (Fig. 2.1). Individual cells group together to form tissues, tissues group to form organs, and organs group to form organ systems. The nine organ systems can be categorized as **primary** and **supportive**, based on the length of time a person can live if they cease to function and, consequently, the importance of their contribution to basic body survival. The primary organ systems are the **circulatory** and **respiratory**, the supportive systems are the **digestive, urinary, skeletal, muscular, nervous, cutaneous,** and **reproductive**. Because of their close association, the urinary and reproductive systems are frequently referred to as the genitourinary system.

The primary organ systems function and interact with two major purposes: to carry oxygen, food, and other essential materials *to* and remove waste products *from* each cell.

The **circulatory system** consists of a "pump," the heart; a set of "pipes," the blood vessels; and fluid to fill the pipes, the blood. It is a closed system composed of two circuits. In the first, or **systemic circuit**, the heart pumps blood through increasingly smaller vessels to the smallest vessels—the **capillaries**—which lie so close to the individual cells that oxygen, nutrients, carbon dioxide, and other waste products

can be transferred easily between the blood and the cells. The blood then flows back to the heart through increasingly larger vessels. It enters the right side of the heart from which it is pumped into the second, or **pulmonary circuit**. In this circuit, the blood flows through the lungs where it takes on oxygen and gets rid of carbon dioxide. The oxygen-rich blood then enters the left side of the heart, from which it is pumped into the systemic circuit again. The wastes are delivered to the kidneys, where they are excreted in the urine.

The **respiratory system** brings air into the lungs, where it comes into close contact with the blood. There, oxygen is transferred from the air to the red blood cells, and carbon dioxide is removed from the blood and expelled into the outside air.

The **digestive system** takes food and water into the body, breaks the food down into simpler nutrient substances that can be absorbed into the blood, and expels the indigestible residue as feces. The blood in the intestinal capillaries absorbs the water and nutrients.

The **urinary system** is the major cleanser of the blood. This system removes the waste products of cellular metabolism and excretes them in the urine.

The **skeletal system** provides protection, form, and support to the body and permits an upright stance.

The **muscular system** acts together with the skeletal system to permit body movement.

The **nervous system** collects and processes stimuli from the environment and controls and coordinates the activities of the other major organ systems.

The skin and subcutaneous tissues make up the **cutaneous system**, which protects the internal body parts and keeps them from drying out. It also helps control body temperature and contains the special organs responsible for sensations of pain, touch, and temperature.

The **reproductive system** provides the means for producing successive generations of offspring.

The Work of The Cell

Living cells have both **basic** and **specialized functions**. All cells convert food to **heat** and **energy** through a complex process that requires oxygen and breaks down carbohydrates, fats, and proteins into water, carbon dioxide, and simple waste compounds. The capacity of food to produce heat and energy in the body is expressed as its **calorie** content. The same amount of water, carbon dioxide, heat, energy, and wastes would be produced if the food were set on fire outside the body, but the heat and energy would be produced in large, uncontrolled, wasteful amounts over a short period of time.

Fig. 2.1 *Typical Cell and its Parts*

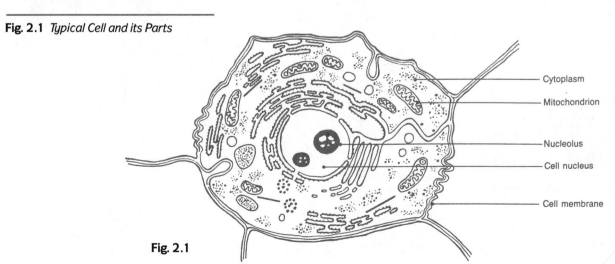

Cytoplasm

Mitochondrion

Nucleolus

Cell nucleus

Cell membrane

Fig. 2.1

Cells use a series of complicated chemical reactions regulated by substances called **enzymes** to produce energy in small, controlled, usable amounts. Because these enzymes work best at or slightly above normal human body temperature, body temperature must be regulated carefully for normal metabolic activity.

Energy is used by cells to fuel basic tasks such as the vital processes of growth, repair, tissue maintenance, reproduction, and storage of energy as fat and carbohydrate.

Most cells also have specialized, energy-requiring functions (Fig. 2.2). For example, cells lining the trachea and other parts of the respiratory tract produce mucus and have hair-like projections called cilia that move with a coordinated wave-like motion to clear the lungs of impurities in the air that have been trapped in the mucus. Muscle cells contain contractile proteins that allow them to shorten, causing the muscle to contract and permitting body movement. Nerve cells are able to transmit electrochemical impulses rapidly through their cytoplasm to other nerve cells. Cells that line the stomach and small intestine produce enzymes and other substances that break down food so it can be absorbed into the bloodstream. Liver cells are able to produce and store the complex carbohydrate **glycogen** within their cytoplasm.

All of these processes are part of the body's **metabolism**, i.e., the chemical reactions that produce or use energy. The rate of metabolism is controlled in part by the hormone **thyroxin**, produced by the thyroid gland. A vital requirement for metabolism is **oxygen**, which is so important that an oxygen-deprived cell can die within minutes. Different body

Skin Cells

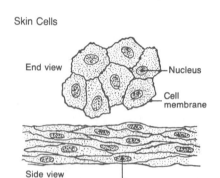

Trachea Cells

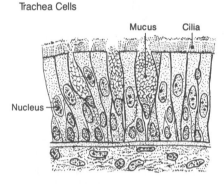

Striated Muscle Cells

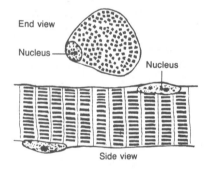

Nerve Cells

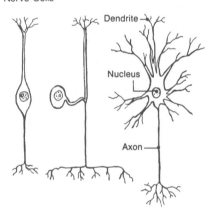

Fig. 2.2 *Specialized Cells*

Fig. 2.3 *An oxygen debt must be paid after strenuous exercise.*

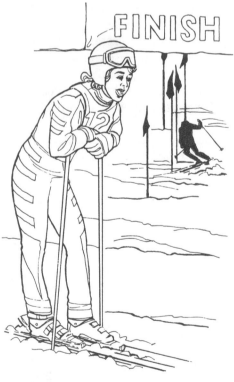

Stomach Cells

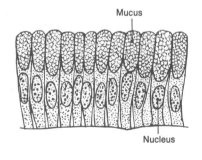

Fig. 2.2

Liver Cells

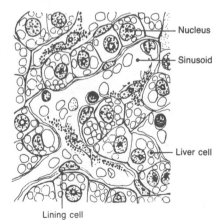

Fig. 2.3

cells may vary in sensitivity to lack of oxygen: heart cells are injured if deprived of oxygen for more than a few seconds, brain cells for more than four to six minutes. Muscle cells can withstand oxygen deprivation much longer and can even incur an **oxygen debt**.

During short periods of very strenuous activity, the muscles use fuel so rapidly that the circulatory and respiratory systems cannot supply the muscles with enough oxygen to completely metabolize their principal fuel, glucose. Without

oxygen, glucose is broken down into an intermediate product, lactic acid, which accumulates in the blood and the muscle tissues during exercise. The oxygen debt is paid after exercise when lactic acid production drops and oxygen delivery is again sufficient to break down both glucose and the remaining lactic acid all the way to carbon dioxide and water (Fig. 2.3). Although a certain amount of lactic acid accumulation is safe, it is one of the causes of muscle pain during and after strenuous exercise.

Because oxygen is so vital to life, techniques to assist and reestablish the function of the respiratory and

circulatory systems assume central importance in emergency care.

Vocabulary

Before examining the nine organ systems in more detail, it is necessary to present a few important anatomical terms used in this text (Fig. 2.4). The terms refer to the human body standing *erect* and *facing* the examiner with the arms held so that the palms of the hands face forward. They permit the rescuer to talk intelligently with members of the emergency medical services (EMS) system, describe observations accurately, and avoid confusion.

Fig. 2.4 *Anatomical Terms for the Human Body*

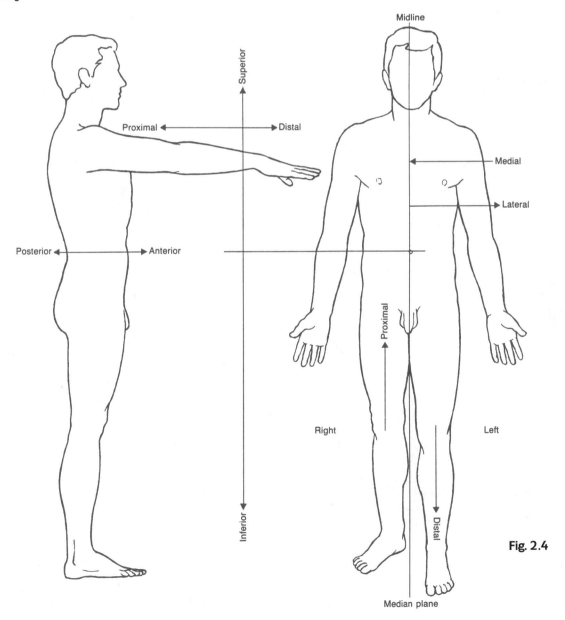

Fig. 2.4

The terms **right** and **left** refer to the *patient's* right and left. The body is considered to be divided into right and left halves by an imaginary plane, the **median plane**. The intersection of this plane with the surface of the body in front and in back is known as the **midline** of the body. Keeping this in mind, there are three pairs of relative terms that can be used to express the relationship of any given structure to another.

The term **anterior** means *nearer* to the *front* surface of the body, while **posterior** means *nearer* to the *back* surface of the body. **Medial** means *nearer* to the **midline** of the body; **lateral** means *farther* from the midline of the body. *Superior* means *nearer* to the **top of the head**, while **inferior** means *nearer* to the **soles of the feet**.

One final pair of terms also is important: **proximal** means *closer* to the **trunk of the body**; **distal** means *closer* to the **tips of the extremities**.

The Circulatory System

The circulatory system consists of the **heart, arteries, capillaries,** and **veins**. These are linked together to form a closed, hollow system (Fig. 2.5) that is filled with the blood. The system has two loops, the **pulmonary** and **systemic circuits**. The heart (Figs. 2.5, 2.6, 2.7) lies between the lungs in the chest. It is divided into a right and left side. Each side contains two muscular chambers, an **atrium** and a **ventricle**. The atria are smaller than the ventricles and have less muscle in their walls because they only have to pump blood a short distance into their respective ventricles. The ventricles have thick walls of powerful muscle. The right side of the

heart is smaller than the left because it pumps blood into the smaller, lower-pressure pulmonary circuit.

Blood returning to the heart enters the **right atrium**. It is pumped from there into the **right ventricle**, which pumps it in turn into the **main pulmonary artery**. This divides into right and left branches, the **right** and **left pulmonary arteries**, which enter the respective **right** and **left lungs**. These branches divide into progressively smaller arteries, terminating as the **pulmonary capillaries**, which run in the walls of the smallest air sacs, the **alveoli**. In the alveoli, the blood picks up oxygen from the air and loses carbon dioxide to the air, as described in Chapter 1. The pulmonary capillaries empty into tiny

---

Fig. 2.5 *Schema of the Heart and Circulatory System*

Fig. 2.6 *Anatomical Position of the Heart in the Chest*

Fig. 2.7 *Heart and the Roots of the Great Vessels*

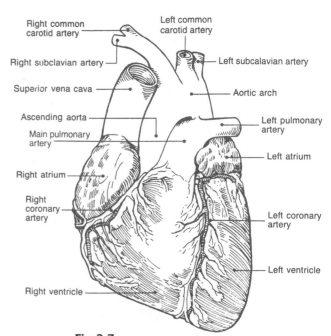

Fig. 2.6

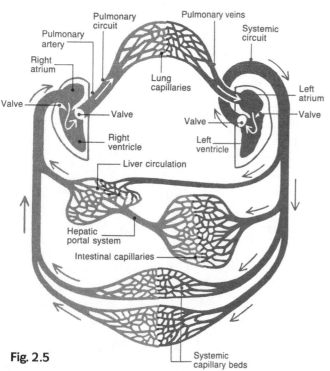

Fig. 2.5

For clarity, the two sides of the heart are shown separated

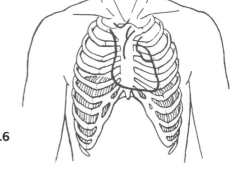

Fig. 2.7

veins that join to form progressively larger veins, eventually emptying into the **left atrium** of the heart. The blood is pumped from the left atrium into the **left ventricle** and then into the major artery of the body, the **aorta**.

The heart, like any pump, contains valves. There are four of these: 1) the tricuspid valve, between the right atrium and right ventricle, 2) the pulmonary valve, between the right ventricle and the pulmonary artery, 3) the mitral valve, between the left atrium and the left ventricle, and 4) the aortic valve, between the left ventricle and the aorta.

The aorta curves up over the heart and then runs down through the body, branching off into a number of large **arteries** (Fig. 2.8a): the **coronaries**, which supply the heart; the **carotids** (common carotids), which supply the head and neck; the **subclavians**, which supply the upper extremities; the **superior** and **inferior mesenterics**, which supply the digestive tract; the **renals**, which supply the kidneys; and the **iliacs** (common iliacs), which supply the lower extremities. These arteries divide into smaller and smaller branches, eventually forming capillaries that interlace around the individual cells. Although most cells *extract* nutrients *from* the blood, in the intestines and liver, nutrients from digested food and glucose from the breakdown of glycogen are also *delivered to* the blood.

Deoxygenated blood containing waste products is conducted back to the heart through larger and larger veins, many named to correspond with the arteries (Fig. 2.8b). Eventually, the returning blood empties into the two major veins of the body, the **inferior** and **superior venae cavae**. The superior vena cava drains the upper body (head, neck, upper extremities, and chest); the inferior vena cava drains the lower body (abdomen, pelvis, and lower extremities). Both of these large veins drain into the right atrium.

In general, the deeper veins of the body run close to the corresponding arteries, while the veins of the skin do not.

The walls of both arteries and veins contain muscle fibers that allow these vessels to vary their size, becoming larger or smaller in response to nerve impulses from the control center in the brain. The control center reacts to changes in the blood pressure, cardiac output, and amount of blood available. These muscles normally stay in a state of chronic slight contraction called **tone** that can be altered by disease or injury as well as nerve impulses.

Blood circulation is a continuous process. The heart normally beats 60 to 90 times a minute in an adult, pumping about 2.5 ounces (80 milliliters) of blood into the aorta with each beat. The heart of an average-sized adult male at rest pumps blood at the rate of about 6 quarts (5.5 liters) per minute. Since the total blood volume in the body of this typical

---

Fig. 2.8 *Major Blood Vessels*

Fig. 2.9 *Microscopic Appearance of the Blood*

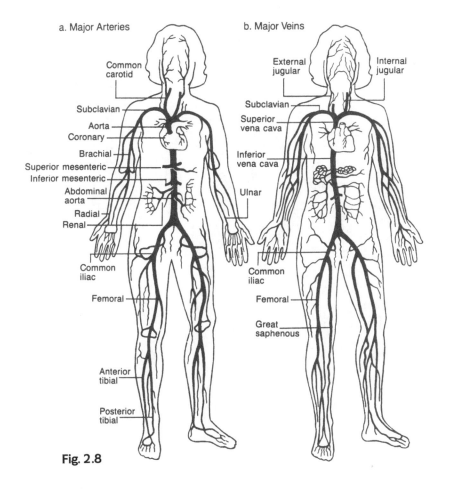

a. Major Arteries

Common carotid
Subclavian
Aorta
Coronary
Brachial
Superior mesenteric
Inferior mesenteric
Abdominal aorta
Radial
Renal
Common iliac
Femoral
Anterior tibial
Posterior tibial

b. Major Veins

External jugular
Internal jugular
Subclavian
Superior vena cava
Inferior vena cava
Ulnar
Common iliac
Femoral
Great saphenous

Fig. 2.8

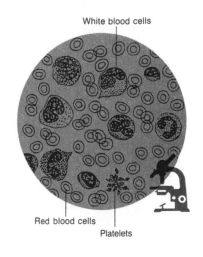

White blood cells

Red blood cells

Platelets

Fig. 2.9

male is only about 5.5 liters, a major injury to the aorta or other large blood vessel can lead to death by hemorrhage within a very short time. Therefore, in emergency care, considerable emphasis is placed on the detection and control of bleeding. On the other hand, the donation of a pint of blood at a blood transfusion center represents a loss of only one-eleventh of the blood volume—an amount the body will tolerate easily and replace quickly.

The Blood

The blood is a thick, red fluid made up of cells suspended in a liquid called **plasma** (Fig. 2.9). There are three types of cells in blood: **red cells**, which carry oxygen; **white cells**, which fight infection; and **platelets**, which aid in blood clotting. Plasma consists of water and a remarkable number of different minerals, inorganic compounds, and organic compounds such as proteins, simple sugars, and fats. It contains *transient* materials such as nutrients and waste materials that are transported to and from cells, and *component* materials such as proteins and other complex substances involved in immunity and blood clotting.

The Respiratory System

The respiratory system includes the organs responsible for bringing outside air into the body and placing it in close contact with the blood. From above downward, the components of the respiratory system (Fig. 2.10) are organized into the **upper airway** (upper respiratory tract), which includes the nose, mouth, nasal cavity, and pharynx; and the **lower airway** (lower respiratory tract), which includes the larynx, trachea, and lungs. The lungs contain the bronchi, bronchioles, and alveoli.

When a person breathes in, air enters the **nasal cavity** through the nose, where it starts to warm as it passes over the convolutions of the turbinate bones. The sensory receptors for smell (olfactory organ) are located at the top of the nasal cavity. From there, the air enters the upper part of the **pharynx**, called the nasopharynx. The pharynx is also part of the digestive system—it is a sac-like organ continuous above with both the nose and mouth. It separates air from food, conducting the air into the **larynx** (below and anterior) and the food into the **esophagus** (below and posterior). A valve at the top of the

Fig. 2.10 *Components of the Respiratory System*

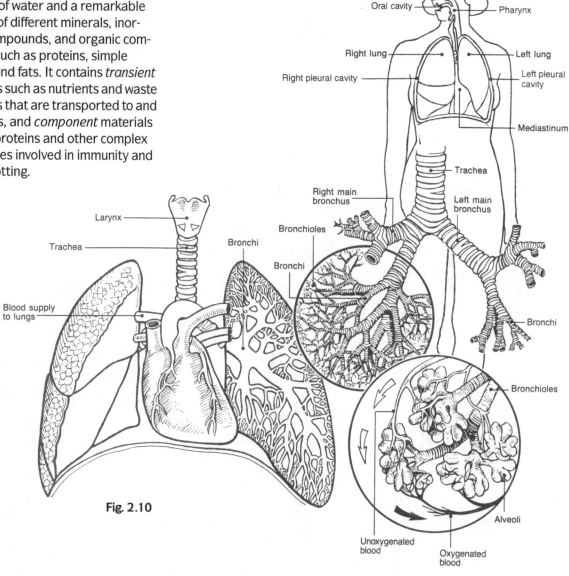

Fig. 2.10

larynx, the **epiglottis**, closes upon swallowing so that food does not enter the lower airway and cause choking.

In the larynx, the air passes across the two **vocal cords** and down into the **trachea**. The trachea runs from the lower part of the neck into the mid-chest where it divides into the left and right **main bronchi**. Each bronchus enters its respective lung, where it divides into smaller and smaller bronchi, and finally into the smallest, the **bronchioles**. The **alveoli** are attached like bunches of grapes to the bronchioles (Fig. 2.10). Lung capillaries in the walls of the alveoli bring the blood to within a few microns of the air in the alveoli. Because the lungs contain elastic tissue, they can expand and contract without tearing or breaking as the air moves in and out.

In emergency care, the term "airway" (as in "clearing the airway") usually refers to the upper airway. The upper airway is located in the head and neck; the lower airway in the neck and chest. Infections of the respiratory system frequently are divided into those of the upper respiratory tract (upper respiratory infections), and those of the lower respiratory tract (laryngitis, tracheitis, bronchitis, and pneumonia).

The Breathing Process

The **chest** is a hollow, cage-like structure whose semi-rigid wall surrounds and encloses a large cavity, the **chest cavity** (also called the thoracic cavity). The outer layer of the chest wall consists of skin, subcutaneous tissue, and the muscles that move the arms and shoulders. The main part of the chest wall (Fig. 2.11) is made up of 12 pairs of ribs that are attached to the spine in back and, except for the last two pairs, to the breastbone (sternum) in front. Between each pair of ribs are several layers of **intercostal muscles**. The chest blends with the neck above and the abdomen below. The chest cavity is separated from the abdominal cavity by

the muscular **diaphragm**. When the outer intercostal muscles contract, the ribs move up and out; when the inner muscles contract, the ribs move closer together. Contracting the outer intercostal muscles and the diaphragm together enlarges the space within the chest cavity as the ribs move up and out and the diaphragm moves down.

The chest cavity contains two smaller cavities, the right and left **pleural cavities**, separated by the **mediastinum**. The right pleural cavi-

---

Fig. 2.11 *Chest Wall*

Fig. 2.12 *Lungs, Pleura, and Pleural Spaces*

Fig. 2.13 *Mechanics of Breathing*

ty contains the **right lung**; the left pleural cavity the **left lung**. A continuous, thin membrane, the **pleura**, lines the inside of each cavity and is continued over the outer surface of each lung, forming a closed sac (Fig. 2.12). The area inside this sac is called the **pleural space**. Normally, the pleura lining the pleural cavity and the pleura covering the outside of the lung are separated only by a thin film of fluid, so that the pleural space is a *potential* rather than an *actual* space. This fluid lubricates the motion of the two layers of pleura across each other as the chest cage and lungs expand and contract during breathing.

The motion of the lung within the chest during breathing is normally

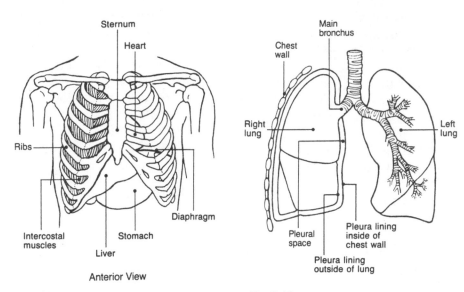

Fig. 2.11

Fig. 2.12

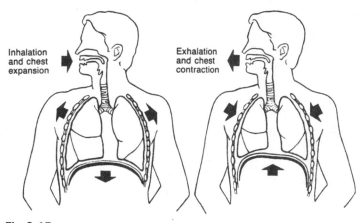

Fig. 2.13

smooth, effortless, and pain-free. In illnesses such as infection of the pleura (pleurisy), pneumonia, or congestive heart failure, and in severe chest injury, the pleural space may become an actual space filled with air, pus, edema fluid, or blood. The pain of pleurisy or pneumonia is caused by inflamed and roughened parts of the pleura moving across each other during breathing or coughing.

When a person breathes in (inhales), the chest expands, enlarging the pleural cavities and tending to drop the pressure in the pleural space below that of the outside air. The greater outside air pressure causes air to flow into the upper and lower airways, enlarging (expanding) the lungs so that they follow the movement of the chest wall and pleural cavities (Fig. 2.13). Note that the lungs expand because they are *pushed out from within* rather than *pulled out* as the chest expands.

Breathing out (exhaling) is normally a passive process—the elastic recoil of the lungs and the chest wall returns them to their previous size and shape. This drives air out of the lungs and allows the pressure inside the pleural space to rise until it is again equal to that of the outside air. Forced exhalation can be performed by contracting the inner intercostal muscles and making the chest cavity smaller by narrowing the spaces between the ribs or by forcing the diaphragm up, as in the Heimlich maneuver (described in Chapter 4 and Appendix B).

The depth, rate, and rhythm of breathing are controlled by the respiratory center in the brain. This center responds to either too little oxygen or too much carbon dioxide in the blood by *increasing* the depth and rate of breathing. It responds to too much oxygen or too little carbon dioxide in the blood by *decreasing* the depth and rate of breathing.

Normally, breathing is automatic. It is possible to hold one's breath voluntarily or to breathe very rapidly for a short time only. When the normal amounts of oxygen or carbon dioxide in the blood are sufficiently altered, the respiratory center will automatically override the strongest voluntary efforts.

The Digestive System

The digestive system consists of the **digestive tract**, a tube that conducts food through the body from mouth to anus, and **associated organs** that produce substances to aid digestion. This system ingests, digests, and absorbs food and fluid, and eliminates wastes. **Ingestion** means to take into the body. **Digestion** is the breakdown of food into simpler substances that can be more easily absorbed into the bloodstream. **Absorption** is the transfer of digested substances through the intestinal wall into the blood. **Elimination** is the expulsion of indigestible residues through the feces.

Starting from above downward, the digestive tract (Fig. 2.14) includes the **mouth, pharynx** (oropharynx),

Fig. 2.14 *Digestive Tract*

esophagus, stomach, small intestine, appendix, large intestine, rectum, and anus. Associated organs include the salivary glands, liver, gallbladder, and pancreas.

Food enters the **mouth**, where it is chewed into small pieces by the **teeth** and mixed with **saliva**. Saliva moistens the food and starts the

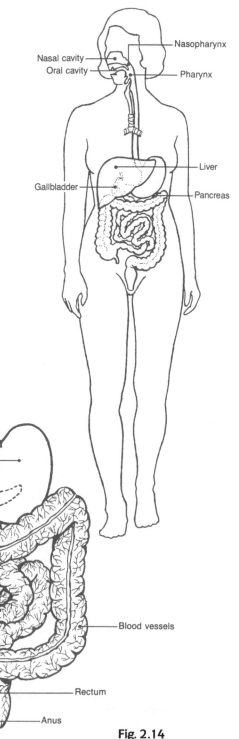

Fig. 2.14

digestive process with an enzyme that breaks down starch. The **tongue** helps move the food and contains **taste buds** that provide the perception of bitter, salty, sweet, and sour **tastes**. The different **flavors** of food are perceived by the **olfactory organ** in the nose; people actually smell the flavor of food rather than taste it.

The chewed and moistened food then passes through the **pharynx** and **esophagus** into the **stomach**, where it is mixed with gastric juice containing hydrochloric acid and a protein-digesting enzyme. Next, the partly digested food enters the first part of the small intestine—the duodenum—where it is mixed with **bile** and **pancreatic juice**. Bile is produced by the **liver** and stored in the **gallbladder**. It contains an emulsifying agent that prepares fat for digestion. Juice produced by the **pancreas** contains enzymes that digest fat, starch, and protein. The rest of the **small intestine** is about 20 feet long and contains additional enzyme-secreting glands in its wall to complete digestion.

Most of the digested food is absorbed into the body through the small intestine. The unabsorbed residue enters the **large intestine**, which concentrates the residue by removing most of its water. The large intestine is about 6 feet long. The resulting fecal matter is stored in the lower part of the large intestine until it can be expelled through the **anus**. The **appendix**, a worm-sized organ that has no obvious useful purpose, is attached to the beginning of the large intestine.

During digestion, the body produces up to 1.6 quarts (1,500 milliliters) of saliva, 3.2 quarts (3,000 milliliters) of gastric juice, 1.6 quarts (1,500 milliliters) of pancreatic juice, and 1 pint (500 milliliters) of bile a day, most of which is **reabsorbed** by the small and large intestines. Vomiting and diarrhea interfere with reabsorption of these fluids and can cause serious dehydration.

The liver has many functions besides bile production. It converts sugars into **glycogen**, a complex carbohydrate that it stores; manufactures proteins; helps metabolize fat; and detoxifies drugs and other substances. In addition to its role in digestion, the pancreas also makes the hormone **insulin**, which is necessary for the metabolism of glucose, the body's chief source of energy.

The Urinary System

The urinary system (Fig. 2.15) consists of the two **kidneys**; the two **ureters**, which drain **urine** from the

Fig. 2.15 *Urinary System*

Fig. 2.16 *Female and Male Genitourinary Systems*

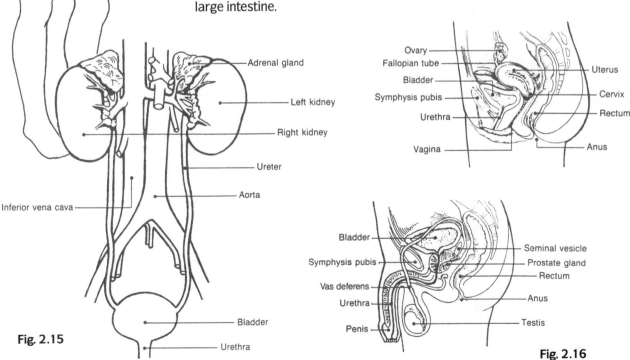

Fig. 2.15

- Adrenal gland
- Left kidney
- Right kidney
- Ureter
- Aorta
- Inferior vena cava
- Bladder
- Urethra

- Ovary
- Fallopian tube
- Bladder
- Symphysis pubis
- Urethra
- Vagina
- Uterus
- Cervix
- Rectum
- Anus

- Bladder
- Symphysis pubis
- Vas deferens
- Urethra
- Penis
- Seminal vesicle
- Prostate gland
- Rectum
- Anus
- Testis

Fig. 2.16

kidneys; the **bladder**, which stores urine; and the **urethra**, which drains urine to the outside.

The kidneys lie on either side of the spine against the upper part of the posterior abdominal wall and contain a complicated system of filters and collecting tubes. They are supplied with blood by the renal arteries, which are large vessels that branch directly from the aorta and bring 25 percent of the heart's output of blood to the kidneys. The kidneys make urine by filtering waste products of cellular metabolism from the blood, processing about 19.8 gallons (75 liters) of blood per hour. During this activity, about 2 gallons (7,500 milliliters) of fluid per hour is filtered from the blood along with the wastes. As this fluid travels through the kidneys, essential minerals and most of the water are reabsorbed by the blood. Thus, the kidneys conserve the body's content of water and essential minerals, producing only about 2 ounces (60 milliliters) of urine per hour and returning the remainder of the filtrate to the blood. In some types of kidney failure, the kidneys are unable to concentrate the urine by removing enough water, and the patient is in danger of rapid dehydration.

The body of a 150-pound (70-kilogram) young adult male is about 60 percent water, which amounts to 11 gallons (42 liters). Of this, 7.4 gallons (28 liters) are within the cells and 3.7 gallons (14 liters) outside the cells, including about 1.5 gallons (5.5 liters) in the blood.

The kidneys carefully guard the content and relative proportions of the body's water and minerals by regulating the excretion of water and minerals such as sodium and potassium. If the diet contains enough fluid,

Fig. 2.17 *Human Skeleton*

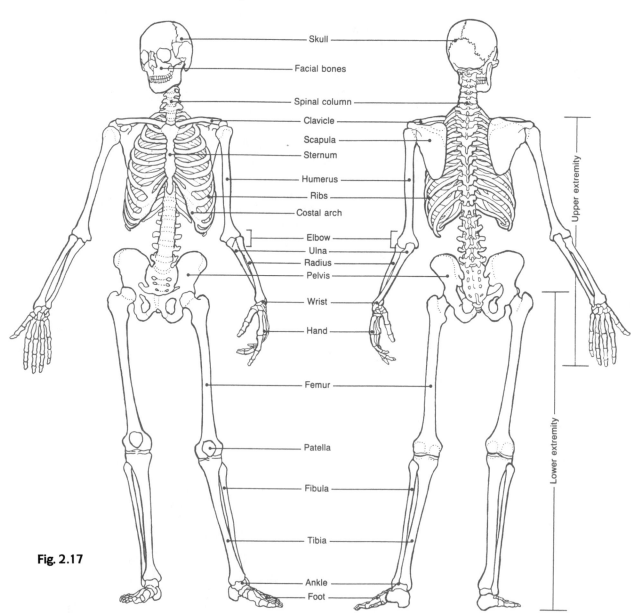

Fig. 2.17

Skull
Facial bones
Spinal column
Clavicle
Scapula
Sternum
Humerus
Ribs
Costal arch
Elbow
Ulna
Radius
Pelvis
Wrist
Hand
Femur
Patella
Fibula
Tibia
Ankle
Foot

Upper extremity
Lower extremity

an average adult excretes about 1.3 quarts (1,200 milliliters) of light-yellow urine daily. Any excess fluid is excreted, producing a large amount of pale urine. Insufficient fluid intake—or excessive fluid loss caused by vomiting, diarrhea, or perspiration—triggers conservation of fluid, with as little as 10 to 14 ounces (300 to 400 milliliters) of concentrated, dark urine being produced each day. If the diet contains too much or too little sodium or potassium, the kidneys will vary the excretion of these minerals. In kidney failure, the kidney loses the ability to excrete wastes and to regulate the body's water and minerals.

Urine drains from each kidney into its funnel-shaped **renal pelvis** at the upper end of its **ureter**, a muscular tube that runs down along the back of the abdominal cavity and empties into the **bladder**. The bladder, a hollow organ with muscular walls, lies in the pelvic cavity behind the pubic bones (Fig. 2.16). The bladder is drained by a tube, the **urethra**. In males, this tube passes through the penis and is about 8 inches long; in females the urethra is about 1 inch long and exits just above the vaginal opening.

The Skeletal System

The skeletal system, made up of 206 **bones** and their associated **ligaments** (Fig. 2.17), provides a rigid framework to protect and support

the softer tissues, gives form to the body and, together with the muscular system, allows body movement. The inner part of bone (the marrow) produces blood cells.

Looking at a dry, dead bone, it is hard to appreciate that normal bone is a living tissue composed of a protein matrix containing deposits of a complex salt made of the important minerals calcium and phosphorus. Bones have many small cavities filled with living cells responsible for bone growth and maintenance. Because bones are richly supplied with blood vessels and nerves, injury to bone can cause severe pain and bleeding. All bones have an outer casing of hard, compact, bony tissue and an interior cavity of spongy bone containing the marrow. There are three major types of bones (Fig. 2.18): **long bones**, found in the limbs; **flat bones**, found in the skull and pelvis; and **irregular bones**, such as the vertebrae.

The bones of young children are less brittle than the bones of adults because they contain relatively more protein matrix. When injured, a child's bone will occasionally bend (greenstick fracture) rather than break completely through. As the body ages, calcium and matrix are gradually lost so that the bones become weaker and more brittle. Even minor falls can cause fractures in the elderly.

Muscles are attached to bones by tough, fibrous structures called **tendons**. Each tendon usually attaches to a bone at a prominent point or ridge.

The area of contact between two bones is called a **joint**. Joints may be **freely movable**, **slightly movable**, or **immovable** (Fig. 2.19). The joints of the limbs are freely movable, while the joints between the vertebrae are only slightly movable. The joints of the skull and pelvis are examples of immovable joints. In general, the more complex, freely movable joints are more prone to damage from trauma than the simpler, less movable joints. At immovable joints, bones are bound directly to each other by tough, fibrous tissue.

In movable joints, the opposing surfaces of bone are covered by cartilage, which provides a smooth riding surface. The joint is surrounded by a sac of fibrous tissue, the **joint capsule**, which is tight in some areas and loose in others to permit joint motion. Parts of the capsule that are thicker and stronger are called **ligaments**, which serve as important attachments between the bones that form the joint. The inner part of the joint capsule is lined by the **synovial membrane**, which produces a fluid that lubricates and nourishes joint tissues.

The two major types of movable joints are the **ball-and-socket joint** and the **hinge joint** (Fig. 2.20). Ball-and-socket joints can bend in any direction and rotate around a central axis; examples are the hip and shoulder joints. Hinge joints usually move in only one plane; examples are the elbow and ankle joints. The knee joint,

Fig. 2.18 *Three Major Types of Bones*

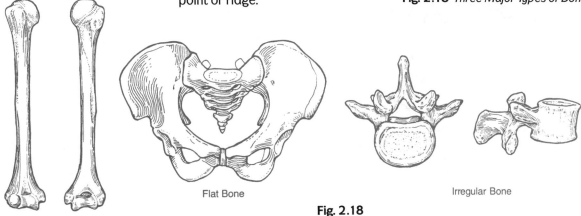

Long Bone

Flat Bone

Fig. 2.18

Irregular Bone

which is discussed in Chapter 11, is a special type of hinge joint that allows both bending and a small amount of rotation around a central axis.

The Skull

The skull (Fig. 2.21) is made up of the **cranium** and the **face**. The cranium is composed of several flat bones tightly fused together to form a rounded container for the brain. The face consists of a number of irregularly shaped bones that support the nose and other facial features. The **maxilla**, or upper jaw, contains the upper teeth. The **mandible**, or lower jaw, contains the lower teeth and is attached to the rest of the skull at the two **temporomandibular (TM) joints**.

The Spine

The spine, or **vertebral column** (Fig. 2.22), which is composed of 33 **vertebrae** (Fig. 2.23), forms the main support for the body and protects the spinal cord. Between each pair of vertebrae is a plate-like **intervertebral disc**, composed of a ring of fibrous cartilage with a soft center. The vertebrae are connected to each other by the discs, by a series of ligaments, and by two pairs of small joints—an arrangement that permits some spinal movement.

Each vertebra has three major parts: the **body**, the **arch**, and the **processes**. The posterior processes are also called **spinous** processes;

Fig. 2.19 *Three Major Types of Joints*

Fig. 2.20 *Two Major Types of Movable Joints*

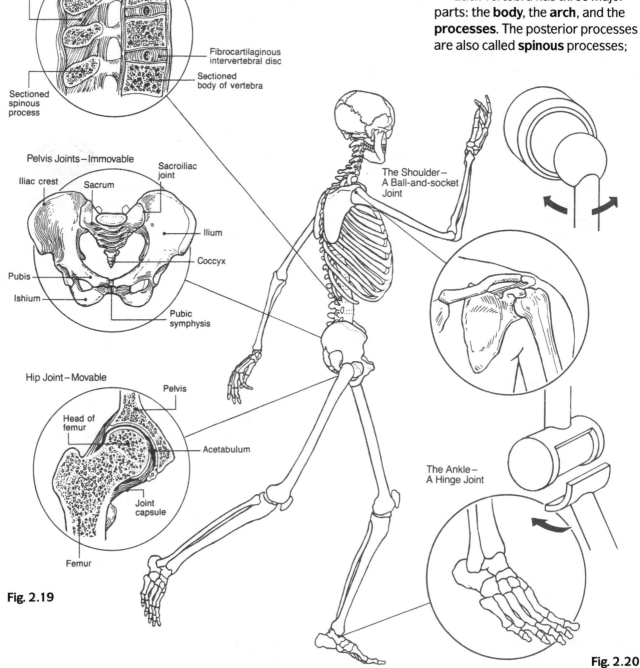

Vertebral Joints—Slightly Movable

Interspinal ligament

Fibrocartilaginous intervertebral disc

Sectioned body of vertebra

Sectioned spinous process

Pelvis Joints—Immovable

Iliac crest   Sacrum   Sacroiliac joint

Ilium

Coccyx

Pubis

Ishium

Pubic symphysis

Hip Joint—Movable   Pelvis

Head of femur

Acetabulum

Joint capsule

Femur

Fig. 2.19

The Shoulder— A Ball-and-socket Joint

The Ankle— A Hinge Joint

Fig. 2.20

the lateral processes are also called **transverse** processes. The **articular processes** form joints with the corresponding processes of the vertebrae above and below. When posture is erect, the vertebral bodies are *anterior* and the arches *posterior*. The processes form attachment points for ligaments and tendons.

The successive vertebral arches form the **spinal canal** (Fig. 2.24), which runs like a tunnel from the top to the bottom of the spine and contains the **spinal cord**. At regular intervals, pairs of **spinal nerves** branch off from the cord and exit through notches between the vertebrae.

The spine is divided into five regions (see Fig. 2.22): **cervical, thoracic, lumbar, sacral,** and **coccygeal**. The cervical spine consists of the seven cervical vertebrae, the thoracic spine consists of the 12 thoracic vertebrae, and the lumbar spine consists of the five lumbar vertebrae. The five sacral vertebrae are fused together to form a single bone, the **sacrum**, and the last four vertebrae are fused to form the vestigial, tail-like **coccyx**. The cervical and lumbar regions of the spine are more mobile and more prone to injury than the thoracic, sacral, and coccygeal regions.

The skull rests on the first cervical vertebra. The spinal cord passes through a large hole (the **foramen magnum**) at the base of the skull and attaches to the base of the brain.

Fig. 2.21 *Bones of the Skull*

Fig. 2.22 *Spine or Vertebral Column*

Fig. 2.23 *Parts of a Typical Vertebra*

Fig. 2.24 *The spinal cord lies in the spinal canal.*

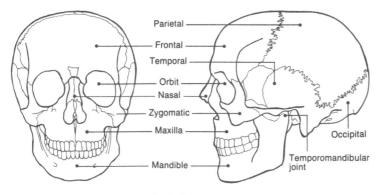

Parietal
Frontal
Temporal
Orbit
Nasal
Zygomatic
Maxilla
Mandible
Occipital
Temporomandibular joint

Fig. 2.21

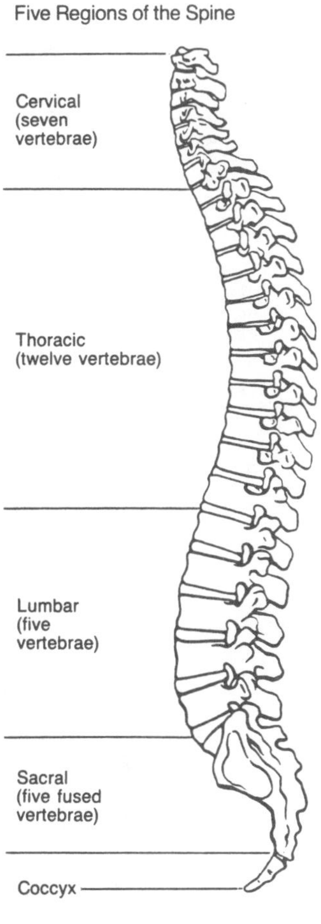

Five Regions of the Spine

Cervical (seven vertebrae)

Thoracic (twelve vertebrae)

Lumbar (five vertebrae)

Sacral (five fused vertebrae)

Coccyx

Fig. 2.22

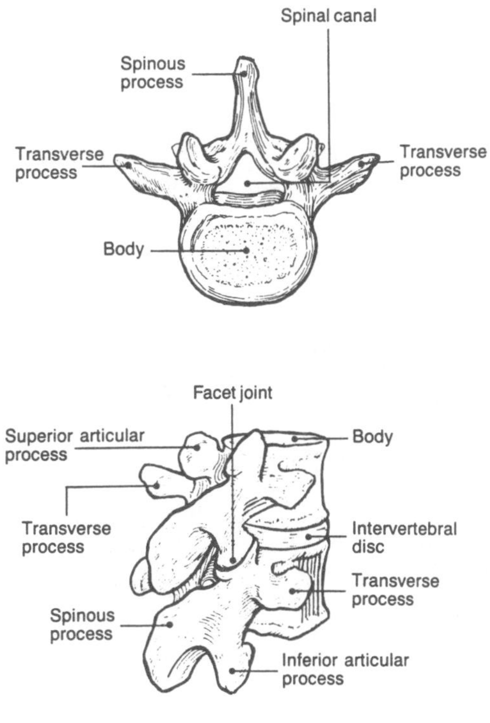

Spinal canal
Spinous process
Transverse process
Transverse process
Body

Facet joint
Superior articular process
Body
Transverse process
Intervertebral disc
Transverse process
Spinous process
Inferior articular process

Fig. 2.23

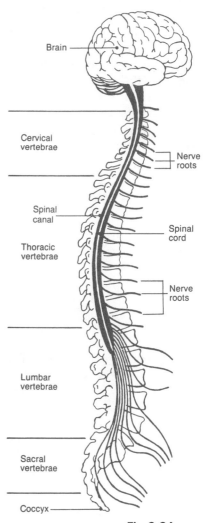

Brain
Cervical vertebrae
Nerve roots
Spinal canal
Spinal cord
Thoracic vertebrae
Nerve roots
Lumbar vertebrae
Sacral vertebrae
Coccyx

Fig. 2.24

The Chest (Thorax)

The bones of the chest wall (Fig. 2.25) are the 12 pairs of **ribs**, the 12 **thoracic vertebrae**, and the **sternum** (breastbone). The chest was discussed previously in the section on the respiratory system (see Fig. 2.11). Each pair of ribs is attached in back to one of the thoracic vertebrae. The upper 10 pairs of ribs also have attachments in front. The two lower pairs lack frontal attachments and are known as the "floating ribs."

The front end of each rib is composed of cartilage. The junction between the bony rear portion and the cartilage is weak and easily sprained. Such sprains are a frequent cause of minor chest pain.

The first through fifth ribs connect directly to the sternum in front, while the sixth through tenth ribs are connected by cartilage to form the **costal arch**, which is attached to the lower end of the sternum. Important features of the sternum include the **sternal angle**, a bony ridge at the junction of the upper and lower parts of the sternum where the second ribs attach, and the **xiphoid process**, a tail of cartilage that hangs from the lower end of the sternum.

Fig. 2.25 *Important Parts of the Thorax*

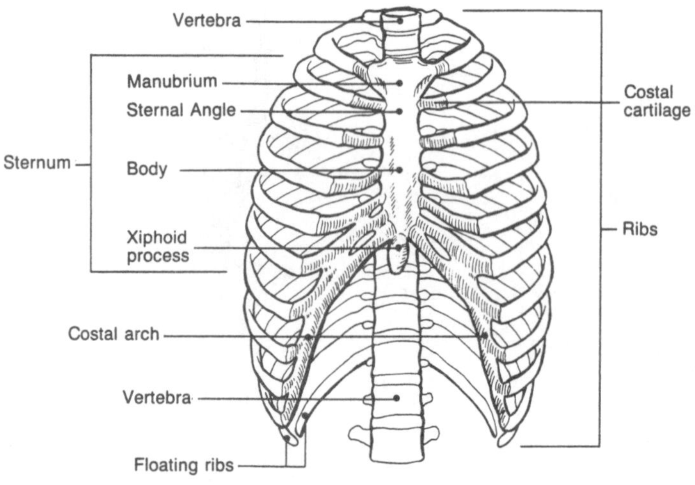

Fig. 2.25

The Upper Extremity

The upper extremity is composed of the **shoulder, arm** (upper arm), **forearm**, and **hand** (Fig. 2.26). The upper part (**shoulder girdle**) contains three bones (Fig. 2.27): the **clavicle** (collarbone), the **scapula** (shoulder blade), and the **humerus** (upper arm bone). Each shoulder girdle also contains three joints: the **sternoclavicular joint**, the **acromioclavicular (AC) joint**, and the **shoulder joint**. Because the upper extremity is directly attached to the rest of the skeleton only by the sternoclavicular joint and because the shoulder joint is a ball-and-socket joint, the upper extremity has a wide range of motion. The cup of the shoulder joint is very shallow (Fig. 2.27), making it unstable and easy to dislocate.

The **clavicle** is a long, thin bone that attaches medially to the sternum and laterally to the acromion process of the scapula. The **scapula**, a large, flat, triangular bone, is held by large muscles against the posterior chest wall. At its outer angle, the head of the **humerus** fits into the shoulder joint socket.

The lower end of the humerus is connected to the two forearm bones

Fig. 2.26 *Upper Extremity Bones*

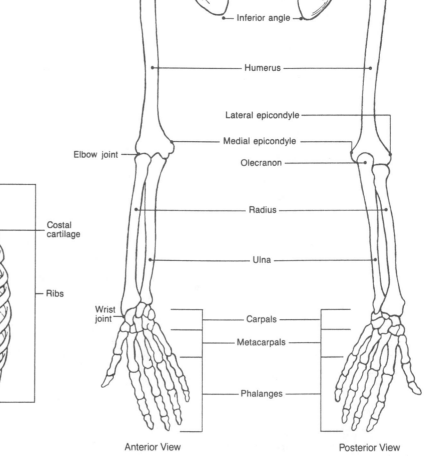

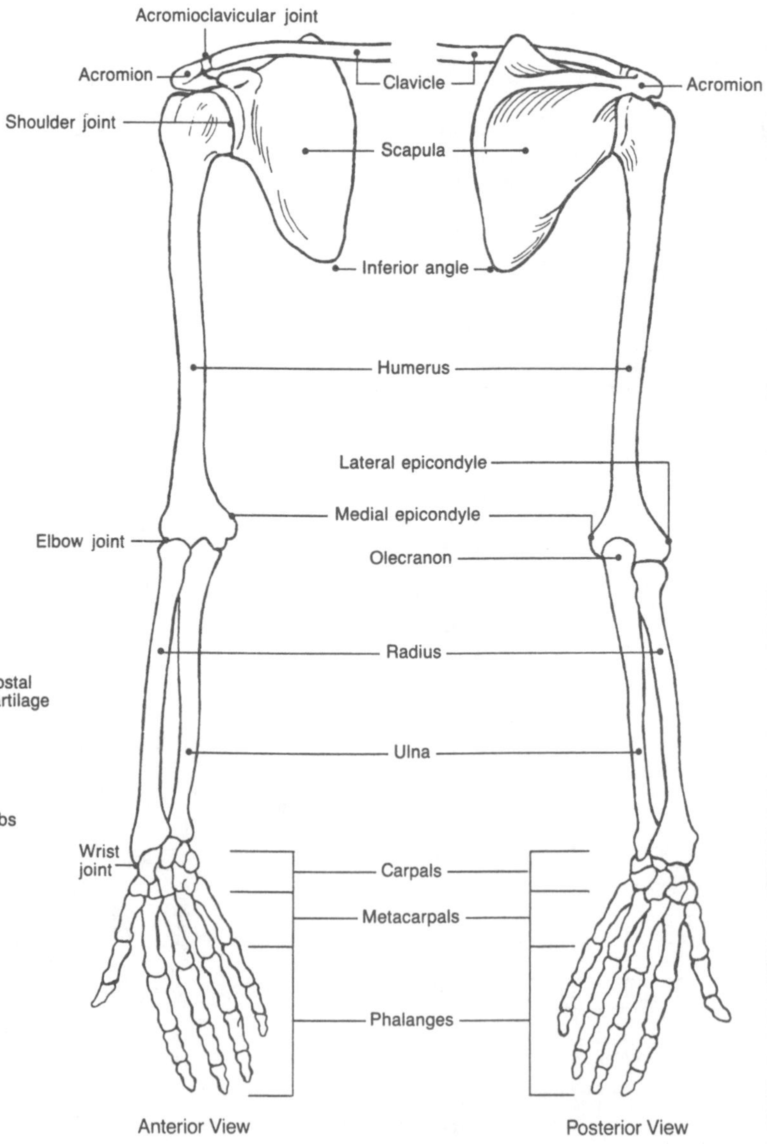

Anterior View   Posterior View

Fig. 2.26

at the **elbow joint**. When a person stands with palms facing forward, the **radius** is lateral and the **ulna** is medial. The elbow joint (Fig. 2.28) is actually made up of two separate joints. The main part is a simple hinge joint formed by a spool-like **condyle** on the medial part of the distal end of the humerus that fits into a notch on the proximal end of the ulna. The other joint is a pivot joint where the proximal end of the radius fits against a round knob on the lateral aspect of the distal end of the humerus and is held in place by a

fibrous ring. This arrangement not only allows the elbow to be bent and straightened but permits the forearm to rotate (Fig. 2.29) so that the palm of the hand can face either forward or backward.

The distal ends of the radius and ulna are connected to the **carpal** (wrist) **bones** at the **wrist joint** (Fig. 2.30). The most distal of the eight carpal bones connect with the five **metacarpal bones**, which are found in the palm of the hand and form a base for the fingers and thumb. Each

finger contains three small bones, called **phalanges**; the thumb has only two phalanges. The phalanges of the thumb and fingers are connected to each other by simple hinge joints. Much of the wide range of motion of which the fingers and thumb are capable, however, is due to the nature of the joints between the metacarpals of the fingers and their proximal phalanges (metacarpophalangeal joints), and between the metacarpal of the thumb and its carpal (carpometacarpal joint). These joints enable each finger and the thumb to

Fig. 2.27 *Shoulder Girdle*

Fig. 2.28 *Detail of the Elbow Joint*

Fig. 2.29 *Forearm Movements*

Fig. 2.30 *Detail of the Wrist and Hand*

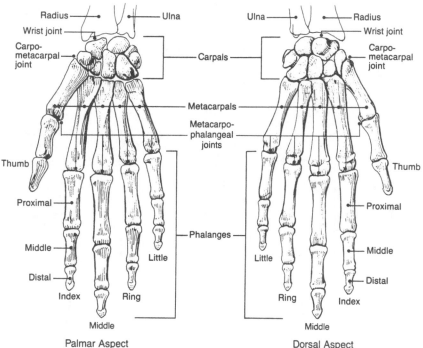

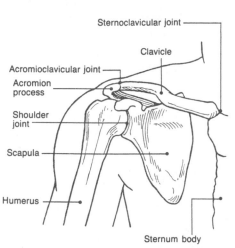

Fig. 2.27

Fig. 2.28

Fig. 2.29

Palmar Aspect   Dorsal Aspect

Fig. 2.30

move in and out (**adduct** and **abduct**) and up and down (**extend** and **flex**). That is because this special type of hinge joint can hinge in more than one direction (but still cannot rotate around a single axis like a ball-and-socket joint). The wrist joint also is this type of joint.

The Pelvis

The pelvis (Fig. 2.31) is a cone-shaped, bony ring made up of the right and left **pelvic bones**, which are joined together in front at the **pubis**. In back, the pelvis and sacrum join at the **sacroiliac joints**. Each pelvic bone consists of three separate bones—the **ilium, ischium,** and **pubis**—joined by immovable joints to form a wing-like structure. The ilium is superior, the pubis anterior, and the ischium posterior. The main feature of the ilium is the long, curving iliac crest. The medial part of the pubic bone is easily felt just above the genitals. The **ischial tuberosities** are the large, bony knobs that can be felt deep in each lower buttock. The pelvis is a rigid structure that encloses and protects the organs in the pelvic cavity—the **bladder, rectum**, and **female reproductive organs** (Fig. 2.32)—and adds support to the body. There is a cup-shaped depression, the **acetabulum** (Fig. 2.33), where the three pelvic bones join laterally. The head of the femur fits into the acetabulum to form the hip joint, a ball-and-socket joint that allows both bending and rotation. Because this socket is much deeper than the shoulder joint socket, the hip is much harder to dislocate.

The Lower Extremity

The lower extremity (Fig. 2.34) consists of the **thigh, leg**, and **foot**. The thighbone, or **femur**, is quite strong and is the longest bone in the body. It joins with the two lower leg bones at the **knee joint**. This joint, a complex one important in skiing and other outdoor activities, is discussed in detail in Chapter 11. The **patella**, or kneecap, lies in the tendon of the quadriceps muscle, which extends the knee. The patella's presence and location increase the efficiency of the knee joint.

The two lower leg bones are the **tibia** and **fibula**. The main weight-bearing of the two is the tibia, which lies medially. Its edge can be felt beneath the skin, and its distal end—the **medial malleolus**—can be felt

Fig. 2.31 *Pelvic Bones*

Fig. 2.32 *Pelvic Organs*

Fig. 2.33 *The three pelvic bones join laterally to form a cup-shaped cavity, the acetabulum.*

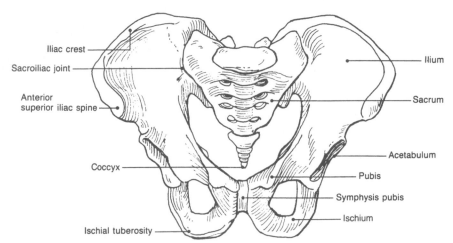

Fig. 2.31

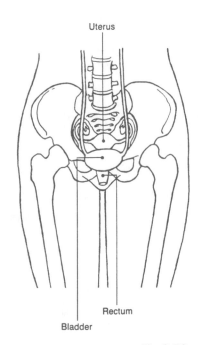

Fig. 2.32

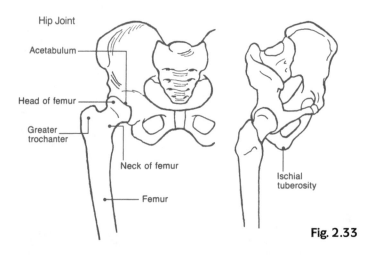

Fig. 2.33

where it forms the *inside* part of the ankle joint. The fibula lies laterally; its head can be felt on the outside of the knee joint, and its distal end—the **lateral malleolus**—can be felt where it forms the *outside* part of the ankle joint (Fig. 2.35).

The **ankle joint** is a hinge joint formed by the lower ends of the tibia and fibula proximally and one of the foot bones, the **talus**, distally. Another important foot bone is the

---

Fig. 2.34 *Lower Extremity Bones*

Fig. 2.35 *Foot and Ankle Bones*

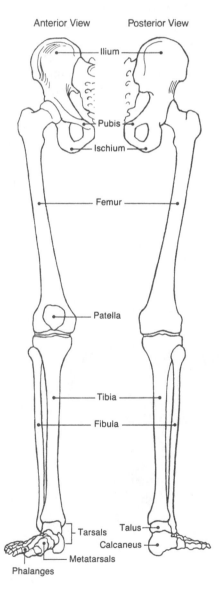

Fig. 2.34

calcaneus, or heel bone, to which the large, rope-like **Achilles tendon** is attached. The other bones of the foot are similar to their counterparts in the hand; they include the five **tarsals**, the five long, slender **metatarsals**, which form the arch of the foot, and the **phalanges**, or toe bones. The great toe has two phalanges, and each of the smaller toes has three.

The Body Cavities

The **chest cavity** has been described previously in the sections on the respiratory system and the chest. Its walls (Fig. 2.36) are formed by the thoracic spine and adjacent muscles posteriorly, the sternum anteriorly, and the sweeping curve of the ribs and their muscles laterally. The chest cavity is limited by the structures of the neck above and is separated from the abdominal cavity below by the diaphragm. It contains the **right** and **left pleural cavities** and the central area between them, the **mediastinum** (Fig. 2.37). The right and left pleural cavities contain the lungs and pleural spaces.

The mediastinum contains the heart, its enclosing sac (the pericardium), the main pulmonary artery

and its two branches, the arch of the aorta, the thoracic aorta, and the first parts of the large arteries supplying the upper body. It also contains the superior and inferior venae cavae, the trachea, the two main bronchi, the esophagus, the vagus nerves, which help regulate the heart rate and digestive tract function, the phrenic nerves, which supply the diaphragm, and other major nerves.

The Abdominal and Pelvic Cavities

The walls of the **abdominal cavity** (Figs. 2.36, 2.38) are formed by the lumbar spine and its associated muscles posteriorly, the abdominal muscles anteriorly, and the flank muscles and upper ilium bones laterally. The abdominal cavity is separated from the chest cavity above by the diaphragm. Below, the abdominal cavity is continuous with the pelvic cavity at the **pelvic brim**, located at the level of the pubis and upper sacrum. The abdominal aorta and inferior vena cava run through the back of the abdominal cavity, which also contains major arteries and veins that supply the abdominal

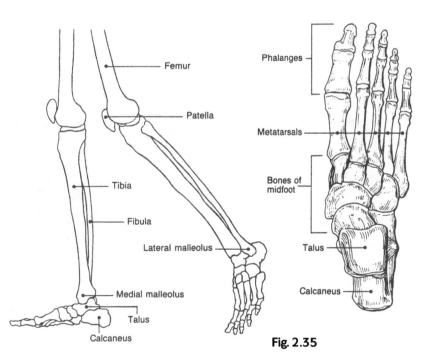

Fig. 2.35

organs. The cavity is lined with a thin membrane, the **peritoneum**, which is continuous with the outer coverings of the organs within the cavity, forming a closed sac similar to the pleural cavities.

Organs of the digestive system (Fig. 2.39) that lie *within* the abdominal cavity are the stomach, duodenum, small intestine, colon, appendix, liver, and gallbladder. The pancreas, kidneys, and ureters lie *behind* the abdominal cavity against the muscles of the back. The **spleen**, an organ that filters the blood, lies in the upper-left part of the abdominal cavity. The exact locations of these organs are discussed in Chapter 3.

Fig. 2.36 *Three Major Body Cavities*

Fig. 2.37 *Contents of the Chest Cavity*

Many of the organs within the abdominal cavity are suspended from its walls by thin sheets of connective tissue called **mesentery**. This arrangement allows organs of the digestive system such as the large and small intestines to move around the cavity to some extent as the contraction of their muscular walls mixes the intestinal contents and propels them forward (peristaltic activity).

The **pelvic cavity** (Figs. 2.36, 2.40) is continuous with the abdominal cavity. Its sides and floor are formed by the pelvic bones and muscles, and it is lined with a continuation of the peritoneum. The pelvic cavity contains the bladder, rectum, and, in females, the reproductive organs.

The peritoneum contains nerves that, when infected or irritated, cause pain. Because the nerves and nerve endings are different from those in the skin, intra-abdominal or pelvic pain is harder to localize than pain arising in the skin.

In general, abdominal and pelvic organs are either **hollow** or **solid** (Fig. 2.41). Hollow organs are shaped like tubes or sacs and contain liquid or semisolid material; examples include the stomach, intestines, gallbladder, urinary bladder, ureters, and uterus. Solid organs include the liver, spleen, pancreas, adrenal glands, and kidneys. Injury to or disease of hollow organs can cause their contents to spill into the peritoneal cavity, causing **peritonitis** (infection or irritation of the peritoneal cavity). Injury to solid organs can cause serious bleeding with shock plus abdominal pain because of irritation of the peritoneum by the blood. The location of early infection or bleeding corresponds fairly well, but not completely, to the location of the pain or tenderness. As the infection or bleeding progresses, pain and tenderness frequently expand to involve the entire abdomen.

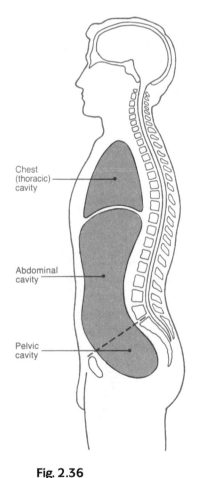

Chest (thoracic) cavity

Abdominal cavity

Pelvic cavity

Fig. 2.36

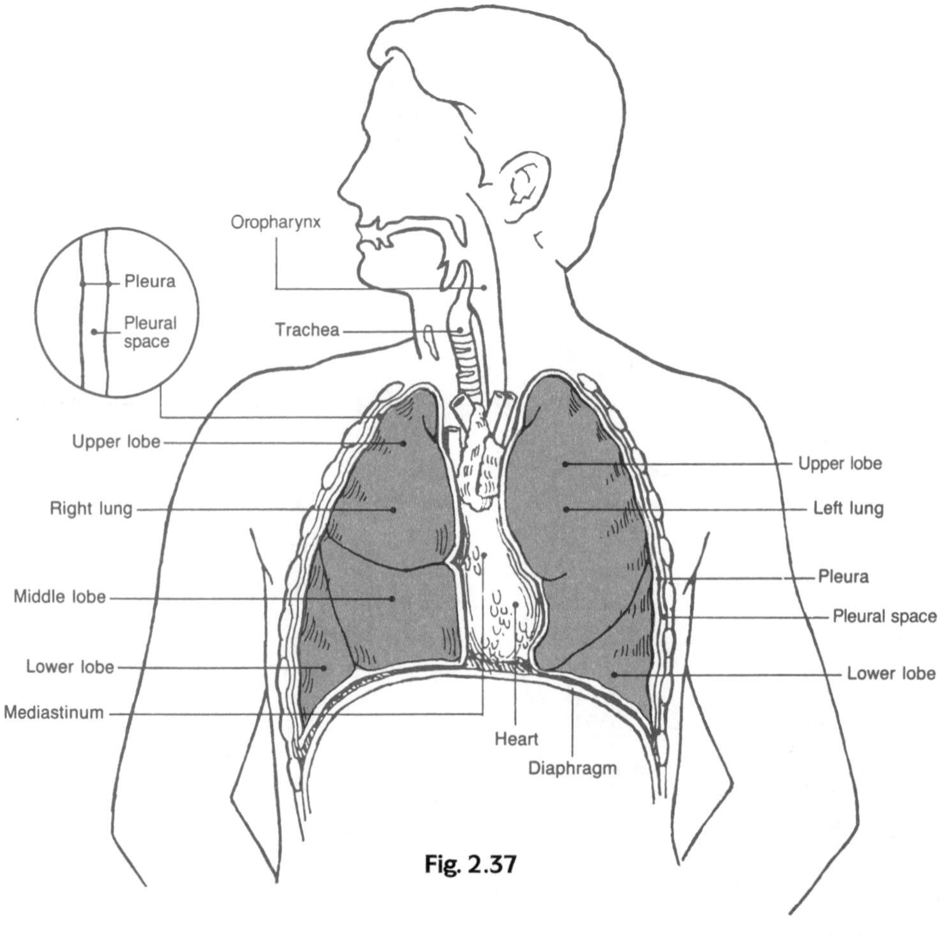

Oropharynx

Pleura

Pleural space

Trachea

Upper lobe

Right lung

Middle lobe

Lower lobe

Mediastinum

Upper lobe

Left lung

Pleura

Pleural space

Lower lobe

Heart

Diaphragm

Fig. 2.37

Fig. 2.38 *Abdominal Cavity*

Fig. 2.39 *Contents of the Abdominal Cavity*

Fig. 2.40 *Pelvic Cavity and its Contents*

The Muscular System

Muscle is a special tissue composed of cells that can shorten, or **contract**, and lengthen, or **relax**. Muscle contraction is an active, energy-requiring process; relaxation is a passive process requiring little energy. There are three types of muscles: **skeletal**, **smooth**, and **cardiac** (Fig. 2.42).

The **skeletal muscles**, which allow body movement, are generally arranged in opposing sets extending across the joints and are attached at points proximal and distal to the joints. Various types of joint movement are produced when opposing sets of muscles are alternately contracted and relaxed.

Skeletal muscles are called **voluntary muscles** because they are under conscious control and can be contracted or relaxed at will. The **motor area** of the brain's **cerebral cortex** controls this function. Nerve fibers travel from this area through the brain and spinal cord to reach the muscles via the **peripheral nerves**.

Muscles are covered by a sheath of tough, fibrous tissue called **fascia**. At the ends of the muscle, the fascia extends into strong cords called **tendons** that attach directly to bone at points above and below the joints (Fig. 2.43).

Smooth muscle gets its name because when viewed under a microscope it lacks the striations, or crosshatches, seen in skeletal and cardiac muscle. Smooth muscle usually forms in sheets rather than fibers and is under automatic rather than voluntary control. It is found in many important organs of the body, particularly the hollow organs of the respiratory, circulatory, digestive, urinary, and reproductive systems. Smooth muscle helps carry out much of the body's automatic internal work.

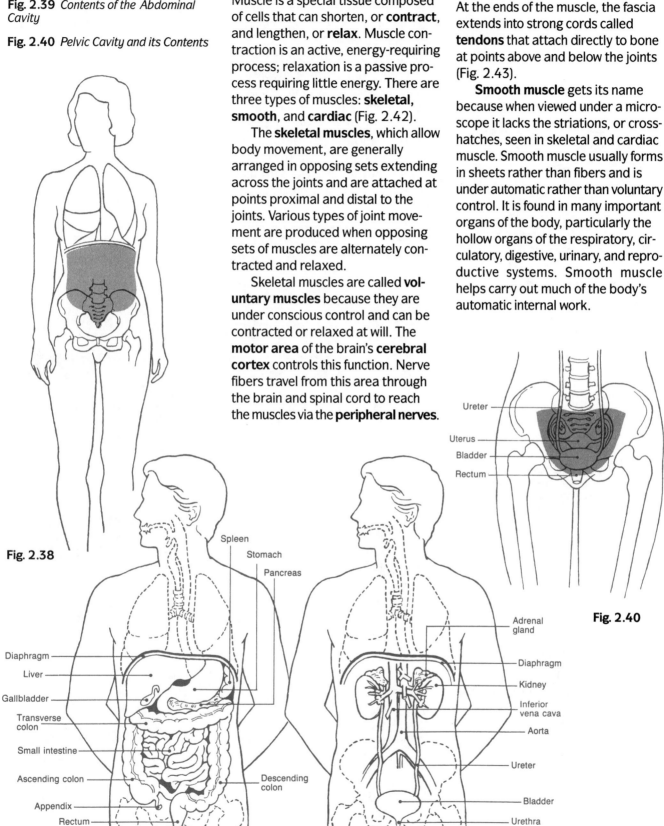

Fig. 2.38

Ureter
Uterus
Bladder
Rectum

Fig. 2.40

Spleen
Stomach
Pancreas

Diaphragm
Liver
Gallbladder
Transverse colon
Small intestine
Ascending colon
Appendix
Rectum

Descending colon

Adrenal gland
Diaphragm
Kidney
Inferior vena cava
Aorta
Ureter
Bladder
Urethra

Organs of the Abdominal Cavity

Organs Behind the Abdominal Cavity

Fig. 2.39

Fig. 2.41 *Organs of the Abdominal and Pelvic Cavities*

Hollow Organ

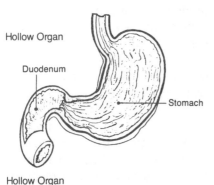

Duodenum

Stomach

Hollow Organ

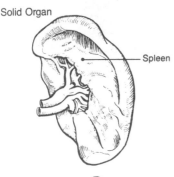

Large intestine

Rectum

Solid Organ

Spleen

Solid Organ

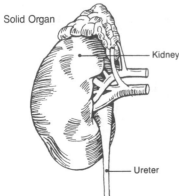

Kidney

Ureter

Fig. 2.41

Cardiac muscle is a special type of striated muscle also under automatic control. Unlike other striated muscles, it never stops working and rests only between heartbeats. To meet these special demands, the heart requires a constant supply of oxygen and nutrients furnished by an uninterrupted blood flow. The coronary arteries (Fig. 2.44), which are the first branches of the aorta, supply the heart with blood. The heart, an organ about the size of a fist that represents less than 1 percent of the

Fig. 2.42 *The Three Types of Muscle Tissue and their Microscopic Appearance*

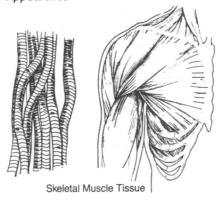

Skeletal Muscle Tissue

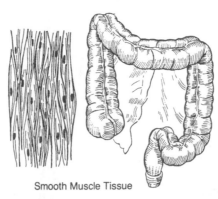

Smooth Muscle Tissue

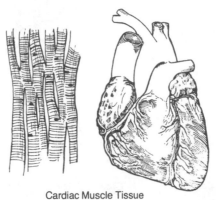

Cardiac Muscle Tissue

Fig. 2.42

body's weight, is nourished by 5 percent of the blood pumped each minute.

To some extent, the diaphragm also is a specialized striated muscle. Although breathing can be voluntarily controlled for short periods, it is mostly under automatic control.

Of the scores of voluntary muscles in the human body, only a few will be described here (Fig. 2.45). First, several new words that describe joint motions must be defined. The term **flex** is used when a joint is *bent*, the term **extend** is used when it is *straightened*. **Adduct** (a term

Skeletal Muscle Tissue

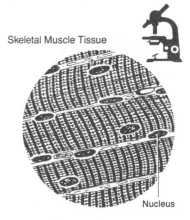

Nucleus

Smooth Muscle Tissue

Blood capillaries

muscle cells

Nucleus

Cardiac Muscle Tissue

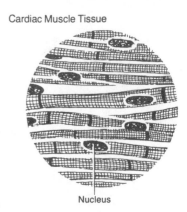

Nucleus

Fig. 2.43 *Skeletal muscles attach directly to bones at points above and below the joints.*

Fig. 2.44 *Coronary Arteries*

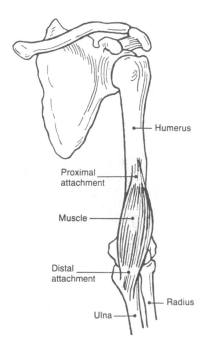

Fig. 2.43

derived from two Latin words meaning "pull toward") means to bring an extremity *toward* the midline, or medially. **Abduct** (a term derived from two Latin words meaning "pull away from") means to bring an extremity *away* from the midline, or laterally. When referring to the feet, which normally are positioned at right angles to the legs, the term **dorsiflex** is used when the foot is bent *upward*, or dorsally; the term **plantarflex** is used when the foot is bent *downward*, or in the direction of the sole of the foot. (In Latin, *planta* means "sole of the foot.")

The head is almost completely covered with muscles, some of which open and close the eyes and mouth and produce facial expression. The large, powerful **masseter** and **temporalis muscles** close the jaws. The **trapezius muscles** are attached to the shoulder girdles laterally and to the spine and base of the skull medially. They strengthen the shoulder girdles and lift the shoulders. The strap-like **sternomastoid muscles**

(sterno-cleidomastoid muscles) on either side of the front of the neck help turn the head and flex the neck. Back movement is provided by a complicated series of long, powerful muscles that run on either side of the spine from the base of the skull to the sacrum. For simplicity, these groups can collectively be called **paraspinous** or **paravertebral muscles**. The **latissimus dorsi muscles**, extending like wings from the shoulder girdles to the spine posteriorly, adduct the upper extremities.

The **intercostal muscles** between the ribs already have been described. Deep muscles in the neck are attached to the clavicles and first ribs, and lift them during deep breathing. The **pectoralis muscles** beneath the breasts help adduct the upper extremities. The muscles covering the front of the abdomen include the strap-like **rectus muscles**, which support the abdomen and flex the lumbar spine. The **iliopsoas muscles**, which flex the hip joints, lie at the back of the abdominal and pelvic cavities on either side of the spine.

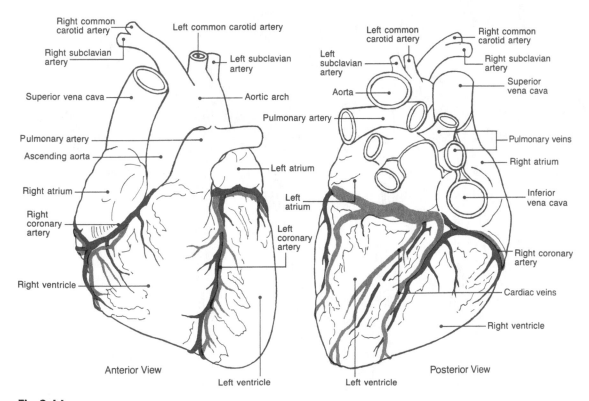

Fig. 2.44

The **gluteus muscles** form the buttocks and extend and abduct the hips. The major muscles of the thighs are the **quadriceps** anteriorly, which extend the knees, and the **hamstrings** posteriorly, which flex the knees. Other muscles located on the inside of the upper thigh adduct the hips. In the lower leg, the anterior muscles dorsiflex the ankle and toes, and the calf muscles plantarflex them.

In the upper extremity, the **deltoids** form the rounded outer part of the shoulders and are the main muscles that lift the extremities to the side and forward. Beneath each deltoid muscle, three small muscles form the rotator cuff, which is a strong, curved band of tendon and muscle that holds the head of the humerus firmly in the shoulder joint socket. These muscles and tendons can become irritated by overuse, causing shoulder motion to be painful, a condition known as bursitis.

The major muscles of the upper arm are the **biceps** anteriorly, which flexes the elbow, and the **triceps** posteriorly, which extends the elbow. The forearm muscles are similar to those in the lower leg, consisting of anterior muscles that flex the wrist and fingers, and posterior muscles

Fig. 2.45 *Major Muscles*

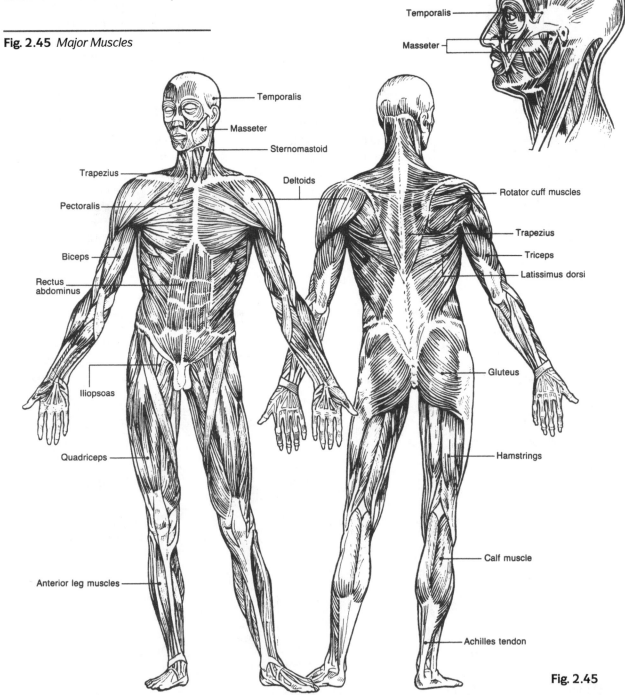

Temporalis

Masseter

Temporalis
Masseter
Sternomastoid
Trapezius
Deltoids
Pectoralis
Biceps
Rectus abdominus
Iliopsoas
Quadriceps
Anterior leg muscles

Rotator cuff muscles
Trapezius
Triceps
Latissimus dorsi
Gluteus
Hamstrings
Calf muscle
Achilles tendon

Fig. 2.45

that extend them. The hands contain a number of small muscles that abduct and adduct the fingers and thumb and aid in flexing and extending them.

The Nervous System

The nervous system contains special cells called **neurons** (Fig. 2.46) that react to stimuli and are able to conduct impulses rapidly through their cytoplasm. Each neuron has a **body**, several short processes called **dendrites**, and a long process called an **axon**. The processes connect with the processes of other neurons at junctions called **synapses**, allowing nerve impulses to be transmitted from one neuron to another. Nerve impulses are basically electrical in nature, although transmission between neurons is accomplished by chemical mediators. Brain cell axons that run into the spinal cord may be more than 2 feet long. Axons are enclosed in a fatty substance called **myelin**, which acts much like the insulation that prevents short circuits in electric wires. Chains of neurons linked by synapses form complicated, computer-like circuits.

The nerve cells and their supporting tissues are grouped into the organs that make up the nervous system: the **brain, spinal cord**, and **nerves**. The brain and spinal cord form the **central nervous system**, and the nerves and their branches form the **peripheral nervous system** (Fig. 2.47). The brain lies within the cranial cavity of the skull; the spinal cord within the spinal canal of the spine. The brain and spinal cord are covered by three layers of protective membranes called **meninges** (Fig. 2.48). The outermost of these protective membranes is a tough, fibrous layer, the **dura mater**, which lines the inside of the skull and the spinal canal. The other meninges are the **arachnoid** and the **pia mater**. The **cerebrospinal fluid**, a clear, colorless fluid resembling water, circulates in the spaces between these membranes. If the skull is fractured, the meninges may be torn and cerebrospinal fluid may leak from the wound. In a patient with a head injury, clear or pink fluid coming from the nose or ear may indicate a fracture of the

Fig. 2.46 *Neurons*

Fig. 2.47 *Central and Peripheral Nervous Systems*

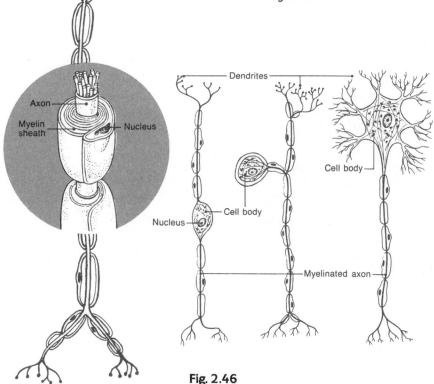

Fig. 2.46

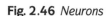

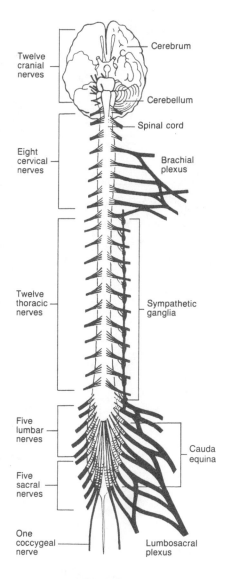

Twelve cranial nerves

Eight cervical nerves

Twelve thoracic nerves

Five lumbar nerves

Five sacral nerves

One coccygeal nerve

Cerebrum

Cerebellum

Spinal cord

Brachial plexus

Sympathetic ganglia

Cauda equina

Lumbosacral plexus

Fig. 2.47

base of the skull with a spinal fluid leak. A serious hazard in this instance might be the introduction of infection into the nervous system through the open fracture site, causing inflammation of the meninges (meningitis) or a brain abscess.

Because most of the arteries that supply blood to the brain and spinal cord lack cross-connections, blockage of one by an injury or blood clot usually will cause the area it supplies to die.

The nervous system is divided into the **somatic** and **autonomic** nervous systems. The somatic nervous system controls voluntary activities such as eating, walking, and talking. The autonomic nervous system controls all bodily activities not under con-

scious control, such as the functions of the heart and blood vessels, digestion, perspiration, and shivering.

The **brain** (Fig. 2.49) is divided into three major parts: the **cerebrum, cerebellum**, and **brain stem**. The cerebrum, which is responsible for the most advanced (higher) functions, consists of the outer right and left **cerebral hemispheres** and the inner **thalamus** and **hypothalamus**. The thalamus is involved in the expression of emotion and, together with the cerebral hemispheres, is responsible for recognition of pain, temperature, and touch. The hypothalamus controls automatic functions such as regulation of the heartbeat, circula-

tion, digestion, and blood pressure. It also regulates pituitary gland activity, water balance, sexual function, sleep, appetite, and body temperature.

The cerebral hemispheres, which are the largest part of the brain, are most highly developed in man and other primates. They control conscious functions, including voluntary movement and the perception of sensations transmitted by the sensory organs for sight, hearing, touch, taste, and smell.

The cerebellum, which lies below and to the rear of the cerebrum, regulates posture, balance, and muscle tone, and coordinates body movement.

The brain stem lies at the base of the brain and contains centers that help regulate breathing, heart function, and blood pressure. It also contains the reticular activating system, an area, which is partly responsible for the awake state. Long nerve fibers from upper parts of the brain pass through the brain stem on their way to the spinal cord.

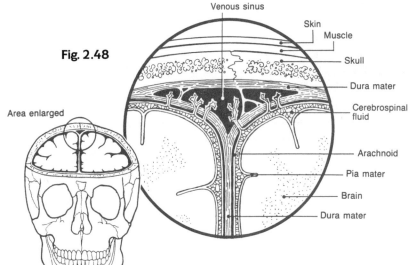

Fig. 2.48

Area enlarged

Venous sinus
Skin
Muscle
Skull
Dura mater
Cerebrospinal fluid
Arachnoid
Pia mater
Brain
Dura mater

Fig. 2.48 *Meningeal Coverings of the Brain*

Fig. 2.49 *Midsagittal View of Brain*

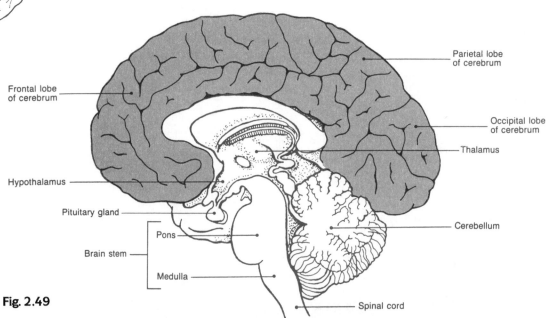

Parietal lobe of cerebrum
Frontal lobe of cerebrum
Occipital lobe of cerebrum
Thalamus
Hypothalamus
Pituitary gland
Pons
Brain stem
Medulla
Cerebellum
Spinal cord

Fig. 2.49

Cranial nerves originate at the base of the brain and leave the skull through openings called **foramina**. They slow the heart; increase peristalsis; supply sensation and motor function to the head, tongue, neck and throat; and are responsible for hearing, taste, smell, sight, eye movement, and action of the pupil of the eye.

The cranial cavity is divided into an upper two-thirds and a lower one-third by a horizontal sheet of tough, fibrous tissue, the **tentorium** (Fig. 2.50). The upper part contains the cerebrum and the lower part the cerebellum. The brain stem, which is attached to the cerebrum above, the cerebellum behind, and the spinal cord below, lies in a notch in the anterior part of the tentorium. The cranial nerve responsible for regulating the size of the pupil also runs through this notch to reach the eye. The importance of these relationships will be emphasized in Chapter 3 and in the section on head injuries in Chapter 12.

Higher mental functions such as consciousness, thought, memory, and intelligence are not localized, but depend upon the integrated activity of large areas of the brain. Consciousness, in particular, depends upon normal function of both cerebral hemispheres and the reticular activating system of the brain stem. The state of consicousness is determined by testing the individual's ability to **respond** to stimuli provided by the examiner, such as the human voice, touch, or mild pain. An individual with a normal level of consciousness is **responsive**, i.e., oriented, talks coherently, and can answer correctly when questioned about name, address, location, day, date, and time of day.

Consciousness can range from this normal state to a completely **unresponsive** (unconscious) state in which only the activity of the circulatory and respiratory systems can be detected. Disturbances of consciousness can be caused by injuries that range from a light blow to the head—which appears to disturb normal brain function by causing a temporary "shorting out" of the normal electrical activity—to serious injuries that cause permanent damage to brain tissue. They also can be caused by inadequate oxygen reaching the brain cells due to such causes as low oxygen in the outside air, malfunction of the circulatory and/or respiratory systems (see Chapter 1, Table 1.2), or increased pressure inside the skull (increased intracranial pressure) due to bleeding or brain swelling. Interference with brain metabolism, as in infection, poisoning, or a general body metabolic body metabolic disturbance such as uncontrolled diabetes, can disturb consciousness also.

Lack of oxygen and other disturbances in brain metabolism affect the higher mental functions first; impaired memory and alteration in the ability to reason and to speak coherently may be early signs of these conditions. Primitive functions such as regulation of breathing and circulation are among the last to be affected.

Any state of consciousness other than the completely normal state is often referred to as "altered mental status." The terms **responsiveness** and **unresponsiveness** are probably preferable to the terms **consciousness** and **unconsciousness** for use in emergency care, since the former terms document what the examiner

Fig. 2.50 *Cranial Cavity*

Fig. 2.51 *Diagram of Nerve Pathways from the Brain to the Spinal Cord*

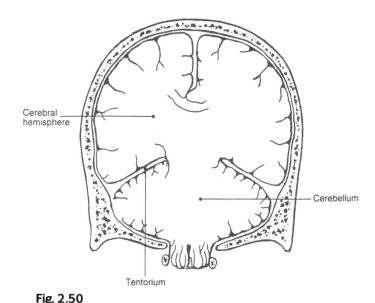

Fig. 2.50

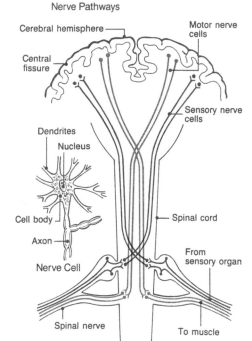

Fig. 2.51

actually observes and do not imply any assumptions or connotations. The preferred terms will be used in succeeding chapters of this textbook, although the reader should understand that the terms consciousness and unconsciousness are widely used in the emergency medical services literature.

The **spinal cord** is a long, rope-like organ that lies in the spinal canal. It is attached to the brain above at the **foramen magnum**, a large hole at the base of the skull, and ends below in a fan-like arrangement of peripheral nerves called the **cauda equina** (Latin for "horse's tail"). At regular intervals, a pair of **spinal nerves** leaves the cord and exits through holes, or foramina, between the vertebrae on either side. These nerves form the **peripheral nervous system** (Fig. 2.47), which consists of 31 pairs of nerves originating from the spinal cord (spinal nerves) plus 12 pairs of nerves originating from the base of the brain (cranial nerves). The cranial nerves exit the brain through foramina in the skull. Most nerves contain both motor and sensory fibers.

Voluntary movement is controlled by special cells called **motor neurons** located in the motor area of the frontal lobe of each cerebral hemisphere. The axons of these neurons form a series of fibers called **motor fibers**. These fibers pass from the frontal lobes through the inner parts of the cerebrum, brain stem, spinal cord, and peripheral nerves, ending in the muscles (Fig. 2.51) and transmitting impulses from the motor neurons to the individual muscles. Injury at any point in this long pathway can cause weakness or paralysis of the corresponding muscle or muscles. The higher a spinal cord injury, the more the disability. Injury to the highest part of the spinal cord may weaken or paralyze all four extremities, the intercostal muscles, and the phrenic nerves that control the diaphragm so that the patient is unable to breathe. Lower injuries may paralyze all four extremities but spare the phrenic nerves; still lower injuries may paralyze only the lower extremities.

Sensory fibers are more complex than motor fibers. They transmit impulses to the brain from the sensory organs responsible for sight, hearing, taste, smell, touch, pressure, pain, and temperature. These organs include eyes, ears, taste buds, the olfactory organ in the nose, and special organs in the muscles, joints, blood vessels, pleura, peritoneum, and dermis of the skin. Sensory nerves constantly supply the brain with information about the relation of the body to its external and internal environments.

The part of the brain that is responsible for sight is the occipital lobe of each hemisphere; for hearing, the temporal lobe; for smell, the olfactory bulb on the inferior surface of the frontal lobe; and for touch, the sensory area of the cortex just posterior to the motor area. Pain and temperature depend on the thalamus as well as the sensory area of the cortex. Injury at any point in these sensory pathways causes loss of the corresponding sensation in the area supplied by the injured nerve fibers.

The motor and sensory fibers that run from the brain into the spinal cord **cross over** (Fig. 2.51) to the **opposite side** during their long path to or from the brain, so that the left side of the brain receives sensations of pain and touch from the right side of the body and vice versa. Similarly, the left side of the brain controls the muscles of the right side of the body and vice versa. In a right-handed person, the left side of the brain is said to be **dominant**, while in a left-handed person, the right side of the brain is dominant. The centers for speech, reading, and writing are located in the dominant cerebral hemisphere.

Peripheral nervous system nerve cells differ from those of the central nervous system in their reaction to

Fig. 2.52 *Reflex Arc*

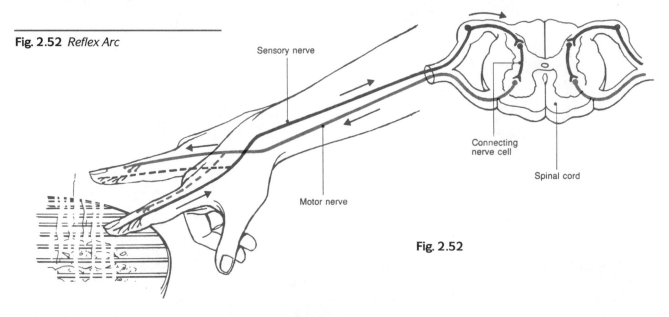

Sensory nerve

Motor nerve

Connecting nerve cell

Spinal cord

Fig. 2.52

injury. If a spinal nerve or its branch is cut, the cut axons usually will regenerate and eventually restore nerve function. A similar injury to the brain or spinal cord will not heal because these axons cannot regenerate, which is why brain and spinal cord injuries are generally permanent.

The spinal cord has many short connections between motor and sensory nerve fibers. These connections, called **reflex arcs**, bypass the brain and generate an immediate reaction to noxious stimuli. For example, a person who touches a hot stove will immediately withdraw his or her finger before thinking about it (Fig. 2.52).

The **autonomic nervous system** controls the automatic functions of the body and consists of two parts with opposing functions: the **sympathetic** and **parasympathetic nervous systems**. Many of the neurons of the autonomic nervous system lie outside the spinal cord in small clusters called **ganglia** (see Fig. 2.47). The sympathetic nervous system prepares the body for action in response to stress. Its fibers cause the pupils of the eyes to enlarge (dilate), hairs to stand erect, the heart rate to increase, perspiration to occur, and body sphincter muscles to tighten. These changes are sometimes called the autonomic stress reaction. The parasympathetic nervous system causes the pupils to constrict, the heart rate to slow, and sphincter muscles to relax.

Some of the body's important nerves will be discussed briefly. The cranial nerves were mentioned earlier in this chapter. The five major nerves of the upper extremity originate in the **brachial plexus**, which lies in the neck behind the clavicle (Fig. 2.53). They are the **radial, ulnar, median, axillary**, and **musculocutaneous** nerves (Fig. 2.54).

The radial nerve supplies the muscles that extend the elbow, wrist, and metacarpophalangeal joints of the fingers and thumb. It runs from the brachial plexus into the armpit and around the back of the humerus into the forearm, where its location exposes it to damage when the humerus is fractured. This causes a condition called "wrist drop."

The ulnar nerve runs through the upper arm, entering the forearm behind a bony knob on the medial end of the humerus. It supplies sensation to the little finger and medial side of the ring finger and controls the muscles responsible for abducting and adducting the fingers and extending the joints between the phalanges.

The lateral side of the ring finger and most of the thumb and first two fingers are supplied with sensation by the median nerve. (As discussed earlier in this chapter, *medial* and *lateral* always refer to the hand held with the palm facing forward.) The median and ulnar nerves supply the muscles that flex the wrist, enable the hand to form a grip, and enable most fine movements of the fingers and thumb.

The axillary nerve supplies the deltoid muscle, which abducts the shoulder, and the musculocutaneous nerve, supplies the biceps and other muscles responsible for flexing the elbow. The axillary nerve can be injured when the shoulder joint dislocates.

The major nerves of the lower extremity, the **sciatic** and **femoral nerves**, originate in deep-lying plexuses in the pelvis (Figs. 2.53, 2.55).

Fig. 2.53 *Important Nerves*

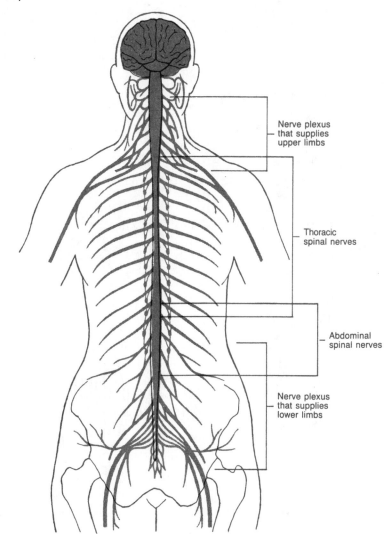

Nerve plexus that supplies upper limbs

Thoracic spinal nerves

Abdominal spinal nerves

Nerve plexus that supplies lower limbs

Fig. 2.53

The sciatic nerve provides sensation to the lateral leg and foot and supplies the muscles that extend the hip, flex the knee, and move the ankle and foot. The sciatic nerve is the largest nerve in the body. It runs from the plexus into the buttock and down the back of the thigh, where it divides into the **tibial** and **peroneal nerves**. The peroneal nerve winds around the head of the fibula before entering the lower leg, where it divides into superficial and deep branches. The peroneal nerve at the head of the fibula and its superficial branch near the lateral surface of the leg are vulnerable to damage from trauma to the side of the upper leg or from too tight a splint.

The femoral nerve enters the front of the thigh just lateral to the femoral artery and provides sensation to part of the front of the thigh and the inner leg. It also supplies the muscles that flex the hip and extend the knee.

The Cutaneous System

The cutaneous system consists of the skin and underlying subcutaneous tissues. The skin (Fig. 2.56), the largest organ in the body, is made up of an outer layer, the **epidermis**, and an inner layer, the **dermis**.

The epidermis is composed of many layers of flat, closely adhering cells and forms a water-tight covering for the body. Its outermost layer consists of dead cells that are constantly being shed. The cells of the innermost (germinative or basal) layer multiply to continually renew the outer layers and replace the shed cells. The dermis contains hair follicles, oil glands, sweat glands, blood vessels, nerves, and the sensory organs that perceive pain, touch, and temperature.

Fig. 2.54 *Upper Extremity Nerves*

Fig. 2.55 *Lower Extremity Nerves*

Fig. 2.56 *Components of the Skin*

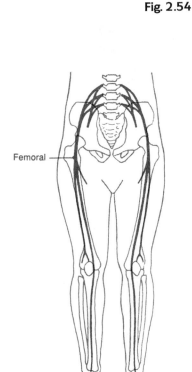

Fig. 2.54

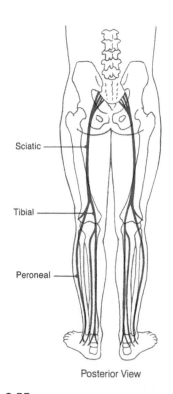

Anterior View   Posterior View

Fig. 2.55

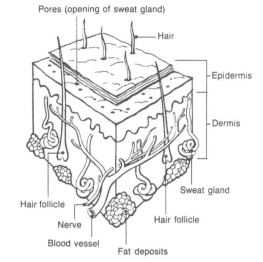

Fig. 2.56

The cutaneous system keeps the body from drying out and protects it from invasion by bacteria and other infectious organisms. It is the major organ system that regulates body temperature, which it controls by producing sweat and adjusting the flow of warm blood through the surface vessels.

The Reproductive System

The male and female reproductive systems continue the human species by creating new life. The female reproductive organs (Fig. 2.57) include two **ovaries**, two **fallopian tubes**, and the **uterus, vagina**, and associated glands. The male reproductive organs (Fig. 2.58) include two **testi-** cles, two **vasa deferentia**, two **seminal vesicles**, and the **prostate gland** and **penis**. Both male and female reproductive systems are controlled by the **pituitary gland** at the base of the brain. The male reproductive organs lie outside the body, except for the prostate, seminal vesicles, and part of the vasa deferentia. The apparent reason is that sperm develop better at a temperature slightly lower than internal body temperature. The female reproductive organs lie entirely inside the body, in the pelvic cavity.

During the female's reproductive years (approximately age 12 through age 50), the ovaries release an egg, or **ovum**, about once every 28 days. The ovum travels through the fallopian tube to the uterus, whose lining has been prepared to receive it by becoming thicker and richer in blood vessels. If a sperm fertilizes the ovum, the resulting **embryo** implants and grows in the lining of the uterus. Otherwise, the ovum dies, and the lining of the uterus breaks down and is expelled through the vagina. This flow, consisting of blood and tissue

---

Fig. 2.57 *Female Reproductive System*

from the lining of the uterus, normally lasts for 5 to 7 days and is called the **menstrual period**. The menstrual period normally begins 14 days after the ovum is released from the ovary. The ovary produces female hormones as well as ova.

The uterus, which lies between the bladder and the rectum, is continuous with the vagina, a muscular tube that opens to the outside at the **vulva**. The ovaries are located on either side of the upper uterus and are connected to it by wide ligaments. The fallopian tubes collect the ovum and conduct it to the uterus.

During the nine months of a normal pregnancy, the fetus grows and develops inside a fluid-filled sac, the **amniotic sac**. The fetus is attached to the wall of the uterus by the **umbilical cord** and the **placenta** (afterbirth), which provide it with oxygen and nourishment from the mother. During birth, the fetus is expelled from the uterus through the vagina to the outside by strong contractions of the uterine muscles.

In the male, the testicles are formed inside the body cavity during embryonic life and pass through canals in the body wall before birth into the sac-like **scrotum**, where they normally lie. The canals sometimes

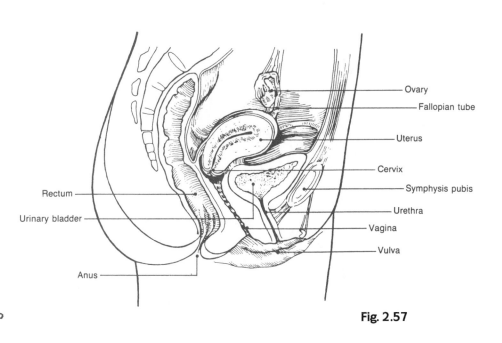

Rectum

Urinary bladder

Anus

Ovary

Fallopian tube

Uterus

Cervix

Symphysis pubis

Urethra

Vagina

Vulva

Fig. 2.57

remain after birth, forming a weak spot in the body wall where an **inguinal hernia** may develop. The testicles produce both sperm and male hormones. The mature sperm travel through the vasa deferentia to be stored in the seminal vesicles, which lie within the pelvic cavity at the base of the bladder. The first part of the urethra passes through the prostate gland, which lies just below the opening of the bladder. The prostate and seminal vesicles together produce the **seminal fluid**, which nourishes and helps transport the sperm. In elderly men, the prostate gland may enlarge and partly block the urethra, causing difficulty in urinating.

The penis is called an **erectile organ** because it contains sinuses that are normally collapsed but can fill with blood to enlarge and stiffen the penis. Erection occurs so that during sexual intercourse the normally soft penis will be able to enter the vagina. At ejaculation, the muscular walls of the prostate and seminal vesicles expel the sperm, mixed with seminal fluid, out through the urethra. When sperm enter the vagina, they travel up into the uterus to fertilize the ovum.

Certain diseases and injuries can cause **priapism**, a long-lasting and painful type of erection. Priapism in a patient with a back or neck injury is almost always a sign of severe damage to the spinal cord.

Fig. 2.58 *Male Reproductive System*

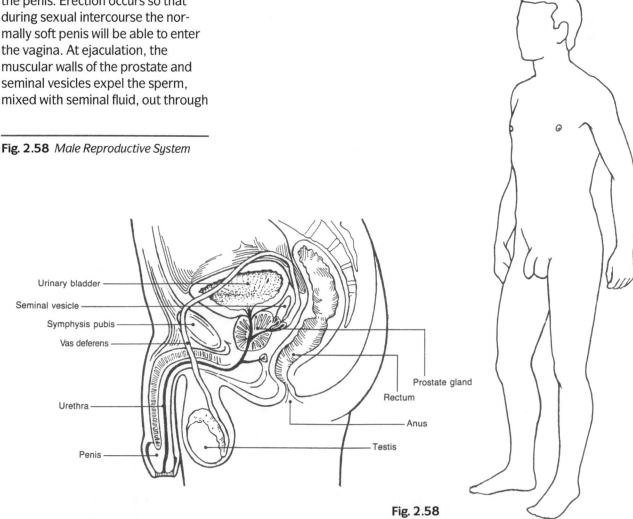

Urinary bladder

Seminal vesicle

Symphysis pubis

Vas deferens

Urethra

Penis

Prostate gland

Rectum

Anus

Testis

Fig. 2.58

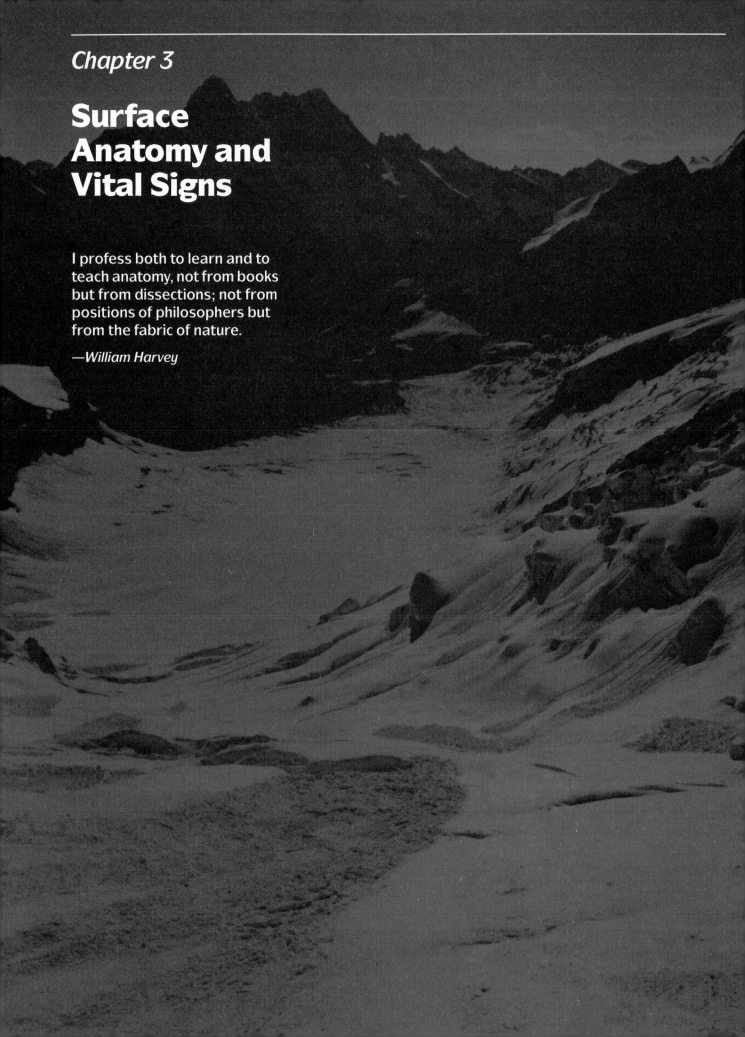

Chapter 3

Surface Anatomy and Vital Signs

I profess both to learn and to teach anatomy, not from books but from dissections; not from positions of philosophers but from the fabric of nature.

—*William Harvey*

The surface of the human body has many characteristic features that most people have been aware of all their lives without realizing their significance. When studied in a systematic manner, these surface features provide clues to understanding the normal body and the changes produced by disease and injury.

The human body is **bilaterally symmetrical.** This means that each half is a mirror image of the opposite half. During patient examination, which in emergency care is called **assessment,** one half of the body can be compared with the other to detect differences that suggest disease or injury. While reading this chapter, consult the illustrations and locate each landmark on your own body or on a companion's body. In the next chapter, you will learn about the part of assessment called the **secondary survey,** a careful examination of each part of the body, *always in the same order* to avoid missing anything important. In general, the order of examination is from top to bottom and from front to back. This order will be followed in presenting the surface features of the head, neck, chest, abdomen, pelvis, lower extremity, upper extremity, and back.

Fig. 3.1 *Surface Anatomy of the Head*

Certain surface characteristics are very important in assessing the patient's state of health. These are the five **vital signs: pulse, respiration, temperature, blood pressure,** and **level of responsiveness.** Five other important characteristics include **skin temperature, moisture,** and **color; capillary refill time; appearance of the pupils of the eyes; ability or inability to move on command;** and **reaction to touch and pain.**

The Head

The head (Fig. 3.1) is divided into the **cranium** and the **face.** With the exception of the forehead, the skin over the cranium (the **scalp**) is covered by hair. The forehead covers the **frontal** part of the cranium. From anterior to posterior, the **temporal, parietal,** and **occipital** parts of the cranium are covered by the corresponding parts of the scalp (see Chapter 2, Fig. 2.21). The face contains the **eyes, ears, nose, mouth, cheeks,** and **lower jaw.** The **orbits** are the bony sockets that contain and protect the eyes; the **eyebrows** lie over the prominent upper part of the orbits. The proximal one-third of the nose is bone; the distal two-thirds are flexible cartilage. The **cheekbone** is the bony ridge of the zygoma below the orbit and above the soft part of the cheek. The external ear, or **pinna,** is made of cartilage covered by skin; it

surrounds the **ear canal,** which leads to the **middle** and **inner ear.** The pulse of the **temporal artery** can be felt just anterior to and above the opening of the ear canal.

The **upper teeth** lie in the maxilla and are covered by the **upper lip,** which is just below the **nostrils.** The **lower teeth** lie in the **mandible,** or jawbone, which is attached to the base of the skull at the **temporomandibular (TM) joints.** You can feel the TM joints move as you open and close your mouth by placing your fingers just in front of and slightly below the ear canal on either side. Just below and behind the external ear is the bony **mastoid process.** The **angle of the jaw** can be felt below the ear where the long lower border of the mandible bends sharply upward toward the TM joint.

Using a flashlight, look in a companion's mouth, nose, and ears. The roof of the mouth is the **palate,** consisting of the bony **hard palate** anteriorly and the **soft palate** posteriorly. A fleshy tail, the **uvula,** hangs down from the back of the soft palate. The **tonsils** are visible on either side of the back of the mouth; they are larger in younger persons (unless they have been removed surgically). Look at the inside of the cheeks. There is a small fleshy tab in the middle of each cheek where the duct of the **parotid salivary gland** opens into

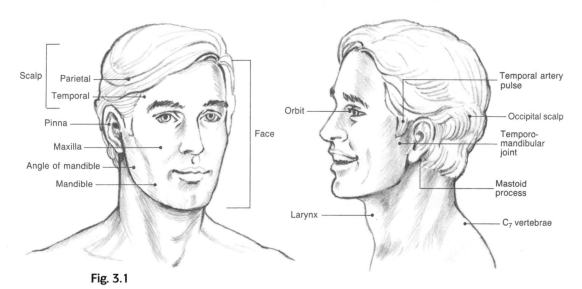

Fig. 3.1

the mouth. The tongue lies in the floor of the mouth. Ask your companion to say "Ah!" This raises the soft palate and you may be able to see the back of the throat (Fig. 3.2).

By looking in the nostrils, you should be able to see part of the internal nose, or **nasal cavity.** A bony plate (the **septum**), divides the two sides of the nasal cavity. Most nosebleeds are caused by bleeding from blood vessels in the septum. Laterally, you may be able to see one or more pink ridges, which are the bones that throw the side of the nasal cavity into waves to provide a larger surface to warm the inhaled air.

Without a special instrument (otoscope) you will not be able to see much in the ear canal, except perhaps a piece of wax. When assessing an injured patient, it is important to look for blood or fluid coming from the ear.

The Neck

The neck (Fig. 3.3) contains many important structures, some of which can be seen or felt. Posteriorly, some of the **spinous processes** of the seven cervical vertebrae can be felt in the midline just under the skin. The most prominent of these is the seventh cervical spinous process at the base of the neck. Moving anteriorly, the wide **trapezius muscles** form the upper shoulders. The **sternomastoid** (sterno-cleidomastoid) **muscles** are attached to the mastoid processes above and run medially to the sterno-clavicular joints below.

In the anterior midline of the neck, portions of the **larynx** and **trachea** can be seen and felt. The visible upper part of the larynx, the **thyroid cartilage,** or "Adam's apple," is more

---

Fig. 3.2 *The Mouth*

Fig. 3.3 *Major Features of the Anterior Neck*

prominent in males than in females. With the neck extended, move your finger downward over the larynx until you reach a soft spot, the **cricothyroid ligament.** Just below this ligament is a curved, horizontal, bony ridge, the **cricoid cartilage.**

The pulsations of the large **common carotid arteries** can be felt between the sternomastoid muscle and the thyroid cartilage on each side.

The **trachea** is attached to the cricoid cartilage and can be felt below it in the midline of the neck. Place a fingertip on either side of the trachea and push gently. The width of the soft space between the trachea and the sternomastoid muscle should be the same on both sides. If the space is unequal, the trachea is said to be deviated. Deviation of the trachea usually is a sign that disease or injury to one of the thoracic cavities has caused a shift in the mediastinum away from the midline. The esophagus runs directly behind the trachea.

The two lobes of the **thyroid gland** are found on either side of the lower larynx and upper trachea. The thyroid generally cannot be felt unless it is enlarged, forming a goiter.

The Chest

The chest (Fig. 3.4) has many bony landmarks. From above downward, the **clavicles** lie just beneath the skin and can be felt from their junction medially with the **sternum** at the **sternoclavicular joint** to their lateral

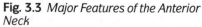

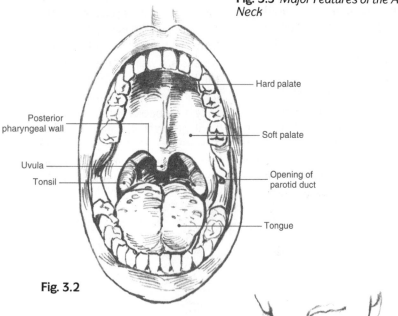

Posterior pharyngeal wall

Uvula

Tonsil

Hard palate

Soft palate

Opening of parotid duct

Tongue

Fig. 3.2

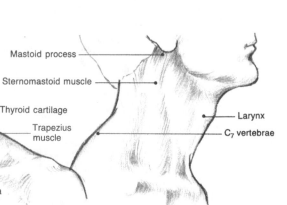

Sternomastoid muscle

Carotid arteries

Cricothyroid ligament

Cricoid cartilage

Sternal notch

Mastoid process

Sternomastoid muscle

Thyroid cartilage

Trapezius muscle

Larynx

C$_7$ vertebrae

Trachea

Fig. 3.3

connection with the **acromion** of the **scapula** at the **acromioclavicular (AC) joint.** The top of the sternum forms a notch, the sternal notch. In the midline of the chest, the flat surface of the sternum can be felt just beneath the skin and, in many persons, the cartilaginous tail of the sternum, the **xiphoid process,** also can be felt. At the junction of the upper one-third and lower two-thirds of the sternum is a prominent horizontal ridge, the **sternal angle,** which lies where the second ribs attach to the sternum. The sternal angle serves as a useful landmark to number the ribs, which can be located one after another downward from the second ribs in slender people. The first ribs cannot be felt because they lie behind the clavicles.

The spaces between the ribs, the **intercostal spaces** or **interspaces,** are numbered according to the rib *above,* i.e., the *second* interspace lies *below* the *second* rib. The lower chest forms an inverted V where the two **costal arches** join the sternum medially. The ends of the floating ribs occasionally can be felt in slender people.

The nipples of the **male breasts** lie at the level of the fourth interspaces. The centers of the **female breasts** also lie at this level but, because a woman's breasts are larger, the nipples usually lie somewhat lower.

The interior of the chest contains many important organs, including the heart, great vessels, esophagus, trachea, lungs, diaphragm, nerves, and lymph nodes. Only the **heart** and **aortic arch** can be located from surface signs. The heart lies behind and to the left of the sternum, at the level of the second to sixth ribs. In slender people, the heartbeat can be felt in the fifth interspace at the **midclavicular line,** an imaginary line running perpendicular to the midpoint of the left clavicle. The aorta arches to the left beneath the upper part of the sternum and, as it descends, lies just to the left of the spine in the posterior chest. In many people, the pulsations of the aorta can be felt in the sternal notch, especially after exercise. Both sides of the chest expand and contract equally during normal breathing. In some types of chest injuries, one side will expand less than the other.

The Abdomen and Pelvis

Visible landmarks on the anterior abdominal wall (Fig. 3.5) include the **costal arches, umbilicus** (navel), **iliac crests,** and **pubis.** The prominent knob at the anterior end of each iliac crest is the **anterior superior iliac spine.** The **inguinal ligament** passes between this spine and the pubis on each side. The pulses of the **femoral arteries** can be felt just below the midpoint of the inguinal ligaments.

The **abdomen** contains the major parts of the digestive and urinary

Fig. 3.4 *Anterior Chest*

Fig. 3.5 *Surface Anatomy of the Abdomen with Quadrants and Landmarks*

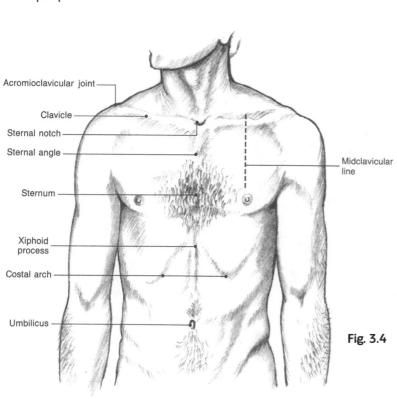

Acromioclavicular joint

Clavicle

Sternal notch

Sternal angle

Sternum

Xiphoid process

Costal arch

Umbilicus

Midclavicular line

Fig. 3.4

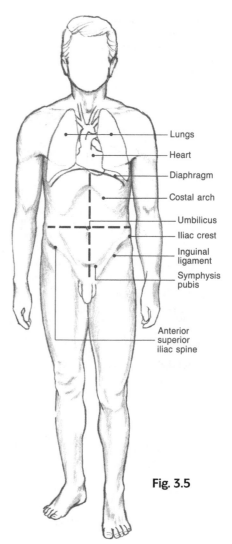

Lungs

Heart

Diaphragm

Costal arch

Umbilicus

Iliac crest

Inguinal ligament

Symphysis pubis

Anterior superior iliac spine

Fig. 3.5

systems. The organs of these systems are customarily located by using two imaginary lines—the midline and a line perpendicular to it that crosses the midline at the umbilicus—to divide the abdomen into four quadrants: the **right** and **left upper quadrants** and the **right** and **left lower quadrants** (see Figs. 3.5, 3.6). When pain or other symptoms arise in one of these quadrants, disease or injury of the underlying organs should be suspected.

Figure 3.6 illustrates the important organs in all four quadrants. The right upper quadrant contains the liver, gallbladder, and the upper right side of the colon. The liver normally lies above and behind the right costal arch, but when the liver is enlarged it can be felt below and parallel to the arch. The gallbladder is located just

below the costal arch at its midpoint; tenderness in this area suggests gallbladder disease. Part of the right colon lies just below the gallbladder. Gaseous distention and certain diseases of the colon can cause tenderness at that location. Injuries to the right upper quadrant or lower right chest frequently involve the liver; tenderness there following trauma suggests a **ruptured liver.**

The left upper quadrant contains the spleen, stomach, and the upper left side of the colon. Following trauma, tenderness above and behind the left costal arch suggests a **ruptured spleen,** particularly if ribs are broken. Gaseous distention of the hairpin bend of the left side of the colon is a frequent cause of pain in the left upper quadrant and in the lower left chest under the ribs.

The right lower quadrant contains the lower right side of the colon and the appendix. **Appendicitis** is a frequent cause of nontraumatic pain

and tenderness in this quadrant. The left lower quadrant contains the lower left part of the colon.

A number of important organs lie in more than one quadrant. The colon begins in the right lower quadrant, travels up into the right upper quadrant, across the midline into the left upper quadrant, and then turns down into the left lower quadrant. The small intestine also occupies parts of all four quadrants. The pancreas is a horizontal organ that lies in both upper quadrants against the posterior abdominal wall. The urinary bladder and uterus normally lie in the pelvis, but, when the bladder is distended or the uterus is enlarged, they may extend into the midline of the lower quadrants of the abdomen.

The kidneys lie in the upper quadrants against the posterior abdominal wall and are drained by the ureters, which run through the lower quadrants into the pelvis where they enter the

Fig. 3.6 *Important Abdominal Organs in the Four Quadrants*

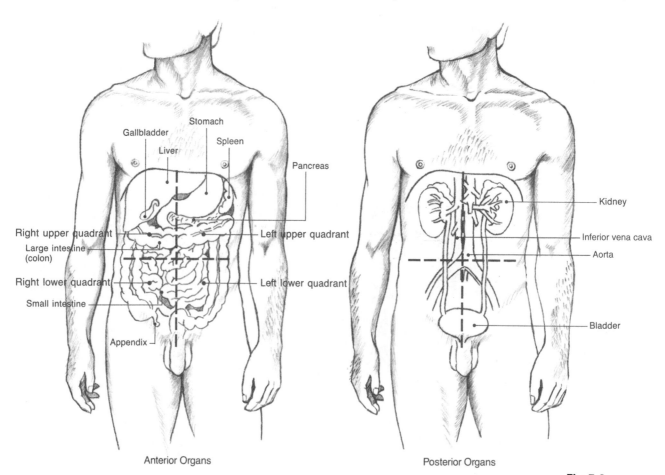

Anterior Organs

Posterior Organs

Fig. 3.6

bladder. (The kidneys are discussed again as part of the external anatomy of the back).

The **pelvis** is separated from the abdomen by an imaginary plane running from the top of the pubis in front to a ridge on the upper sacrum in back. The pelvis contains the bladder, urethra, lower ureters, lower colon, rectum, the female reproductive organs (vagina, uterus, fallopian tubes, and ovaries), and the internal parts of the male reproductive system (part of the vasa deferentia, the prostate, and the seminal vesicles).

The Lower Extremity
(Fig. 3.7)

The bony prominence on the outside of the upper thigh is the **greater trochanter** of the femur. Many people mistake the greater trochanter for the hip joint, which is located below the midpoint of the inguinal ligament just behind the femoral artery. Trauma can cause the **bursa** that separates the greater trochanter from its overlying muscles to become inflamed and tender. Trochanteric bursitis may occur in beginning skiers who hit their trochanters when they fall sideways in the snow. The shaft of the femur is buried within the thigh muscles and cannot be felt.

Many of the components of the knee joint can be felt just beneath the skin. The major landmark is the **patella,** or kneecap, in front of the joint. A broad, strong tendon attached to the major muscle of the anterior thigh, the **quadriceps femoris,** surrounds the patella. The continuation of this tendon, the **patellar ligament,** extends from the patella to the **tibial tuberosity.** As the knee joint moves, the patella glides up and down in a groove between the two rounded projections of the distal femur called the **femoral condyles.** The joint line of the knee is about an inch below the lower border of the patella and can be felt when the knee joint is flexed to a right angle. The **medial** and **lateral femoral condyles** can be felt above the joint line on either side. The **medial** and **lateral hamstring tendons** can be felt on either side of the hollow behind the knee where they attach to the head of the fibula just below the joint line of the knee laterally and the upper tibia medially.

The **peroneal nerve** is a sensitive, cord-like structure that can be felt in the indentation below the head of the fibula. Because of its exposed position, the peroneal nerve is susceptible to damage from a blow to the side of the knee or from too tight a splint. Damage to the

peroneal nerve can cause foot drop (inability to dorsiflex the foot).

The **tibia** is triangular in cross-section; its anteromedial side lies just beneath the skin and can be felt throughout its length to the point where it forms the inner part of the ankle joint at the **medial malleolus** (Fig. 3.8). The pulse of the **posterior tibial artery** can be felt just below and behind the medial malleolus.

Fig. 3.7 *Easily Felt Features of the Lower Extremity*

Fig. 3.8 *Major Surface Features of the Foot*

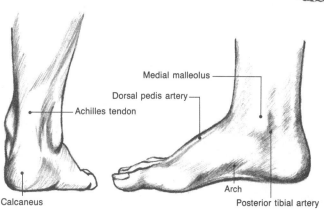

Fig. 3.7

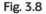

Fig. 3.8

Most of the fibula is buried in the leg muscles, but the lower fourth can be felt to the point where it forms the outer portion of the ankle joint at the **lateral malleolus.**

The subcutaneous tissues of the ankle and foot are so thin that their underlying structures can be felt easily through the skin. The tendons of the muscles that dorsiflex the foot can be felt when the muscles on the front of the leg are tightened. Easily felt features (see Fig. 3.8) include the posterior part of the calcaneus, which forms the **heel;** the **Achilles tendon,** which is attached to the calcaneus; the **arch** of the foot, made up of the calcaneous, talus, and tarsal bones; the five slender **metatarsals;** and the five toes, or **digits,** with their respective **phalanges** and **joints.** The pulse of the **dorsalis pedis artery** can be felt on the top of the foot, between the first and second metatarsals. Because of their prominence and thin skin covering, the medial and lateral malleoli should be well-padded during splinting to avoid excessive pressure and skin damage.

The Upper Extremity
(Figs. 3.9, 3.10)

In the upper chest and shoulder, the entire **clavicle** can be felt from the **sternoclavicular joint** to where it connects with the acromion of the scapula to form the **acromioclavicular (AC) joint** at the point of the shoulder. The head of the **humerus,** which lies just below the AC joint, is covered by the **deltoid muscle** to form the rounded part of the shoulder. The medial margin and part of the spine of the **scapula** can be felt in back of the shoulder.

Most of the humerus is covered by muscles, principally the **biceps** and **triceps,** but its lower end can be felt at the elbow where it has two rounded points, the **medial** and **lateral epicondyles.** An important nerve, the **ulnar nerve,** can be felt in the groove behind the medial epicondyle. This nerve is called the "crazy bone" because bumping it causes a tingling sensation in the medial forearm and hand. Another important nerve, the **radial nerve,**

winds around the humerus at its mid-point. Because of its location, the radial nerve can be injured if the humerus is fractured. The pulse of the **brachial artery** can be felt beating against the humerus on the medial side of the upper arm, midway between the shoulder and elbow.

The **olecranon,** the large upper end of the **ulna,** is found between the medial and lateral epicondyles posteriorly. The **triceps tendon,** which is attached to the olecranon, can be felt when the triceps muscle is tightened. The main tendon on the front of the elbow is the **biceps tendon,** which attaches to the **radius.** If the biceps muscle is tightened, the tendon can be easily felt just medial to the soft hollow at the front of the elbow.

In the forearm, the entire posterior border of the ulna can be felt just below the skin. The lower ends of the **radius** and **ulna**—the two bones of the forearm—form the upper part of the wrist joint. The pulse of the **radial artery** can be felt anterior to the

Fig. 3.9 *Surface Anatomy of the Upper Extremity*

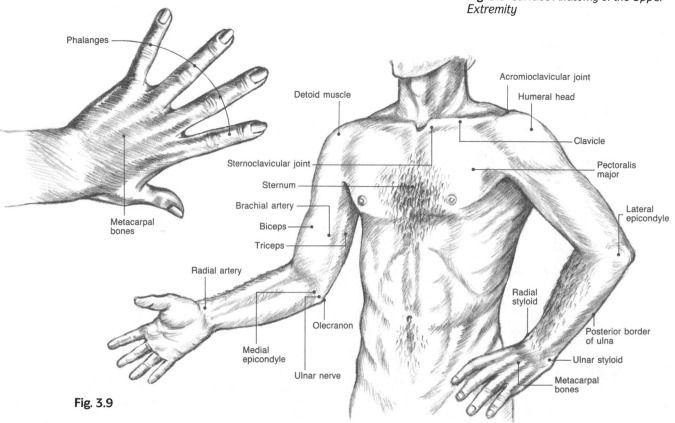

Phalanges

Metacarpal bones

Radial artery

Medial epicondyle

Ulnar nerve

Olecranon

Detoid muscle

Sternoclavicular joint

Sternum

Brachial artery

Biceps

Triceps

Acromioclavicular joint

Humeral head

Clavicle

Pectoralis major

Lateral epicondyle

Radial styloid

Posterior border of ulna

Ulnar styloid

Metacarpal bones

Fig. 3.9

lower end of the radius and above the base of the thumb. Many of the muscles, bones, and tendons of the wrist and hand can be seen as well as felt. The more obvious features include the long, slender **metacarpal bones,** which are easy to feel on the backs of the hands, and details of the **digits** and their **phalanges** and **joints.** Tendons of the muscles that extend the wrist can be seen and felt, especially over the knuckles. On the palmer (anterior) surface, the tendons of the muscles that flex the wrist can be seen in the middle of the wrist.

The Back

The major features of the back (Fig. 3.10) will be covered starting from the large **trapezius muscles** that form the "web" of the neck on either side and are used to raise the shoulders.

The trapezius muscles are attached to the spinous processes of the cervical and upper thoracic vertebrae medially and the scapula laterally.

The spinous processes of the **cervical, thoracic,** and **lumbar vertebrae** can be felt beneath the skin in the midline. The flat, triangular surface of the **sacrum** lies below the lowest lumbar vertebra. The sharp **coccyx,** which hangs like a short tail from the lower end of the sacrum, can sometimes be felt. The sacrum is joined to the iliac bones at the two **sacroiliac joints,** which can be felt just beneath the skin on either side. From these joints, the **iliac crests** curve up and around toward the front. The **ischial tuberosities,** on which we sit, are the rounded knobs that can be felt deep on either side just below the buttocks. The two **sciatic nerves** descend from the buttocks into the thighs just lateral to these tuberosities. Sitting in certain positions puts pressure on these nerves, causing the foot to "fall asleep."

The two wing-like **latissimus dorsi muscles,** which adduct the upper arms, can be felt as they extend downward from the armpits on the sides of the chest. These muscles are attached to the humerus laterally

and the spinous processes of the vertebrae medially. The large, prominent, strap-like **paraspinous (paravertebral) muscles** that lie on either side of the spine are used to flex, extend, and bend the spine sideways. The triangular space formed between the lowest rib and the spine on each side is called the **costovertebral angle (CVA).** The kidneys lie anterior to the costovertebral angles at the back of the peritoneal cavity. Tenderness produced by tapping the muscles of the costovertebral angle may indicate disease or injury of the underlying kidney.

Vital and Other Important Signs

As emphasized in Chapter 2, proper functioning of the circulatory and respiratory systems is vital to life. Death will occur within a few minutes if one or both of these systems fails completely, and serious damage will occur even if failure is only partial. Proper functioning of the nervous system is only slightly less important.

Fig. 3.10 *Major Features of the Back*

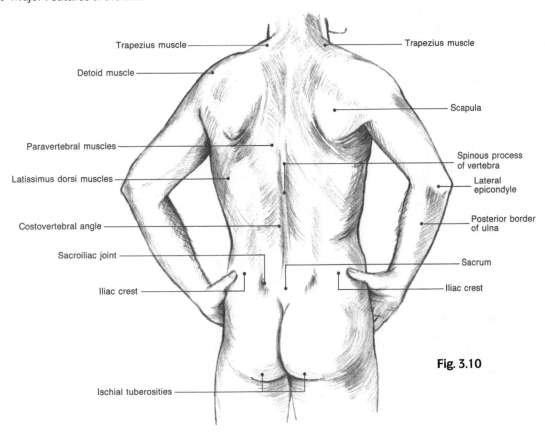

Trapezius muscle

Detoid muscle

Trapezius muscle

Scapula

Paravertebral muscles

Latissimus dorsi muscles

Spinous process of vertebra

Lateral epicondyle

Costovertebral angle

Posterior border of ulna

Sacroiliac joint

Sacrum

Iliac crest

Iliac crest

Ischial tuberosities

Fig. 3.10

The internal workings of the three systems cannot be examined directly in the living body outside of a hospital; however, techniques have been developed for obtaining information indirectly by looking for surface clues to system functioning in the form of signs and symptoms.

Certain signs are so important that they are called "vital signs." Three of the vital signs—**pulse, respirations, and blood pressure**—evaluate the circulatory and respiratory systems; **level of responsiveness** evaluates the nervous system; and **temperature** evaluates the state of the body as a whole. Five additional important signs are **skin temperature, moisture, and color,** which evaluate the circulatory system and the body as a whole to some extent; the **capillary refill time,** which evaluates the circulation locally and to some extent in general; and the **state of the pupils, ability to move,** and **response to pain and touch,** which evaluate the nervous system.

A **sign** is an important characteristic that the *observer* notes by looking, feeling, listening, or smelling. Signs can be normal or abnormal; the latter suggests the possibility of illness or injury. Signs are distinguished from **symptoms,** which are important characteristics that the *patient* notes and discusses with the observer.

Table 3.1

The Five Vital Signs

    Pulse
    Respiration
    Temperature
    Blood Pressure
    Level of Responsiveness

The Pulse

The pulse is the surface expression of blood being propelled through blood vessels by the heart's contractions. It is a rhythmic, expanding tap felt when the fingers are placed over an artery lying close to the body surface. The pulse represents the pressure wave propagated in the arteries each time the heart beats.

The presence of a pulse means that the heart is beating, it is beating strongly enough for the beat to be transmitted to the examiner's fingers, and the arterial channel is open between the heart and the examiner's fingers. The absence of a pulse means that the heart is beating very weakly or not at all, the arterial channel is blocked (especially important information if the pulse is being recorded in an injured extremity), or, too frequently, the examiner is searching for the pulse in the wrong place!

The normal resting heart rate is 60 to 90 beats per minute in an adult and 90 to 110 beats per minute in a child. Although the pulse normally has a regular rhythm, young people and the aged may exhibit sinus arrhythmia, a pulse rate that increases slightly on inhaling and decreases slightly on exhaling. The pulse rate is controlled by a center in the brain stem through two sets of nerves containing autonomic fibers that have opposing effects: the **vagus nerves,** which slow the heart, and the **sympathetic nerves,** which speed it and increase the strength of the heart's contractions.

The important features of the pulse are its **rate, rhythm,** and **strength.** The rate and rhythm indicate how many heart beats there are per minute and whether or not they are regular. The strength indicates to some extent how strong the heart muscle is contracting and whether the blood vessel tone is normal or decreased. Many injuries and illnesses will affect the heart rate, the strength of the heart's contractions, the tone of the blood vessels, or any combination of the three. Therefore, in the injured or ill patient, the exact type of pulse produced may depend on which of these effects predominate.

There is a close relationship between the rate and strength. If the heart muscle is normal, the pulse is usually stronger when the rate is slow and weaker when the rate is very fast, because more blood is pumped if the heart has more time to fill with blood between beats. There is also a close relationship between pulse strength, blood vessel tone, and the strength of the heart muscle. If the tone is low and the blood vessels are relaxed (as in certain types of shock), the pulse will tend to be weak unless the heart muscle contraction is strong enough to compensate. If the tone is high and the blood vessels are contracted, the pulse may be relatively strong even though the strength of the heart's contraction is weaker than normal. If the heart muscle is weak and the blood vessel tone low (as in advanced shock) the pulse may be so weak that it can barely be felt.

During physical activity and in response to pain or emotions such as excitement or fright, the increased activity of the sympathetic nerves and the action of adrenalin increase the pulse rate and strength. With fever alone, the pulse rate increases five to 10 beats per minute for each degree (Fahrenheit) the body temperature rises. The pulse rate also is faster if the basal metabolic rate is increased by overactivity of the thyroid gland. In early heat stroke, before the heart muscle has weakened, the pulse will be both fast and strong. If the heart muscle is weak, the regulatory center in the brain speeds up the heart rate to increase the amount of blood being pumped. This is what produces a fast, weak pulse in patients with serious infections, some types of heart attacks, and other diseases that weaken the heart muscle.

The pulse rate is slow during sleep. It also is slow in those with hypothermia, because of the effect of cold; in those with a decrease in metabolic rate, due to underactivity of the thyroid gland; and in those who have fainted or have certain head injuries, because of increased vagus nerve activity. Certain types of heart disease also can slow the pulse because of blockage of the electrical pulse wave as it travels from one part of the heart to another.

A slow pulse is normal in well-conditioned athletes. The normal heart rate may be as low as 45 to 50 beats per minute in marathon runners and nordic ski racers.

An irregular pulse may be due to sinus arrhythmia but usually is caused by heart disease with atrial fibrillation or frequent extra beats.

Often the state of the pulse will change over time as the patient's condition changes. For example, in early shock, the pulse may be normal, later it becomes fast and strong, and finally fast and weak as the tone of the blood vessels relaxes and the heart muscle weakens.

In a head-injured patient with increasing intracranial pressure, initially the pulse may be normal and strong, later slow and strong, and finally slow and weak (occasionally fast and weak).

In an emergency, the best places to find the pulse are the large, easily located vessels such as the **carotid artery** in the neck or the **femoral artery** in the groin. When extremities are injured, the extremity pulses can be used to determine whether circulation *distal* to the injury is intact.

Important pulse points are shown in Figure 3.11. The easiest pulse to find in the upper extremity is the **radial pulse,** located just *proximal* to the base of the thumb at the wrist. The **brachial pulse** can be felt at the midpoint of the inside of the upper arm. In the lower extremity, the **dorsalis pedis pulse** is on the *dorsum* (top) of the foot between the first and second metatarsals, and the **posterior tibial pulse** is *posterior* to the medial malleolus of the tibia. These pulses usually are easy to find on young, previously

Table 3.2

Causes of Pulse Changes *

Normal pulse
  Healthy person
  Uncomplicated high blood
    pressure
  Early shock (patient lying
    down)

Strong, slow pulse
  Normal sleep
  Simple fainting
  Early increased intracranial
    pressure
  Well-conditioned athlete
  Underactive thyroid gland

Weak, slow pulse
  Hypothermia
  Late increased intracranial
    pressure

Strong, fast pulse
  Early heat stroke
  Fever
  Overactive thyroid gland
  Early shock
  Excitement or fright
  Strenuous physical activity

Weak, fast pulse
  Overwhelming infection
  Late heat stroke
  Late shock
  Diabetic coma
  Some types of heart disease

Irregular pulse
  Sinus arrhythmia
  Heart disease

* Please note that you may see any one of the above six categories in the patient with heart disease.

healthy people, but may be very difficult to find in those who are elderly, ill, severely injured, or who have arteriosclerosis or other blood vessel disease.

Practice locating the six important pulses shown in Figure 3.11 on yourself and fellow students until you can find them within a few seconds. Use the first three fingers to feel the pulse (Fig. 3.12). Never use the thumb, which has a strong pulse of

its own that can be mistaken for the patient's pulse. Count the pulse for 30 seconds and multiply by two to calculate the rate in beats per minute.

The **rate** and **characteristics** of the pulse of a seriously ill or injured patient should be recorded at regular intervals (every 10 to 15 minutes). In a patient with a severely injured extremity, record the presence or absence of a pulse distal to the injury initially and again before and after alignment or splinting.

Respiration

Normal breathing is noiseless, effortless, and regular. The normal respiratory rate is 12 to 20 breaths per

Fig. 3.11 *Locations of the Important Pulses*

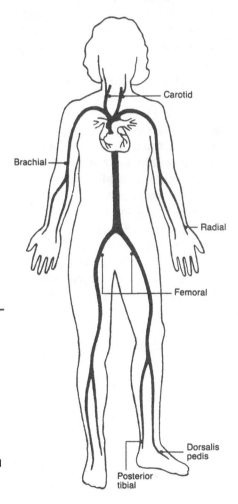

Fig. 3.11

minute for adults and somewhat higher for children and infants. Respirations may be changed by disease or injury, becoming slower or faster, deeper or shallower, noisier than normal, or a combination of these. Breathing that is abnormal and associated with obvious distress is called **labored breathing.**

Abnormal breathing may reflect changes in the upper or lower respiratory tract, the thoracic cage, the blood, the breathing control center in the brain, or the body as a whole as interpreted by special sense organs that send impulses to the breathing control center.

For example, a patient with fractured ribs or inflammation of the pleura (pleurisy) will have shallow, rapid respirations because it is painful to breathe deeply. A change in lung stiffness due to pneumonia or pulmonary edema will cause labored breathing regardless of whether the patient is getting enough oxygen. A rise in either blood **temperature** (fever) or blood **acidity** (acidosis) increases the rate and depth of breathing. A fall in blood temperature (hypothermia) slows the breathing rate. A head injury that damages the respiratory control center may lead to either rapid, shallow breathing or slow, deep breathing. In an unconscious patient who develops an altered breathing pattern, always think first of *obstruction of the upper airway.*

When the blood's oxygen content falls or carbon dioxide rises, there is an increase in the rate and depth of breathing. Common causes include high altitude, suffocation, pneumonia, pulmonary edema, heart failure, and shock. In an unconscious patient, noisy breathing may be caused by relaxation of the tissues of the pharynx, partial obstruction of the upper airway by the tongue, or accumulation of secretions the patient cannot expel by coughing. Bronchitis, pneumonia, asthma, and other lung diseases cause characteristic coughs, wheezes, and rattles.

Abnormal breath odors may be caused by poor oral hygiene, recent ingestion of alcohol or pungent foods, or indigestion. The breath may have a fruity odor in patients with diabetic acidosis and a urinous odor in patients with kidney failure.

Temperature

Normal body temperature is usually 98.6°F (37°C), when measured by a thermometer placed under the tongue. (In 95 percent of normal young adults, there is a range of 97.3 to 98.8°F [36.3 to 37.1°C]). Body core temperature, measured rectally, is a degree higher, and the temperature measured in the armpit is a degree lower. Normally, body temperature varies slightly during the day, with the lowest temperature occurring after midnight and the highest temperature occurring in the evening.

During assessment, the body temperature is taken to determine whether it is normal (**normothermic**), low (**hypothermic**), or high (**hyperthermic**). Most patients with acute injuries or non-infectious illnesses will be normothermic. Hypothermia, which frequently can be diagnosed only by taking the patient's temperature with a low-reading thermometer, requires special care (see Chapter 18). Hyperthermia is almost always caused by **fever,** a condition in which the normal mechanisms of heat regulation are still working but the body's thermostat appears to be reset at a level higher than normal. Fever usually is caused by an infection, occasionally by an injury. In some cases, such as heat stroke (see Chapter 18), hyperthermia is due to breakdown of the normal body heat-regulating mechanisms.

Temperatures as high as 104 to 105°F (40 to 40.6°C) or higher can be seen in some infections, especially in children. Temperatures as high as 106 to 110°F (41 to 43°C) can occur in heat stroke. Wide variations in temperature can be seen in severe head injury because of damage to the temperature regulating center in the brain.

Body temperature usually is taken by placing the bulb of an oral thermometer under the tongue and leaving it in place, with the lips closed around it, for three minutes. If the patient is a child or a disoriented adult, the temperature may be read more reliably and safely by placing a thermometer in the armpit (axilla) and leaving it in place for 10 minutes.

Rectal temperatures, although quite accurate, often are inconvenient or difficult to obtain, especially out-of-doors in severe environments. In general, rectal thermometers can be distinguished from oral thermometers by differences in their bulbs: the bulb of a rectal thermometer is shorter, wider, and more round, while the bulb of an oral thermometer is longer and thinner. Frequently, the top end of a rectal thermometer is flat (Fig. 3.13).

An ordinary clinical thermometer contains mercury and is graded from

Fig. 3.12 *Technique of Feeling the Radial Pulse*

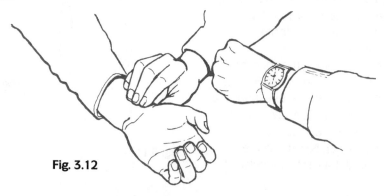

Fig. 3.12

94°F to 106 or 108°F. Thermometers that read in centigrade also are available, as well as electronic thermometers with digital readouts, although they are more expensive than standard thermometers. If an oral temperature reading is 94 to 95°F (34.4 to 35°C), the temperature should be repeated with a special thermometer capable of documenting the lower body temperatures that occur in hypothermia.

Blood Pressure

Blood pressure is the pressure transmitted to the walls of the arteries by the blood as it is propelled by the rhythmic contractions of the heart. Thus, blood pressure is closely related to blood flow. The body has a complicated feedback system by which the regulatory center in the brain stem constantly monitors the blood pressure and varies the action of the heart and the blood vessels to ensure adequate blood pressure for maintaining blood circulation.

Because blood circulates in a closed system, a change in one component of the system affects the other components. Therefore, blood pressure varies depending on the **pulse rate, cardiac output, blood volume,** and the **tone** of the **blood vessels.** An increase in any one of these tends to *raise* the blood pressure; a decrease tends to *lower* it. For example, an injury that causes blood loss tends to lower blood pressure because less blood is expelled with each beat of the heart. Pressure monitors in the circulatory system respond to a fall in blood pressure by signaling the brain to increase the heart rate and narrow the blood vessels. If bleeding stops, these adjustments usually will restore adequate blood pressure. If bleeding continues, the blood pressure eventually will drop despite them. A marked fall in blood pressure is one of the characteristics of the later stages of **shock** (discussed in Chapter 6).

Abnormally high blood pressure also is dangerous, because it can strain the heart and damage or even rupture blood vessels. When blood pressure is high, the brain tends to slow the heart rate. It is important to

have a physician diagnose and treat the causes of both high and low blood pressure.

The pressure in the aorta and arteries rises when the heart muscle contracts and falls when the heart muscle relaxes. This produces a wave-like pressure curve (Fig. 3.14); the highest point of the curve corresponds to the **systolic pressure** and the lowest point to the **diastolic pressure.** Blood pressure is measured by an instrument called a sphygmomanometer, which consists of a cuff that is wrapped around the arm, a rubber bulb to inflate the cuff, and a pressure gauge (Fig. 3.15). A stethoscope also should be available. The width of the cuff's bladder should be 40 to 50 percent of the circumference of the patient's arm, and the length should be 80 percent of the arm's circumference. Therefore, different-sized cuffs are needed for adults, children, and obese individuals. Cuffs that are too small may give false high readings; cuffs that are too large, false low readings. Because blood pressure readings can vary depending on the patient's emotional state, readings usually are more accurate when taken *early* in the assessment *before* painful or anxiety-producing procedures are carried out.

Fig. 3.13 *Standard rectal and oral thermometers are shown on the left. A low-reading hypothermia thermometer is on the right.*

Fig. 3.14 *Relation of the Systolic and Diastolic Pressures to the Pulse Curve*

Fig. 3.15 *Blood Pressure Cuff and Stethoscope*

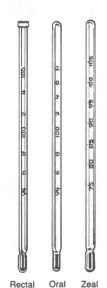

Rectal   Oral   Zeal

Fig. 3.13

Pressure (mm Hg)

120

70

Systolic pressure

Mean pressure
Diastolic pressure

0   1   2   3   4
Time (sec.)

Fig. 3.14

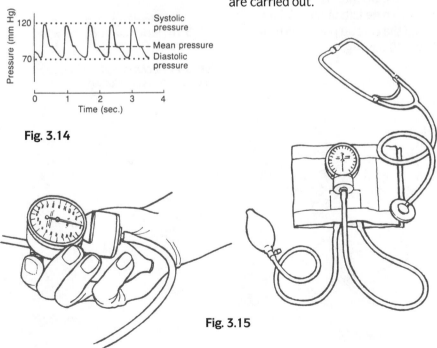

Fig. 3.15

To measure blood pressure, wrap the cuff snugly around the arm (Fig. 3.16) so that its lower edge is 1 inch above the bend of the elbow. Place the center of the cuff (marked with an arrow) over the brachial artery. Blood pressure can be taken either by feeling (**palpation**) or by listening (**auscultation**). Traditionally, the blood pressure is measured in millimeters of mercury (mm Hg), corresponding to the height a column of mercury is raised within a glass tube. Many sphygmomanometers use such a mercury tube. Aneroid sphygmomanometers use a gauge to record air pressure directly from the cuff, with the readings translated into millimeters of mercury by the gauge. Electronic digital readout sphygmomanometers are available also, but are generally more expensive, less durable, and less reliable than the more simple mechanical ones.

It is difficult to read blood pressure by auscultation in noisy places and in moving vehicles; under these circumstances, palpation may have to be used. If no sphygmomanometer is available, blood pressure can be estimated by feeling for important pulses. If the radial pulse can be felt, the patient's systolic blood pressure is at least 80 mm Hg; if the femoral pulse can be felt, at least 70 mm Hg; and if the carotid pulse can be felt, at least 60 mm Hg.

To take the blood pressure by palpation (Fig. 3.16) locate the patient's radial pulse (for technique, see **The Pulse** above). Inflate the cuff for an additional 30 mm Hg after the pulse disappears, then slowly deflate the cuff until the pulse reappears. The reading on the gauge at the point the pulse reappears is the systolic pressure. Because the palpation method is less accurate than auscultation, record it by following the systolic pressure reading with a slash P, i.e., 120/P. Diastolic pressure cannot be obtained by palpation.

To take blood pressure by auscultation (Fig. 3.17), first put on the stethoscope so that the rubber-tipped ear pieces face forward (toward the nose) in your ears. Next, locate the brachial artery pulse at the bend of the elbow, and place the end piece of the stethoscope over it. Inflate the cuff while listening with the stethoscope. You can begin to hear the pulse beat when the pressure in the cuff reaches about 80 mm Hg.

Continue to inflate the cuff until the audible pulse disappears and for about 30 mm Hg above that point. Then, slowly deflate the cuff until the audible pulse reappears. The gauge reading at that point is the systolic

---

Fig. 3.16 *Technique of Taking Blood Pressure by Palpation*

Fig. 3.17 *Technique of Taking Blood Pressure by Auscultation*

blood pressure. Continue to slowly deflate the cuff until the audible pulse disappears. The reading at this point is the diastolic pressure. Record the systolic and diastolic pressure readings obtained by auscultation separated by a slash, e.g. 120/80, and indicate the patient's position while the reading was being taken, i.e., lying, sitting, or standing.

The blood pressure of a healthy, young adult usually is about 120/80; pressures from 85/50 to 140/90 are within the normal range. Blood pressure tends to rise slowly with age and can vary widely in the same individual in response to pain, emotion, or even the minor stress of having the blood pressure taken. An isolated abnormal blood pressure reading means little, but repeated values over 140/90 or below 80/50 are abnormal at any age and should be investigated by a physician.

Any seriously ill or injured patient should have the blood pressure taken and recorded every 10 to 15 minutes.

Level of Responsiveness

An individual with a *normal* level of responsiveness (level of consciousness or LOC) responds fully when questioned by the examiner and appears alert when observed, i.e., is oriented, talks coherently, and can easily answer questions about identity, location, day, date, and time of day. Respon-

Palpation

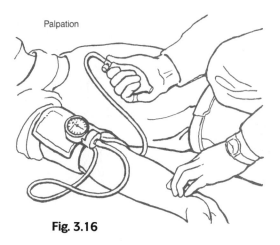

Fig. 3.16

Auscultation

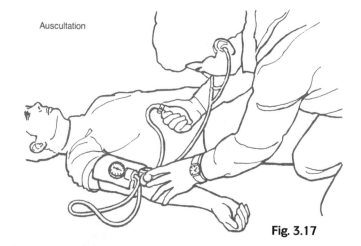

Fig. 3.17

siveness can range from this normal state to a completely unresponsive state where only the activity of the circulatory and respiratory systems can be detected. Any state of responsiveness other than the completely responsive state is often referred to as "altered mental status." As mentioned in the previous chapter, the terms **responsiveness** and **unresponsiveness** are preferable to the terms **consciousness** and **unconsciousness** for use in emergency care, because the former terms document what the examiner actually observes and do not include any assumptions or connotations.

Impaired responsiveness can be caused by head injury, shock, poisoning, drug use, stroke, hypothermia, hyperthermia, alteration of brain metabolism by severe illness, or damage to the circulatory or respiratory systems. When caring for an injured patient, it is important to record the level of responsiveness initially and at regular intervals (every 10 to 15 minutes). This is done by repeatedly asking the patient simple questions such as "How do you feel now?" "Are you doing all right?" and "Can you remember your name and where you are?" Responsiveness also may be determined by gentle stimulation, if necessary, such as pinching a fold of skin on the inside of the patient's upper arm or pinching the patient's fingernail with your finger and thumb.

The level of responsiveness usually is recorded with the aid of the AVPU Scale (Table 3.3), which grades the patient's responsiveness from normalcy to complete unresponsiveness.

The Glasgow Coma Scale (Table 3.4) is another useful but more complicated scale. It is based on three types of response (eye, motor, and verbal), and catalogs what happens to each as a patient's condition deteriorates or improves.

Table 3.3

AVPU Scale

Alert: The patient appears normal, talks coherently to the examiner, knows his or her own identity, location, address, telephone number, day, and date.

Responds to Verbal Stimuli: The patient is not alert, the eyes do not open spontaneously, but the patient responds in some way when spoken to.

Responds to Pain: The patient does not respond to verbal stimuli, but moves or cries out in response to pain, i.e., a firm pinch. This response is not valid if the extremity is numb or paralyzed.

Unresponsive: The patient responds neither to verbal stimuli nor to pain.

Table 3.4

Glasgow Coma Scale

		Score
Eyes:	Opens eyes **spontaneously**	4
	Opens eyes to **examiner's speech**	3
	Opens eyes to **painful stimuli**	2
	Does not open eyes	1
Motor:	Follows **simple commands** to move hand or foot	6
	Pulls **examiner's hand** away when pinched	5
	Pulls **body part** away when pinched	4
	Flexes body or body part when pinched	3
	Extends body or body part when pinched	2
	No motor response to pinching	1
Verbal:	Talks **appropriately,** knows name, date, location	5
	Speech intelligible, but **confused and disoriented**	4
	Talks, but makes **no sense** at all	3
	Makes **sounds** but no words	2
	Makes **no sounds** at all	1

Table 3.5

Five Other Important Signs

Skin temperature, moisture, and color
Capillary refill
Pupillary reaction
Reaction to touch and pain
Ability to move

In addition to the five vital signs, five other important signs must be evaluated: **skin temperature, moisture and color; capillary refill time; appearance of the pupils of the eyes; reaction to touch and pain;** and **inability to move on command.**

Skin Temperature, Moisture, and Color

Skin temperature is the net result of the difference between the temperature of the environment and the temperature of the blood. Skin wetness depends on the activity of the sweat glands (moisture from the environment excepted). Skin color depends on the state of the surface blood vessels and the blood within them. However, in dark-skinned people, skin pigment may mask color changes, and examination of the whites of the eyes or the nailbeds may be more reliable.

As the blood flows through the capillaries in the skin, oxygen is extracted and the blood changes from bright red to a more bluish red. If the blood vessels are **dilated** (widened) there is an increase in the volume and speed of blood flow through the skin, less oxygen is removed from each unit of blood, and the skin is redder and warmer. If the blood vessels are **constricted** (narrowed), there is a decrease in the volume and speed of blood flow through the skin, more oxygen is removed from each unit of blood, and the skin becomes bluer and cooler. If blood vessels are markedly constricted, very little blood reaches the surface capillaries and the skin appears pale, ashen or grey, and cool or cold. The skin also can appear pale in anemia, a condition characterized by too few red blood cells.

Sweat production is an efficient method of losing heat by evaporation, but also can occur in response to mental or physical stress. Conversely, when the body is trying to conserve heat, sweat production is reduced.

In patients with an injury, illness (such as low blood sugar from too much insulin), or a mental state that elicits a stress reaction from the autonomic nervous system, the skin is pale, clammy, and cold because of narrowing of the surface blood vessels and increased sweating. In shock, the skin is pale, clammy, and cold because of stress plus the body's efforts to maintain core circulation by shutting down skin circulation.

Redder, warmer, moist skin typically is seen in association with fever, a warm environment, when the body is trying to lose heat, in thyroid gland overactivity (**hyperthyroidism**), and in certain other metabolic diseases such as diabetic coma. In heat stroke, the skin is hot and red but may be dry if the sweating mechanism is not functioning well. Red, warm skin may be a sign of chronic high blood pressure or too many red blood cells (polycythemia) due to high altitude or blood disease. Since alcohol increases blood flow through the skin, it may also be a sign of chronic alcohol overuse. Occasionally the skin is red in patients with carbon monoxide poisoning, also.

Cold exposure, hypothermia, and thyroid gland underactivity (hypothyroidism) produce pale or bluish, cool or cold, dry skin. When there is inadequate oxygen in the blood because of high altitude or disease of the heart or lungs, the skin is a bluish color (a condition called **cyanosis).** Hepatitis and other types of liver disease can lead to an accumulation of bilirubin in the blood, which causes the skin and the whites of the eyes to turn yellow. This condition, called jaundice, should not be confused with carotenemia, which is yellowing of the skin caused by eating large quantities of foods, such as tomatoes and carrots, that contain high levels of the vitamin A precursor carotene.

Even though examination of the skin does not always tell you what is going on in the body, it does furnish important clues regarding oxygenation, metabolic state, general body stress, and whether the body is trying to conserve or lose heat.

Table 3.6

Skin Temperature, Moisture, and Color

Red, moist, warm skin
  Hot environment, some cases of heat stroke, hyperthyroidism, strenuous exercise, diabetic coma

Red, dry, warm skin
  Alcoholism, polycythemia, high blood pressure, some cases of heat stroke

Pale, moist, cool skin
  Shock, autonomic stress reaction, exercising in a cold environment, heat exhaustion, hypoglycemia (low blood sugar)

Pale, dry, cool skin
  Cold environment, hypothermia, anemia, hypothyroidism

Blue skin
  High altitude, heart or lung disease, hypoxia, shock

Yellow skin
  Jaundice, carotenemia

Capillary Refill Time

Capillary refill time is the time it takes the circulatory system to refill small vessels after blood has been squeezed out of them (Fig. 3.18). Using the thumb and forefinger, squeeze a finger or toe tip until the nail blanches, then release the pressure. The tissues under the nail should return to their normal pink color within *two seconds* (count "one-and-two-and" or say "capillary refill"). If longer than two seconds, the test is abnormal, or positive.

This test measures skin perfusion in the tested area. It is roughly correlated with blood pressure, general blood vessel tone, and the state of the body circulation. Capillary refill is prolonged or absent in cases of serious illness or injury, particularly shock, but also may be prolonged in an injured extremity when the circulatory system as a whole is normal. Therefore, an abnormal capillary refill time can mean either local or general circulatory dysfunction.

A normal capillary refill time indicates that the blood circulation to the skin in the area tested is normal and, by implication, that the circulatory system as a whole is functioning normally or close to that. Unfortunately, the test is unreliable in the cold, when circulation in the skin and extremities is normally slowed.

Fig. 3.18 *Technique of Testing Capillary Refill Time*

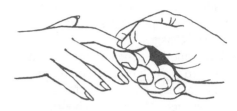

Fig. 3.18

Reaction of the Pupils

The pupils are normally round and equal to each other in diameter. Ten percent of normal individuals have unequal pupils. An artificial eye, changes causes by prescription drugs or eye drops, eye injury, or eye surgery, e.g., for a cataract, also can cause differences in pupil size. Conditions causing pupillary change can be divided into those that change both pupils and those that change only one pupil.

Shining a bright light into one eye normally causes both pupils to **constrict** (become smaller). Both pupils will constrict in response to strong glare or opiates. **Dilation** (enlargement) of both pupils occurs normally in dim light. Abnormal dilation occurs in response to certain drugs (e.g., marijuana and barbiturates), in individuals with an autonomic stress reaction due to pain or fright, and with lack of oxygen to the brain as in suffocation, shock, or cardiac arrest. Patients who are in cardiac arrest generally have dilated pupils that do not constrict in response to a bright light. The pupillary response to light also is lost quickly after death.

In a patient with a head injury, unequal pupils (one pupil is normal and the other dilated) frequently indicate a serious injury involving the brain, usually on the same side as the dilated pupil. The injury causes swelling of the cerebral hemisphere on that side, increasing the pressure inside the cranial cavity and pushing part of the brain down through the opening in the tentorium. This compresses the nerve that controls pupil size, the third cranial nerve, which also runs through this opening (see **The Nervous System** in Chapter 2). When a patient has a head injury or altered responsiveness, it is important to *recheck* and *record* the pupil size and equality at regular intervals (every 10 to 15 minutes). Figure 3.19 illustrates common pupillary changes.

Reaction to Pain and Touch

Reaction to pain and touch can be either general or local. The general reaction to pain was discussed earlier in **Level of Responsiveness.** Local reaction to pain and touch usually is tested after determining the patient's level of responsiveness. In the responsive patient, test for a normal pain reaction by gently pinching the skin or scratching it with a fingernail (Fig. 3.20) while asking "Can you feel this?" Always compare the two sides of the body. An inability to feel pain or touch usually means damage to the nerve pathways running from that body part to the brain. The site of damage can be anywhere on this path and may or may not be obvious. Lack of sensation is frequently, but not always, accompanied by impaired ability to move the affected body part.

Fig. 3.19 *Normal Pupils and Pupillary Changes*

Fig. 3.20 *Testing for Pain and Sensation*

Fig. 3.21 *Testing for Impaired Movement*

It is difficult to test for pain and touch in the unresponsive patient, since a general inability to respond to pain and touch will overshadow a local inability to respond. A firm fingernail or toenail pinch or a pinch of the sensitive skin of the inner arm or thigh is usually required to detect lack of response. Careful comparison of the two sides of the body will sometimes reveal a difference in response from one side to the other.

Ability to Move

To test for impaired movement, ask the patient to move the fingers of both hands and the toes of both feet, and to squeeze your hands with both hands (Fig. 3.21). A conscious patient who is unable to comply is said to be **paralyzed.** Paralysis can involve a single extremity, one side of the body, or both sides of the body. Record exactly what the patient can or cannot do.

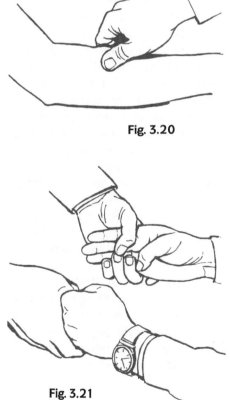

Fig. 3.20

Fig. 3.21

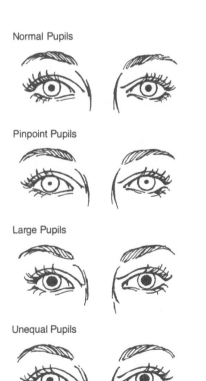

Normal Pupils

Pinpoint Pupils

Large Pupils

Unequal Pupils

Fig. 3.19

Paralysis of a single extremity most often is caused by nerve damage resulting from injury to that extremity. Paralysis can be caused by severe injury without nerve damage if motion is so painful that the patient refuses to try to move. Test motion in an injured extremity initially and again before and after any attempt to align or splint the extremity. Do *not,* however, ask the patient to move the part of an extremity that has a fracture or other serious injury.

Paralysis of one side of the body is most often caused by a stroke, but can also follow a head injury, usually to the *opposite* side of the head. The paralysis can be due either to direct brain injury or to compression of the motor pathways in the brain stem by the same mechanism that causes the pupil to enlarge on that side (see **Reaction of the Pupils** above). Injury to the spinal cord in the neck may result in paralysis of all four extremities and the body below the neck; spinal cord injury below the neck may paralyze only the legs.

If the patient is unresponsive, it is more difficult, but also more urgent, to assess the ability to move. Observe the patient for spontaneous movement of both sides. If there is none, test for movement in response to pain by firmly pinching the skin or a finger or toenail in all four extremities. It is significant if, in one or more extremities, there is a delay in response, a different type of response, or the need for a stronger stimulus to get a response. Especially significant is evidence of weakness of both extremities on one side or the other, which is called **lateralized extremity weakness.**

In a patient with altered responsiveness due to an injury, the **level of responsiveness** (level of consciousness), **state of the pupils,** and presence or absence of **lateralized extremity weakness** are three important signs that may indicate the presence of a serious head injury. They should be looked for initially and rechecked at frequent intervals (every 10 to 15 minutes). If the patient is becoming more and more unresponsive and has an enlarging pupil and increasing weakness on one side, a **neurosurgical emergency** exists and the patient must be taken to a hospital with a neurosurgeon as soon as possible.

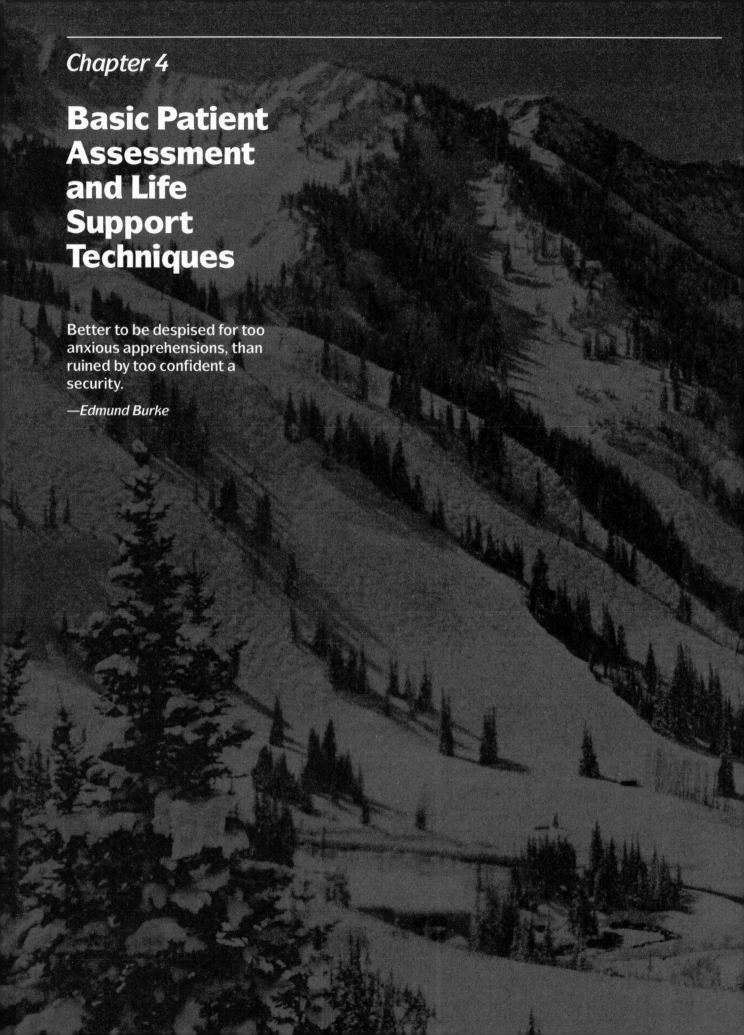

Chapter 4

Basic Patient Assessment and Life Support Techniques

Better to be despised for too anxious apprehensions, than ruined by too confident a security.

—*Edmund Burke*

The overall purpose of this book is to provide information about how to give correct emergency care to the injured and ill. But before emergency care can be given, the rescuer must determine what is wrong with the patient by means of a type of examination called **assessment** (Fig. 4.1).

This chapter will describe **basic assessment**, which consists of a series of actions that must be performed correctly and in the proper order each time. The essentials of these actions and the order in which they are performed have been perfected through many years of experience by expert clinicians. They form the core of every course in emergency care and are remarkably similar from one course to another.

Most emergency care courses have been developed to improve the level of care given to injured patients at the accident scene and during transport to a hospital or other medical facility. Therefore, basic assessment has traditionally been **trauma assessment**. However, illnesses such as infection, cancer, and degenerative disease of the circulatory and respiratory systems disable and kill many more Americans than do accidents. Hence, it is equally important to understand the basics of assessment of a patient with an **illness**.

The objectives of assessment are
1. to detect and treat life-threatening injuries and illnesses rapidly;
2. to find out if anything else is wrong; and
3. to miss nothing significant.

Rescuers must learn the techniques of assessment thoroughly and practice them repeatedly so they can perform these actions accurately and in the right order despite distractions or a hostile environment. Most mistakes in emergency care are caused by lack of thorough or systematic assessment rather than lack of knowledge. Perhaps because of the stress of the moment, some rescuers may perform patient examination too hurriedly or haphazardly to find the true nature of the problem.

Because one of the purposes of assessment is to discover life-threatening conditions and treat them immediately, assessment may have to be interrupted periodically while certain emergency care measures are performed. These measures are directed largely toward reestablishing the proper function of the respiratory and circulatory systems and include, among others, the techniques that make up **basic life support**. The emergency care measures are
1. to support respiration by opening a blocked airway, giving rescue breathing, assisting ineffective respirations, stabilizing a flail chest, or sealing an open chest wound, and
2. to support circulation by controlling hemorrhage, caring for shock, and providing closed chest cardiac resuscitation.

When caring for an injured patient, the rescuer should always suspect the possibility of a neck or back injury and act to minimize the danger of additional spinal cord injury.

This chapter will outline the main elements of basic life support as they are included in basic assessment. These elements are considered in detail in Appendix B.

It is important to remember that assessment means more than examination alone. In addition to using the eyes, ears, hands, and nose, the rescuer also must use the brain to make accurate observations, ask appropriate questions, evaluate the information gathered, understand its significance, pursue fruitful leads,

Fig. 4.1 *Thorough patient assessment is the foundation of emergency care.*

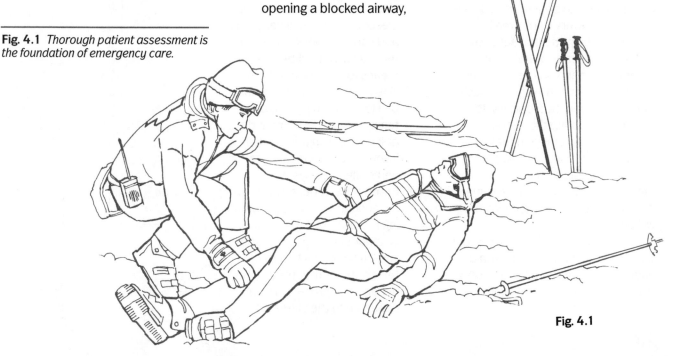

Fig. 4.1

and take appropriate action. Although assessment is relatively easy to learn and perform under classroom conditions, *it may be very difficult to conduct under severe environmental conditions.* For example, cold and wind may numb the examiner's fingers and prevent undressing the patient.

Assessment is divided into three major categories, which are performed in the following order: the **first impression**, the **primary survey**, and the **secondary survey**.

The first impression is entirely automatic and almost instantaneous. It includes recognizing obvious characteristics of the *scene*, such as the presence of possible hazards to the patient or the rescuer; whether there is a need for extrication; and the probable mechanism(s) of injury (see Chapter 9). The first impression also includes recognizing obvious characteristics of the patient, such as whether the person is obviously responsive and whether there is obvious bleeding.

The primary survey is conducted semi-automatically and consists of a rapid and systematic, but not hasty, evaluation of the level of responsiveness (level of consciousness) and the condition of the respiratory and circulatory systems. A rigid protocol is followed so that, first, all life-threatening problems will be looked for in the proper order and treated immediately, and second, every body area indicated by the patient or suspected by the examiner as a site of pain or other abnormality will be assessed.

The secondary survey is conducted more slowly and methodically. It includes evaluating the vital signs and other important signs, taking a brief history, and assessing the remaining organ systems, always in the same order and with the same protocol so that nothing important will be overlooked.

As mentioned before, the rescuer arrives at the patient's side with a number of important intrinsic "tools": the brain, eyes, ears, hands, and

nose. A watch with a second hand, a small flashlight, a pair of heavy-duty scissors, a seam ripper, and a notebook and pencil should be available as well. The rescuer should *think, look, listen, feel,* and occasionally even *smell.* The rescuer must be familiar with the normal appearance and function of the components of the organ systems and search for signs and symptoms that indicate deviations from the normal state.

As an aid in remembering the components of the primary and secondary surveys, it is customary in the emergency medical services (EMS) system to follow the sequence of the **ABCDE mnemonic:**

A Open the <u>A</u>irway, while guarding the cervical spine, if indicated, and briefly assess the level of responsiveness by testing the response to the verbal stimulus "<u>A</u>re you okay?"

B Assess for the presence of spontaneous <u>B</u>reathing. Estimate its adequacy, and provide rescue breathing or bag-valve-mask assistance, if indicated. Immediately search for causes of abnormal breathing and manage accordingly.

C Assess for the presence of <u>C</u>irculation, meaning the presence of a carotid pulse. Provide care for severe, obvious bleeding, give CPR, if necessary, and care for shock, if present.

D Assess for <u>D</u>isability, which means to look for additional illnesses and injuries that may be life-threatening or cause temporary or permanent disability. These injuries usually involve the musculoskeletal and/or nervous system.

E <u>E</u>xpose the patient by removing enough clothing so that all injuries are identified. In the outdoor environment, "exposure" also serves to remind the examiner that the patient needs to be protected from exposure to the elements.

It is crucial to conduct assessment properly and in the right order to avoid missing a significant sign or symptom; therefore, the rescuer must review and practice assessment constantly. It is particularly useful to review and practice assessment when introduced to injuries or illnesses involving a new body area or organ system in subsequent chapters of this book.

Psychology of Dealing With the Ill or Injured

Two things should be firmly in mind when approaching a patient: your initial reaction to the patient and the patient's initial reaction to you as the rescuer. Everyone responds to outside events both emotionally and intellectually. The emotional reaction to a patient who is hysterical, in pain, or injured is to *do something*, e.g., provide emergency care, tell a hysterical patient to calm down, summon

Fig. 4.2 *While approaching a patient, consider the person's emotional reaction.*

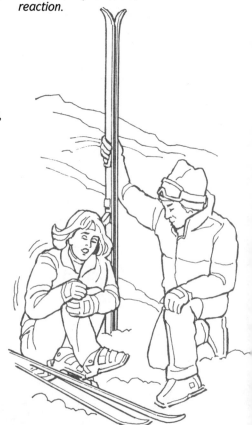

Fig. 4.2

assistance, or even to vomit or run away. Each of these reactions is normal. Fortunately, with training and experience, the initial reaction to an emergency can be managed so that the intellect rather than the emotions predominates (Fig. 4.2)

In most Western countries, a person's body is inviolate, and interfering with it or even touching it without permission is discouraged or even illegal. During training for emergency care, the rescuer must gradually overcome the normal hesitation to touch another person during an assessment.

Most, though not all, patients will be reasonable and cooperative. Any severe stress tends to cause regression to a more infantile, dependent state. Take advantage of this reaction by assuming a calm demeanor of trustworthiness, competence, professionalism, kindness, and authority. The patient's concerns should be taken seriously. Avoid making jokes and uttering banalities such as "There is nothing to worry about." The patient knows very well that there may be something to worry about.

Make eye contact with the patient, introduce yourself as a trained rescuer and emergency care provider, and ask, "May I be of help?" or "May I help you?" In some cases, help will be refused. A rational, informed adult with a normal mental status has a legal right to refuse care if he or she so desires. A refusal always should be *documented* and *witnessed,* even if the patient has a normal mental status and appears to have minor injuries. For the refusal to be "informed," the patient must be told what may happen if care is refused; this also must be documented. Members of ski patrols and other rescue organizations frequently carry special forms for the patient or other responsible person to sign, acknowledging that care has been offered and refused (an example is provided in Appendix E).

Even if the patient refuses help, stay with the person until you are satisfied that everything is under control. A person with a significant illness or injury may soon realize that he or she will need help after all. If an irrational patient refuses help, you may have to provide necessary care despite the refusal; this also should be documented and witnessed, and you should consider contacting law enforcement personnel.

Giving care to a seriously ill or injured child may be difficult and emotionally taxing, especially for rescuers who have children of their own. The child often will be frightened and may be hysterical, but children usually respond to an adult who behaves in a kind and parental manner. Always secure permission from the parent or other responsible adult, if present, before caring for a child. Children are often more modest than adults, and assessment may be difficult. Move slowly, use simple terms, make eye contact, and explain procedures, especially painful ones, before they are carried out. When parents or siblings are present they may be helpful in calming the child and explaining what is happening.

When conducting the secondary survey on a child with a minor illness or injury, tell the child what you are going to do and why, then begin at the feet and move toward the head. Painful procedures and examination of obvious injuries are best left until after a trusting relationship has been established. A seriously ill or injured child, however, should be assessed in the same order as an adult.

Always think before speaking, since statements are easily misinterpreted by uncomfortable patients and their concerned friends and relatives at the scene. Explain each action to the patient *before* it takes place. Do not lie to the patient, particularly about a procedure that will be painful. Rescuers should *never* argue or criticize each others' actions within hearing of the patient or bystanders (Fig. 4.3). Discuss plans for emergency care and evacuation privately; inform the patient after the arrangements are complete.

Remember, rescuers are not physicians. It is inappropriate for

---

Fig. 4.3 *Don't be guilty of this!*

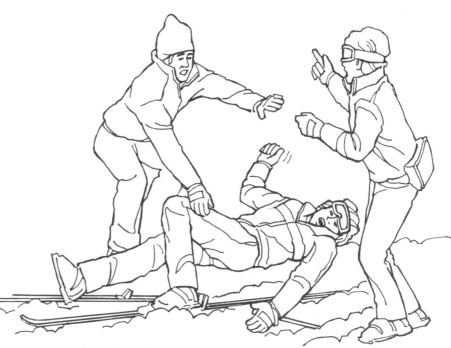

Fig. 4.3

rescuers to offer detailed information on possible further treatment or outcome. In particular, avoid guessing how soon the patient will be well again. First aid and emergency care is an inexact science. Even the best assessment is imperfect; diagnostic facilities outside of a medical center are primitive; and a serious injury or illness may not be obvious in the field. Remember that more than one condition can be present, and avoid the temptation to attribute all signs and symptoms to the most obvious injury.

People who are under the influence of alcohol or other drugs are more prone to injury. It is important not to overlook these injuries or attribute all signs and symptoms solely to the effects of the drug. People under the influence of alcohol or drugs and those who are senile or psychotic must sometimes be protected from injuring themselves or others. They may behave erratically, and their normal judgment and usual protective reflexes may not be functioning. They may fall and injure themselves, wreck their vehicles, wander into danger, promote fights, and become belligerent and obnoxious. Occasionally, they may become violent and dangerous.

The rescuer must remain calm, patient, nonjudgmental, nonthreatening, and reassuring. Approaching the patient from the side may be preferable to a head-on approach,

which the patient may interpret as an act of aggression. Refrain from arguing and—except in an emergency and preferably with plenty of help and witnesses present—do not attempt forceful restraint. Do not leave any patient with an altered mental status alone until he or she has been turned over to the EMS system or another responsible agency.

For an example of the type of psychological reaction the rescuer may have to face, read **Scenario #1** at the end of this chapter. It is based on an actual experience.

In the rest of this chapter, the steps of assessment will be discussed in considerable detail. To keep in mind the overall picture of the primary survey, repeatedly refer to the algorithms of the Primary Survey of the Unresponsive Patient (Table 4.5) and the Primary Survey of the Responsive Patient (Table 4.6).

First Impression

While approaching the patient, the rescuer forms an immediate first impression of the situation (also called the "global assessment" or "scene survey"), which takes less time to do than to read about here. The first impression begins to take form when you receive information via the first radio call or other notification and continues from when you first catch sight of the patient until arriving at the patient's side (Fig. 4.4). It includes

the following bits of information, which are registered almost simultaneously.

1. Is there any *danger* to the rescuer(s), the patient, or others at the scene (from terrain, rockfall, avalanche, other skiers, snow vehicles, etc.)? Is the patient in danger of falling from an insecure location?
2. Will *disentanglement* or *extrication* from an awkward or difficult location be required?
3. Does the patient appear to have an *injury* or an *illness*?
4. What most likely has occurred, as indicated by the patient's location, position, probable *mechanism of injury*, etc.?
5. Is the patient obviously *responsive* or *unresponsive*?
6. Is the patient obviously *breathing*? *Talking*?
7. Are there signs of obvious *bleeding*?

If there is a chance of exposure to the patient's blood or other body fluids, be sure to institute **universal precautions** before making physical contact with the patient. (See Appendix F for a discussion of how to prevent transmission of blood-borne pathogens). This means putting on *disposable rubber gloves as a minimum*.

Fig. 4.4 *The first impression is formed while approaching the patient.*

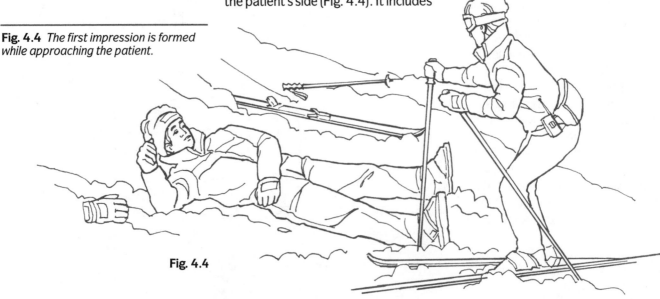

Fig. 4.4

Table 4.1

First Part of Primary Survey

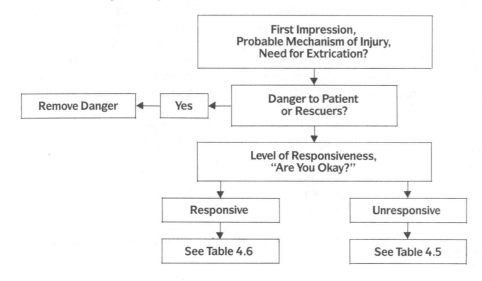

Primary Survey

After registering the first impression, proceed rapidly to the primary survey, whose purpose is to immediately identify and treat life-threatening emergencies. The techniques described here are those used for the adult patient; techniques used for children and infants are summarized in Tables 4.2 and 4.3 and detailed in Appendix B.

In emergency care, it is important to know the three anatomical terms used to describe the various positions of a patient lying down. **Prone** means the patient is lying face down; **semiprone** means the patient is lying face down but on one side, usually with the opposite knee drawn up; and **supine** means the patient is lying face up.

Shortly after reaching the patient, you should have a good idea of whether the patient is responsive or unresponsive. If not, gently shake the patient and ask loudly, "Sir, (Ma'am or Miss) are you okay?" To avoid aggravating a possible spine injury, shake the patient's shoulder while steadying the head with your other hand on the patient's forehead. Beyond this point, how you the conduct the survey will depend on the answer to this question.

Assessment of the Unresponsive Patient

If the patient does not answer, the patient is considered unresponsive and the situation is a genuine emergency. First, shout or radio for help. Then, unless the patient is obviously breathing normally, *immediately* open the airway and determine the presence or absence of breathing and its adequacy.

Although the airway can be opened, it is difficult to perform the assessment or other required emergency procedures if the patient is lying prone or semiprone. Therefore, unresponsive patients not found supine must be turned to the supine position. A constant worry is the possibility of aggravating a neck or back injury in a patient who is unresponsive due to trauma; therefore, *usually you should wait to turn a normally breathing patient until enough help arrives to use safe turning techniques* (see Chapter 13). However,

there is great danger in delaying resuscitative efforts in the patient with labored breathing who does not improve rapidly with the jaw-thrust technique (described below) or who is in respiratory or cardiac arrest. The single rescuer must immediately turn the patient to the supine position unless competent help is available on the spot to assist with repositioning the patient.

To turn the patient to the supine position without the assistance of others, kneel by the patient's shoulder, far enough away so the patient can be rolled toward you. Cross the patient's far ankle over the nearer one and move both of the patient's arms to the sides to help splint the spine (Fig. 4.5). With one hand, grasp the patient's neck just below the back of the head. Place your other hand under the patient's far armpit so that your hand is against the anterior part of the patient's shoulder. Gently roll the patient toward you with a minimum of bending or twisting of the patient's neck or back.

Opening the Airway

In the unresponsive patient, the muscles of the upper airway may relax, allowing the tongue to fall back and close the airway by obstructing the pharynx. After positioning the patient supine, the rescuer's next step is to make sure the airway is open. In any patient with a possible head or neck injury—which includes all patients unresponsive due to trauma—the airway should be opened in a way that causes minimal bending or twisting of the neck to prevent worsening of a possible neck fracture. However, because the patient will die if breathing is not restored, it is acceptable to bend the neck slightly, if necessary, to open the airway.

Because the tongue is attached to the lower jaw, any movement that brings the lower jaw forward will move the tongue forward and away from the airway. In the unresponsive patient where trauma is unlikely, the preferred technique of opening the airway is the simple and effective **head tilt/chin-lift** technique (Fig. 4.6). Place one hand on the patient's forehead and tilt the head back. At the same time, place several fingertips of your other hand under the tip of the patient's chin, just behind the point of the jawbone, and lift to bring the chin forward. The patient's mouth should be partly open. If it is necessary to open the patient's mouth, use the **crossed-finger** technique (Fig.

4.7). If the patient is wearing dentures that remain in place, leave them in place. Remove any visible foreign material using a hooked finger or piece of cloth.

If the head-tilt/chin-lift technique does not open the airway, or if a neck injury is suspected, use the **jaw-thrust** technique (Fig. 4.8). This maneuver is very effective in opening the airway, but is technically more difficult than the head-tilt/chin-lift. If CPR is needed, the jaw-thrust will slow this procedure, especially if the patient is lying on the ground rather than on a cot or

---

Fig. 4.5 *One-person Logroll*

Fig. 4.6 *Opening the Airway with the Head-tilt/Chin-lift Method*

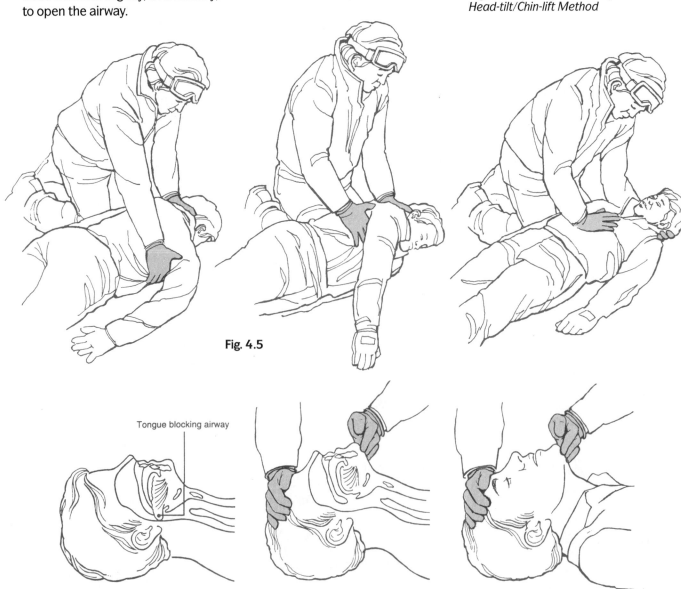

Fig. 4.5

Tongue blocking airway

Fig. 4.6

hospital litter. To perform the jaw-thrust, kneel at the patient's head, place the ring finger and little finger of each hand behind the angles of the patient's mandible (jawbone), and thrust the jaw forward by lifting your hands, at the same time stabilizing the patient's head and neck with your thumbs, palms, and the index and middle fingers of each hand. During this maneuver, rest your elbows on the surface on which the patient is lying. With practice, you may be able to do the jaw-thrust technique with only one hand (the hand nearest the patient's head) while kneeling at the patient's side, a position that makes it much easier to perform rescue breathing, if needed.

When you practice the jaw-thrust technique on a volunteer, it may be painful and difficult for the "patient." Remember that the jaw muscles of an unresponsive patient are relaxed, making the maneuver much easier and more effective.

Assessing Breathing

Once the airway is open, assess breathing by *observing* whether the chest rises and falls, *listening* for the escape of air (place your ear next to the patient's mouth and nose), and *feeling* for the flow of air (Fig. 4.9). If the patient is breathing adequately, continue to monitor the airway to make sure it remains open. If the patient has no gag reflex, insert an oral airway (oropharyngeal airway) to help keep the airway open (see Chapter 5). If breathing is present but inadequate, begin rescue breathing (described below) or use a bag-valve-mask (Chapter 5) as needed. If the patient is not breathing, begin rescue breathing.

Fig. 4.7 *Open the patient's mouth with the crossed-finger technique and remove visible foreign material with a hooked finger.*

Fig. 4.8 *Opening the Airway with the Jaw-thrust Maneuver*

Fig. 4.9 *Determine if the patient is breathing spontaneously.*

Fig. 4.10 *Use a mouth shield or pocket mask when performing rescue breathing.*

Rescue Breathing

Rescue breathing is done by the **mouth-to-mouth** technique, which is more efficient than older techniques of artificial respiration and is effective because exhaled air retains sufficient oxygen (16 percent) to support life, at least at low-to-moderate altitudes (below 10,000 feet/2,743 meters).

The acquired immunodeficiency syndrome (AIDS) epidemic has raised concern about giving mouth-to-mouth breathing. Hepatitis and other contagious diseases also are possible dangers. Even though no case of AIDS or hepatitis is known to have been transmitted in this manner to date, both viruses have been found in human saliva. Consequently, using your unprotected mouth during basic life support *should be avoided if at all possible*. Rescuers should carry mouth shields or, preferably, pocket masks (Fig. 4.10) to use when performing rescue breathing or CPR. These should be made of soft plastic that does not become rigid or brittle in the cold, and they should have a one-way valve. Pocket masks should be made of clear plastic. The use of these devices is described in Chapter 5.

Maintain the patient's airway, and if you are using your unprotected mouth or a mouth shield, pinch the patient's nostrils closed to prevent air from escaping through the nose.

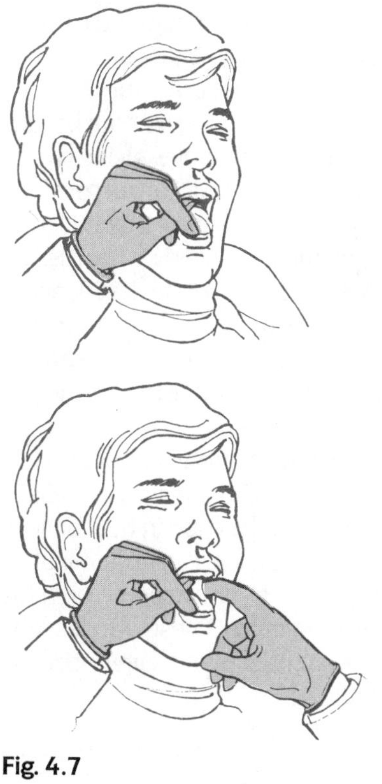

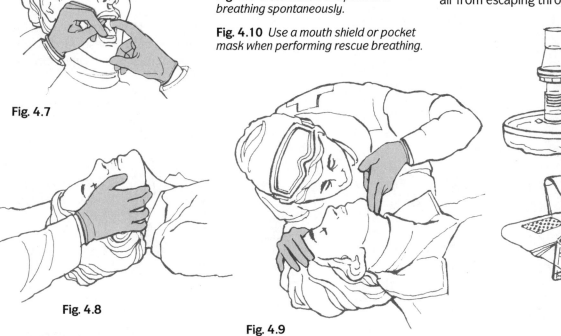

Fig. 4.7

Fig. 4.8

Fig. 4.9

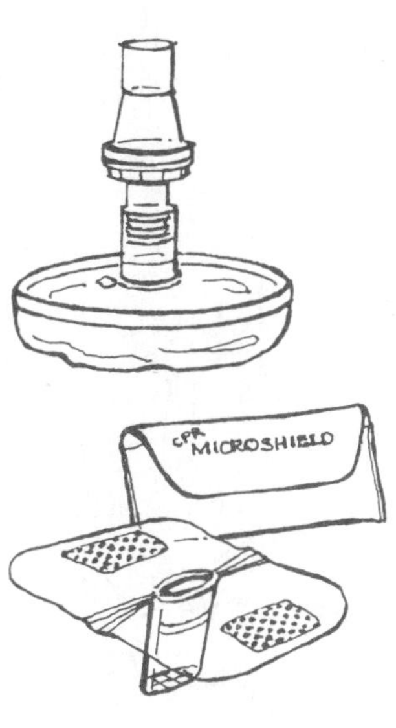

Fig. 4.10

If the airway is being maintained with the head tilt/chin-lift technique, use your thumb and index finger of the hand on the patient's forehead to pinch the nostrils closed. If the jaw-thrust technique is used, you may have to press your cheek across the patient's nostrils to prevent air from escaping through the nose. If you are using a pocket mask, it will cover the mouth and the nose and you will not need to pinch or block the nose. Take a deep breath, seal your lips around the patient's lips or the mouth-piece of the device, and blow into the patient's mouth (Fig. 4.11). Give two rescue breaths of one-and-a-half to two seconds each (count "one and two" at a normal speaking rate). Take a deep breath before each rescue breath. The patient's chest should rise and fall with each breath and you should hear and feel air escaping during exhalation. If this is unsuccessful, the patient's airway is probably still not open. Reposition the patient's head and chin (or jaw) and repeat the attempt at rescue breathing. If successful, assess circulation next (see **Assessing Circulation**). If a second set of two breaths is not successful, a foreign body may be blocking the airway.

Relieving Airway Obstruction Caused By a Foreign Body

The Heimlich maneuver is the technique for relieving upper airway obstruction in the adult. Quickly kneel astride the patient's thighs,

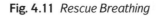

Fig. 4.11 *Rescue Breathing*

Fig. 4.12 *Performing the Heimlich Maneuver on a Supine Patient*

Fig. 4.13 *Mouth-to-nose Technique of Rescue Breathing*

facing the patient's head (Fig. 4.12). Place the heel of one hand on the patient's abdomen midway between the xiphoid process and the navel, and place your other hand, the second hand, on top of the first. Press into the abdomen with a quick, upward thrust. Repeat up to five times, and then open the patient's mouth by grasping the tongue and lower jaw between your thumb and fingers and lifting the mandible. This draws the tongue forward. Insert the index finger of your other hand along the inside of the cheek and deeply into the throat at the base of the tongue. The foreign body, if felt, can be brought up into the mouth and removed with a hooking motion. Be careful not to force the foreign body deeper, and remember that you may be in danger of being bitten.

Then, open the patient's airway again and attempt rescue breathing as described above, giving two rescue breaths. If still unsuccessful, repeat the Heimlich maneuver up to five times, followed by another finger sweep. Continue these sequences until the airway is clear, or until you are relieved by another responsible person, are exhausted, or the patient is pronounced dead.

Some modifications of the Heimlich maneuver are required for relief of airway obstruction in the conscious adult, adult with an abdominal injury, pregnant or obese adult, or in the child or infant. These are described in Appendix B and summarized in Table 4.2.

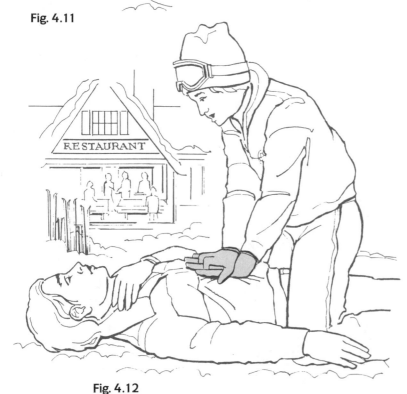

Fig. 4.11

Fig. 4.12

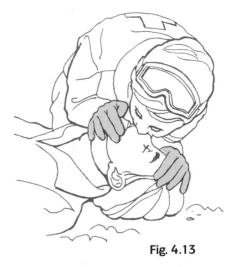

Fig. 4.13

Table 4.2

Techniques for Relieving Upper Airway Obstruction

	Adult	Pregnant or Obese Adult	Child	Infant
Rescuer's body position	Conscious: Stand or sit behind patient. Lying: Kneel astride patient's thighs.	Conscious: Stand or sit behind patient. Lying: Kneel at patient's side.	Conscious: Same as adult Lying: Same as adult	Conscious: Seated Unconscious: Seated
Hand position	Conscious, standing or sitting: Thumb side of one fist in midline just above navel. Grasp fist with other hand. Lying (unconscious): Heel of hand in midline just above navel with second hand on top of first.	Conscious, standing or sitting: Same as adult, except midsternum instead of abdomen. Lying: Same hand position as standing/sitting but use heel of hand.	Conscious, standing or sitting: Same as adult Lying: Same as adult	Conscious or unconscious: Infant prone on forearm with head lower than body. Support head by grasping jaw with fingers. Give four back blows between scapulae with heel of other hand. Turn infant over on thigh. Give four chest thrusts (same hand position as infant CPR).
Direction of thrust	Upward	Backward	Upward	Backward
Blind finger sweeps?	Yes	Yes	No, visual sweeps only	No, visual sweeps only
Back blows?	No	No	No	Yes
Number of thrusts before repeating rescue breaths	Up to five	Same	Same	Four

The **mouth-to-nose** technique (Fig. 4.13) may be more effective than the mouth-to-mouth technique in patients with facial injuries or when you do not have a pocket mask and cannot open the patient's mouth or achieve a tight seal around the mouth. Maintain an open airway, except this time keep the patient's mouth tightly closed. Take a deep breath, seal your lips around the patient's nose, and blow into the nose. Avoid excessive pressure on injured tissues.

In smaller children and infants, perform rescue breathing with your mouth over both the mouth and nose of the child.

Assessing Circulation

After two successful rescue breaths, assess circulation by determining the presence or absence of the carotid pulse. To find the pulse, feel over the carotid artery for five to 10 seconds with two or three fingers (Fig. 4.14).

This artery lies between the trachea and the sternomastoid muscle, just lateral to the Adam's apple. It is important not to miss a weak or slow

Fig. 4.14 *Locate the carotid artery lateral to the Adam's apple and check for a pulse.*

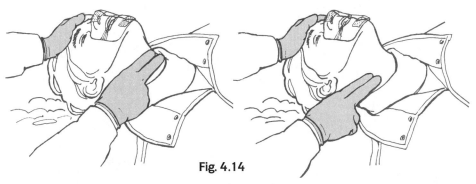

Fig. 4.14

pulse, because serious complications can be caused by performing external chest compressions on a patient with a pulse. If there is any question, continue checking the pulse for several more seconds. Check for up to two minutes in a patient with hypothermia, if necessary, because the pulse may be very slow and weak.

If the patient has a pulse but is not breathing spontaneously, continue rescue breathing at a rate of one breath every five seconds (12 breaths per minute—say *"one* and *two* and *three* and *four* and *breathe* and *one...")*. Each breath should last one and one-half to two seconds. Mouth-to-nose rescue breathing is given at the same rate as mouth-to-mouth.

If there is no pulse, the patient is in **cardiac arrest**, and external chest compressions should be started along with rescue breathing ("full" CPR).

CPR can be given by either one or two rescuers. One-rescuer CPR (Fig. 4.15) can be started immediately and maintains adequate circulation and ventilation but is more exhausting than two-rescuer CPR. When a second rescuer arrives, two-rescuer CPR can be substituted.

One-rescuer Adult CPR

To give external chest compressions, apply pressure over the lower half of the sternum in a regular, rhythmic manner. The cardiac output produced in this way, though only 20 to 30 percent of normal, is enough to sustain life. Because blood flow to the brain is below normal, the patient's head should not be above chest level. For chest compressions to be effective, the patient should be lying supine with the arms at the sides on a firm, flat surface such as the floor, the ground, a spine board, or a toboggan.

The proper hand position is important. Using the middle and index fingers of the hand nearest the patient's feet (called the "first hand"), locate the nearest of the two costal arches. Slide the fingers medially up the arch until your middle finger is in the notch between the two arches (Fig. 4.16a). Then place your index finger so that it is next to your middle finger, on the lower end of the sternum (Fig. 4.16b). Place the heel of your other hand (the

---

Fig. 4.15 *One-rescuer CPR*

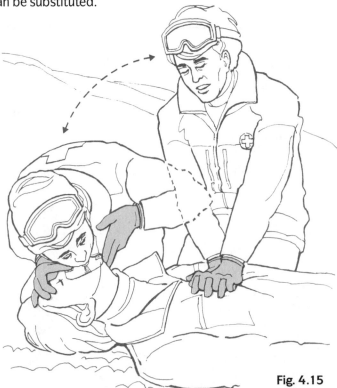

Fig. 4.15

"second hand") on the lower half of the sternum, next to the index finger of the first hand (Fig. 4.16c). Then, move the first hand so that it is on top of and parallel to the second hand (Fig. 4.16d). Your fingers should be pointing across the sternum and should be kept lifted off the patient's chest.

Start compressions by straightening your arms and locking your elbows into an extended position. Keep your shoulders above your hands so that the thrust for each compression is directed straight down (Fig. 4.17). Rock forward at the hips and knees, thrusting down so that the heel of your hand depresses the patient's sternum 1 ½ to 2 inches with each compression. Release pressure on the chest completely by rocking back between compressions, but do not lift your hands completely off the patient's chest. Perform compressions at a rate of 80 to 100 per minute. To aid in timing, count briskly, *"one* and *two* and *three* and...,"* giving a compression each time you say a number.

In one-rescuer CPR, maintain a ratio of 15 compressions to two breaths. After completing 15 chest compressions, move quickly to the patient's head, open the airway, and deliver two rescue breaths of one and one-half to two seconds each as described above. Move quickly back to the patient's chest, locate the proper hand position, and give another set of 15 chest compressions (Fig. 4.17). Give four complete cycles of 15 chest compressions interspersed with two rescue breaths, and then reevaluate the patient by checking the carotid pulse for five seconds. If it is absent, resume CPR. If a pulse is present, check breathing for three to five seconds. If breathing is absent, continue rescue breathing at the rate of one breath every five seconds, and monitor the pulse closely. If breathing and pulse are both present, stop CPR and monitor breathing and pulse closely. If CPR must be continued, check for the return of a spontaneous pulse and spontaneous breathing every few minutes. Do not interrupt CPR for more than seven seconds except in special circumstances (see below).

Two-rescuer Adult CPR

The first rescuer is positioned at the patient's head and the second rescuer is on the opposite side at the patient's chest (Fig. 4.18). The first rescuer is responsible for rescue breathing, maintaining an open airway, and monitoring the carotid pulse for adequacy of chest compressions and for return of spontaneous heart action. The second

rescuer is responsible for chest compressions. The ratio of compressions to ventilations is 5:1 rather than 15:2, with a pause of one and one-half to two seconds between each set of five compressions to allow for ventilation. If the rescuer responsible for compressions becomes fatigued, the two should switch positions.

The rescuer responsible for rescue breathing checks the pulse during compressions to evaluate their effectiveness. Stop chest compressions for five seconds after one minute and every few minutes thereafter to see if a spontaneous pulse and/or respirations have returned.

The technique for administering CPR to children and infants is somewhat modified because of their

smaller size, faster heart rate, and faster breathing rate. These modifications are described in detail in Appendix B and summarized in Table 4.3. When to discontinue or withhold CPR is discussed in Appendix B also.

Assessing and Managing Serious Hemorrhage

Severe bleeding, where blood is spurting or flowing rapidly from a wound, is almost as life-threatening as cardiac or respiratory arrest, since a patient can bleed to death within minutes from an injury to a large artery. Bleeding should be controlled as rapidly and effectively as possible by direct pressure (Fig. 4.19). A single rescuer can sometimes use a pressure dressing to continue

Fig. 4.16 *Locating the Proper Hand Position for Chest Compressions*

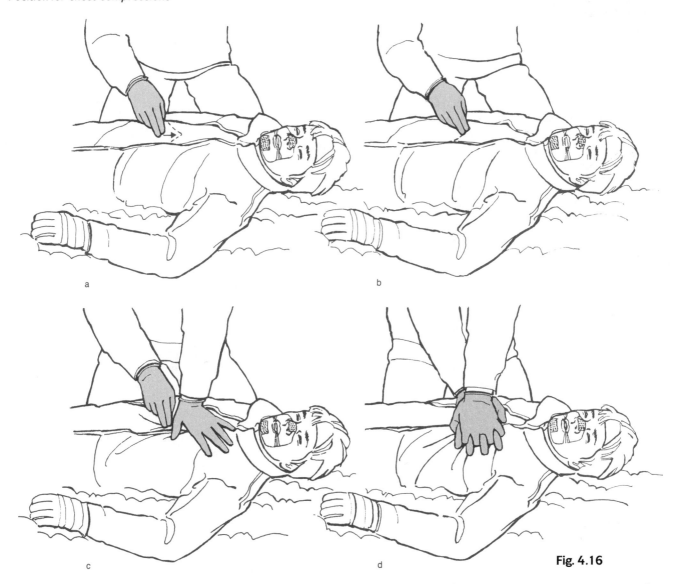

a

b

c

d

Fig. 4.16

Table 4.3

CPR Techniques for Patients of Different Ages

	Adult	Child	Infant
Hand position	Middle finger in notch of costal arch, index finger on lower sternum, heel of second hand next to index finger on lower end of sternum. First hand then placed on top of second.	Same as adult	Draw imaginary line between infant's nipples, place index finger of hand closest to infant's feet on sternum, just below this line. Area of compression is at location of middle and ring fingers.
Part of rescuer's hand(s) on chest	Heel of second hand with first hand on top (fingers off chest)	Heel of one hand only	Two or three fingers
Depth of compression of sternum	1½ to 2 inches	1 to 1½ inches	½ to 1 inch
Rate of compressions	80 to 100/min.	80 to 100/min.	>100/min.

Ratio of breaths to compressions
  a. One rescuer
  b. Two rescuers
	2:15
	1:5
		1:5
		1:5
			1:5
			—

Rescue breathing rate: ("one and" equals 1 second)	12/min. (one every 5 seconds)	15/min. (one every 4 seconds)	20/min. (one every 3 seconds)
Rescue breathing duration	1½ to 2 seconds	1 to 1½ seconds	1 to 1½ seconds
Artery monitored for pulse	Carotid	Carotid	Brachial
Recheck carotid pulse for 5 seconds	a. One rescuer: after 1 minute (four cycles), then every few minutes b. Two rescuer: after 1 minute (10 cycles), then every few minutes	a. One rescuer: after 1 minute (10 cycles), then every few minutes b. Two rescuer: Same as adult	Same as child —
Preferred technique of opening airway	Head-tilt/chin-lift or jaw-thrust	Same as adult, avoid over-extension of neck	Head-tilt/chin-lift only, avoid over-extension of neck
Rescue breathing	Mouth (occasionally nose)	Mouth (mouth and nose in small child)	Mouth and nose
Special considerations		One rescuer CPR usually requires both head-tilt and chin-lift, so relocate hand position visually rather than manually to maintain adequate chest compression rate.	To maintain adequate chest compression rate, try to maintain open airway with head-tilt only without losing finger position on chest. If head-tilt and chin-lift both required, relocate hand position on chest visually rather than manually.

direct pressure on the bleeding wound (see Chapter 6 for techniques) if there are other urgent things to do. If two rescuers are present, one can control bleeding while the other performs the rest of the primary survey. However, since a little blood frequently looks like a lot, especially on snow, rescuers should avoid delaying other, more important resuscitative measures in order to stop minor, non-life-threatening bleeding.

In the unresponsive patient who is breathing normally, severe bleeding should be controlled as soon as breathing has been assessed. In the patient who requires rescue breathing, severe bleeding should be controlled after the first two successful breaths. Speed is essential, so that the rescue breathing can be resumed

Fig. 4.17 *Proper Arm Position for Chest Compressions*

Fig. 4.18 *Two-rescuer CPR*

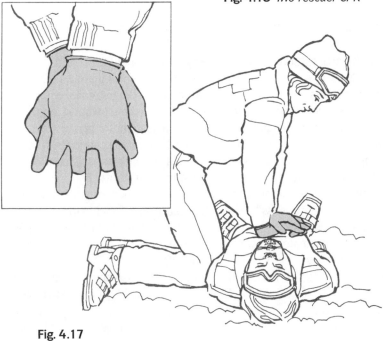

Fig. 4.17

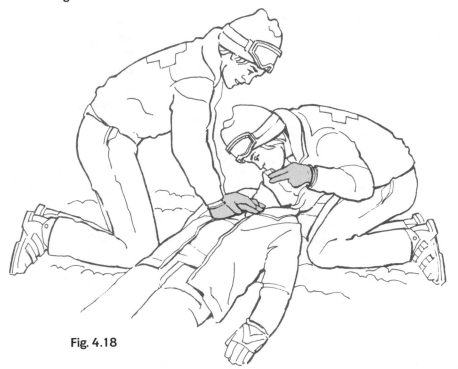

Fig. 4.18

again as soon as possible. In the patient requiring CPR, the lack of circulation will inhibit bleeding, which will begin again after CPR is started. If two rescuers are available, one rescuer can control bleeding while the other gives CPR. If only one rescuer is available, one cycle of two breaths and 15 chest compressions should be given, the hemorrhage should be controlled as swiftly as possible, and the CPR resumed.

Unresponsive Patient Not Requiring Rescue Breathing or CPR

If the unresponsive patient is breathing normally and has a carotid pulse, put an oral airway in place, continue to monitor the upper airway, and stabilize the cervical spine *manually* and with a rigid collar ("C-collar" or extrication collar) as soon as one can be applied, unless the patient's condition is clearly unrelated to trauma. Whenever a patient is unresponsive following trauma or from an unknown cause, assume that the cervical spine has been injured, either during the original trauma or from a fall following the trauma. If not handled properly, such injuries can lead to spinal cord damage and possible permanent dis-

Fig. 4.19 *Find and control major sources of bleeding.*

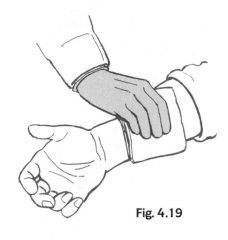

Fig. 4.19

ability; therefore, the cervical spine *must* be stabilized as soon as possible and the stabilization maintained throughout the primary and secondary surveys.

If more than one rescuer is available, the second rescuer can maintain stabilization while the first assesses the patient (Fig. 4.20). If only one rescuer is available, he or she will usually have much to do and cannot be tied up with manual stabilization while waiting for help. If the patient is in a secure position, the head and neck usually can be considered stabilized in place if the patient does not move or is not moved. Otherwise, the head and neck can be immobilized with a first aid belt, backpack, blanket, parka, rocks, branches, or by piling snow or dirt on both sides of the head. Once the primary survey is completed, the single rescuer can stabilize the head and neck manually until help arrives, if appropriate. In the partly responsive, uncooperative patient who refuses to remain still, the rescuer may have to stabilize the head and neck manually until help arrives, realizing that interfering with the patient's ability to move in any way may make the patient even more upset and disturbed.

Severe bleeding, if present, must be controlled as soon as possible after the airway is opened and breathing

Table 4.4

AVPU Scale

Alert: The patient appears normal, talks coherently to the examiner, and knows his or her own identity, location, address, telephone number, day, and date.

Responds to Verbal Stimuli: The patient is not alert, the eyes do not open spontaneously, but the patient responds in some way when spoken to.

Responds to Pain: The patient does not respond to verbal stimuli, but moves or cries out in response to pain, i.e., a gentle pinch. This response is not valid if the stimulated extremity is numb or paralyzed.

Unresponsive: The patient does not respond to either verbal stimuli or to pain.

and circulation are assessed and found to be present. In many cases, breathing may be present but is too slow, too shallow, or too fast (labored breathing). A pulse also may be present but too slow, too fast, too weak, or irregular. If the patient's breathing is labored and does not improve after you reposition the airway, and/or the pulse is abnormal, immediately assess the neck and chest. If the neck and chest appear normal, immediately assess the abdomen and pelvis for signs of injury that may indicate internal bleeding. Also assess the extremities for major fractures and bleeding wounds you might have missed. Assessment of these areas should be conducted as described below in **Secondary Survey of the Unresponsive Patient.**

Any abnormalities uncovered should be cared for immediately, i.e., stop external bleeding, stabilize a flail chest, seal an open chest wound, and/or treat the patient for shock. Patients with inadequate breathing may require rescue breathing or assistance by bag-valve-mask (Chapter 5).

In all unresponsive patients, assess the head next, looking for signs of injury that may explain the unresponsiveness. (This includes assessing the state of the pupils.) Then, reassess the level of responsiveness (level of consciousness or LOC) according to the AVPU Scale (Table 4.4). The Glasgow Coma Scale is more sensitive to minor changes in LOC but also is more complicated and harder to remember (See Chapter 3, Table 3.3). You should establish the habit of assessing and reassessing the state of the pupils and the ability to move both sides of the body along with the level of responsiveness in the head-injured patient. This will help you detect the triad of decreasing level of responsiveness, progressive enlargement of one pupil, and decreasing ability to move on one side, which indicate increased bleeding or swelling of one side of the brain, a neurosurgical emergency.

At this point, it is time to catch your breath and make sure the patient's temperature is stabilized. In cold and/or windy weather, this

Fig. 4.20 *Manual stabilization is applied to the head and neck when the patient is unresponsive.*

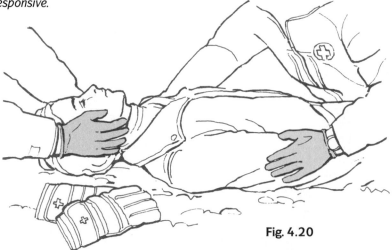

Fig. 4.20

usually requires placing windproof insulating material such as spare clothing over *and under* the patient. On the ski hill, you may need to put your parka, jacket or vest over the patient while waiting for the toboggan with its blankets or sleeping bag. In hot weather, protect the patient from the direct rays of the sun by using clothing or natural materials to make a sun shield.

Secondary Survey of the Unresponsive Patient

The secondary survey is best done in the aid room or some other shelter where the patient can be undressed. It can be started while waiting for a toboggan or other transportation; however, do *not* delay transportation of a seriously ill or injured patient to conduct a detailed secondary survey in the field.

The first step in the secondary survey is to assess and record the vital signs: pulse, respiratory rate, body temperature, and blood pressure. Note the color, temperature, and degree of wetness of the skin, and check skin perfusion with the capillary refill test. While assessing the vital signs, note any noises or movements the patient makes. It is especially important to note and record whether all four extremities move spontaneously and, if all four do not, which move spontaneously and which do not. It is also important to assess and record the response of each extremity to pain. The body temperature should be taken rectally. If no blood pressure apparatus is available, you can estimate the blood pressure by locating the major pulses (see **Blood Pressure**, Chapter 3). If you can feel the radial pulse, the patient's systolic blood pressure is at least 80 millimeters of mercury (mm Hg); if you can feel the femoral pulse, at least 70 mm Hg; and if you can feel the carotid pulse, at least 60 mm Hg.

With a responsive patient, the next step in the secondary survey would be to interview the patient to find out what happened, reconstruct the mechanisms of illness and injury, and obtain pertinent information about the patient's hisory. Although an unresponsive patient cannot be interviewed, you may obtain this information from companions, witnesses, or family members. Interview these bystanders as outlined below in **Secondary Survey of the Responsive Patient.**

Whole Body Survey

The rescuer then conducts a thorough examination of the patient's body from the head down. If there is no obvious external bleeding, but changes in the pulse, skin color, blood pressure, and/ or capillary refill time make you suspect impending shock, it is particularly important to examine the chest, abdomen, pelvis, and thighs for evidence of injuries that could produce internal bleeding (discussed in Chapter 6). It is also important to identify any fractures and dislocations of the extremities so you can splint them before transporting the patient. In severe weather, expose only one small area of the patient's body at a time. Although the patient should be shielded from the eyes of bystanders, misguided modesty is no excuse for missing a significant illness or injury. All unresponsive injured patients are assumed to have a spine injury and should be transported on a long spine board (see Chapters 8, 10, 11, and 13).

Procedure for Examination

The examination is performed by *looking* (inspection), *feeling* (palpation), *listening*, and *smelling*. Usually these techniques are performed simultaneously. The patient should be in the supine position. If the patient is found prone and there is any chance of a back or neck injury, logroll the patient into the supine position as described in Chapter 13. Before logrolling the patient from the prone position, however, assess the back.

The Head

Starting at the top of the head and proceeding downward, look at the scalp, face, and jaw for abnormal skin color, moisture, obvious perspiration, bleeding, open and closed wounds, scars, swelling, depressions, and asymmetry. Inspect the eyes, especially the area around them, for bruising.

Using a flashlight, inspect the pupils again for shape, size, equality, and response to light (Fig. 4.21). It is generally safe to leave contact lenses in place, even if the patient is unresponsive, as long as the eyes are kept closed, by taping if necessary (described below), and the patient can be transported to a hospital within two to three hours. Alert hospital personnel by writing "Contact Lenses" on a piece of tape and sticking it to the patient's forehead. Never remove a contact lens if the patient has sustained an injury to the eye. However, in injuries to the face, remove contact lenses before the eyes swell shut.

Using a flashlight, inspect the ears and nose for bleeding or a clear, colorless, or pink discharge that may represent spinal fluid leaking from a skull fracture. If uncertain whether spinal fluid is present, allow a few drops of

---

Fig. 4.21 *Assessment of the Head*

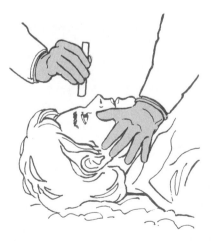

Fig. 4.21

Table 4.5

Primary Survey of Unresponsive Patient

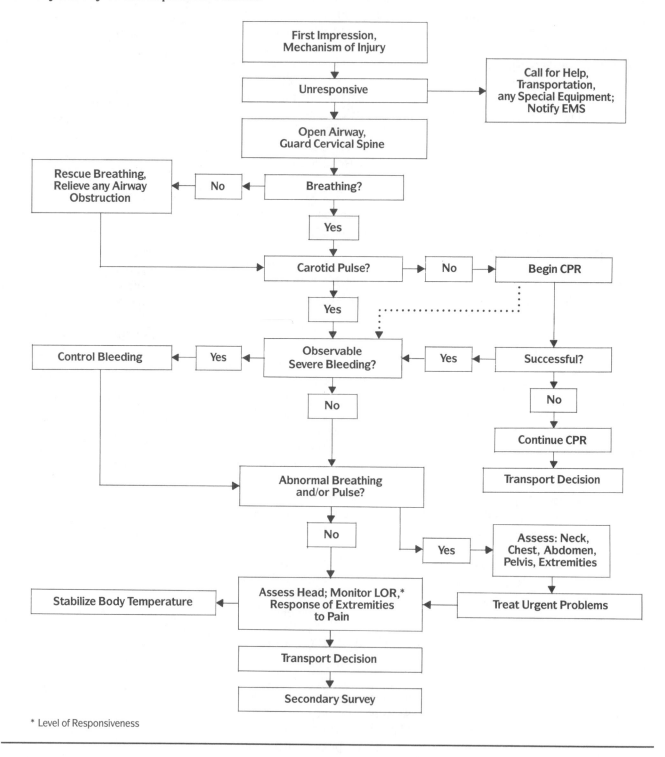

* Level of Responsiveness

the discharge to fall on a white hand-kerchief. A bulls-eye pattern with a red center and a pink rim indicates blood mixed with spinal fluid. Make sure that blood in the ear canal is coming from the canal and is not merely blood trickling down from a scalp injury.

Using a flashlight and tongue blade or spoon handle, inspect the mouth for dentures, foreign objects, broken teeth, bleeding, and wounds. Inspect the teeth for obvious injury and disturbed alignment. Note whether the lower jaw is properly aligned under the upper jaw when the patient's mouth is closed.

Starting at the top of the head and proceeding downward, feel the scalp, face, and jaw for bumps, tenderness, swellings, and the type of spongy, soft depression that may indicate a depressed skull fracture. If blood has matted the hair, palpate against the direction that the hair is matted.

Listen for abnormal noises in the nose and throat, such as gurgles, wheezes, and crowing sounds. Also, smell the breath for unusual odors such as alcohol, the fruity/acetone smell of diabetic acidosis, or the urinous smell of kidney failure.

Technique for Removing Contact Lenses

Hard contact lenses are difficult to remove without a special suction cup made for this purpose. Most individuals who travel to remote areas carry this equipment. If a hard lens cannot be removed, it sometimes can be slid from the clear part of the eye (cornea) onto the white of the eye.

Some soft contact lenses are designed to be left in place for weeks and are unlikely to injure the eye as long as they remain moist. This can be assured by taping the eyelids shut. To do this, pull the eyelids closed, lay a gauze pad firmly but gently over each eye, and tape over the gauze. Never apply tape directly to the eyelid or eyebrow. If it is necessary to remove soft contact lenses, you can usually lift them by pinching them gently between your thumb and index finger. Rescuers who wear contact lenses are used to doing this and can help.

The Neck

Starting just below the jaws and moving downward, look for variation from normal skin color and moisture, open and closed wounds, scars,

bleeding, swelling, lumps, engorged neck veins, asymmetry, abnormal position, or deformity. Look for a Medic-Alert tag on a chain.

Starting below the jaw and moving downward, feel the front, sides, and back of the neck for tender areas, lumps, swellings, deformities, and the impression of "Rice Krispies" produced by air under the skin (subcutaneous emphysema). Check just above the sternal notch to see whether the trachea is in the midline. This is done by pushing your index finger inward just medial to each sternomastoid muscle. The resistance should be the same on each side. If it is less on one side than the other, the trachea is *deviated* (being pushed or pulled to the opposite side).

The Chest

The rescuer must open or remove the patient's clothing to adequately assess the chest (Fig. 4.22). Starting at the clavicles and proceeding downward, look for open and closed wounds, bleeding, scars, lumps, swellings, asymmetry, and deformities. Note the breathing rate, the effort required for breathing, and any obvious pain produced by breathing or coughing.

Fig. 4.22 *Assessment of the Chest*

Fig. 4.23 *Assessment of the Abdomen and Pelvis*

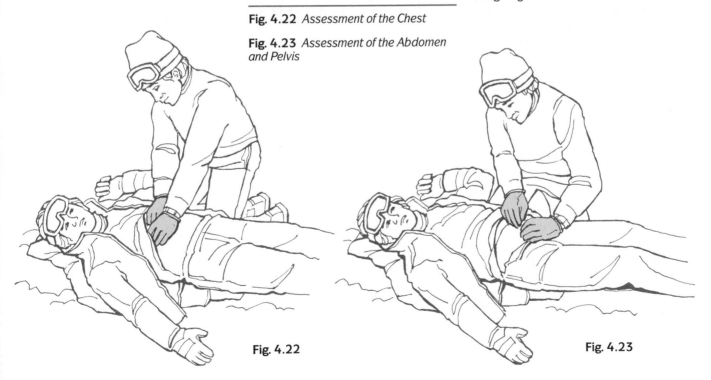

Fig. 4.22   Fig. 4.23

Again, start at the clavicles and proceed downward, feeling the sternum and all the ribs in turn to detect swellings, tenderness (especially over the ribs), and subcutaneous emphysema. Examine both sides of the chest simultaneously so that they can be compared with each other. Place one hand on each side of the lower, anterior chest to see whether both sides are expanding equally with inhalation. Listen for audible wheezes, rattles, squeaks, and other abnormal sounds.

The Abdomen and Pelvis

To adequately assess the abdomen and pelvis, the rescuer must open or remove the patient's clothing (Fig. 4.23). Starting at the costal arches and moving downward, look for open and closed wounds, scars, lumps, local swellings, and general abdominal swelling (distension). Try to always assess the abdomen from the same side of the patient, if possible. If you are right-handed, assess from the patient's right side because it is easier to detect enlargement or tenderness of the spleen, liver, or gallbladder with the hand nearest to the patient's feet. If left-handed, assess from the patient's left side. In a female, look for evidence of vaginal bleeding; in a male for priapism or bleeding from the penis. (Have a witness of the same sex as the patient present when you do this).

Using the pads of your fingertips, examine the four quadrants of the abdomen in a clockwise manner, starting with the right upper quadrant. Gently palpate the abdominal wall to check for tenderness, rigidity, local swelling, masses, and tightening of the abdominal muscles overlying a tender area ("guarding"). If there has been trauma, gently press the sides of the pelvis toward the midline with a rotary motion to see if this causes pain or a grating feeling (**crepitus**), a sign of a possible frac-

tured pelvis. If this is negative, push each side of the pelvis backward to see if this causes pain or crepitus. Listen for audible gurgling noises, and smell for abnormal odors, such as the fecal odor resulting from incontinence.

The Lower Extremities

The two lower extremities should be compared with each other during this assessment (Fig. 4.24). Since it is difficult to expose the thighs and legs adequately in patients wearing several layers of tight clothing, the rescuer can examine the extremities on the ski hill by feeling for swelling, tenderness, and deformity through the clothing. If abnormalities are found and a significant injury is suspected, use a seam-ripper or heavy scissors (bandage or trauma scissors) to expose the area. Remove the shoes, boots, and socks to assess the feet and ankles. This is usually done in the aid room or other sheltered area. (See Chapter 21 for a discussion of the indications for ski boot removal.)

Again, start with the groin area and move downward, looking at the thighs, knees, legs, ankles, and feet for open and closed wounds, scars, swelling, bleeding, deformities, and

unusual positions. If in doubt, carefully compare the injured extremity with the opposite normal extremity, particularly if you suspect abnormal shortening of one extremity.

In the same order, feel the skin and muscles for tender areas, swellings, and depressions, and for the grating feeling of crepitus, which indicates a fracture. Locate and palpate the femoral, dorsalis pedis, and posterior tibial pulses, and check capillary refill in the toenail of each big toe. Check the sensation of both thighs and legs by gently scraping the skin with a fingernail. Next, check for response to pain by gently pinching the responsive patient's skin; pinch the skin or toenail of the unresponsive patient a bit harder. Compare the reactions of the two extremities.

It is especially important to assess circulation by feeling for the pulses and checking the capillary refill time, and to check for motion and sensation in the extremity *distal* to a fracture or other serious injury. Remember that the capillary refill time may not be reliable in cold weather.

Fig. 4.24 *Assessment of the Lower Extremity*

Fig. 4.25 *Assessment of the Upper Extremity*

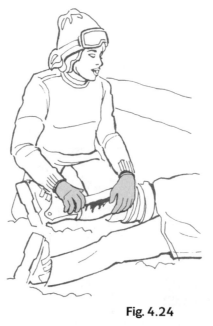

Fig. 4.24

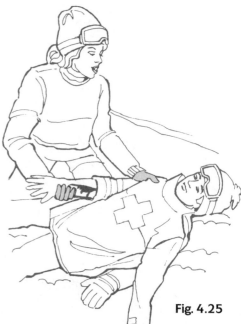

Fig. 4.25

In the responsive patient, ask the individual to move the hips, knees, and ankles, and to wiggle the toes; also ask the patient if the legs or feet feel numb or "tingly." Do not ask the patient to move the injured part of an extremity. Note any differences in skin color, temperature, or moisture between the two extremities. Smell any open wounds to detect abnormal odors, which may indicate the presence of infected or gangrenous tissue.

The Upper Extremities

The two upper extremities should be compared with each other during this assessment (Fig. 4.25). Starting at the shoulders and moving distally, look at the skin for abnormal color, texture, and moisture. Look at each shoulder, arm, elbow, forearm, wrist, and hand for open and closed wounds, scars, bleeding, swelling, deformities, abnormal shortening, and unusual positions. Again, if in doubt, compare the injured extremity with the opposite normal extremity. Look for a Medic-Alert bracelet.

In the same order, starting at the shoulder and moving distally, feel the shoulder, arm, elbow, forearm, wrist, and hand, looking for abnormal swellings, tender areas, and depressions. Feel the radial pulse at each wrist,

and test the capillary refill time in a fingernail. (It is good to get in the habit of checking the pulse and capillary refill time together, whether assessing circulation in general or the circulation in an injured extremity.) Remember that the capillary refill time may not be reliable in cold weather.

In the responsive patient, ask the individual to move the shoulder, elbow, wrist, and fingers, and to tell you whether the fingers and hands feel numb or tingly. Ask the patient to squeeze both your hands simultaneously so you can compare the grip of one hand with the other and test the patient's strength; however, do *not* ask the patient to move the injured part of an extremity. Check sensation by gently scraping the skin of the arms and forearms with a fingernail. Check for response to pain by gently pinching the responsive patient's skin; pinch the skin or fingernail of the unresponsive patient a bit harder. Compare the reactions of both extremities.

Note any crepitus at the site of an injury, which may indicate a fracture. Compare the two extremities for differences in skin color or temperature. Remove all jewelry from an injured extremity as soon as possible,

documenting what was removed, what was done with it, and to whom it was turned over. Smell any open wounds to detect abnormal odors, which may indicate the presence of infected or gangrenous tissue.

The Back

To allow adequate examination of the back, logroll the patient onto the side (see Chapter 13 for technique) and open his or her clothing (Fig. 4.26). If the mechanism of injury, location of pain, or abnormalities detected during examination of the lower or upper extremities makes you suspect a spine injury, you may want to assess the back at the time the patient is placed on a spine board to avoid unnecessary logrolling.

While waiting for a spine board to arrive, you may begin assessment of the back with the patient supine. Slide your hand (while wearing rubber gloves) under the neck and back, feel each spinous process in turn from above downward for swelling, tenderness, and deformity, especially an abnormal prominence or the "step off" type of deformity that may mean a fracture or dislocation of the spine. At times, bleeding can be detected in this way as well.

Fig. 4.26 *Assessment of the Back*

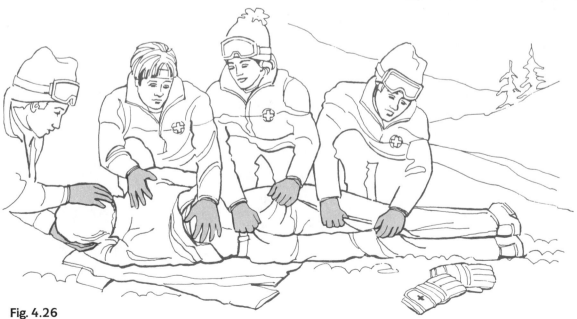

Fig. 4.26

If the patient is found in the prone or semiprone position, you may have time to examine the back before turning the patient into the supine position, unless circumstances require you to turn the patient over rapidly to give basic life support. (In the responsive patient, if the mechanism of injury or abnormalities found during assessment of the back make you suspect a back or neck injury, the patient should not be turned until enough help arrives so that the patient can be safely logrolled into the supine position).

Starting at the neck and moving downward, look at the skin of the neck, back, and buttocks for open and closed wounds, scars, lumps, swelling, bleeding, deformities, or unusual positions.

In the same order, beginning with the neck, feel the neck, back, buttocks, and, especially, the spinous processes for swellings, tenderness, deformities such as a "step-off deformity," unusual prominence, or unusual positions.

Assessment of the Responsive Patient

To be responsive, the patient must have some function of the circulatory and respiratory systems as well as the nervous system. Consequently, there is rarely a need for the formal type of primary survey used in the unresponsive patient. A responsive patient, however, may be developing airway obstruction, may have severe bleeding, may be having a heart attack, or may be in the early stages of shock or some other serious condition. Each of these conditions is considered a medical emergency, and you must provide immediate care if you suspect any of them. Severe complications that compromise the circulatory, respiratory, and/or nervous systems may lead to unresponsiveness (such as cardiac arrest in a patient with a heart attack).

Approach the patient, make eye contact, and introduce yourself as a person trained in emergency care by giving your name and the name of your organization (e.g., a ski patrol or mountain rescue group). Next, ask if you can be of help. If the patient accepts your help, put on rubber gloves, and proceed immediately to control any obvious hemorrhage. Otherwise (or after the hemorrhage is controlled) ask, "What happened to you?" or "What is wrong?" If possible, the patient should be sitting or lying down in a protected area for assessment. Continue eye contact during questioning and examination to detect the patient's reactions. Ask appropriate questions, and follow leads to determine the patient's main problem(s). An important question to ask of a patient who has been injured is "Do you hurt anywhere?" Ask the patient to describe what happened in detail, so that you can use the mechanism of injury (see Chapter 9) to predict possible injuries—particularly neck, back, and internal injuries.

If you suspect a neck or back injury and the patient's position is stable, instruct the patient not to move while you are performing the primary survey. If the patient is uncooperative or in an unstable position, you may have to stop at that point and stabilize the patient's head and neck manually until more help arrives.

Next, grasp the patient's wrist and assess the rate, rhythm, and strength of the radial pulse (Fig. 4.27). Check the capillary refill time and the skin temperature, color, and moisture. Note the respiratory rate and whether the patient is having trouble breathing. This tends to separate the more critical patient with a rapid and weak pulse and/or abnormal respirations from the less critical patient with a normal pulse and/or normal respirations. Checking the pulse also identifies you as a medically oriented person and helps establish trust, reliance, and a beneficial giver-receiver relationship.

Observe the patient's face for unusual expression, color changes, and excessive perspiration. Then, examine the major problem site(s) identified by the patient, looking for bleeding wounds, in particular, and any other abnormalities. In a patient with labored breathing, and/or a rapid or weak pulse, expose and assess the neck and chest. If you do not find any abnormalities there, move rapidly to assess the head, abdomen, pelvis, and ex-

Fig. 4.27 *Check the radial pulse to separate a critical patient from a noncritical patient.*

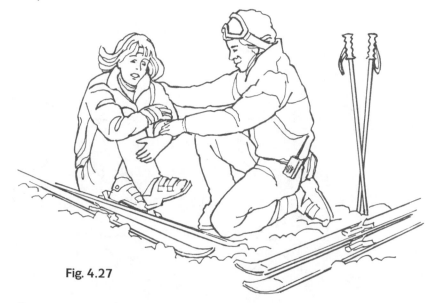

Fig. 4.27

Table 4.6

Primary Survey of Responsive Patient

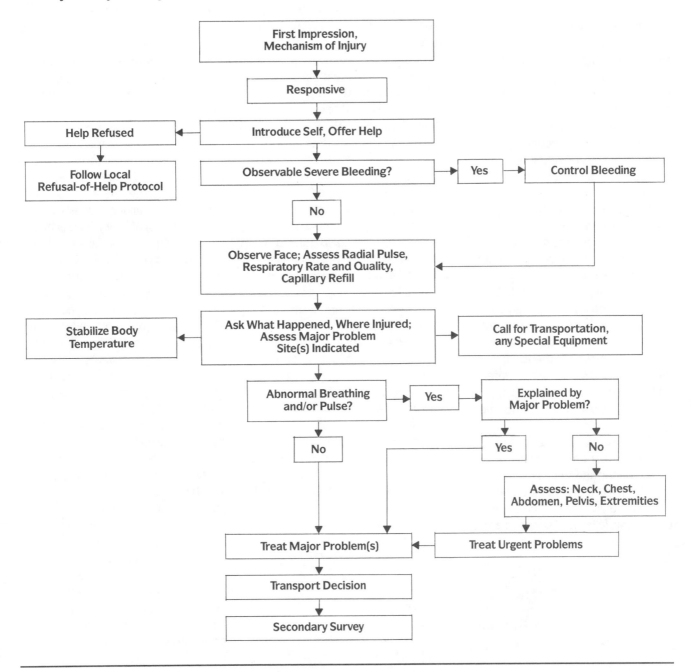

tremities. The assessment of the major problem site(s) the patient has indicated or you suspect should be conducted as outlined above in the appropriate anatomical section of **Secondary Survey of the Unresponsive Patient.** When finished, *always* ask,

"Is there anything else wrong?" Every body area indicated by the patient as a site of pain or other abnormality should be assessed before you conduct the secondary survey.

Scenario #2 at the end of this chapter provides an example of how to conduct the primary survey and

prepare a patient for toboggan transport. The primary survey of a seriously injured, responsive patient is depicted in **Scenario #3**.

Secondary Survey of the Responsive Patient

The secondary survey can begin while waiting for the toboggan or other transportation to arrive. In inclement weather, however, transport of a responsive patient to a warm, dry aid room or other shelter should not be delayed so that the rescuer can perform a detailed secondary survey. *A patient who is obviously critically injured should be transported off the ski hill as soon as the rescuer completes the primary survey, identifies critical injury sites, and performs necessary emergency care procedures.*

The extent of the secondary survey depends partly on the nature of the primary injury or illness. It is always carried out completely when the patient is unresponsive (as outlined above in **Secondary Survey of the Unresponsive Patient**), has an altered mental status, has suffered multiple, serious injuries, or appears to be seriously ill, unreliable, or mentally impaired.

The secondary survey can be abbreviated or postponed if the injuries are minor and the patient can *clearly* indicate that no additional problems exist. For example, if a patient has fallen and sprained a knee

at an alpine ski area and has a normal level of responsiveness (see **Scenario #2**), it is more important to prevent hypothermia by transporting the patient to a warm aid room than to perform a secondary survey on the ski slope (Fig. 4.28). Similarly, because it is important to maintain spinal stabilization, do not unstrap a patient from a spine board to do a secondary survey. Otherwise, the rescuer should take every opportunity to perform a detailed secondary survey, since constant practice is the only way to develop and maintain efficient and accurate techniques of assessment.

In conducting the secondary survey, the rescuer should think, ask questions, listen to the patient's answers, and examine the patient by looking, feeling, listening, and occasionally even smelling. Always carry a small notebook and pencil to record the patient's history and other important information. Many ski patrols and other rescue organizations have developed special forms for the purpose of recording the patient's history, vital signs, condition, and care given (see Appendix E for an example).

The first step is to record the pulse, respiratory rate, body temperature, and blood pressure; grade the

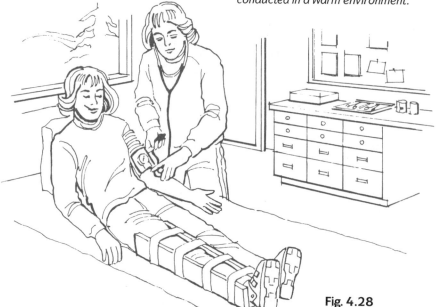

Fig. 4.28 *The secondary survey is best conducted in a warm environment.*

Fig. 4.28

level of consciousness by the AVPU scale (Table 4.4); check the reaction of the pupils; and observe the skin of the face for abnormal temperature and moisture. Then, interview the patient to find out in more detail the events surrounding the chief complaint, or main problem of the moment. This requires exploring and documenting in detail exactly *what* happened, *how* it happened, *when* it happened, *why* it happened, and to *whom* it happened. Try to reconstruct *in chronological order* the events leading up to the illness or injury. In the case of an injury, reconstruct the mechanism(s) of injury, if possible.

Make sure all painful and possibly injured areas have been identified. Avoid asking leading questions, and listen carefully to what the patient tells you, at the same time noting abnormal sounds, particularly in the respiratory system. Important things to question injured patients about include general body weakness or excessive fatigue; headache, dizziness, and loss of consciousness (even momentary); double vision or inability to see normally; numbness, tingling, weakness, paralysis, pain or pain on motion of an extremity; chest pain, shortness of breath, cough, blood in sputum, pain on breathing or coughing; nausea, vomiting, abdominal pain or cramps, blood in the feces or in the urine; and trouble urinating.

If the patient complains of pain, ask the person to describe the time of onset and location at onset; any change in location or severity with time; and the radiation, severity, and character (dull, aching, crushing, sharp, burning, stabbing, crampy, constant, intermittent). Also note whether the pain changes in response to breathing, coughing, motion, or change in position and whether the patient has had similar pain in the past.

If the patient appears to have an *illness* rather than an injury, the approach is somewhat different. The most important signs and symptoms of illness are fever, pain in some area (including headache), and variations from the normal functions of the circulatory, respiratory, gastrointestinal, and genitourinary systems. Significant symptoms that arise from these variations include fever or chills (usually described as the sensation of being hot or cold), sore throat, runny nose, earache, cough, chest pain, shortness of breath, wheezing, pus in the sputum, palpitations, pain or difficulty on swallowing, heartburn, sour stomach, nausea, vomiting, vomiting blood, diarrhea or other change in bowel habits, abdominal pain or cramps, painful urination, or blood in the bowel movements or urine.

After discussing the patient's chief complaint thoroughly, seek information about the patient's medical history. Emergency medical technicians (EMTs) commonly use the **AMPLE mnemonic** to help them remember the sequences of questioning for the important elements of the patient's history.

A: **A**llergies

M: **M**edicines or drugs, both legal and illegal

P: **P**ast medical history

L: **L**ast meal

E: **E**vents prior to the incident in question

The most important elements of the patient's medical history are

1. whether there has been pre-existing illness or previous injuries, especially those to the same area. Prompt the patient by asking if there are any chronic medical problems such as diabetes, epilepsy, or heart disease.

2. whether the patient has allergies to any particular drugs or medicine

3. what medicines or drugs are taken regularly

4. if there is any other useful information. Always ask, "Is there anything else about your health that I should know?"

After completing the interview, thoroughly examine the patient's body from the head down. Look for open and closed wounds, bleeding, scars, swellings, lumps, depressions, discharges, abnormal positions, deformities, abnormal odors, asymmetry, loss of motion, loss of sensation, abnormal sensations such as "pins and needles," changes in skin color, or moisture, tenderness, and crepitation. Check pulses and capillary refill times in all four extremities. If in doubt, compare the area in question with the opposite, normal area. Assess the body in the same order each time. The sequence for assessment of an adult is: head, neck, chest, abdomen and pelvis, lower extremity, upper extremity, and back. For a child, it is: lower extremity, abdomen and pelvis, upper extremity, chest, neck, head, and back.

The details of examination are described above in **Secondary Survey of the Unresponsive Patient**. If the patient has a medical illness, however, you may need to add a few techniques to your examination of the symptomatic areas. Using a flashlight and a tongue blade or spoon handle, check the patient's throat and tonsils by pressing down on the tongue and asking the patient to say "Ah." Palpate the upper neck under the sides of the jaw to check for tender and/or enlarged lymph nodes. The rattles of bronchitis, the wheezes of asthma, the bubbles of pulmonary congestion, and the gurgles of gastroenteritis frequently can be heard by the unaided ear, but the sounds are better heard when the ear or a stethoscope is placed directly against the skin of the patient's chest or abdomen.

Examine the abdomen for distension, tenderness, rigidity, and scars of previous operations or injuries (Fig. 4.29). If you suspect a urinary infection, palpate the costovertebral angles for kidney tenderness. Inspect wounds for swelling, redness, tenderness, or discharge. Inspect the ankles for swelling, particularly pitting edema, which is characterized by a depression or pit that remains after a finger is pressed into a swollen area. If the patient complains that an extremity is weak, compare its strength with that of the opposite, normal extremity by having the patient squeeze both your hands or push the feet against your hands.

In any seriously ill or injured patient, the patient's condition changes over time. Prepare a written record of serial vital signs and major events such as a change in level of responsiveness or a change in location or quality of pain. Record the time of each observation.

Fig. 4.29 *It is important to assess a patient's symptomatic areas.*

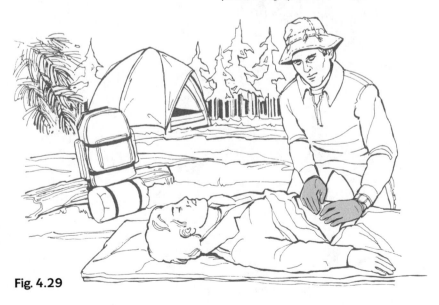

Fig. 4.29

Scenario #1 (Fig. 4.30)

The following scenario provides an example of a psychological reaction that is stressful to the rescuer and may be difficult to deal with.

You have just brought a toboggan down to an accident. As you approach the site, you see a young woman lying on the snow crying loudly. One leg and foot, with the ski attached and binding unreleased, is doubled under her other leg at an abnormal angle. Several of her friends surround her. You stop the toboggan below her and anchor it with your skis. As you approach the patient, you see a fellow patroller, Mike, coming over the rise and heading for the site also.

You: "Miss, I'm Charlie Dole of the High Range Ski Patrol. Can I help you?" (You reach for her wrist to check her pulse, but she pulls her hand away and continues to cry.) "Miss, I'm here to help you. What's happened?"

Patient: "Don't touch me! My leg is hurt. Get me an orthopedic surgeon right away. Call a helicopter!"

You: "Miss, if you'll let me and Mike help you, we can get your ski off and take a look at your leg."

Patient: "Who are you? How do I know you have any training? I'm a nursing student and I can tell if you know what you're doing."

You: "Miss, I've been trained in Winter Emergency Care to take care of ski accidents, and I've been patrolling at High Range for 20 years. It looks like you've hurt your leg. We can put a splint on it and take you to the bottom of the mountain in just a few minutes, then get you to a hospital, if necessary." (The patient cries louder.)

"The first thing we'd better do is get that ski off your boot. I'm sure it is making your leg hurt worse than it would otherwise."

Patient: "Don't touch me! I want you to call me a helicopter right now. My father is a lawyer."

You: "I'm sorry, Miss. We can't land a helicopter where we are. The slope is too steep and the trees are too close together. If you'll let us put a splint on your leg, it will feel much better."

(At this point, you try to calm the patient down by distracting her attention from her injury.) "By the way, what's your name?"

Patient: "Sue Happy."

You: "Where do you live, Sue?"

Patient: "Dust Bin, Oklahoma."

You: "Where do you go to nursing school?"

Patient: "The One-Horse Hospital and Health Center in Dust Bin."

You: "What year are you in?"

Patient: "My first year."

You: "I'm sure you know a lot about anatomy. Show me where your leg hurts."

Patient: "Right there" (pointing).

You: "Can you feel your toes? Can you wiggle your toes?"

Patient: "Yes."

You: "Let me check your pulse." (This time she lets you palpate her radial pulse and check her capillary refill time. They are both normal.) "Have you ever studied any first aid?"

Patient: "Not since the Girl Scouts."

You: "If we're careful, we can straighten your leg and get a splint on it. You know that will help."

Patient: "Well, maybe, but you're going to hurt me."

You: "It will only hurt temporarily while we're straightening it. It will feel better as soon as we get the splint on. Let's get that ski off. Mike, will

Fig. 4.30 *Scenario #1*

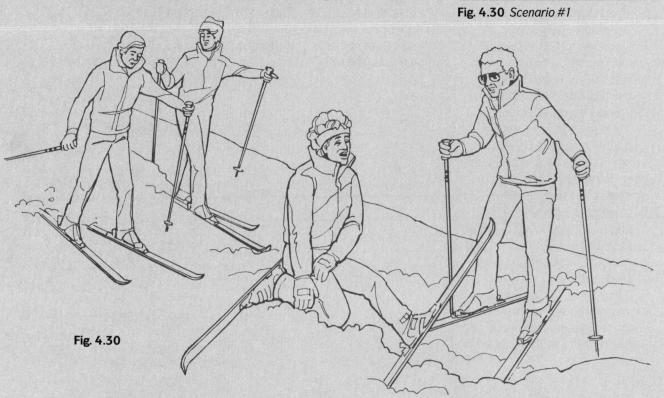

Fig. 4.30

you steady the boot, please?" (Mike does so. You release the binding and remove the ski.) "That's better, isn't it?"

Patient: (reluctantly) "Maybe. What are you going to do next?"

You: (You take charge a bit more, ignoring the question.) "Did you hurt yourself anywhere else? Did you hit your head or hurt your neck or back?"

Patient: "No."

You: "This is the splint we're going to use." (You take a quick splint from the toboggan and open it on the snow beside her.) "You can see it's padded and won't pinch your leg. It will keep the leg from moving and prevent any further damage. It goes on very quickly and uses Velcro straps."

Patient: "Do you have to move my leg?"

You: "We will have to straighten it to get the splint on, but it should be straightened anyway to help the circulation." (Sue starts to cry again.)

"We'll show you how we do it and we'll tell you everything we're going to do before we do it. This is the type of thing you need to know how to do as a nurse, too."

Patient: "I'm getting cold. I feel dizzy."

You: (You recheck her pulse. It is strong and about 90 beats per minute.) "The sooner we get you off the hill the better you'll feel."

You and Mike are able to straighten her injured leg and apply the splint, although not without further tears from the patient. She clearly feels

better with the splint on, and you are able to get her into the toboggan and to the aid room. After she gets there, she is seen by Dr. Bill Osler of the Doctor's Patrol. She asks him for his credentials, refuses to let him examine her because he is not an orthopedist, and is persuaded with difficulty to have her obviously fractured leg x-rayed and splinted at a local hospital rather than make the two-day nonstop trip back home in the ski bus with a temporary splint on.

Scenario #2 (Fig. 4.31)

The following scenario provides an example of how to conduct the primary survey and prepare a patient for transport in a toboggan.

You are answering a radio message from the base to help a skier who fell on Big Elk Run just below its juncture with Little Elk Run. As you ski up, you see a teenage girl sitting in the snow, holding her right knee. Both skis are off and she is surrounded by six of her friends. There is no sign of any blood on the snow.

You: "Hi, I'm Ben Schussen of the High Range Ski Patrol. Can I help you?" (You talk while taking off your skis and approaching the girl.)

Patient: "I'm glad to see you. I'm Betty Winsome. I fell and really hurt my knee."

You: (You observe her face, noting that the skin is dry and pink.) "Excuse me a minute, Miss Winsome, I'm going to put your skis up in the snow to warn uphill skiers to ski around us." (You form an X with the patient's skis uphill from the accident. Then, you radio for a toboggan and return to the patient.)

"You hurt your right knee?" (You grasp her wrist and note that her pulse is strong, regular, and about 80/minute. Her breathing is normal.)

Fig. 4.31 *Scenario #2*

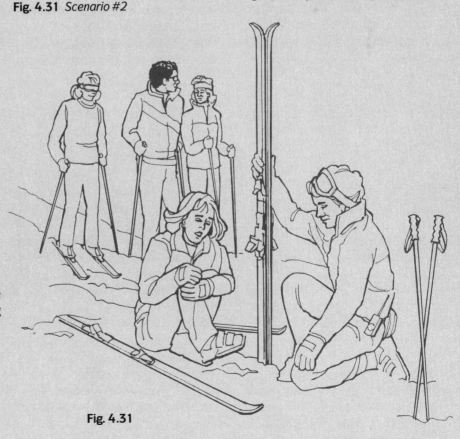

Fig. 4.31

Patient: "Yes. I was trying a turn, and one ski went one way and one went the other. I fell down between them."

You: (You take off her glove and check her capillary refill time in a finger.) "Did your bindings release?"

Patient: "Yes, both of them, but my knee got twisted when I fell down."

You: "Did you feel a pop in your knee when you fell?"

Patient: "No."

You: "Did you hurt yourself anywhere else besides your knee?"

Patient: "No."

By this time, you have established that Betty's airway, breathing, circulation, and level of responsiveness are normal, and that there is no obvious severe bleeding. You have assessed her pulse, capillary refill time, and the warmth, color, and moisture of her wrist, all of which are normal. The mechanism of injury does not suggest that anything else is wrong. Now it is time to examine the site of major complaint.

You: "I've called for a toboggan so we can give you a ride down the hill. Let me put my jacket around you to keep you warm. I also want to loosen your boots" (doing so). "While we're waiting, I'll take a look at your knee. Can you feel your toes okay?"

Patient: "Yes."

You: "Can you wiggle them?"

Patient: "Yes."

You: (You examine her knee through her ski pants, noting that there is no swelling, no tears in that area of the pant leg, and no sign of blood. You palpate the major ligaments around the knee.) "Does your knee hurt here? How about here? Here?" (Betty indicates that the medial ligament is tender.)

"Here comes the toboggan. We're going to put a splint on your leg to stabilize your knee and make you more comfortable while we give you a ride down to the patrol room."

Scenario #3 (Fig. 4.32)

In another scenario, the primary survey of a more seriously injured but still responsive patient might proceed as follows.

You are patrolling the upper part of High Range Mountain when you intercept a radio message that there is a skier down in the trees on the left side of upper Big Elk Run. You notify the base that you can handle the call. As you approach the scene, you see several skiers gathered at the side of the run. A skier is lying supine with his right side against a large tree about 10 feet off the run. You see a set of ski tracks leading from the edge of the run to the skier. Both bindings have released. As you get nearer, you see that the skier's eyes are open and that his breathing is fast and shallow. You quickly get out of your skis and approach the skier.

You: "Hi, I'm Ben Schussen of the High Range Ski Patrol. Do you need some help?"

Patient: (panting) "Yes, thanks. I'm hurting bad..." (panting) "in my right side and..." (panting) "can't breathe."

You: (You reach over and perform the jaw-thrust technique; it doesn't improve the patient's breathing.)

"What happened to you?" (While talking, you grasp the patient's wrist and feel the radial pulse. The pulse is strong, and regular—130 beats per minute. The patient's face is pale and there are beads of perspiration on his forehead.)

Patient: "Not sure..." (panting). "Was skiing the powder..." (panting) "along the side and lost it..." (panting). "Went in the woods and hit this tree."

You: (You take off the patient's glove and check the capillary refill. It is delayed.) "What's your name?"

Patient: "Mark Sitz."

You: "Did you hit your head or neck? Does your back hurt?"

Patient: (panting) "No, just my side."

By this time, you have determined that the patient's airway is open, he is breathing, has a pulse, and a normal level of responsiveness. However, his breathing is labored and his pulse is rapid. Something serious is probably going on.

Fig. 4.32 *Scenario #3*

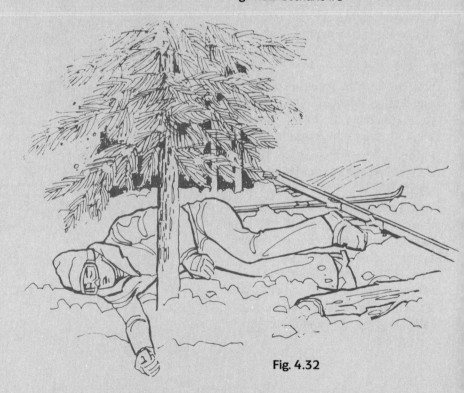

Fig. 4.32

You: "Excuse me a minute, I'll call for a toboggan to get you off the hill" (keying the radio transmission button). "Schussen to Summit, copy?" (Summit replies.) "I have an accident at location M-5 on upper Big Elk Run. I need a toboggan, oxygen, suction, a spine board, and some help."

Patient: "Tell them to hurry..." (panting), "I'm feeling worse."

You: "Keep still right where you are. I need to check you some more to see what is wrong."

You assess the patient's neck quickly. There are no areas of tenderness, particularly over the spinous processes, nor is there subcutaneous emphysema or other abnormalities. The trachea is in the midline. Moving quickly, you open the patient's jacket and pull up his turtleneck and longjohn top. Assessing the chest from the top down, you note that the right side of the chest is not moving as well as the left side. There is a large bruise over the lower right ribs laterally, extending down onto the upper right lateral abdomen. Palpation reveals some crepitus to light pressure over several ribs and a crackling sensation (air in the skin or subcutaneous emphysema) over these ribs. You then pull the patient's clothing back down over his chest and expose his upper abdomen. The patient is

quite tender in the right upper quadrant. The rest of the abdomen is soft and non-tender.

You now have a good idea of what has happened. Mark was traveling quite fast and collided with a tree, hitting his right chest and abdomen. As a result, several ribs are broken and there is some air in the tissues, indicating injury to the underlying lung. The patient also has right upper quadrant abdominal tenderness, raising the possibility of liver injury. He is in respiratory distress and appears to be in early shock, probably from internal bleeding, since there is no obvious external bleeding and no other cause of shock evident. Although you can proceed with the rest of the secondary survey while waiting for the toboggan to arrive, the patient should be transported off the ski hill without delay. He is obviously seriously injured and needs to be taken to a hospital as soon as possible.

You: (keying the transmitter button) "Schussen to hill chief, copy?" (The hill chief replies.) "We need an ambulance to meet us at the bottom of the hill as soon as we get down. Would you also please page Dr. Smith of the Doctors' Patrol and ask her to meet us at the ambulance?" (The hill chief affirms.)

(Turning back to the patient) "Do you hurt anywhere else besides your chest and right side? Does your head

hurt?" (Meanwhile, you slide your hand behind the patient's back and run it down the center of his back to the sacrum. There is no sign of swelling or deformity and no tenderness of the spinous processes.)

Patient: "No."

You: "Were you knocked out?" (You check the patient's pupils. They are round, regular, and equal.)

Patient: "I don't think so."

You: "Can you move your arms?" (The patient does so.) "Squeeze my hands." (The patient does so.) "Can you move your legs and feet and wiggle your toes?" (The patient says he can.) "Can you feel this?" (You gently pinch the skin on the backs of both the patient's hands.) "This?" (You gently pinch the skin of the patient's anterior thighs through his ski pants. The patient indicates that he can feel both.)

You have now established that, despite the serious nature of the accident, there is probably no head, neck, or back injury. Nevertheless, the patient should be placed on a long spine board because of the mechanism of injury.

You: "I'll loosen your boots so you'll be more comfortable. Here comes the toboggan. We'll be on our way in a few minutes."

Scenario #4 (Fig. 4.33)

The following scenario describes how to assess a responsive patient with a minor medical illness.

You and three climbing friends have just finished a two-day ski mountaineering trip from the roadhead into Diorite Peak (13,000 feet), the highest summit in the Granite range. Your plan is to spend the night in a snow cave at about 11,000 feet and do a winter climb of the 1,500

foot south face the next day. Your alarm watch goes off at 4 a.m., and you awake to hear your friend Lucky coughing. You reach for a match to light a candle. The light reveals your friend's face, and he looks ill.

You: "Lets get moving. We want to hit the face at first light."

Patient: "I don't feel so good."

You: "What's the matter?"

Patient: "My throat was starting to feel scratchy after we ate last night. I've been hurting all over and feeling

hot and cold. I didn't sleep at all. Now my throat is so sore I can hardly swallow, my head hurts, my chest hurts, and I'm coughing up some nasty stuff."

You: "Have you had any nausea, diarrhea, or painful urination?" (While talking, you place your hand on his forehead. The skin is hot. You next check his pulse; it is strong, regular, and faster than normal, consistent with fever. His capillary refill time is normal.)

Patient: "I feel bad enough without anything else." (You note that he is breathing at a normal rate and without difficulty.)

You: "Where does your chest hurt?"

Patient: "Right in the middle" (pointing to his sternum).

You: "All the time or mainly when you breathe or cough?"

Patient: "All the time, but worse when I cough."

You: (You get the first aid kit and a flashlight.) "Open your eyes wide and look straight ahead." (His pupils are round, regular and equal, and both respond to light.) "Open your mouth. That's good. Say 'Ah!'" (Using the flashlight and a spoon from the cooking kit as a tongue blade, you inspect his mouth and throat. You can see that his throat is red. His tonsils are swollen and red with white spots on them, and his uvula is swollen.)

"I'm going to take your temperature." (The thermometer registers 100.6 °F.) "You've got a fever."

Patient: "Yeah, I feel hot."

You: "Does this feel sore?" (You feel under both sides of Lucky's jaw and down both sides of his neck. There is a tender, almond-sized enlargement under the right jaw angle.)

Patient: "Yes, on that right side."

You: "Put your chin on your chest." (Lucky does so easily, indicating that

---

Fig. 4.33 *Scenario #4*

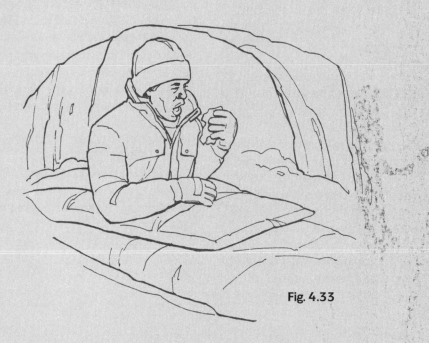

Fig. 4.33

his neck is not stiff.) "Let me listen to your chest." (You open his shirt and pull up his undershirt, laying your ear on the anterior chest, then the posterior chest, upper and lower parts. You hear a few rattles on both sides as he breaths in and out. He coughs and the rattles clear.)

It is now clear that Lucky has a significant infection—probably tonsillitis and bronchitis. There is no suggestion of gastroenteritis or a urinary tract infection, which are other common causes of fever on backcountry trips. You are worried that the altitude might worsen his illness. Fortunately, his pulse and respirations are good, and his level of responsiveness is normal.

There will be no climbing for him today. He needs to stay in base camp, in his sleeping bag, with one of the other party members to take care of him. He will need water, simple food, and some mild pain medicine such as aspirin or acetaminophen. If one of the party is carrying an antibiotic, Lucky should probably take it. With luck, he will be better the next day and will be able to ski back out, although part of his pack may have to be distributed among other party members. Without luck, he will be worse, and consideration should be given to moving the camp to a lower altitude while two party members ski out to get help. (The party is probably too small to carry him out on an improvised toboggan.)

Scenario #5 (Fig. 4.34)

Another scenario illustrates the care of a more serious medical condition.

You are sitting in the patrol room having a cup of hot tea after bringing a patient with an injured knee down by toboggan. The telephone rings; it is the cafeteria manager, who says, "Ski patrol? We need someone up here in the cafeteria to help a man who has passed out." You grab your radio and patrol belt and run outside, across the snow to the cafeteria. Inside, a crowd of onlookers is gathered around a portly elderly man lying on the floor. As you approach, you see a distraught woman kneeling at the patient's side. There is a tray on the floor with overturned dishes and spilled food. The patient is obviously breathing, and his respirations are deep, slow, and noisy. He is breathing through his mouth, and as he exhales, his right cheek puffs out more than his left. His eyes are closed, and his face is flushed. You notice that the right side of his face seems smoother than the left.

You: "Hi, I'm Bonnie Waydell of the High Range Ski Patrol. What's happened?"

Patient's Wife: "It's my husband. He was eating lunch and he just slumped down in his chair and slid onto the floor. I can't get him to say anything."

You: "Sir, are you okay?" (You steady his forehead with one hand, while shaking his shoulder gently with the other. The patient moans slightly. You note that the skin of his forehead is dry and warm, and his color is normal. You perform the jaw-thrust maneuver with the one-handed technique. The patient's respirations become noticeably less noisy.)

"Has he ever had anything like this happen before?"

Patient's Wife: "No."

You: (You radio the patrol room, requesting a litter, oxygen, suction, and some help. As you remove your hand from the patient's jaw, you notice that his respirations remain easier and quieter.) "What's your husband's name?"

Patient's Wife: "Sid Entarry."

You: (You assess his carotid pulse. It is strong and regular at a rate of 100.) "How old is he?"

Patient's Wife: "Sixty-two."

You: "Does he have any medical conditions that we should know about?"

Patient's Wife: "He's had high blood pressure for years, but he takes medicine for it. I believe it's called chlorothiazide."

You: (You assess capillary refill in a fingernail; it is normal.) "Any heart disease, diabetes, or strokes?"

Patient's Wife: "He has some mild diabetes, but he controls it with diet."

You: "Is he taking any other medicine?"

Patient's Wife: "No."

You: (You assess the patient's pupils with a flashlight. They are both round, the same size, and react to light.) "Does he have any allergies?"

Patient's Wife: "No."

You: "I'm going to check his arms and legs to see if he moves them normally." (You take each of his hands into you own.) "Sid, squeeze my hands." (Nothing happens. You then pinch the index fingernail of each hand between your thumb and forefinger. The patient withdraws his left arm but not his right. Then you pinch the skin of his leg on both sides. He withdraws his left leg but not his right.)

You can now sum up the situation as follows: An elderly man with a history of high blood pressure and mild diabetes collapses suddenly while eating. He is partly responsive, with a V rating on the AVPU scale. His airway is open, so this is not a case of food aspiration. His circulation is good. He appears to move less well in response to pain on the right side than the left. He probably has suffered a stroke and has a paralyzed right side (right hemiplegia).

You: "Is there anything else about your husband that we should know?"

Patient's Wife: "No, I can't think of anything. He's always been so healthy."

You: "Here come some of our people with a stretcher. We're going to give him some oxygen and take him down to the aid room. We'll call an ambulance and get him to the hospital."

Patient's Wife: "What do you think has happened?"

You: "I'm not sure, Ma'am, but we'll take good care of him until the paramedics come."

Fig. 4.34 *Scenario #5*

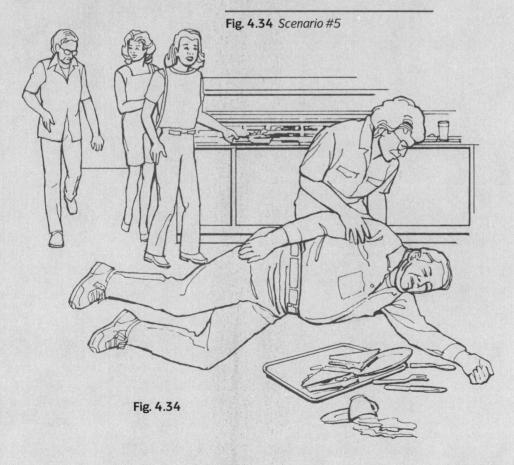

Fig. 4.34

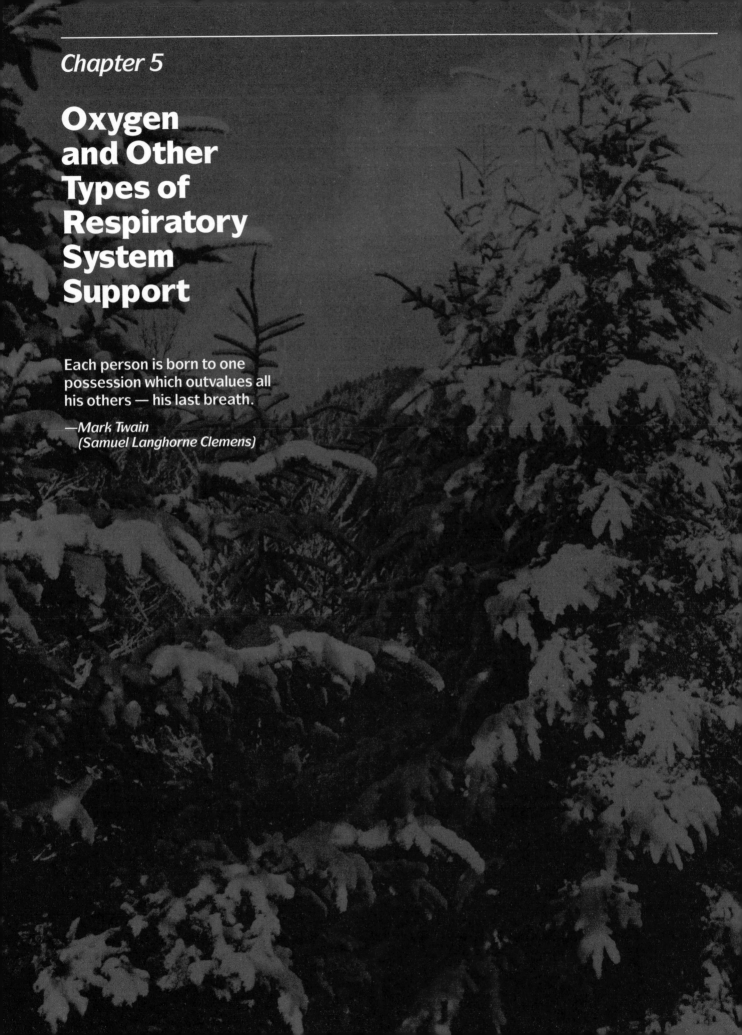

Chapter 5

Oxygen and Other Types of Respiratory System Support

Each person is born to one possession which outvalues all his others — his last breath.

—*Mark Twain*
(Samuel Langhorne Clemens)

Earlier chapters of this textbook stressed that oxygen is needed for living cells to function properly. This textbook also examines the ways in which oxygen's pathway to the lungs and cells can be disrupted. A large part of emergency care consists of re-establishing this pathway.

Aside from standard emergency care techniques—such as opening the airway, giving rescue breathing or CPR, closing a sucking chest wound, and stopping hemorrhage—tissue oxygenation can be improved by adding oxygen to the inhaled air. Giving supplemental oxygen ensures that the blood carries the greatest possible amount of oxygen to the tissues; however, giving oxygen is *not* so urgent a need that it takes precedence over *standard* emergency care techniques such as those listed above. If the oxygen in ordinary air cannot get to the tissues, neither will added oxygen.

Inhaled air contains 21 percent oxygen, which is more than enough for normal body function. The lungs extract about 25 percent of the oxygen in the inhaled air, so that exhaled air contains 16 percent oxygen. Rescue breathing and CPR can be effective because, at altitudes below 9,000 to 10,000 feet (2,743 to 3,048 meters), even this amount of oxygen is enough to sustain life. However, patients who are ill or injured have increased oxygen requirements. At the same time, their respiratory and circulatory systems may be compromised so that they are unable to take up and transport oxygen at the normal rate. Adding oxygen to the inhaled air increases the amount of oxygen that can be taken up by the blood and transported to the cells, thereby improving chances of survival and recovery of normal function.

The ability to provide supplemental oxygen and to use respiratory support devices is an essential component of modern emergency care. Illnesses and injuries that interfere with tissue oxygenation are common in urban society and not rare in the outdoors. Although supplemental oxygen and respiratory support devices are not available to the casual outdoor traveler, they are found in most ski patrol first aid rooms, wilderness search and rescue caches, and U.S. Forest Service and National Park Service emergency vehicles.

Oxygen Equipment

Basic oxygen equipment (Fig. 5.1) includes medical oxygen cylinders, pressure-reducing valves, pressure gauges, flowmeters, tubing, masks, nasal cannulas, oral (oropharyngeal) airways, nasal (nasopharyngeal) airways, bag-valve-mask (BVM) devices, and suction equipment. In addition, ambulances, helicopters, and hospital emergency departments are equipped with sophisticated ventilators and other complicated oxygen delivery equipment. Most emergency vehicles and many search and rescue units also have equipment for bypassing obstruction of the upper respiratory tract and supporting breathing in critically injured patients, by introducing tubes into the trachea through the nose or mouth (nasotracheal or orotracheal intubation), and through the membrane between the thyroid and cricoid cartilages (cricothyroidotomy). These latter devices are used

Fig. 5.1 *Basic Oxygen Equipment*

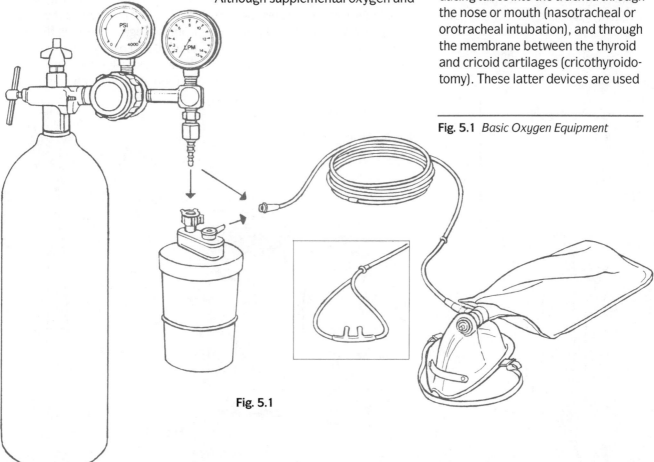

Fig. 5.1

only by people who have special training, such as physicians, nurses, paramedics, and EMT-I's.

The following are general guidelines on the assembly and operation of basic oxygen equipment. No attempt has been made to list all available options, as these vary widely across the country. The equipment chosen should be compatible with the protocols of local EMS units. The value of choosing equipment carefully and becoming thoroughly familiar with its use through frequent practice cannot be overemphasized. Most important, after reading this chapter you should *not* assume that you can operate this equipment before you have actual hands-on training under the supervision of an experienced instructor.

Figure 5.2 illustrates three different sizes of oxygen cylinders. The most practical oxygen cylinders for field use are D cylinders (approximately 20 inches high, weighing 10¼ pounds empty, and containing 360 liters of oxygen) and E cylinders (approximately 30 inches high, weighing 15 pounds empty and containing 625 liters of oxygen). At a flow rate of 10 liters per minute, a full D cylinder will last 36 minutes and a full E cylinder will last 62½ minutes. (This is calculated by dividing the tank capacity in liters by the flow rate.) The large M cylinders, which contain 3,000 liters of oxygen, are useful as stationary units in ski patrol aid rooms and other permanent first aid facilities. In deciding on the tank sizes and the number of tanks to be stocked, take into account the number of people served by your rescue group, transport times involved, and experience with the amount of oxygen used per week or month. As a rule, field units need a minimum of two portable tanks on hand; ski patrols need one tank at the summit of each mountain and two in the patrol aid room.

In the United States, federal regulations require that cylinders containing oxygen be painted green or have green markings to distinguish them from cylinders containing other gases. Cylinders can be purchased or rented from hospital supply companies; however, oxygen is considered by the federal and state governments to be a drug, so a physician's prescription may be required to purchase oxygen for emergency care use.

The pressure gauge reading provides an estimate of the oxygen remaining within a cylinder. When fully loaded, the pressure within a cylinder is 2,000 pounds per square inch (psi). If the gauge shows 1,000 psi, the cylinder is about half full. When the gauge reads less than 200 psi, the cylinder should be replaced by a full cylinder since, for all practical purposes, it is empty.

Cylinders smaller than D size are impractical when patient transport times are long. EMS supply houses carry special backpacks that will hold one or two cylinders (usually D size) with their accompanying attachments, a hand-suction unit, and a bag-valve-mask device. Rescuers can easily carry these on foot or on skis to the site of an emergency (Fig. 5.3). Since aluminum cylinders weigh about half as much as steel cylinders, they are recommended for portable units.

To deliver oxygen, each cylinder must be fitted with a pressure-reducing valve, a pressure gauge, and a flowmeter, which together are commonly called a **regulator**. The regulator reduces the pressure of the oxygen from the high level within the cylinder to about 50 psi as it reaches the patient, and allows the flow rate to be regulated between 1 and 15

Fig. 5.2 *Three Sizes of Oxygen Cylinders*

Fig. 5.3 *Example of an Oxygen Backpack*

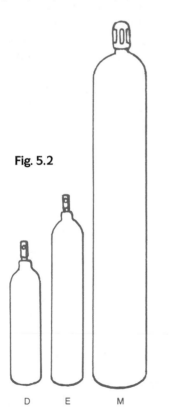

Fig. 5.2

D   E   M

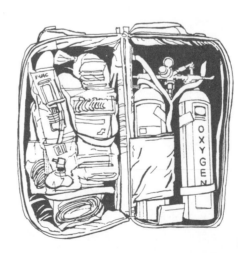

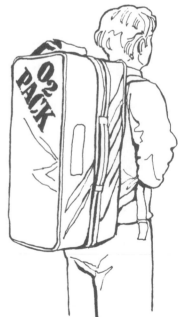

Fig. 5.3

liters per minute. Regulator systems are designed so they cannot be attached to the wrong size or type of tank by mistake. This is to prevent patients from accidentally receiving nitrous oxide, acetylene, or some other gas instead of oxygen. D and E cylinders both accept a yoke-style regulator (Fig. 5.4a) that uses a keyed pin system to ensure that the yoke will fit only the cylinder for which it is designed. The larger M, H, and K cylinders usually are equipped with DISS threaded outlet valves, which accept screw-on regulators (Fig. 5.4b).

The most practical regulator for field use is one that contains a Bourdon gauge flowmeter (Fig. 5.5a), which is unaffected by position, altitude, or gravity. However, because it measures pressure rather than flow, the reading will be affected if the tubing has a kink or is obstructed. Another satisfactory field regulator is the fixed orifice flowmeter (Fig. 5.5b). Flowmeters that use a graduated glass tube containing a steel ball (Fig. 5.5c) are more accurate but depend on gravity to register flow rate and work correctly *only in the upright position.* Therefore they are not practical for portable oxygen units.

Patients who require oxygen can be divided into two general categories: those who are breathing spontaneously and those who are not. Patients breathing spontaneously are then categorized into those breathing adequately and those breathing inadequately.

Patients breathing adequately are given supplemental oxygen with disposable, transparent delivery devices such as a non-rebreather mask or a nasal cannula (Fig. 5.1). Patients who are not breathing or who are breathing inadequately are resuscitated or assisted with supplemental oxygen attached to the oxygen input nipple of a mouth-to-mask device (pocket mask) or a bag-valve-mask device. In emergency care, almost without exception, oxygen should be given *in high concentration and at a high flow rate.*

The best mask for delivering a high flow rate of oxygen is the non-rebreather reservoir mask (Fig. 5.6a). This is a transparent mask fitted with a plastic reservoir bag and a one-way valve so that the patient can inhale oxygen from the bag but cannot "rebreathe," i.e., cannot exhale into the bag. This type of mask can provide 80 to 90 percent oxygen at flow rates of 10 to 15 liters per minute; flow rates of less than 6 liters per

minute should not be used. The reservoir bag should be kept one-third to one-half full of oxygen so that it will not collapse completely when the patient inhales.

A nasal cannula (Fig. 5.6b) delivers lower concentrations of oxygen at lower flow rates, but may be preferred for field use in some cases because it allows the patient to talk, drink, and eat, making it better tolerated by the responsive or partly responsive patient. It also is preferred when oxygen supply is limited, in patients who are likely to vomit, and in patients with chronic obstructive disease (COPD, or emphysema). The nasal cannula can provide 25 to 40 percent oxygen at flow rates of 2 to 6 liters per minute.

The nasal cannula and non-rebreather mask will be sufficient for most occasions when supplemental oxygen must be administered at alpine ski areas or in the outdoors in general. Other types of masks and special oxygen equipment are necessary only in special situations; their use is usually confined to ambulances, helicopters, and hospitals.

Oxygen from a tank is very dry and has an undesirable drying effect on the tissues of the respiratory tract.

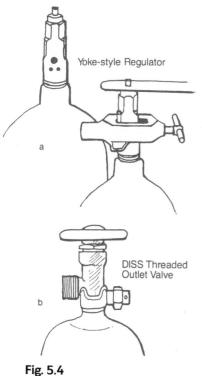

Yoke-style Regulator

a

DISS Threaded Outlet Valve

b

Fig. 5.4

Fig. 5.4 *Yoke-style Regulator and DISS Threaded Outlet Valve*

Fig. 5.5 *Examples of Flowmeters*

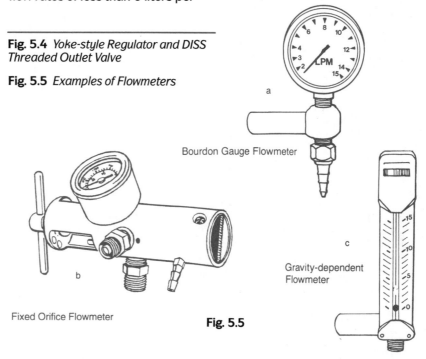

Bourdon Gauge Flowmeter

a

Fixed Orifice Flowmeter

b

Gravity-dependent Flowmeter

c

Fig. 5.5

A humidifying device should be used during prolonged administration of supplementary oxygen. Usually, a small jar of sterile water is attached to the tank so that the oxygen bubbles through the water before reaching the patient (Fig. 5.7). However, humidification is difficult to use outdoors, particularly at subfreezing temperatures, and is unnecessary if the patient can be transferred to an ambulance or hospital within 60 minutes or so.

Indications for Oxygen Use

Administer oxygen to
1. All patients with labored breathing or who are cyanotic, except possibly those who are hyperventilating obviously (see Chapter 16). Theoretically, patients with chronic obstructive pulmonary disease (emphysema) should be given oxygen at a flow rate of no more than 2 liters per minute. Because the breathing center in the brain is driven by hypoxia, too much oxygen may curb the drive and cause the patient to stop breathing. In practice, this is more likely to occur during long-term oxygen use and probably is irrelevant in an emergency situation, especially if the emphysematous patient is injured.
2. All patients with chest injuries other than the most trivial.
3. All patients who are seriously ill, i.e., those suffering from cardiac arrest, heart attack, or stroke.
4. All patients who are seriously injured, particularly with head or spinal cord injuries; femur, hip or pelvic fractures; multiple injuries; or severe burns, particularly of the respiratory tract.
5. All patients who are unconscious or in shock, or in whom shock is anticipated.
6. All patients with suspected diseases of altitude.
7. All patients with more than minor injuries or illnesses at altitudes above 8,000 feet (2,438 meters).
8. Any patient who, in the opinion of the experienced rescuer, would benefit from supplementary oxygen.

Procedure For Giving Oxygen
(Fig. 5.8)
1. Place the cylinder upright and position yourself to the side. Open and close the tank valve slowly with a wrench to clean debris from the outlet. This process is called "cracking" the tank.
2. Close the regulator flow valve and attach the regulator to the tank, making sure that the "O" ring gasket is in place and that the key prongs and oxygen outlet are lined up correctly. Tighten it securely by hand.
3. Open the tank valve slowly to one-half turn beyond the point where the regulator becomes pressurized. Note the tank pressure registered on the pressure gauge of the regulator (in pounds per square inch, or PSI).
4. Attach the plastic delivery tubing to the regulator output nipple, and attach the mask or cannula to the other end of the tubing. (The tubing that comes attached to the mask or cannula may be long enough by itself.)

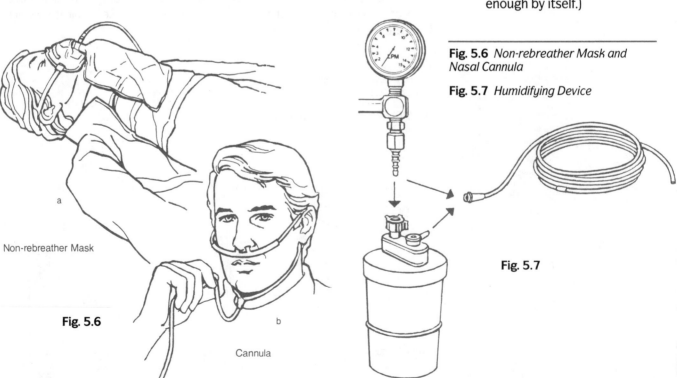

Fig. 5.6 *Non-rebreather Mask and Nasal Cannula*

Fig. 5.7 *Humidifying Device*

Non-rebreather Mask

a

Fig. 5.6

b

Cannula

Fig. 5.7

5. Open the regulator flow valve until the desired flow rate in liters per minute (LPM) registers on the flow gauge. Some regulator flow valves will select only low (2 to 4 liters), medium (4 to 8 liters), and high (10 to 15 liters) readings. The valve may turn in a direction opposite from what you expect. Remember that the flow rate for a non-rebreather mask should not be less than 6 LPM, and the flow rate for a nasal cannula should not be more than 6 LPM.

6. Explain to the patient why oxygen is needed and what you are going to do. If using a cannula, test the output by feeling it on the back of your hand. If using a reservoir non-rebreather mask, set it at 10 LPM and, with your finger, occlude the hole between the reservoir bag and the mask until the bag is partially inflated. Then, adjust the liter flow to the desired rate, position the mask on the patient's face, and adjust the elastic strap.

7. When you have finished administering oxygen, remove the mask or cannula from the patient. Turn the regulator flow valve until the rate on the flow gauge registers zero.

8. Shut off the main tank valve and remove the delivery tubing from the regulator output nipple.

9. Bleed the valves and gauges by opening the regulator flow valve again until the flow rate stays at zero.

10. Close the regulator flow valve. Be sure that the valve wrench is secured to the tank or regulator in such a way that it cannot be lost. Discard the cannula or mask, since these are *not* designed for reuse.

Precautions

1. Remember that oxygen tanks contain oxygen under very high pressure and can be as lethal as explosives if mistreated. Do *not* position any part of a rescuer's or patient's body directly over the tank valve, because a loose-fitting regulator can be blown off the top of the cylinder with enough force to maim or kill. Do *not* expose oxygen tanks to excessive heat, and always secure them so there is no danger that a tank can topple over and knock off the valve. *Never* drop a tank.

2. *Never* use an oxygen tank without a proper fitting regulator. *Never* use tape and other "foreign" material on oxygen equipment.

3. Close all valves when a tank is not in use, even if it is empty.

4. Oxygen will not explode when exposed to fire but *will* cause a burning object, such as a cigarette, to flare up, with the danger of setting other combustibles on fire. Smoking and other sources of open flame are prohibited where oxygen is being used. Flammable materials such as oil or grease should not come in contact with oxygen equipment.

5. *Never* move an oxygen cylinder by rolling it on its side or its bottom.

6. Inspect valve seat inserts and gaskets regularly. Do *not* lose your "O" rings. Have extra "O" rings on hand.

7. Store oxygen cylinders in cool, ventilated areas. Avoid expos-

Fig. 5.8 *Sequence of Administering Oxygen*

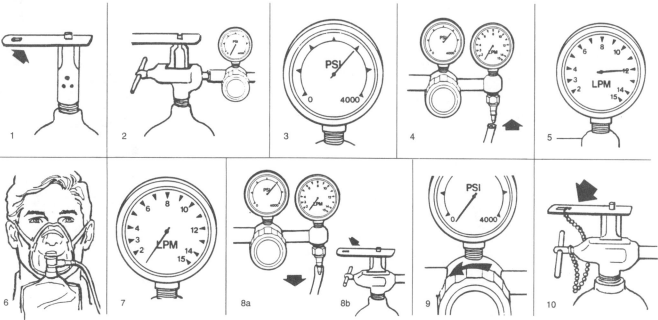

Fig. 5.8

ing cylinders to temperatures below freezing and above 125°F (52°C).

8. Have oxygen cylinders hydrostatically tested at regular intervals. The dates of previous tests are stamped on the top of the cylinder near the valve stem.

Other Equipment

Universal precautions should be instituted whenever using equipment or techniques that may allow contact with a patient's saliva or vomitus (see Appendix E). This means wearing disposable rubber gloves at a minimum.

A **pocket mask with an oxygen inlet** can be used for mouth-to-mask ventilation (Fig. 5.9). It should be made of transparent plastic that does not become brittle or rigid in the cold. The mask must be soft enough that a good seal can be maintained and should

have a one-way valve to protect the rescuer from the patient's saliva or vomitus. An oxygen inlet nipple on the mask allows the patient to be ventilated with air from the rescuer's lungs enriched by oxygen added from a tank. (If no inlet nipple is provided, oxygen can still be added by slipping the tip of the oxygen tubing under the edge of the mask.) The mask should have an elastic cord to slip over the patient's head and help hold the mask in place.

There are a number of pocket masks available; some are made of semi-rigid, clear plastic and look like ordinary oxygen masks. One, the SealEasy, has a soft bladder that conforms to the patient's face and provides a tight seal with less hand pressure than that required with an ordinary mask (Fig. 5.10).

The **mouth shield** (Fig. 5.11) is an inexpensive, compact, disposable device that fits easily in a first aid kit

or patrol aid belt and is designed for CPR only. The mouth shield has no oxygen inlet nipple. It consists of a rectangular piece of plastic that fits over the patient's nose and mouth, and a mouthpiece with a ventilation tube that fits into the patient's mouth. The mouthpiece has a one-way valve to prevent the rescuer's mouth from contacting the patient's saliva.

It is almost as easy to perform one-rescuer CPR with a pocket mask or mouth shield as without; rescue breathing alone or two-rescuer CPR is not a problem with these devices.

To use a pocket mask, attach the oxygen tubing to the mask, kneel at the patient's head, and open the airway with the jaw-thrust maneuver (Fig. 5.9). Place the mask over the patient's nose and mouth, with the apex over the bridge of the nose and the base in the groove between the lower lip and chin. Place your hands at the sides of the patient's head, with your thumbs and index fingers

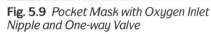

Fig. 5.9 *Pocket Mask with Oxygen Inlet Nipple and One-way Valve*

Fig. 5.10 *SealEasy Pocket Mask*

Fig. 5.11 *Mouth Shield*

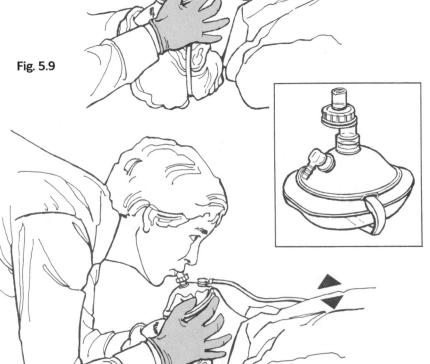

Fig. 5.9

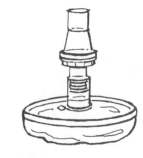

Fig. 5.10

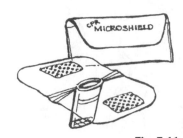

Fig. 5.11

pressing on the sides of the mask to maintain an airtight seal. Place your remaining fingers along the lower edge of the jaw and behind its angle to maintain the forward jaw-thrust. Place your lips on the intake valve mouthpiece of the mask. Perform rescue breathing at the same rate as with the standard mouth-to-mouth technique, watching between breaths to make certain the patient's chest is rising and falling. Once ventilation using expired air is in progress, turn on the oxygen to 10 LPM.

To use a mouth shield, open the sealed package and read the enclosed directions. Position the shield so that the side with the word "Chin" is over the patient's chin. Open the airway and place the ventilation tube in the patient's mouth so that the plastic barrier is flush against the patient's lips and face. Place your fingers under the top of the shield to pinch the patient's nostrils closed. Place your mouth on the barrier over the patient's mouth, pressing hard enough to maintain a seal. Provide rescue breathing at the usual rate, watching between breaths to make sure the patient's chest is rising and falling.

Oral (oropharyngeal) airways (Fig. 5.12) are designed to keep the tongue from falling back and occluding the upper airway. Airways are made in six to nine graded sizes ranging from infant to adult. They are used *only in unresponsive patients without a gag reflex.* They will cause fully or partially responsive patients or unresponsive patients with a gag reflex to vomit. If, on insertion, the patient gags, immediately withdraw the airway.

Oral airways should be carried in every first aid kit and used on every unresponsive patient without a gag reflex. They do not eliminate the rescuer's responsibility to see that the airway remains open, but they do relieve the rescuer from having to constantly maintain the patient's airway manually, a benefit when manpower is limited.

To choose the proper size, hold the airway against the side of the patient's face. It should extend from the corner of the mouth to the angle of the jaw (Fig. 5.12a). To insert, open the patient's mouth with the crossed-finger technique (Figs. 4.8, 5.12b), and insert the airway with the tip up or to the side to avoid pushing the tongue

backwards (Fig. 5.12c). When the airway is inserted halfway, rotate it slowly into position (Fig. 5.12c) so that, when fully inserted, its tip will point down and its curve will lie along the curve of the tongue, holding the tongue forward. An alternative way is to use a tongue blade to depress the tongue and slide the airway in with the tip pointing down. The flange of the airway should be resting against the patient's lips (Fig. 5.12d). To remove the airway, simply pull it out gently. In infants and children, the airway should *not* be inserted upside down and rotated 180 degrees because of the danger of injuring the teeth or soft tissues. Use a tongue blade to depress the tongue and insert the airway right side up, sliding it gently into place over the tongue.

Suction devices include mechanical suction apparatus (Fig. 5.13) that can be either fixed, semi-portable, or portable. For outdoor emergency care, a high-quality, battery-operated, rechargeable, portable device such as the Laerdal or Ohmeda is ideal. A portable suction unit can be kept on the recharge setting in a first aid room or rescue cache and used on-

Fig. 5.12

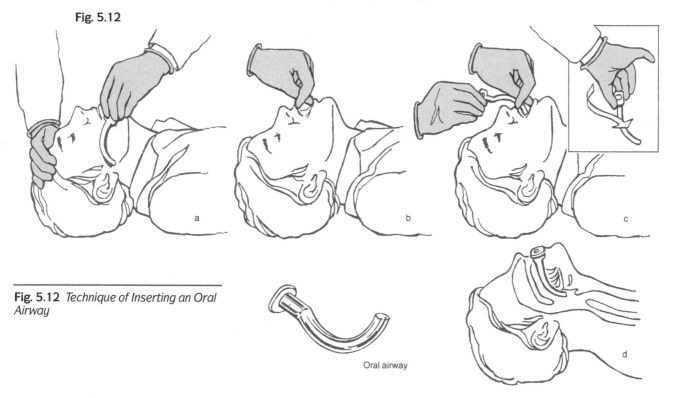

Fig. 5.12 *Technique of Inserting an Oral Airway*

Oral airway

site or unplugged and transported on a moment's notice to the site of an emergency. The unit should have a wide-bore, non-kinking rubber tube and a rigid, plastic pharyngeal suction tip (Yankauer or "tonsil" tip). A supply of water also will be needed to frequently rinse the suction tip and tubing during use.

Hand-operated suction devices such as the V-Vac, Res-Q-Vac, and Vitalograph work well and are less expensive and much lighter than the battery-operated devices, although not quite as effective. Foot-operated devices also are available. Hand-operated suction bulbs and bulb syringes similar to turkey basters are better than nothing and are small enough to be carried in a first aid belt or other small aid pack.

In the cold, suction tubing should be insulated during use. Do not use small-bore tubing because it plugs and freezes too easily. The active battery life of battery-operated units is reduced when they are used in the cold, so they should be insulated during transport to the accident site.

Rigid tips are better than flexible ones or tubing without a tip because their rigidity permits them to be easily inserted and controlled. Use them with caution if the patient is fully or partly responsive because they stimulate the gag reflex and may induce vomiting.

If the patient is being ventilated with a mouth-to-pocket mask or a bag-valve-mask, hyperventilate the patient for a few breaths before suctioning. To use a suction device, open the patient's mouth using the crossed-finger technique, and clear out any solid debris with a cloth or your gloved fingers. Interrupt the suction when you insert the suction tip, either by clamping the tubing or using a Y tube with the side-arm of the Y open. Insert the tip with its convex side along the roof of the mouth. Start the suction by releasing the clamp or closing the open end of the Y device with your finger. If using a non-electrical device, begin pumping it with your hand or foot. Because suction removes oxygen from the airway, it should be intermittent and only for 5 to 10 seconds at a time. Suction only as far back as you can see.

It is a serious matter for a patient to vomit and aspirate the vomitus. The aspirated material can cause suffocation from airway blockage or a serious and hard-to-treat case of pneumonia. It is much better to prevent aspiration than to try to treat it with suction. Place all responsive or semi-responsive patients without neck or back injuries in the semiprone position, also called the NATO or stable side position (Fig. 5.14), as soon as you have completed assessment and urgent procedures. All responsive or semi-responsive patients and any responsive patient with a serious illness or injury should be watched carefully. Remember that *the*

Fig. 5.13 *Mechanical Suction Devices*

Fig. 5.14 *Sequence of Turning a Patient to the NATO or Stable Side Position*

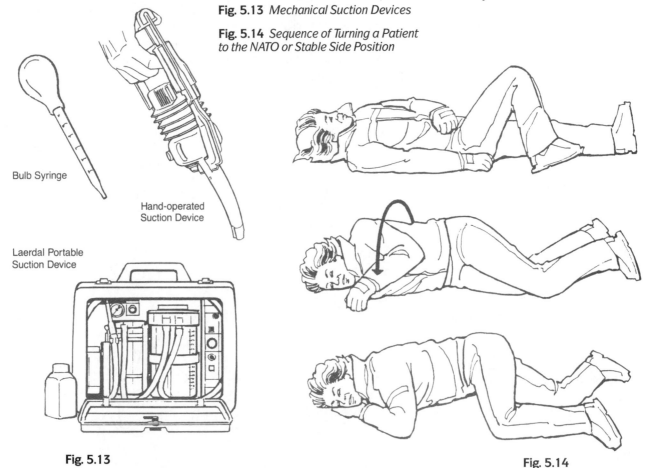

Bulb Syringe

Hand-operated Suction Device

Laerdal Portable Suction Device

Fig. 5.13

Fig. 5.14

rescuer assumes full responsibility for the airway of a patient strapped to a spine board, since the patient is unable to help himself or herself. Be ready at any time to tip the board to one side and apply suction at the slightest indication that the patient is going to gag or vomit.

Suctioning is indicated any time the upper airway is in danger of being blocked by sputum, edema fluid, blood, vomitus, or foreign material such as snow. Persons with impaired responsiveness may lose the gag reflex and the ability to cough and clear their airways, and may suffocate from the normal secretions produced by the nose, throat, and lungs. Listen for danger signs such as snoring, noisy rattling, or crowing sounds coming from the upper respiratory tract.

The **bag-valve-mask** (Fig. 5.15) is an effective device that is used to ventilate a patient who is not breathing or who is breathing inadequately. It consists of a mask attached to a resuscitation bag that the operator squeezes rhythmically to provide ventilation to the patient. A set of one-way valves prevents re-breathing into the bag. An oxygen reservoir attached to the bag permits giving high concentrations of oxygen. The bag-valve-mask can deliver oxygen at a much higher concentration than a pocket mask.

When used by two rescuers—one maintaining the mask seal on the patient's face with both hands and the other squeezing the resuscitation bag with both hands (Fig. 5.16)—the bag-valve-mask is much more effective than rescue breathing or the use of the mouth-to-pocket mask. It is more comfortable for the rescuers, who can sit or stand upright rather than bending over the patient. The device also prevents the rescuer's mouth from coming into contact with the patient's saliva or vomitus.

The bag-valve-mask is difficult for a single rescuer to use because it is difficult to maintain an airtight mask seal on the patient's face with one hand and squeeze the bag with the other. Using this device can be awkward and tiring, especially for rescuers with small hands. The mouth-to-pocket mask technique is usually easier and more effective for a single rescuer, even though better results can be obtained with the bag-valve-mask by squeezing the resuscitation bag between the hand and the opposite forearm, thigh, or chest. Correct use of the bag-valve-mask requires special training, considerable experience, and frequent practice.

The bag-valve-mask is used with an oral airway in place. If the patient is breathing inadequately but is responsive, be sure to explain what you are going to do and why before you start. The procedure for a single rescuer is as follows:

1. Inflate the mask's cushion to improve the seal, if necessary.
2. Attach the oxygen tubing to the intake nipple and set the oxygen flow at 12 to 15 liters per minute. Make sure the reservoir bag is inflated one-third to one-half full.
3. Place yourself close to the patient's head, open the airway with the jaw-thrust maneuver, and, in the unresponsive patient without a gag reflex, insert an oral airway.
4. Place the mask over the patient's mouth and nose, with the apex over the bridge of the nose and the base in the groove between the lip and the chin.
5. Hold the mask firmly on the face with the thumb and index finger of one hand, while placing the other three fingers under the lower edge of the jaw and behind the angle of the mandible to maintain the jaw-thrust maneuver.

Fig. 5.15 *Bag-valve-mask with Oxygen Tubing Attached to the Oxygen Intake Nipple*

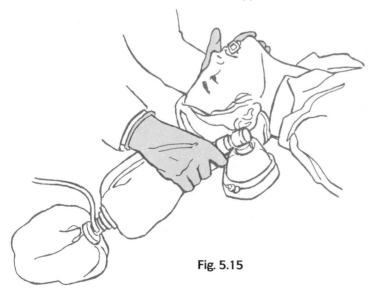
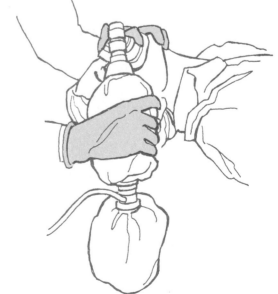

Fig. 5.15

6. In the unresponsive patient who is not breathing, every five seconds compress the bag with your other hand against your forearm, thigh, or side. Observe the patient's chest to be sure it rises and falls. In the unresponsive patient who is breathing inadequately, time the bag compressions with the patient's own respirations.

The procedure for two rescuers is modified as follows:

1. The first rescuer holds the mask firmly on the patient's face with the thumb and index finger of each hand, while placing the other three fingers of each hand under the lower edge of the jaw and behind the angle of the mandible to maintain the jaw-thrust maneuver.

2. The second rescuer uses both hands to compress the resuscitation bag.

As mentioned above, a bag-valve-mask is very difficult, if not impossible, to use during one-rescuer CPR, and squeezing the bag is tiring even with two rescuers. When two rescuers are available, they should trade jobs frequently; if more than two are available, they should relieve each other when necessary.

Fig. 5.16 *Positioning of Two Rescuers Using the Bag-valve-mask*

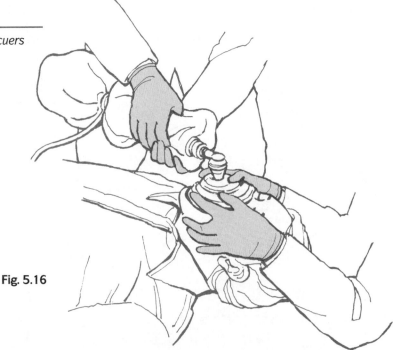

Fig. 5.16

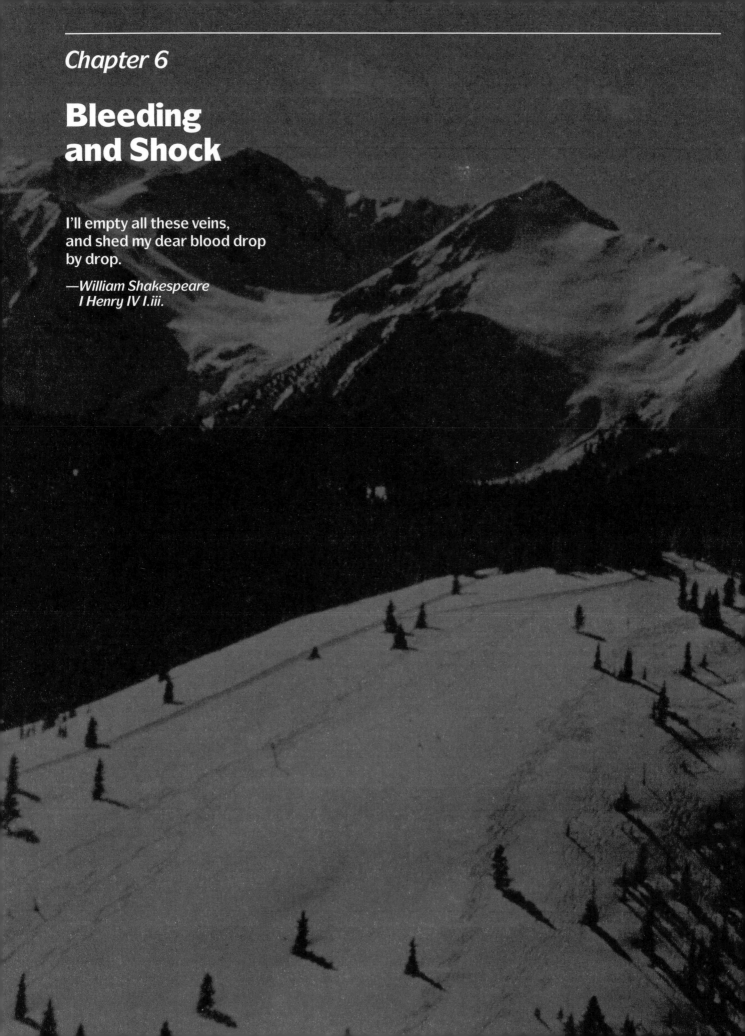

Chapter 6

Bleeding and Shock

I'll empty all these veins,
and shed my dear blood drop
by drop.

—*William Shakespeare*
  I Henry IV I.iii.

The function of the circulatory system in carrying oxygen from the lungs to the tissues requires intact blood vessels and enough blood to fill them. Damage to vessels from illness or injury may cause loss of blood from the system, or **bleeding.** Bleeding can be minimal, moderate, or severe. Severe bleeding (**hemorrhage**) can reduce the blood volume swiftly and significantly. **External** bleeding is bleeding that can be seen coming from a wound, while **internal** bleeding involves bleeding inside the body where it may be hard to detect.

The body of an average 150-pound (70-kilogram) adult male contains about 6 quarts (5,500 milliliters) of blood. Anyone who has donated blood is aware that the loss of 17 ounces (500 milliliters) of blood (11 percent of the blood volume) is of no consequence to a healthy adult. Loss of even 1.1 quarts (1,000 milliliters) may not cause serious difficulty. However, the loss of more than 1.1 quarts can produce the signs and symptoms of **shock,** a type of circulatory failure discussed later in this chapter.

Blood can be lost from arteries, veins, or capillaries; most bleeding is from more than one type of blood vessel. When arteries are damaged, the contractions of the heart and the high pressure within the arteries usually produce intermittent spurts of bright red, oxygenated blood. Venous blood, which is dark red because it is less oxygenated, flows out steadily under lower pressure. Capillary blood, also dark red, oozes out slowly because of the small size and low pressure of the capillaries. If other factors are equal, arterial bleeding is the most dangerous because blood is lost faster.

The rescuer should institute universal precautions against blood-borne infection before caring for a patient who is bleeding (see Appendix E). At a minimum this means putting on a pair of disposable rubber gloves. This precaution is especially important if the skin of the rescuer's hands is broken by cuts, sores, or a rash.

When bleeding is external, blood can be seen on the body surface, although clothing may have to be opened to find it. Bleeding that does not involve arteries or large veins usually will stop spontaneously in 5 to 10 minutes. Even arterial bleeding may stop without treatment, since a torn artery tends to respond to the injury by contracting its muscular walls and retracting back into the tissues. Nonetheless, the rescuer cannot rely on the body's natural protective mechanisms to control bleeding before a dangerous amount of blood is lost. When a patient is hemorrhaging, every minute may count.

Most external bleeding can be controlled by **direct pressure,** which collapses the blood vessels and occludes (closes up) the gaps in their damaged walls until normal clotting mechanisms can seal them. Pressure is applied locally, directly over the wound (Fig. 6.1). Other techniques, which serve only as supplements to direct pressure, include the following:

1. **Elevation and immobilization,** which promote clotting by reducing motion and lowering blood pressure at the injury site. (This technique is suitable mainly for extremity bleeding.)
2. **Pressure on a major artery** proximal to the wound (pressure

point). This technique may decrease bleeding, but rarely stops it entirely because most wounds are supplied by more than one artery.
3. **Pneumatic counterpressure devices,** such as air splints and pneumatic antishock garments (PASGs). The use of the PASG, formerly called the medical antishock trouser (MAST), requires additional training, certification, and in some areas, licensing.
4. **Application of a tourniquet,** used only when all else fails and the patient's life is in danger.

Direct Pressure

To apply direct pressure, select a sterile dressing large enough to cover the wound completely. Place the dressing directly on the wound and press on it with your gloved hand, hard enough to stop the bleeding. This is called **manual pressure.** If the situation is urgent and a sterile dressing is not available, a clean piece of cloth or a clean sanitary napkin may be substituted. If necessary, apply pressure with a finger or hand alone.

After bleeding has stopped, maintain pressure by applying a self-adhering roller bandage such as Kling or Kerlix firmly over the dressing.

If bleeding occurs despite initial direct pressure, place additional dressings over the original ones and apply stronger pressure. Tell the patient not to move, elevate the wound, and if it is on an extremity, immobilize it by splinting. If bleeding still continues, remove all dressings and inspect the wound to make sure pressure is being applied in the right place. Bleeding from a small artery at the edge of a wound may have been overlooked.

Pressure Points

If bleeding continues despite the use of the above techniques, the addition of pressure over a major artery sup-

Fig. 6.1 *Control external bleeding with direct pressure.*

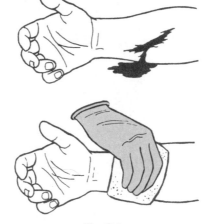

Fig. 6.1

plying the area of injury may slow the bleeding and buy time until definitive medical care can be obtained. The major pressure points are located where large arteries lie close to bone. Examples are the brachial artery in the arm and the femoral artery in the groin (Fig. 6.2). After locating the arterial pulse, use several fingers or the palm of the hand to press the artery against the underlying bone.

Tourniquet

Because a tourniquet completely occludes the blood vessels, it will cause distal tissues to die if left on too long. Even *brief* application of a tourniquet can crush the underlying tissues and permanently damage nerves and blood vessels. Therefore, if a tourniquet is chosen, it should be applied as far distally as possible. Tourniquets are not useful for trunk injuries and should not be used below the elbow or knee because nerves lying close to the surface can be injured so easily. In any case, wounds of the forearms and legs rarely bleed severely enough to require a tourniquet. Remember, *the decision to use a tourniquet is always a decision to risk losing a limb.* Nevertheless, a tourniquet can be lifesaving when a major extremity blood vessel is injured and bleeding cannot be controlled in any other way. Examples of such injuries include high-velocity gunshot wounds and amputations.

Tourniquet Application Technique (Fig. 6.3)

1. Fold a triangular bandage into a band to form a **cravat** 3 to 4 inches wide. Wrap the cravat twice around the extremity and tie the ends with an overhand knot. Position the cravat as far distally as possible while still keeping it above the site of bleeding.
2. Place a 6-inch stick or dowel on top of the overhand knot and

Fig. 6.2 *Major Pressure Points*

Fig. 6.3 *Tourniquet Application Technique*

Brachial

Femoral

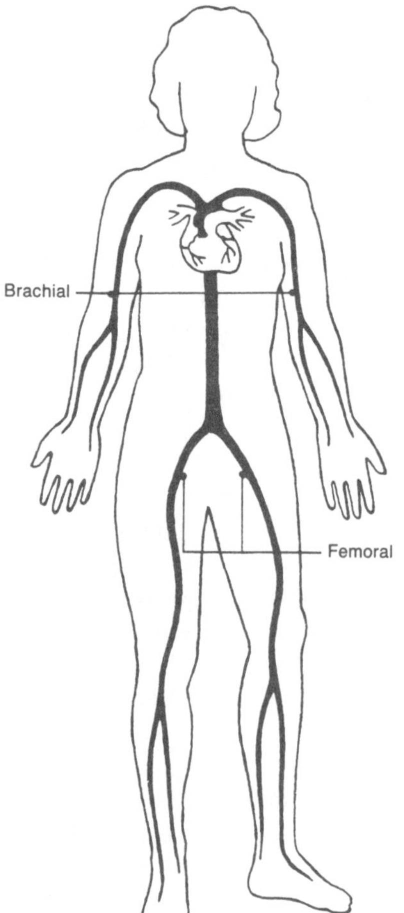

Fig. 6.2

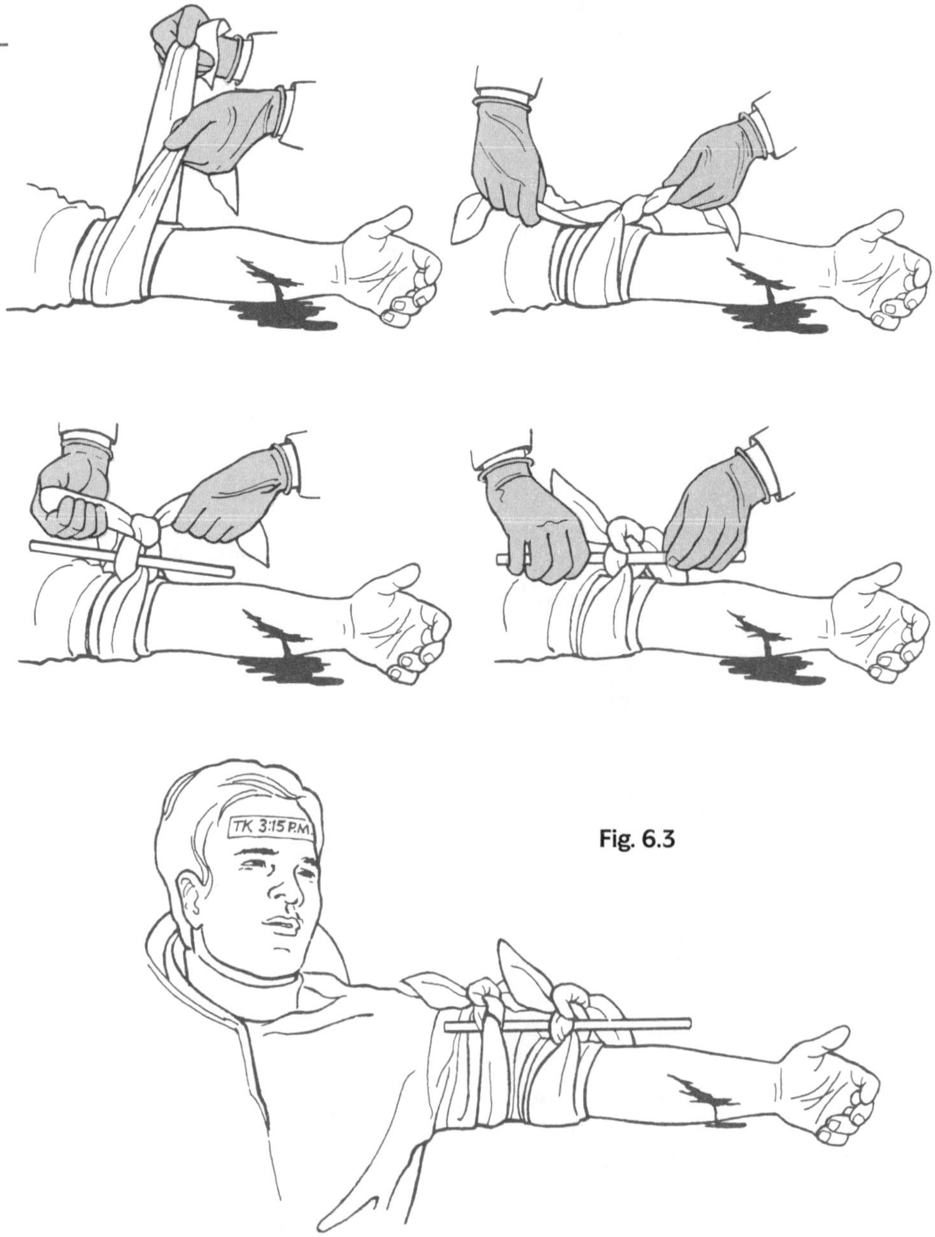

Fig. 6.3

tie a square knot firmly over the stick.

3. Twist the stick until the tourniquet has tightened just enough to stop the bleeding.

4. Secure the stick in place.

5. Write the letters "TK" and the time of application on a piece of tape and fasten it to the patient's forehead. Be sure to inform medical personnel or other members of the EMS system of the tourniquet when they take over care of the patient.

6. If bleeding is severe enough to require a tourniquet, give the patient oxygen, if available, in high concentration and at a high flow rate.

Always leave a tourniquet *in plain view.* Never cover a tourniquet with a bandage or clothing. A blood pressure cuff inflated to above systolic pressure can substitute as a tourniquet, but wire, rope, or other thin materials that may cut the skin or concentrate the pressure in too narrow an area should *never* be used.

Pneumatic Counterpressure Devices

Air splints are useful for extensive skin and soft-tissue extremity injuries with widespread bleeding because they provide direct pressure to an entire extremity (Fig. 6.4). Blood pressure cuffs, inflated to 30 to 40 mm Hg, can provide direct pressure

---

Fig. 6.4 *An air splint can be used to control external bleeding.*

to small wounds. PASGs are useful mainly to control intra-abdominal bleeding or internal bleeding from fractures of the pelvis or femur.

Internal Bleeding

Because internal bleeding is not directly visible, its presence must be suspected based on the mechanism of injury (see Chapter 9) and the effects of bleeding on the function of the involved body part, the circulatory system, and the body as a whole. Theoretically, internal bleeding can involve any body part, but certain types and locations of internal bleeding are more common than others.

Unless a large vessel is torn, bleeding into subcutaneous tissue and muscle usually stops promptly because these tissues contain large amounts of clot-promoting substances and because the local pressure produced by bleeding into dense tissue narrows or collapses the bleeding vessels.

However, neither of these mechanisms operates when there is bleeding into hollow organs or body cavities, or when bleeding occurs from large vessels, ruptured solid vascular organs, or from large or multiple bone fractures. In these cases, hemorrhage can be severe, prolonged, and life-threatening.

Small hemorrhages into important organs, especially those with a limited ability to swell (such as the brain) can be more devastating than larger hemorrhages into less important, more

expandable organs. Internal bleeding into hollow organs may become visible at the body surface. For example, a bleeding ulcer can produce blood in vomitus or bowel movements, and a ruptured kidney can produce bloody urine. Any vaginal bleeding in a pregnant woman may mean a serious complication. Vaginal bleeding in a non-pregnant woman other than during the normal menstrual period may or may not be serious but always should be investigated by a physician.

Examples of Serious Internal Bleeding

1. Bleeding into the brain from a stroke or head injury.

2. Bleeding from a stomach or duodenal ulcer.

3. Bleeding from a fractured femur, fractured pelvis, or from multiple fractures.

4. Intra-abdominal bleeding caused by trauma-induced damage to the liver, spleen, kidney, pregnant uterus, or large vessels.

5. Intra-thoracic bleeding caused by trauma-induced damage to the lung, heart, aorta, or other large vessels.

6. Bleeding into the pelvis caused when a fetus develops in a fallopian tube instead of in the uterus (ectopic pregnancy).

Signs and Symptoms of Some Types of Serious Internal Bleeding

1. A suitable mechanism of injury (see Chapter 9), such as a blunt or penetrating injury to the head, neck, chest, abdomen, pelvis, thigh, or multiple sites.

2. A history of indigestion and/or abdominal pain, accompanied by abdominal tenderness and associated with signs and symptoms of shock.

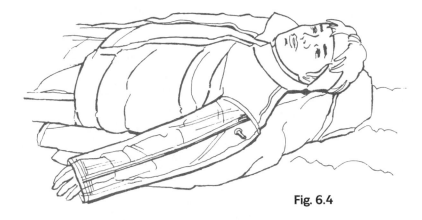

Fig. 6.4

3. Progressive pain, tenderness, nausea, vomiting, rigidity, and enlargement of the abdomen following abdominal trauma.
4. Progressive respiratory distress following chest trauma.
5. Progressive enlargement, pain, tenderness, dysfunction, and possible loss of pulses in an injured limb.
6. Blood in vomitus, sputum, feces, or urine.
7. Signs and symptoms of shock following trauma when there is no external bleeding or other obvious cause of shock, or when the severity of shock is not explained by the extent of obvious injuries.
8. Progressive abdominal pain, tenderness, and enlargement in a woman of child-bearing age who has missed several menstrual periods.
9. Progressive ecchymosis (bluish-purple skin discoloration) of the involved area (not an acute sign).

Emergency Care of Internal Bleeding

A patient with significant internal bleeding may go quickly into shock and die. Field emergency care for internal bleeding is not very effective unless intravenous therapy is available. However, proper splinting of a fractured extremity will decrease bleeding into the limb, thereby tending to prevent shock. If equipment and trained personnel are available, a PASG is useful to treat intra-abdominal hemorrhage and internal bleeding from pelvic and lower-extremity fractures. The most important outdoor emergency care measure for internal bleeding is to *suspect the bleeding early and evacuate the patient rapidly to a hospital.* Care for shock should be given (see below) and high flow oxygen should be administered, if available.

Table 6.1

Classes of Hemorrhage

	I (Blood Donor)	II (Compensated Shock)	III (Decompensated Shock)	IV (Preterminal)
Percent of blood lost	<15%	15 to 30%	30 to 40%	>40%
Average blood loss (ml) *	Up to 500	600 to 1,500	1,500 to 2,000	>2,000
Pulse	Slight rise	>100	Fast	Very fast
Respirations	Normal	Slight increase	Fast	Fast
BP	Normal	Normal (lying)	Low	Low or unobtainable
*Pulse pressure** *	Normal	Slight decrease	Moderate decrease	Marked decrease
Capillary refill test	Normal	Positive	Positive	Refill absent
Mental status	Normal	Anxious	Significantly altered	Markedly altered
How serious?	Usually not serious	May need transfusion	Probably needs transfusion	Life threatening —needs rapid transfusion and surgery

*Based on average 150-pound (70-kilogram) male
**Pulse pressure = difference between the systolic and diastolic pressures

Shock

In emergency care, the term shock refers to a form of rapid failure of the circulatory system that frequently accompanies severe illness or injury. The signs and symptoms of shock are caused both by lack of effective circulation to the tissues and by the body's attempts to compensate for the failing circulation.

Three components are essential for normal blood circulation: adequate blood to fill the blood vessels, a heart capable of pumping blood, and blood vessels that can adjust the tone of the muscles in their walls. When a person is in shock, one or more of these components is not normal. The names of the three major categories of shock—**hypovolemic, cardiogenic,** and **vasogenic** (vascular)—reflect the failure of each respective component (Fig. 6.5).

Shock can be either **reversible** or **irreversible.** If its causes and effects are treated promptly, the body's compensation efforts usually can restore circulation. However, the longer a patient remains in shock, the longer the vital organs are deprived of oxygen. After a certain period, they are irreversibly injured by lack of oxygen, and the mechanisms that control vascular tone are paralyzed by toxic substances produced by altered metabolism. This state is called irreversible shock because even the best treatment started at this point cannot reestablish effective blood circulation or produce organ recovery.

Shock also can be **compensated** or **decompensated**. In compensated shock, the body's response efforts keep the circulatory system functioning at a normal or near-normal level. In decompensated shock, the circulatory system begins to fail, despite the body's best response efforts.

Hypovolemic shock is caused by a decrease in circulating blood volume significantly below normal. The fall in volume, which usually is rapid, may result from the loss of *whole blood* (as

in external or internal hemorrhage), or of the *fluid portion of the blood* (as in dehydration from vomiting, diarrhea, or severe burns). Hemorrhage is classified from Grade I to IV based on severity (Table 6.1). The loss of more than 1.1 quarts (1,000 milliliters) may cause moderate shock, marked by a fast pulse and low blood pressure when the patient sits up or attempts to stand, although the pulse and blood pressure may be normal or near-normal when the patient is lying down. A blood loss of 1.6 quarts (1,500 milliliters) causes clinical shock, marked by a fast pulse and low blood pressure even when the patient is lying down. A blood loss of more than 2.1 quarts (2,000 milliliters) causes severe shock with unconsciousness.

Cardiogenic shock occurs when the pumping function of the heart fails. It is caused by weakness of the heart muscle itself, as in a heart attack or chest injury; from ineffective contractions of a normal muscle, as in a too-rapid or too-slow heartbeat; or from blockage of blood going *from* the heart, as in a blood clot in the lung, or *to* the heart, as in tension pneumothorax or with fluid or blood in the pericardium.

Vasogenic shock occurs when the mechanisms that normally control blood vessel tone fail, causing the vessels to relax and enlarge. Consequently, the normal blood volume becomes inadequate to fill the vessels, and a state of "relative hypovolemia" is created. This state can be caused by conditions that affect the blood

Fig. 6.5 *Schema of the Three Major Types of Shock*

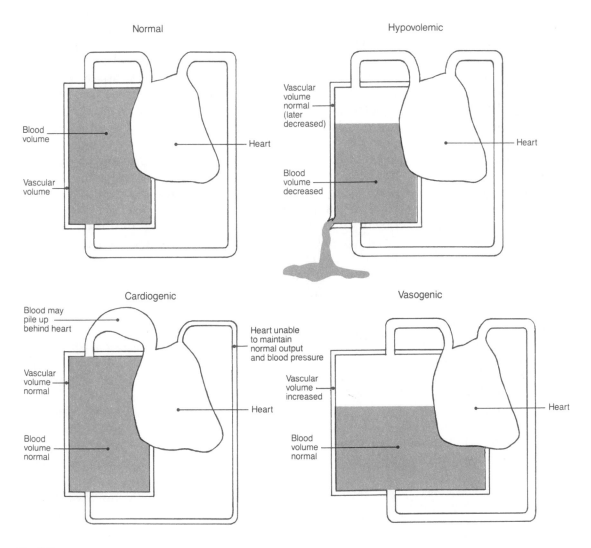

Fig. 6.5

vessel wall directly—such as severe infection, metabolic illness (diabetic ketoacidosis, etc.), or severe allergic reactions—or that interfere with the normal nerve control of the blood vessel walls—such as simple fainting or spinal cord injury. The type of vasogenic shock seen in spinal cord injury is often called **neurogenic shock.**

Shock because of failure of one component alone is rare (except in simple fainting), since the components are interrelated and failure of one eventually affects the others. For example, in a severely hypothermic patient, shock occurs because dehydration lowers the blood volume and the effect of cold weakens heart muscle contraction, slows the heartbeat, and interferes with blood vessel control. In severe infections, the toxic products of bacterial growth injure the heart, cause the blood vessels to leak, and injure the muscles of the blood vessel walls, interfering with the ability to maintain vascular tone. In hemorrhagic shock, lack of oxygen affects the contraction of the heart and the ability of blood vessels to maintain their tone.

The severity of a case of shock depends on whether its causes are treatable and how soon treatment is started. Even treatable shock can be fatal if not attended to promptly. The most common causes of shock in the outdoor environment are trauma with internal or external bleeding, dehydration, and heart attack.

Regardless of the underlying cause, the signs and symptoms of shock tend to be similar because they reflect the effects of hypoxia on the body organs and the body's compensatory attempts to counter this by maintaining circulation to vital organs. The common denominator in all three forms of shock is a *reduction in effective circulating blood volume,* which tends to cause a *fall in blood pressure.* This stimulates corrective changes, which increase heart rate and output per beat to pump more blood; con-

tract blood vessels in the shell (skin, muscles, and extremities) to shunt blood to the core, maintain blood pressure, and maintain circulation to vital organs; and stimulate breathing so that more oxygen can extracted by the lungs and each unit of blood can carry more oxygen.

These changes cause the skin to become cold, clammy, pale, or cyanotic. The patient develops shortness of breath and an increased pulse rate. The pulse becomes weak and thready if shock progresses. The kidneys reduce urine output to conserve the water and salts needed to maintain the plasma volume. Oxygen lack in the brain causes confusion, anxiety, nausea, and mental dullness; oxygen lack in the muscles causes fatigue and weakness.

In the early stages of shock, the compensatory changes may maintain circulation at a close-to-normal level (at least when the patient is lying flat and the heart does not have to pump against gravity). The pulse and breathing rates may increase only slightly or not at all, and the blood pressure may remain normal. Later, as compensatory efforts become more stressed, the classic **signs and symptoms of shock** develop. Early signs of advancing shock are a fall in blood pressure and an increase in pulse rate when the patient sits up. Shock should be *anticipated* when a suitable mechanism of injury or illness exists, so that it can be cared for early before the classic signs and symptoms develop.

Classic Signs and Symptoms of Shock

A. Related to lack of effective organ circulation:
1. Restlessness and anxiety
2. Nausea, occasionally vomiting
3. Weakness and fatigue
4. Cyanosis
5. Dull or lusterless eyes
6. Falling blood pressure
7. Changes in mental status; confusion and mental

dullness may progress to stupor and coma
B. Related to the body's attempts to compensate:
1. Rapid pulse, which later becomes weak and thready
2. Cold, clammy, pale skin
3. Thirst
4. Abnormal respirations, usually rapid at first, then labored, and finally gasping
C. Due to the autonomic stress response:
1. Profuse sweating
2. Dilated pupils
D. Signs and symptoms of the underlying condition that caused the shock

The classic signs and symptoms of shock *may not be present* in the neurogenic type of vasogenic shock, because of damage to the nerve pathways that speed the pulse, control sweating, and constrict the blood vessels. Therefore, in neurogenic shock, the pulse usually is slow rather than fast, and the skin is warm, dry, and pink rather than cool, pale, and wet— at least below the level of spinal cord injury. Respirations may be abnormal because of injury to the spinal cord tracts supplying the intercostal muscles (and occasionally the diaphragm).

Assessment and Emergency Care of Shock

Assessment of the patient in shock or in whom the development of shock can be anticipated follows the procedures outlined in Chapter 4.
1. Reconstruct the mechanism of injury, which will lead you to suspect the presence of injuries or illnesses that may be accompanied by shock.
2. Assess the airway, the presence and adequacy of breathing, and the presence and quality of the pulse. Give rescue breathing, if required.
3. Control obvious bleeding.

4. If the pulse or respirations are abnormal, assess the neck and chest. If no abnormalities are found, assess the abdomen, pelvis, and thighs, and care for any abnormalities found.

5. Administer oxygen at a high concentration and flow rate, if available.

6. Splint fractures and dislocations. Elevate the lower extremities about 12 inches, except in cases of cardiogenic shock or when contraindicated by the type of injury.

7. Maintain the patient's body temperature but avoid excessive warming, which may worsen shock by counteracting constriction of the blood vessels (shell vasoconstriction).

8. As a general rule, keep the patient supine to lessen the work of the heart. In some cases, a shock patient may also have lung congestion from heart failure or lung disease and should be supine because of shock, but may need to sit up because of inability to breathe when lying flat. In this situation, use the Rothberg position, in which the patient's upper body is raised at a 45-degree angle, the abdomen is flat, and the lower extremities are elevated by flexing the hips at about 15 degrees or bending the knees (Fig. 6.6).

9. Do not give the patient anything to eat or drink, unless the patient is in shock due to dehydration.

10. Check and record vital signs at frequent intervals (every 10 to 15 minutes).

11. If shock is caused by a suspected fracture of the pelvis or femur or by intra-abdominal hemorrhage, rescuers who have he proper training, experience, licensing, and equipment can apply a PASG.

Table 6.2

Summary of Emergency Care of Shock

1. Give basic life support, as necessary.
2. Control bleeding, if present.
3. Give oxygen.
4. Elevate lower extremities, except in cardiogenic shock.
5. Maintain body temperature.
6. Keep patient lying down unless patient is short of breath.
7. Splint fractures.
8. Give nothing to eat or drink.
9. Check and record vital signs at regular intervals.
10. Give special care for specific types of shock:
    a. Hypothermia (see Chapter 19)
    b. Use of a PASG for specific types of shock by specially trained rescuers
11. Rapidly transport patient to a hospital.

12. If needed, give other special emergency care for specific causes of shock, e.g., care for hypothermia (Chapter 18).

13. Because there is no specific field of emergency care for most causes of shock, *the patient must be transported to a hospital as soon as possible*. The rescuer always should *anticipate* the development of shock in injuries and illnesses known to frequently lead to shock.

Fig. 6.6 *The Rothberg Position*

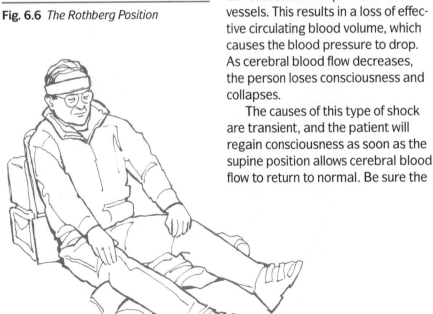

Fig. 6.6

Special Types of Shock

Simple Fainting

Simple fainting, sometimes called psychogenic shock, is a common and benign form of acute vascular shock that can have either physical or emotional causes. Stimuli such as pain, the sight of blood, or a strong emotion such as fear can trigger nerve reflexes that produce sudden enlargement (dilation) of blood vessels. Sitting or standing for a long time without moving, especially in a hot environment, can cause blood to pool in dilated vessels. This results in a loss of effective circulating blood volume, which causes the blood pressure to drop. As cerebral blood flow decreases, the person loses consciousness and collapses.

The causes of this type of shock are transient, and the patient will regain consciousness as soon as the supine position allows cerebral blood flow to return to normal. Be sure the patient is lying flat and, if the fall was hard, assess for injuries. Move the patient to a cool place if the environment is hot. Advise the patient to rest before resuming normal activity. Evaluation by a physician may be advisable, especially if fainting is recurrent.

Anaphylactic Shock

Anaphylactic shock is an emergency that may cause rapid death unless treated promptly. It is an immediate and overwhelming allergic reaction, usually to an insect sting, drug, or food. Common offenders are bee and wasp stings, penicillin, aspirin, seafood, nuts, and berries. Contact with the offending substance (known as the **allergen**) causes the release of histamine and other substances from the injured tissues. This causes blood vessels to leak, the blood pressure to fall, bronchial walls to swell, and smooth muscle in the bronchi and other organs to go into spasm. The patient may develop hives, acute respiratory distress, wheezing, massive swelling of the face and tongue, nausea, vomiting, cramps, and diarrhea. The condition may progress rapidly to convulsions, coma, and death.

The emergency antidote for anaphylactic shock is **epinephrine** (adrenalin) by injection. Rescuers who are not properly trained and licensed cannot legally give injections. However, many people in danger of anaphylactic shock from bee stings or other sources carry kits containing pre-loaded syringes of epinephrine with directions for use (Fig. 6.7). Every minute counts. The rescuer should assist the patient in injecting the drug if necessary. The patient will need a second injection of epinephrine 5 to 10 minutes later if he or she does not improve promptly. The patient a should be taken immediately to a hospital and may require oxygen, rescue breathing, or CPR on the way.

Fig. 6.7 *Example of a Kit Carried by People Subject to Anaphylactic Shock*

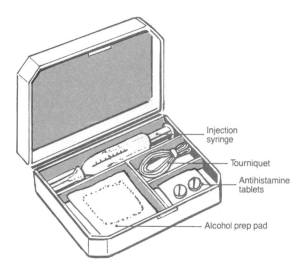

Injection syringe

Tourniquet

Antihistamine tablets

Alcohol prep pad

Fig. 6.7

Scenario #6 (Fig. 6.8)

The following scenario illustrates the assessment and emergency care of an injured skier with shock.

You are about to get on the upper lift at High Range Ski Area when you hear a transmission that a skier is down on Mad Dog, a black diamond run on the lower mountain. You duck under the rope and ski off to the entrance to Mad Dog, 100 yards away off the east cat track. You stop and look down. About two-thirds of the way to the bottom in the center of the run you see two skis stuck in the snow to form an X, with a small group of skiers nearby. A minute later you are close enough to see a skier lying on her side below a large mogul. You do not see any blood on the snow. You remove your skis and approach the downed skier. Her face looks pale and her eyes are closed. Her respirations are easy but about twice the normal rate.

Fig. 6.8 *Scenario #6*

You: (grasping her wrist) "Hello, I'm Bonnie Waydell of the High Range Ski Patrol. Are you okay?" (The radial pulse is strong but about 120 beats per minute.)

Patient: "No, something's wrong, My left side is hurt."

You: (You take off her glove and check the capillary refill in a finger; it is >2 seconds.) "What happened?"

Patient: "I lost an edge on the ice on the downside of that bump and hit my side hard. It hurts to breathe."

You: "Were you feeling okay before that happened?"

Patient: "Yes."

You: (reaching for your radio) "Waydell to Midway, copy?" (Midway replies.)

"I need a toboggan, oxygen, suction, and some help on Mad Dog, two-thirds of the way to the bottom." (Base confirms.) "Do you hurt anywhere else?" (You put your hand on her forehead. It is cool and clammy.)

Patient: "I don't think so."

You: "What's your name?"

Patient: "Helen Wheels."

You: "Did you hit your head?"

Patient: "I may have, I don't know."

You: "Were you knocked out at all?"

Patient: "No."

You: "Did you hit your neck or back?"

Patient: "No."

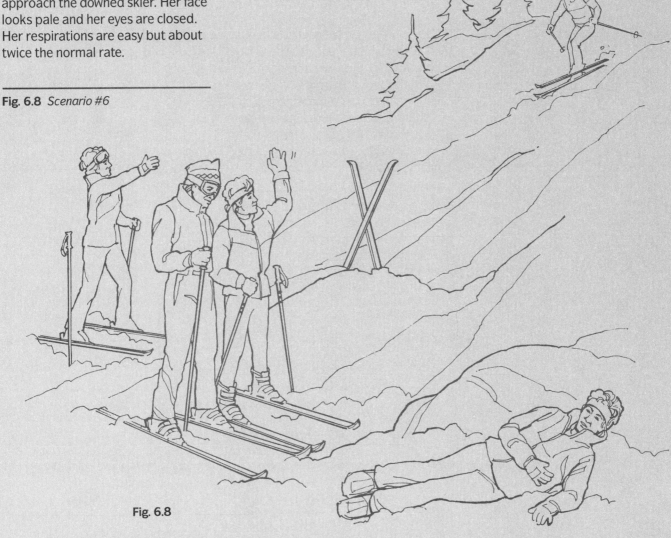

Fig. 6.8

You: "Where are you from?"

Patient: "Dallas."

You: "Do you know today's date and what day it is?"

Patient: "March 13, Friday."

You: "I need to check your chest and side."

The neck looks normal—there are no wounds, tenderness, lumps, or bleeding. In particular, there is no tenderness of the spinous processes. The trachea is in the midline and there are no obvious abnormalities of the upper chest. You pull up her turtleneck and long-john top. Her lower chest also looks normal, and both sides are moving equally. You quickly feel the ribs on both sides one by one. There are no lumps or tenderness. You pull her clothes back down and unloosen the belt of her jeans. The abdomen looks normal. You carefully palpate the abdomen, starting in the right upper quadrant and moving clockwise. She is very tender in the left upper quadrant and the muscles are tight in this area. At this point, she starts to retch and vomits in the snow. The vomitus appears to be the contents of a recent meal; there is no sign of blood.

You stop a moment and think. She is alert and oriented, but her pulse is fast and her breathing is fast but not labored. Her capillary refill is delayed. Her radial pulse is strong so her blood pressure is at least 80 mm Hg. Her chest appears normal, but she is very tender in her left upper abdomen. You recheck the pulse again. It is now 130 beats per minute and seems weaker. Something is going on, possibly internal bleeding causing shock.

You: "The toboggan will be coming in a minute and we'll take you down to the aid room." (You radio the hill chief to request that an ambulance meet you at the aid room.)

Patient: "I'm really feeling weak and dizzy."

You: "I'm going to check some other areas and ask you some more questions while we're waiting, if you don't mind." (You start to assess the head. There are no signs of wounds or bleeding on the face and no swellings, tenderness, or lumps on the scalp).

Patient: "Okay."

You: "I'm going to shine this light in your eyes to check your pupils." (They are round, regular, and equal. There is no bleeding or discharge from the ears.) "Open your mouth." (There is no blood, and the teeth look regular.) "Do you have any chronic medical conditions like diabetes, epilepsy, or heart trouble?"

Patient: "No."

You: (moving on to the pelvis) "Does this hurt?" (pressing on the iliac crests from side to side and the pelvis from back to front).

Patient: "No."

You: "Are you taking any drugs or medicines?"

Patient: "No."

You: "Any allergies?"

Patient: "No."

You: "Anything else about you we should know?"

Patient: "Well, I'm just getting over a case of mono. You know, the doctor told me my spleen was enlarged and I shouldn't ski or play any contact sports."

You: "Oh?"

Patient: "I already had my tickets for here and they aren't refundable. It's spring break, so I decided to come anyway. Maybe I shouldn't have."

You: "Maybe not. Did you hurt your arms or legs when you fell?"

Patient: "No, just my side."

You: "Here's the toboggan. We'll lift you into it and be on our way. We're going to put you in so your head is at the front end so you won't feel so weak and dizzy, and give you some oxygen to help your breathing."

Chapter 7

Skin and Soft-Tissue Injuries, Burns, and Bandaging

But a certain Samaritan went to him, and bound up his wounds, pouring in oil and wine.

—Luke 10:33

This chapter will discuss the general principles of injuries to the **soft tissues**, which include the skin, subcutaneous tissues, and muscles. The hard tissues—bones, joints, and their associated tendons and ligaments—are presented in Chapter 8. Before starting this chapter, review the sections on the skin and muscles in Chapter 2.

One of the major functions of the skin is to *protect the body from infection* by forming a barrier between the underlying tissues and infectious organisms. Bacteria, viruses, and fungi are everywhere in the environment and are found normally on the skin's surface. Any illness or injury that breaks the skin may lead to **infection** as well as bleeding.

Soft-tissue injuries are divided into two types: **closed** and **open.** A closed injury may damage the skin and deeper tissues but does not involve a break in the skin; an open injury involves a break in the skin as well as damage to the tissues beneath it.

Closed injuries include **contusions, hematomas,** and **muscle strains.** Open injuries include **abrasions, lacerations, incisions, avulsions, amputations,** and **punctures.**

Closed Soft-tissue Injuries

Contusions are caused by an impact with a blunt object such as a rock (blunt trauma). The underlying tissues are crushed and small blood vessels are torn, causing local bleeding. Blood accumulates under the skin, producing swelling and a characteristic bluish discoloration known as a bruise or **ecchymosis.** Capillary damage may allow the fluid part of the blood (plasma) to leak into the surrounding tissues, leading to a type of pinkish swelling called **edema.** The body's response to any tissue damage is **inflammation,** which consists of swelling, pain, heat, redness, and loss of function of the injured area. A

severe contusion may damage larger blood vessels and cause a tumor-like collection of blood in the tissues called a **hematoma**. Hematomas also may be found at the site of fractures, strains, and other injuries involving large blood vessels.

Strains, or muscle pulls, occur when a muscle is severely stretched or torn. Strains are caused by a violent movement of an extremity, which creates a pull strong enough to damage the muscle. Injury to small vessels and capillaries causes swelling and ecchymosis.

Emergency Care of Closed Soft-tissue Injuries

Soft-tissue injuries are treated with the application of cold, pressure, elevation, and splinting. Cold causes blood vessels to narrow; pressure and elevation tend to reduce the circulation in the injured area; and splinting prevents further damage by limiting motion. Together these actions reduce the amount of blood and plasma that leaks from the injured vessels, resulting in less pain and tissue injury, less swelling, and shorter healing time.

Apply pressure by wrapping the site of injury firmly with a self-adhering roller bandage or rubberized bandage. A cold pack can be made by putting ice, snow, or a cloth soaked in cold water in a plastic bag. Wrap the bag in a towel and apply it to the injury for about 20 minutes per waking hour for the first 24 hours. Do not apply ice or snow directly to the skin or wrap the injured site so tightly that circulation is restricted. Be sure the patient continues to be able to feel and move the extremity below the injury, and that peripheral pulses remain intact.

Inspect the area under the compress frequently to detect possible cold injury. Cold compresses should not be applied to a patient who is hypothermic or in a cold environment.

If the injury involves an extremity, elevate and splint it or, in the case of

the upper extremity, use a sling. If another part of the body is involved, advise the patient to rest as much as possible for the first 24 hours, with the injured area at or above heart level.

Patients in the backcountry who have severe closed soft-tissue injuries of a lower extremity usually are unable to walk and will need to be evacuated by litter or toboggan. Patients with lesser injuries may be able to walk if the damaged extremity is supported by being wrapped with a rubberized bandage.

Table 7.1

Emergency Care of Closed Soft-tissue Injuries

1. Apply a pressure bandage.
2. Apply a cold compress.
3. Elevate the injury.
4. Immobilize the injury by splinting or have the patient rest.
5. Assist with evacuation as necessary.

Open Soft-tissue Injuries

Abrasions (Fig. 7.1a) are superficial injuries caused by moving contact between the skin and a parallel rough surface. This process, also called planing or shearing, scrapes off the epidermis but usually not the dermis. Abrasions ooze blood and plasma from injured vessels. Large abrasions are very painful because many pain nerves are irritated. Common examples of abrasions are "road burn" in cyclists and "floor burn" in gymnasts.

Lacerations (Fig. 7.1b) are tears in the skin that also may involve deeper tissues. Bleeding may be profuse or mild, depending on the size and number of blood vessels injured.

Incisions (Fig. 7.1c) are "clean" lacerations caused by a knife, ski

Fig. 7.1 *Types of Open Injuries*

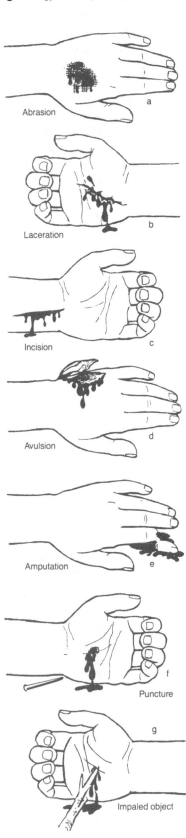

Fig. 7.1

edge, or other sharp object. They are more linear and regular than lacerations and usually bleed more because less tissue-clotting factors are released, and the cleanly cut blood vessels constrict and retract less effectively.

Avulsions (Fig. 7.1d) are pieces of skin torn loose from underlying tissues and left hanging by a flap.

Amputations (Fig. 7.1e) are parts of the body, usually limbs or other appendages, that are torn completely free from the body.

Punctures (Fig. 7.1f) are wounds caused by sharp, narrow objects such as a knife, ski pole tip, or ice pick. Punctures also can be caused by high-velocity blunt objects such as bullets. The apparent damage caused by a puncture is often deceptive: the entrance wound may be small with little bleeding, giving no clue to the extent of damage to organs and blood vessels beneath. Bullets and long, sharp objects may penetrate completely through a body part; thus, the rescuer also should search carefully for exit wounds. An **impaled object** (Fig. 7.1g) is one that protrudes from a wound after an injury.

Tetanus can be a serious complication of open soft-tissue wounds. This disease is caused by soil bacteria that, when introduced into open wounds, grow and produce a toxin that provokes serious muscle spasms and interferes with breathing. Since tetanus organisms flourish in an oxygen-poor environment, puncture wounds and other deep, small wounds that are shut off from contact with the air are particularly dangerous. All open wounds are susceptible, however, especially those contaminated by soil. To prevent tetanus, everyone should be fully immunized in infancy and have a booster immunization of toxoid (usually given in combination with diphtheria toxoid) every 10 years. The decision as to what additional protective measures are needed to care for a fresh wound should be left up to the patient's physician.

The following are general guidelines for whether a booster shot is needed after a soft-tissue injury. If a wound is clean and the patient has had a booster immunization within 10 years, no additional booster is usually needed. If, however, the patient has had no booster within 10 years or has an unknown or incomplete immunization history, a booster should be given within 72 hours. In tetanus-prone wounds (i.e., deep puncture wounds, or severe or heavily contaminated wounds), a booster should be given if the patient has had no booster within five years. If the immunization history is unknown or incomplete, both a booster and an injection of tetanus immune globulin should be given within 72 hours.

Assessment and Emergency Care of Open Wounds

1. To protect against accidental exposure to the AIDS or hepatitis viruses, be sure to institute universal precautions (see Appendix F), which means, at a minimum, putting on rubber gloves when caring for patients with open wounds.
2. Perform a primary survey as outlined in Chapter 4.
3. Inspect the wound. Remove all overlying clothing to fully expose the wound, preferably by cutting or ripping along a seam.
4. Control bleeding by direct pressure. Elevation, splinting, and pressure point control may occasionally be required as well. A tourniquet is rarely needed. Give additional care for shock as necessary.
5. While assessing the wound, guard against contaminating it further.
6. All open wounds are considered contaminated, even though no obvious contamination can be seen. The wounds of skiers and other over-snow travelers usually are free of

dirt, although pieces of cloth or tree bark may be present. If the patient will receive definitive medical care within a few hours, the wound need not be washed, although any loose pieces of dirt, bark, and other foreign matter should be removed with sterile forceps or tweezers from a Swiss Army knife if no forceps are available. Sterilize forceps by heating them over a lit match or cleaning them with rubbing alcohol or an antiseptic such as povidone-iodine solution (Betadine). Next, cover the wound with a sterile gauze dressing, large enough that its edges extend at least 1 inch past the margins of the wound. Hold this in place with a bandage of tape or gauze roller bandage (see **Commonly Used Dressings and Bandages** below).

If it will be more than a few hours before the patient will receive definitive medical care, the wound should be cleaned more thoroughly. Be certain all bleeding is controlled. Cover the wound with a sterile dressing and wash the surrounding skin with 10 percent Betadine, soap and water, or another antiseptic solution. (First, question the patient about allergies to iodine or other chemicals.)

Next, generously irrigate the wound with clean, warm water or, preferably, sterile physiological saline solution. The most effective way to clean a dirty wound is with pressure irrigation—using a clean (preferably sterile) 20 or 30 cc syringe fitted with a 16- or 18-gauge needle to squirt the cleaning liquid under pressure into the wound. Press down firmly on the plunger of the syringe, but use care to avoid being splattered with

bloody saline. Dry the wound with a sterile dressing, and if the wound is small, close it with butterfly bandages or tape sutures (Steristrips). If the wound is large, usually it is best left open. Next, apply a sterile dressing and use a suitable bandage to hold it in place. If the wound is large and painful, splint and elevate it as well. If the patient must walk, small lower-extremity wounds can be supported with an elastic roller bandage. In very cold weather, if evacuation by litter or toboggan will take very long, it is preferable to tape all wounds closed.

Physiological saline solution, also called normal saline solution, is a 0.9-percent solution of ordinary table salt in water. This concentration of salt water has the same osmotic pressure as normal human tissue and causes minimal

pain or injury when used to irrigate an open wound or keep tissue moist. Sterile physiological saline solution can be purchased in bottles or bags and stored in the first aid room or rescue cache. The remainder of the opened container should be discarded after use.

7. Puncture wounds cannot be cleaned adequately and should always be seen by a physician. If there is a suspicion that underlying organs might have been injured, the patient must be transported rapidly to a hospital.

8. Wash all abrasions gently with soap and clean water before bandaging. Sterile dressings that have nonadhesive material on one side (such as Telfa) cause less pain when removed than ordinary dressings.

9. For avulsions, replace the flap of tissue into its normal position before applying direct pressure to control bleeding. If

Table 7.2

Emergency Care of Open Soft-tissue Injuries

1. Use universal precautions.
2. Perform a primary survey.
3. Expose the wound completely and inspect it, removing clothing as necessary.
4. Control bleeding by direct pressure.
5. Prevent further contamination.
6. Close the wound, if appropriate.
7. Apply a sterile dressing and bandage.
8. Advise the patient to have a physician see all but the cleanest and most minor open wounds.
9. Advise the patient to consider obtaining a tetanus shot.
   Additional measures as necessary:
10. Cleanse the wound if the time to definitive medical care will be long.
11. Elevate and splint the injured part.
12. Treat the patient for shock.
13. Considerations for special types of wounds
    a. Wash abrasions with soap and water.
    b. Replace avulsions.
    c. Preserve amputated parts.
    d. Bandage impaled objects in place.

time permits (i.e., bleeding is minimal), first clean the flap and the wound (see 6. above). During bandaging, place the sterile dressing over the repositioned flap rather than directly on the raw wound.

10. With modern surgical techniques, it frequently is possible to reattach amputated parts. Always preserve such parts and send them along with the patient to the hospital. Wrap the part in a sterile dressing moistened with clean (preferably sterile) physiological saline solution, and place it in a clean plastic bag. Put this bag in a second plastic bag containing ice and water. Keep the part cool but *do not allow it to freeze*.

11. Do not remove impaled objects unless they obstruct the airway. Any motion may damage important underlying structures, and removal may cause uncontrollable bleeding. Do not exert pressure directly on an impaled object, or on tissues close to any sharp edges. Large objects that interfere with patient handling may be stabilized and *carefully* cut off with a pipe cutter, tree pruner, or saw. Bandage the wound with a bulky dressing so that the impaled object is immobilized. After it is bandaged, use care to avoid bumping it. Because surgery will be

required to remove the object, give the patient nothing by mouth, and arrange prompt transportation to a hospital.

12. Large or painful extremity wounds and extremity wounds where control of bleeding is difficult should be elevated and splinted.

13. All open wounds, especially puncture wounds, should be seen by a physician. Possible exceptions include clean, small to moderately sized abrasions, and lacerations whose edges come together spontaneously or can be brought together with butterfly bandages or tape sutures such as Steristrips. Most facial wounds should be seen by a physician, because they may cause disfiguring scars if not closed properly.

14. Ask the patient about the status of tetanus immunization. Even if a wound is not serious enough to require medical attention, advise the patient to consult a physician about whether to obtain a tetanus shot.

Burns

A burn is a wound of the skin or mucous membranes caused by excessive thermal, electrical, or radiant energy. Certain chemicals cause similar injuries, which also are called burns. Burns are classified by cause as **thermal**, **chemical**, and

electrical. Eye burns are discussed in Chapter 12; sunburn is discussed in Chapter 18.

Thermal Burns

There are many dangerous sources of heat that can cause burns. In the outdoors, burns can be caused by forest fires, campfires, tent fires, stove explosions, and excessive exposure to the ultraviolet rays of the sun. The amount of damage from heat or ultraviolet light depends on the temperature or intensity, length of exposure, and the size and location of the contact area. To date, nothing better than the human eye has been devised for estimating the seriousness of a burn based on its physical characteristics and the amount of body surface involved.

Burns are divided into first, second, and third degree according to the depth of the damage.

First-degree burns, also called superficial burns, involve the outer layers of the epidermis (7.2a). The skin is red, tender, and painful, and may be swollen. No blisters form.

Second-degree burns, also called partial thickness burns, involve the epidermis and part of the dermis (7.2b). Pain, swelling, and blister formation occur.

Third-degree burns, also called full thickness burns, penetrate the

---

Fig. 7.2 *Three Types of Burns*

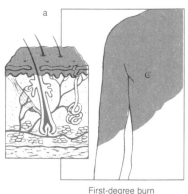
First-degree burn

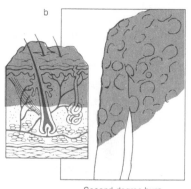
Second-degree burn

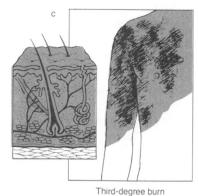
Third-degree burn

Fig. 7.2

epidermis and dermis and extend into the subcutaneous tissue (7.2c). The involved skin is "cooked" and appears to be dead; it is dry, thickened, leathery, and charred or otherwise discolored. Because nerves and blood vessels in the skin are destroyed, no blisters form and the area is numb.

A burned area may contain all three degrees of injury, sometimes with a third-degree burn in the center, surrounded by a second-degree burn and an outer rim of first-degree burn. The *size* of the burned area is very important; size can be roughly estimated by applying the **Rule of Nines** (Fig. 7.3). In adults, the head and neck represent 9 percent of the body surface area; the front and back of the trunk, 18 percent each; each arm, 9 percent; each leg, 18 percent; and the genital area, 1 percent (Fig. 7.3a). In infants and small children, the head is relatively larger and the legs relatively smaller; the head makes up 18 percent and each leg, 13.5 percent (Fig. 7.3b). For irregular burns, remember that one surface of the patient's hand represents approximately 1 percent of his or her body surface. The severity of a thermal burn is classified as **critical, moderate**, or **minor** depending on the extent and depth of the burned area, the age and general health of the patient, the presence of additional injuries, and whether critical areas such as the respiratory tract, hands, feet, or genitals are involved.

Classification of Thermal Burns

1. Critical
   a. Burns of any degree complicated by injury to the respiratory tract, fractures, or other major injuries
   b. Third-degree burns of the face, hands, feet, or genitals
   c. Third-degree burns of more than 10 percent of the body surface

   d. Second-degree burns of more than 25 percent of the body surface (20 percent in children and the elderly)
2. Moderate
   a. Third-degree burns of 2 to 10 percent of the body that do not involve the face, hands, feet, genitals, or respiratory tract and are not accompanied by fractures or other major injuries
   b. Second-degree burns of 15 to 25 percent of the body in adults (10 to 20 percent in children and the elderly)
   c. First-degree burns of 50 to 75 percent of the body surface

3. Minor
   a. Third-degree burns of less than 2 percent of the body surface, if no critical areas are involved
   b. Second-degree burns of less than 15 percent of the body surface (less than 10 percent in children and the elderly)
   c. First-degree burns of less than 50 percent of the body surface

Assessment and Emergency Care of Thermal Burns

1. Put out the fire immediately. If someone's clothing has caught on fire, shout at the person to drop to the ground and roll.
2. Move the patient away from the burning or smoke-filled area;

Fig. 7.3 *Rule of Nines*

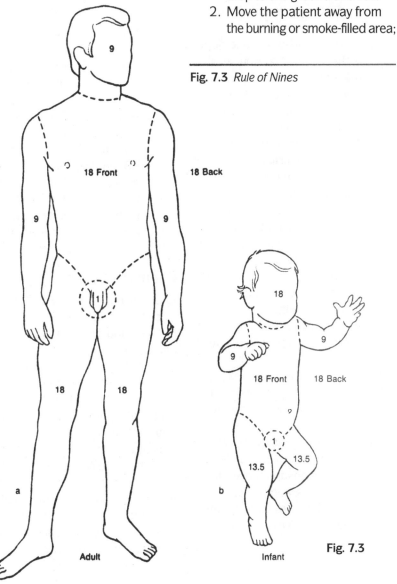

Adult

Infant

Fig. 7.3

cut away smoldering clothing or soak it with cold water.

3. Immerse hot skin in clean, cold water or cover it with a cold, wet, clean cloth for about 10 minutes. This will halt any residual burning of the skin and underlying tissues and relieve pain. Although burns of more than 20 percent of the body surface area can also benefit from cooling, because of their size care must be taken to avoid chilling the patient and inducing hypothermia.

4. Perform the primary survey, with particular attention to the airway and breathing.

5. Burned skin is sterile. Avoid contamination and protect blisters to prevent them from breaking.

6. Estimate the extent and depth of the burn and note any involvement of critical areas.

7. Remove rings, bracelets, and watches from burned extremities, if possible.

8. Assess for fractures and other significant injuries, especially if the patient jumped from a building, was in an explosion, or was exposed to falling debris.

9. Cover the burn with a dry, sterile dressing or, if it is extensive, with a clean sheet or pillowcase. Do *not* put any type of grease, lotion, or antiseptic on burned skin.

10. In extremity burns, place non-adhesive gauze pads between fingers and toes.

11. Splint a burned extremity.

12. Transport the patient promptly to a hospital, unless the burn is minimal.

13. Watch for respiratory distress in patients who have suffered smoke exposure, those with facial burns, and those with burns classified as moderate or critical. Give oxygen, if

---

Table 7.3

Emergency Care of Burns

1. Put out the fire (including smoldering clothing) and/or remove the patient from the heat source.
2. Apply cold water. Use caution if the burn is more than 20 percent of the body surface.
3. Perform the primary survey with attention to the airway and breathing.
4. Avoid contaminating burned skin and rupturing blisters.
5. Estimate the extent and seriousness of the burn.
6. Remove jewelry from a burned extremity, if possible.
7. Assess and care for additional injuries.
8. Cover the burn with sterile or clean material. Do not apply greases or other substances.
9. Watch for respiratory distress and give oxygen as necessary. Consider carbon monoxide poisoning.
10. Immobilize a burned extremity.
11. Treat the patient for shock, if necessary.
12. Transport the patient to definitive medical care.

---

available, in high concentration and high flow rate to such patients. Anticipate and treat shock when burns are extensive (third-degree burns of over 10 percent of body surface, second-degree burns of over 25 percent, first-degree burns of over 50 percent).

14. Anyone trapped in a burning building may have suffered carbon monoxide poisoning. Its emergency care is discussed in Chapter 17.

Chemical Burns

Chemical burns are most often caused by contact with strong acids or alkalis. It is essential to remove the chemical immediately (protecting yourself with rubber gloves). Initial emergency care of a chemical burn consists of immediate, prolonged flushing (for at least 15 minutes) of the involved area with *copious* amounts of water— preferably by a hose or in a shower—unless the substance is not very soluble in water or combines chemically with water. If in doubt, call your local poison control center (see Chapter 23).

Partly soluble organic acids should be sponged off with olive oil or cook-

ing oil before flushing. (The organic acid phenol is preferably rinsed off first with polyethylene glycol, if available.) Dry lime, which combines with water to form a strong alkali, should be brushed off before the site is flushed. Other substances that react with water, such as sulfuric acid and metallic sodium, should not be washed off unless they can be flushed off rapidly with a hose or in a shower. (Refer to **Contact Poisons** in Chapter 23 for more information.)

After removing the chemical, remove any of the patient's clothing that might harbor chemical residue, by cutting it off if necessary. Then, cover the burned area with a sterile dressing and take the patient to a physician or hospital.

Electrical Burns

Electrical injury is discussed in Chapter 18. The local treatment of electrical burns is the same as for thermal burns. Electricity usually produces an entrance and exit burn. The damage caused by electricity usually appears small on the surface, but may be extensive internally, because an electric current tends to penetrate the tissues deeply along the paths of blood vessels. Depending on voltage and other factors, respiratory and/or cardiac arrest may occur, necessitating rescue breathing or CPR. All patients with high-voltage electrical burns should be seen by a physician.

Dressings and Bandages

A dressing or compress is a piece of sterile material placed directly on a wound. A bandage is the material that holds a dressing in place. In popular usage, the term "bandage" frequently refers to the dressing and bandage together, and "bandaging" denotes the process of applying both the dressing and the bandage to a wound.

The ability to tie secure knots is a necessary skill for successful bandaging and splinting. (Eight useful knots are illustrated in Appendix G.)

All open wounds require dressing and bandaging to prevent further contamination, to absorb blood and wound secretions, and to control bleeding. A dressing should extend at least 1 inch beyond the edges of the wound.

In the past, a large amount of class time in first aid courses was devoted to the art of bandaging. Bandaging is easier using modern supplies such as the self-adhering roller bandage, and in modern emergency care, any combination that does the job is acceptable. However, there are a few tricks that help in bandaging geometrically difficult areas such as the head or extremities.

Apply the bandage snugly to keep the dressing on the wound. Most extremity bandaging requires that bandages be wrapped entirely around a body part, which introduces the danger of restricting circulation if the bandage is too tight. Leave the fingers or toes exposed distal to an extremity wound so that signs of poor circulation can be detected.

Special Types of Dressings and Bandages

1. Occlusive dressings
   a. For sucking chest wounds (see Chapter 14), place a universal dressing or several layers of sterile compresses directly on the wound and cover with a sterile, airtight layer of plastic, foil, or Vaseline gauze (gauze impregnated with petrolatum). Seal three of the four edges tightly to the skin with adhesive tape, preferably while the patient holds his or her breath after a maximum exhalation (Fig. 7.4).
   b. Cover open abdominal wounds that expose organs with a universal dressing or several layers of sterile compresses moistened with sterile physiological saline solution. If sterile saline solution is not available, use clean water mixed with one-half teaspoon of table salt per quart (or liter). This will keep the organs from drying out. Cover the moist dressing with a piece of sterile, airtight material taped to the abdomen.
2. Pressure dressings (Fig. 7.5), used to maintain direct pressure on a bleeding wound, consist of one or more sterile dressings held in place by a firmly applied self-adhering roller bandage. A rubberized bandage such as an Ace bandage can be used instead, but the danger of accidentally interfering with circulation is greater.
3. Stabilizing dressings (Fig. 7.6), used to stabilize an impaled object, consist of a thick layer

Fig. 7.4 *Occlusive Dressing for a Sucking Chest Wound*

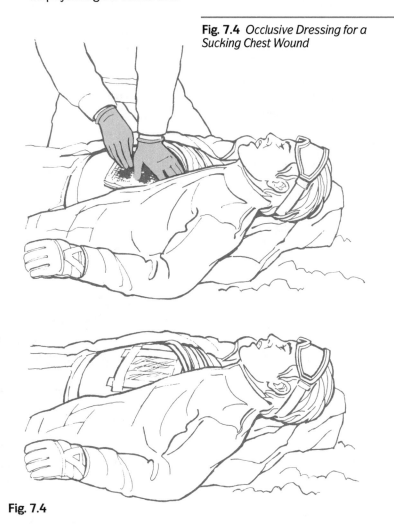

Fig. 7.4

of sterile dressings held firmly in place by tape or self-adhering roller bandages.

Commonly Used Dressings and Bandages

1. Dressings (Fig. 7.7a)
   a. Sterile, nonadhesive pads come in several sizes and are covered on one side by a semipermeable plastic material (Telfa, etc.). These pads are used to cover small wounds or as the first layer for larger wounds.
   b. Sterile gauze pads, available in many sizes ranging from 1-inch by 1-inch to 4- inches by 8-inches, are used to cover small- and medium-sized wounds.
   c. Universal dressings, 9-inch by 36-inch pads made of thick, absorbent material, are used to cover large wounds.

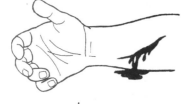

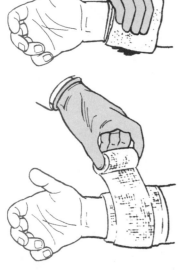

Fig. 7.5

d. Vaseline gauze is available in long, narrow strips used to pack bleeding noses, and in standard-sized dressings. It is airtight and nonadhesive.
e. Handy, small, prepackaged bandage strips (Band-Aids, etc.) are useful for minor cuts and blisters. These strips combine a small dressing with a bandage. They can be improvised by cutting a small square from a larger sterile pad (i.e., with sterile, flamed scissors) and placing it in the middle of a 3- or 4-inch piece of 1-inch tape.

2. Bandages (Figs. 7.7b, 7.7c)
   a. Prepackaged materials such as sterile butterfly bandages and paper tape sutures (Steristrips) are used for wound closure. Butterflies can be improvised in the field from adhesive tape; the part to be laid directly on the wound should be sterilized by holding it over a match flame. The application technique is illustrated in Figure 7.7b.

Fig. 7.5 *Pressure Dressing*

Fig. 7.6 *Stabilizing Dressing for an Impaled Object*

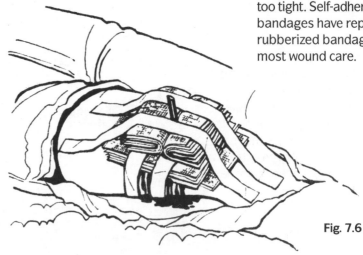

Fig. 7.6

b. Triangular bandages are large, triangular pieces of cloth that measure about 55 inches at the base and 36 to 40 inches along each side. They can be used to form slings or can be folded lengthwise to form long, narrow cravats several inches wide. Cravats can be used as bandages, swathes, splints for fractured ribs, and supports for sprained ankles and knees. They also can be used as tourniquets.
c. Self-adhering roller bandages are useful modern versions of the venerable gauze roller bandages. They are available in several widths. Because the material sticks to itself, extensive taping is not necessary to secure the ends. Self-adhering roller bandages are slightly elastic and, when used as pressure bandages, cause less potential danger to the circulation than rubberized bandages.
d. Elastic (rubberized) bandages in different widths are used as pressure bandages and as supports for sprained wrists, ankles, or knees. Use them with caution on a patient who is not alert enough to complain of pain and numbness if the bandage is too tight. Self-adhering roller bandages have replaced rubberized bandages for most wound care.

e. Adhesive tape comes in several widths. The handiest sizes for field use are the 1- and 2-inch widths; the latter can be torn lengthwise if 1-inch widths are needed. Waterproof tape is preferable if exposure to water or snow is likely. Use cloth tape rather than plastic or paper tape. Some people are allergic to tape; ask the patient before applying it. Adhesive tape is most useful in taping blisters, splinting sprained ankles and fractured ribs, and securing dressings to flat or slightly curved surfaces (such as the chest, back or abdomen) where a roller bandage or cravat is unsuitable. Adhesive tape does not stick well when cold or when the skin is wet. In cold weather, its adherence can be improved by warming it against the rescuer's body or heating it briefly over a lit match. It is best to shave hairy skin before taping it, but if this has not been done, tape can be removed more easily by pulling it off in a distal rather than a proximal direction, or by using tape remover. Never wrap tape completely around an injured extremity, because the tape can act as a tourniquet if swelling occurs.

Improvisation of Dressings and Bandages

In an emergency, dressings can be improvised from any clean cloth, such as pillowcases, sheets, towels, and sanitary napkins (Fig. 7.8). Never place loose cotton directly on an open wound, because the fibers are difficult to remove. Pack straps, belts, strips torn from clothing, cord, or nylon webbing can be used to improvise

bandages. Kerchiefs and bandannas can be used as cravats and triangular bandages. Rolled T-shirts can be used as cravats, and clean socks can be used as hand or foot bandages. Plastic sandwich or garbage bags can be placed over sterile compresses to make an occlusive dressing.

Special Techniques for Problem Surfaces

Moving joints require a special technique because joint motion, even if only occasional, tends to loosen

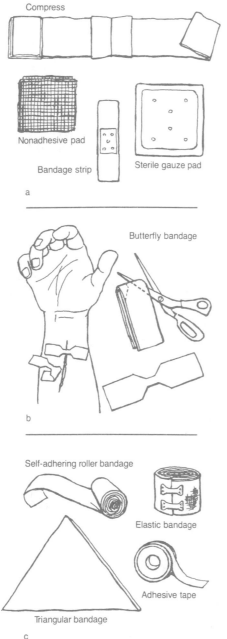

Fig. 7.7

adhesive tape and shift other types of bandages to a position above or below the joint. The preferred bandage material is self-adhering roller bandage, which is elastic enough to stretch with joint motion rather than move. Apply this material in a figure-of-eight (Fig. 7.9). Make several circular turns around the limb above the joint, overlapping the upper end of the dressing. Bring the bandage diagonally across the dressing and make several similar turns around the limb below the joint. Next, bring

Fig. 7.7 *Various Types of Dressings and Bandages*

Fig. 7.8 *Improvised Bandages and Dressings*

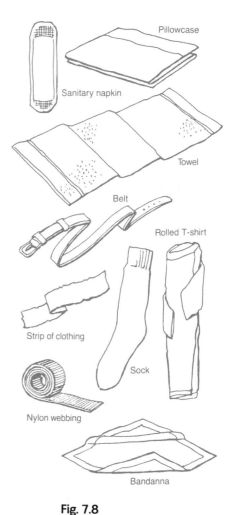

Fig. 7.8

the bandage diagonally back up over the dressing and make several turns around the limb above the joint. Repeat this process until the dressing is snug. Use tape or a safety pin to anchor the loose end above or below the joint, not over or behind it.

Bandage joints in the most comfortable position. Usually, the knee is bandaged while slightly flexed; the ankle and elbow are bandaged while flexed to just under 90 degrees.

Tapering cylinders such as the upper arm, forearm, thigh, or leg are also best bandaged by wrapping with a self-adhering roller bandage (Fig. 7.10). Make several turns around the limb below the dressing, and then continue up, over, and above the dressing, with each turn overlapping the one below by ½ inch to ¾ inch. Complete the bandage by making several overlapping turns above the dressing and anchoring the loose end. If the patient must walk on a

bandaged lower extremity, anchor the bandage to the skin above the dressing with several vertical strips of adhesive tape.

Bandages tend to slip off the **head** because it is spherical. Compresses can be anchored with a bandanna-style triangular bandage or with the patient's hat. Fold a triangular bandage (Fig 7.11) twice along the long side to make a 2-inch hem. Place the bandage on top of the patient's head

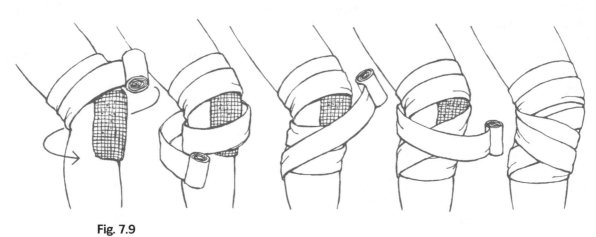

Fig. 7.9

Fig. 7.9 *Application of a Figure-of-eight Bandage to the Knee*

Fig. 7.10 *Application of a Self-adhering Roller Bandage to the Forearm*

Fig. 7.11 *Application of a Triangular Bandage to the Head*

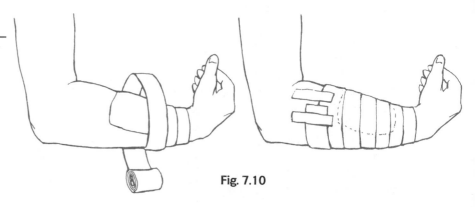

Fig. 7.10

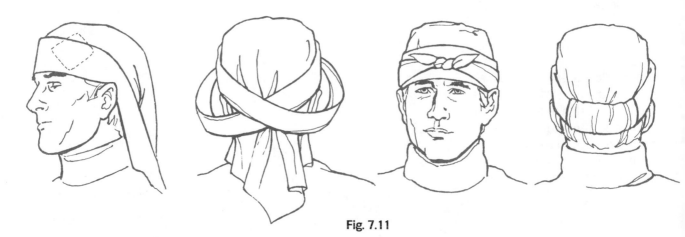

Fig. 7.11

with the triangular tail below the occiput (back of the skull) and the hem across the forehead just above the eyebrows. Wrap the two ends of the hem around the sides of the head above the ears, cross at the occiput, and bring them around the opposite sides of the head to the forehead. Then tie the ends snugly with a square knot. Tuck the tip of the tail into the hem at the occiput. The bandage should be snug and wrinkle-free over the top of the head. Anchor the outer

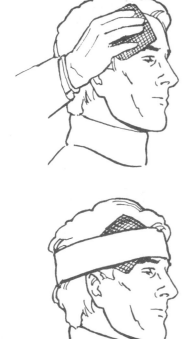

Fig. 7.12

surface of the compress beneath the bandage with a safety pin sterilized over a lit match. Anchoring with the patient's hat works better if the sweatband is directly over the wound, or, if available, use a snug-fitting headband (Fig. 7.12) or ski cap.

Because the **hands** are seldom still, even when injured, bandages tend to work loose easily. An effective technique is to immobilize the hand completely by cupping the fingers over a wad of gauze held in the palm, then wrap the entire hand with a roller bandage or a cravat to form a "bulky hand bandage" (Fig. 7.13). Since the fingers are not exposed, ask the patient at intervals whether the fingertips can be felt and whether they feel numb or tingly.

When the fingers must be free, an alternate technique suitable for wounds of the palm or back of the hand is to make a modified figure-of-eight bandage out of a self-adhering roller bandage (Fig. 7.14). Anchor the bandage with several turns around the wrist, then run it diagonally across the palm or back of the hand to anchor the dressing. Continue making several more turns around the palm and back of the hand, alternating the turns above and below the thumb. Then, run the bandage diagonally across the back of the hand, and make several additional turns around the wrist. Repeat this sequence several times until the compress is firmly anchored, then secure the loose end at the wrist.

Because **fingers** are hard to bandage, bandage strips (Band-Aids, etc.) should be used whenever possible. Large finger wounds can be bandaged with a bulky hand bandage. An alternative is to modify the figure-of-eight bandage used for the hand (Fig. 7.15). Anchor the dressing on the finger with multiple turns of a narrow, self-adhering roller bandage, which can be improvised if necessary by cutting a wider bandage lengthwise. Bring the bandage diagonally across the back of the hand, anchor it with several turns around the wrist, then bring it across the back of the hand again from the opposite side of the wrist to loop the finger. Repeat until the bandage is snug. Secure the loose end at the wrist.

In general, it is best to use a bandage whose width approximates the diameter of the part being bandaged.

  a. Finger: 1 inch wide
  b. Hand, wrist, small foot: 2 inches wide
  c. Forearm, lower leg, foot: 3 inches wide
  d. Upper arm, small thigh: 4 inches wide
  e. Thigh, chest: 6 inches wide

Fig. 7.12 *Use of a Headband to Secure a Dressing*

Fig. 7.13 *Bulky Hand Bandage*

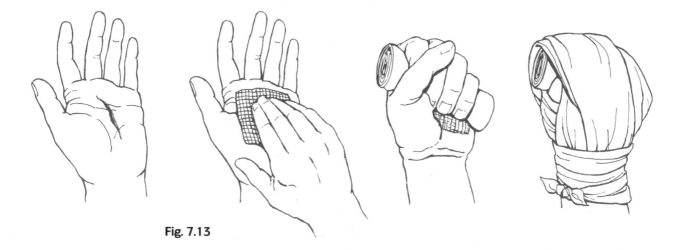

Fig. 7.13

Fig. 7.14 *Figure-of-eight Bandage Modified for the Hand*

Fig. 7.15 *Figure-of-eight Bandage Modified for the Finger*

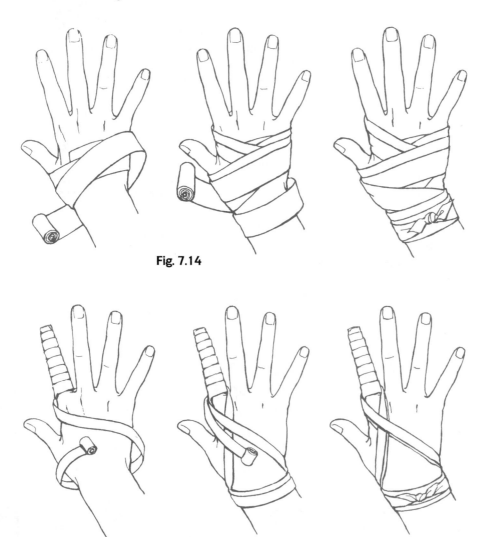

Fig. 7.14

Fig. 7.15

Scenario #7 (Fig. 7.16)

The following scenario illustrates the care of two different types of wounds.

It is a beautiful spring day after a foot of powder the night before. You are getting off the upper lift at the High Range Ski Area when you receive a transmission about a skier hurt and bleeding in the trees on the left side of Autobahn about two-thirds of the way down. You wave to the patroller on duty at the top and radio that you are taking a toboggan down to check it out. As you arrive at the accident site, you see a man lying in the snow at the edge of the run. There is obvious blood in the snow near his head and his skis are still on. You park the toboggan below the skier and anchor it with your skis. As you approach, you can see that the skier's eyes are open and that he is breathing. His hat is off and there is blood dripping onto the snow from a large laceration on the left side of his head. There is also a large tear in his left sleeve with blood on his glove.

You: "Hi, I'm Ben Schussen of the High Range Ski Patrol. Can I help you?"

Patient: "Yes."

You: "What happened?" (grasping the patient's uninjured forearm and assessing the radial pulse; it is strong and 90 beats per minute.)

Patient: "I guess I clipped a tree."

You: "Did you actually hit it head-on or just clip it?"

Patient: "I got too close to it, and I think one of the branches cut my head."

You: "Skiing the powder along the edge, eh? What's your name?"

Patient: "Otto Control."

You: "Did you hit your head at all?"

Patient: "No."

You: "Were you knocked out?"

Patient: "No."

You: "Does your neck hurt?"

Patient: "No."

You: "Do you know where you are and what day it is?" (The patient replies appropriately.) "You're bleeding from a cut on your head. I need to get that stopped."

You take off your fanny pack, open it, and take out a flashlight, a Swiss Army knife, a waterproof match container, three 3-inch by 4-inch sterile packages of Telfa, a tongue blade, a roll of Kling, and a pair of rubber gloves. You put on the gloves and assess the patient's head. There is a 3-inch laceration just above the hairline on the left forehead, bleeding freely. There are several large pieces of bark in the wound. The skin of the patient's forehead is warm and there are a few beads of sweat on it. You light a match and flame the forceps of your knife, then use them to remove the three pieces of bark. You take the compresses out of their packages and place them over the wound. Very carefully, you feel the patient's head through the compresses. The cut is through the scalp, but there is no break in the smoothness of the underlying cranium. Holding pressure on the wound with one hand, you feel

Fig. 7.16 *Scenario #7*

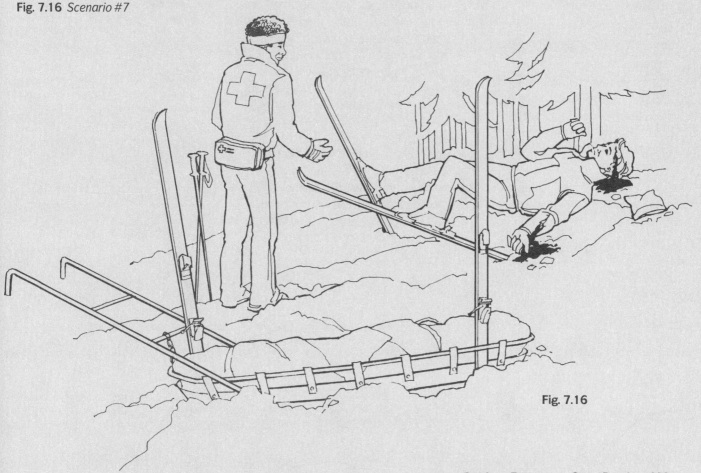

Fig. 7.16

the rest of the scalp carefully; there are no other injuries. After a minute, you note that the bleeding has stopped. Holding the compresses in place, you retrieve the patient's cap and put it carefully back on the patient's head. The compresses stay in place and there is no further obvious bleeding.

You then assess the rest of the patient's head, using the flashlight to check both pupils and to look in the mouth, ears, and nose. The scalp shows no additional abnormalities. The pupils are round, regular, and equal, and there is no bleeding or drainage coming from the nose or ears. You examine the patient's mouth with the assistance of the tongue blade; the mouth appears normal. Moving down to the neck, you assess it and find no wounds, swellings, tenderness, or other abnormalities.

You: "Did you hit your chest or abdomen?"

Patient: "No."

You: "I need to take a look at your arm. There's blood on your sleeve and glove, and your sleeve is torn. Does your arm hurt?"

Patient: "Yes. I didn't even notice that."

You: "Do you hurt anywhere else?"

Patient: "No."

You remove the patient's glove and use a pair of paramedic shears to enlarge the tear in the arm of the patient's windshirt and long-john top to expose the forearm. There is a

1-inch puncture wound with a 2-inch part of a tree branch sticking out of it. It is oozing a little blood, and there is blood over most of the distal forearm. The radial pulse is strong and about 100 beats per minute. The capillary refill is normal.

At this point, a fellow patroller arrives. You ask her to remove the patient's skis. She places them in an X uphill from the accident and loosens the patient's boots.

You: "Can you wiggle your fingers on this hand?" (The patient does so.) "Make a fist, and then spread your fingers like this." (The patient imitates you.) "Does your hand feel numb or tingly?"

Patient: "No."

You pack two more sterile compresses around the branch, covering the wound. You take a cravat and a 3-inch roll of Kling from your first aid belt, form the cravat into a donut, and lay it over the compresses. You wrap the Kling around the patient's forearm, holding the cravat, the compresses, and the impaled object in place.

You can now pause and review the situation. The patient is alert and oriented, and even though he has a scalp laceration, there is no sign of a serious head or neck injury. His breathing and circulation are normal and there is no airway problem. He had significant bleeding from a scalp wound, although it was not enough to produce hypovolemic shock. It is now controlled. He also had another wound in his forearm that did not bleed significantly but has part of a tree branch impaled in it. There is no evidence of damage to nerves and blood vessels from the arm injury, which is now bandaged.

The other patroller has brought the toboggan closer to the patient. Before the patient is moved, however, you need to make sure there are no other significant injuries, especially back injuries and extremity fractures.

You: "Does this hurt?" (using both hands to palpate the arm of the injured extremity, the uninjured arm and forearm, and both thighs and legs. There is no tenderness, swelling, or deformity.)

Patient: "No."

You: "Can you feel your fingers and toes?"

Patient: "Yes."

You: "Can you wiggle them?"

Patient: "Yes" (wiggling them).

You: "Do you have any pain in your back?"

Patient: "No."

You quickly run your hand down the patient's back to his tailbone, asking as you go whether anything feels tender. There are no tender spots, "step-off" deformities, or swellings. It is now time to load the patient into the toboggan and take him to the aid room. The rest of the secondary survey can be carried out there.

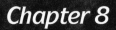

Chapter 8

Emergency Care of Bone and Joint Injuries: General Principles

The broken bone, once set together, is stronger than ever.

—*John Lyly Euphues*

This chapter presents the general principles of the emergency care of bone and joint injuries. The care of specific fractures, dislocations, and sprains of the upper and lower extremities and pelvis will be discussed in Chapters 10 and 11. The care of injuries of the neck and back will be covered in Chapter 13.

Fractures

The term "fracture" is used for any break in the continuity of a bone. A fracture can range in severity from a hairline crack difficult to see on an X-ray film to severe disruption with marked displacement and multiple fragments. The number of separate fragments, or **amount of comminution**, is roughly proportional to the magnitude, type, and direction of the forces involved in the injury.

Fractures can be classified in several ways:

Closed or Open Fractures

A closed fracture is one in which the overlying skin is intact (Fig. 8.1a). Most fractures are closed.

Fig. 8.1 *Types of Fractures*

An open fracture involves a wound of the overlying skin (Fig. 8.1b), which can occur when the sharp ends of the fractured bone break the skin from within or when an object such as a bullet penetrates from the outside. A blunt force that fractures a bone also can produce a wound of the overlying skin that does not necessarily connect anatomically with the fracture. Nevertheless, *any fracture with an overlying skin wound is regarded as open*. The skin wound may be tiny or large, and the bone may or may not be visible in the wound.

Open fractures are very serious injuries. Bleeding is frequently more severe than in closed fractures and, because the fracture site is exposed to outside contamination, there is considerable danger of infection. Infections associated with open fractures may be difficult to treat and can cause life-long disability.

Displaced or Non-displaced Fractures

In a displaced fracture, the bone ends are moved out of their normal in-line position (Fig. 8.1c). Displacement, which is suspected based on the amount of **deformity** at the frac-

ture site, can be minimal to marked. The distal part of the limb may be angulated or rotated, and the entire limb may be shortened because muscle spasm has caused the bone fragments to override.

A non-displaced fracture may or may not be deformed, although there usually is swelling and tenderness at the fracture site. X-ray examination may be required for a definite diagnosis (Fig. 8.1a).

Fractures also can be classified as **simple, comminuted, greenstick, transverse, spiral**, and **stress**.

1. A **simple fracture** has only one fracture line (Figs. 8.1a, 8.1c).
2. A **comminuted fracture** has two or more fracture lines with three or more fragments (Fig. 8.1d).
3. A **greenstick fracture** is a fracture through only part of the bone shaft. Although the bone may be angulated at the fracture site, the bone ends are not separated. Because a greenstick fracture can occur only in elastic bones, it is seen only in the young and is most common in the ankle and distal forearm (Fig. 8.1e).

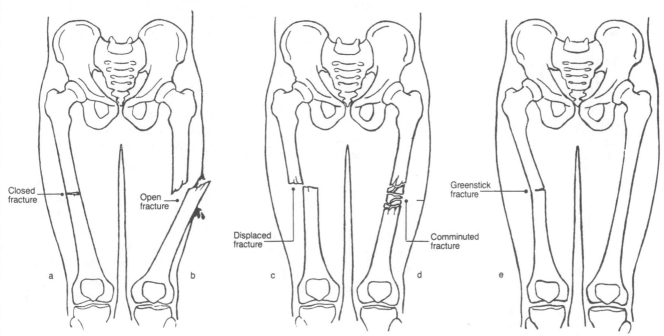

Fig. 8.1

4. In a **transverse fracture** (Fig. 8.1a), the fracture line is at or close to a right angle to the long axis of the bone. A common example is the type of lower leg bone fracture that can occur when a skier's bindings do not release during a forward fall over the ski tips.

5. In a **spiral fracture**, the fracture line spirals around the shaft of the bone. These fractures are caused by rotational (twisting) forces; a common example is the type of lower leg bone fracture that can occur during a rotational fall when the skier's foot is fixed and the rest of the body rotates (Fig. 8.1f).

6. A **stress fracture** is a hairline fracture caused by repeated small traumas to a bone. Stress fractures are common in long-distance runners and should be suspected in joggers and runners who experience chronic, localized pain in the leg, foot, or back made worse by running or hard walking.

When the topic of fractures is first studied, it is easy to focus on the dramatic aspects of bone injury. X-rays

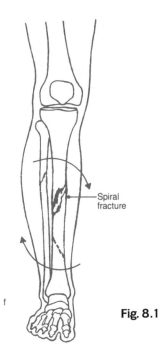

Spiral fracture

f

Fig. 8.1

may reveal interesting and sometimes startling abnormalities. However, do not forget that serious—although less obvious—soft-tissue damage also is present, particularly to nerves and blood vessels. These injuries can be caused both by the initial trauma and by the sharp ends of the fractured bone. Soft-tissue damage contributes greatly to the pain and disability of a fracture.

Signs and Symptoms of Fractures

A fracture should be suspected in any person who complains of continued pain after an injury. A child with a fracture may have *no* signs or symptoms other than pain.

1. A **suitable mechanism of injury** (see Chapter 9). A fracture should be suspected whenever there is trauma of suitable type and magnitude.

2. **Pain**. Pain may be mild but more typically is severe. The patient usually will be able to point to the site of pain with one finger. Pain almost always increases if the injured part is moved.

3. **Tenderness**. Tenderness usually is confined to the injury site and can be found by gentle palpation.

4. **Deformity**. Deformity is not always present or obvious. Compare an injured extremity with the opposite, uninjured one.

5. **Sound**. The patient may have heard the bone snap.

6. **Function**. Usually, the patient loses the use of the limb partly or completely. Occasionally, however, the patient is able to move the limb with little or no pain.

7. **Swelling and ecchymosis**. Bleeding into the tissues from the disrupted blood vessels causes swelling. As the blood

works its way to the skin surface, it causes the bluish-purple discoloration of ecchymosis. These signs take time to develop and may not be present initially.

8. **Crepitus and false motion.** Crepitus is a grating sensation caused by the broken bone ends grinding against each other. Limb motion where there is no joint is called false motion. These signs should *not* be deliberately elicited.

9. **Wounds**. Open fractures involve an open wound; sometimes exposed bone ends can be seen in the wound.

Within a few hours after a bone is fractured, a swelling composed of blood and inflammatory cells forms around and between the bone ends. The blood clots and, within a few days, other types of cells begin to grow out into the clot, eventually uniting the broken bone ends with fibrous tissue. At first, this union is weak, but soon it begins to calcify and gradually becomes stronger. This calcified tissue, called a **callus**, eventually becomes as strong or stronger than the original bone.

Before a strong callus has been formed, motion at the fracture site can rebreak the bone and delay or prevent healing. Thus, a splint or cast must be used to prevent motion, allow proper healing, and control pain.

Dislocations

A dislocation is a type of joint disruption that occurs when the joint is forced to move beyond its normal range. Dislocations may be either complete or incomplete and may be associated with a fracture. During a dislocation, the joint capsule and ligaments are stretched or torn, and the bones of the joint may be completely displaced from their normal positions. Damage to blood vessels and nerves is common. A dislocated joint frequently is locked in the displaced position, making an attempt to move it very painful.

The most commonly dislocated joints are those with less stability and a wide range of motion (e.g., the shoulder, Fig. 8.2), and those whose location and type of use make them more susceptible to forces that can cause dislocation (e.g., the elbow, small joints of the fingers, the patella, and the ankle). Dislocations of the hip (Fig. 8.3) also are fairly common and usually are accompanied by a fracture of the deep hip joint cup (acetabulum). Dislocations of the knee and elbow are serious injuries because important but poorly protected nerves and blood vessels cross these joints. Damage to these structures may lead to permanent disability or even loss of the limb.

Signs and Symptoms of Dislocations

It may be difficult to distinguish dislocations from fractures. However, a bone can be dislocated only where it forms a joint with another bone, but it can be fractured at any point. Fractures and dislocations can occur together. Signs and symptoms of dislocations include the following:

1. The **mechanism of injury** is one that can cause a dislocation (see Chapter 9).

2. **Pain** usually is more severe than would be expected for a fracture in the same area. Pain increases with any attempt to move the joint.
3. Some degree of **deformity** is always present. This is marked with complete dislocations, but in partial ones may be so slight that comparison with the opposite side may be necessary.
4. Normal joint **motion** is lost.
5. There is **swelling** and **tenderness** over the joint.

Sprains

Sprains are produced in the same manner as dislocations, but by weaker forces. Stretching and tearing of the joint capsule and ligaments are less severe. The bones of the joint are not displaced, and any deformity is minimal.

Sprains have three grades of severity, depending on the extent of damage. In **Grade I sprains**, the capsule and ligaments are stretched but not torn; in **Grade II sprains**, they are badly stretched or partly torn; in **Grade III sprains**, they are completely torn. The most commonly sprained joints are the knee, ankle, and shoulder.

Signs and Symptoms of Sprains

1. **Tenderness**, which frequently can be located with a fingertip.
2. **Swelling and ecchymosis**, caused by edema and bleeding from injured small blood vessels.
3. **Pain** at the site of injury, which usually increases with joint motion.
4. Some degree of **loss of joint function** because of pain.

Because the signs and symptoms are similar, it may be difficult to tell a severe sprain from a fracture or dislocation. Because the goal of emergency care is the same for all these injuries—to reduce motion at the injury site—sprains should be splinted the same as fractures and dislocations.

Assessment of Musculoskeletal Injuries

After completing the primary survey and caring for any emergent conditions, examine the patient's injury site or sites. Try to determine the mechanism of the injury (Chapter 9). Decide if the type, direction, and magnitude of the forces involved were sufficient to produce a fracture or dislocation, or only a sprain or minor soft-tissue injury. Open all overlying clothing in all but the most trivial injuries (e.g., minor sprains), preferably by cutting or ripping open a seam, and examine

Fig. 8.2 *Shoulder Dislocation*

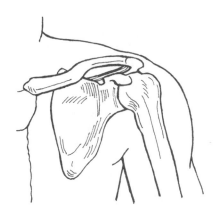

Normal shoulder joint

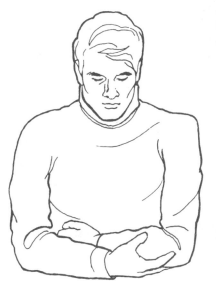

Fig. 8.2

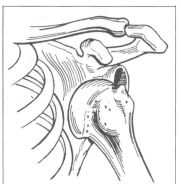

the site for wounds, swelling, tenderness, ecchymosis, and deformity. In very cold weather, it may be preferable to minimize or postpone clothing removal until the patient has been stabilized, splinted, and evacuated to a protected site such as a ski patrol first aid room.

Next, evaluate the state of the circulation and nerve supply below the injury. This is especially important with fractures and dislocations because many important nerves and blood vessels lie close to bones and joints. Test motor function by asking the patient to squeeze your hand and to make a fist and then open it, or to wiggle the toes. Test sensory function by determining whether the patient can feel a gentle pinch or a fingernail scrape. If you suspect a significant injury, do *not* ask the patient to move an extremity at the injury site.

Check the appropriate pulses: the radial pulse in the upper extremity and the dorsalis pedis and posterior tibial pulses in the lower extremity. Check capillary refill time in a fingertip or top of the foot, but remember that this may be unreliable if the extremities are cold. It is difficult to examine the feet without removing shoes or boots; this may be a problem in severe weather, especially with ski injuries. In serious injuries with actual or potential damage to the circulation and nerve supply, such as a dislocated knee or ankle or a fracture above the knee (described in Chapter 11), remove the footgear at the accident site to feel the pulses, test sensation, and watch the patient move parts distal to the injury. With

less serious injuries, such as knee sprains, simply ask if the parts distal to the injury are still comfortable, whether there has been any change in the way they feel, and whether the patient can feel his or her toes wiggle. If the answers to these questions are satisfactory and the patient has a normal mental status, the remainder of the evaluation of circulation and nerve supply may be postponed until shelter is reached. If there is any doubt, however, remove footgear immediately so that a complete assessment can be made. In any case, ski boots and other tight footgear should be unbuckled or loosened, on both an injured and an uninjured lower extremity.

A fractured femur presents a special case, since traction splinting (described below) will be required to control bleeding into the fracture site and prevent shock. Application of a traction splint is done faster and more comfortably if the traction harness is put on over the boot. Many experts feel that circulation and nerve supply can be assessed satisfactorily without removing the boot. Ask the patient whether he or she can move the toes and feel the feet. Even if the answer is "no," any problem with circulation or nerve function that can be improved in the field will respond to traction alone. Transportation becomes a high priority, and removing the boot at the site to check circulation and nerve function would only delay transportation. If the patient is unresponsive or otherwise not able to respond to questions, then transportation also is a higher priority than removing the boot in the field.

If changes in vital signs are not explainable by the major injury alone, expose and assess the neck, chest, abdomen, and pelvis as appropriate. Assess any other sites of pain indicated by the patient.

Unresponsive patients present a special problem because they can-

Fig. 8.3 *Hip Dislocations*

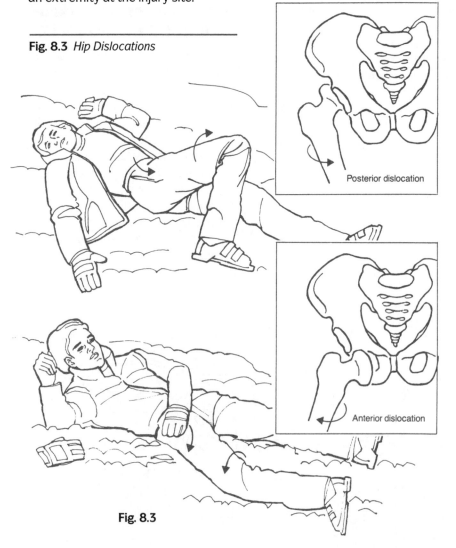

Posterior dislocation

Anterior dislocation

Fig. 8.3

Table 8.1

Summary of Assessment of Musculoskeletal Injuries

1. Perform the primary survey.
2. Determine the mechanism of injury.
3. Expose and assess the site of major injury indicated by the patient.
4. Assess the circulation and nerve supply below the injury.
5. If the pulse is rapid and/or breathing is labored and these changes are not explainable by the major injury, assess the neck and chest (followed by the abdomen and pelvis, if appropriate).
6. Assess any additional pain sites indicated by patient.

not be questioned about sensation or asked to move their fingers and toes. However, the patient's body can be examined for signs of injury, and the pulses and capillary refill time can be assessed. The patient can be watched for spontaneous movement and for withdrawal of an extremity in response to pain. The amount of spontaneous movement and pain response of the two sides should be compared. Every unresponsive, injured patient must be assumed to have a spine injury.

General Principles of Emergency Care for Musculoskeletal Injuries

The basic emergency care for all musculoskeletal injuries is immobilization of the injured site by **splinting**. Fractures, dislocations, and sprains may be difficult to tell apart in the field. If in doubt, *splint*.

Purposes of Splinting

1. To prevent the jagged fragments of broken bones from grinding against each other or causing further damage to nerves, blood vessels, and other tissues.
2. To prevent accidental conversion of a closed fracture to an open fracture.
3. To reduce pain, swelling, and bleeding by preventing motion at the injury site.
4. To prevent shock.
5. To allow greater ease in transport.

6. To speed healing, prevent long-term disability, and decrease rehabilitation time.

With a fracture, proper splinting means immobilizing the **joints** *above* and *below* the injury to prevent motion from being transmitted to the injury site. With a dislocation or sprain, the bones *above* and *below* the injury site are immobilized.

A fractured limb that is markedly deformed cannot be splinted unless the deformity is corrected. This process is called **alignment**. Careful alignment is unlikely to damage the injured area any further. It is performed by gentle *manual axial traction*, meaning traction applied *parallel* to the *long axis* of the extremity with the rescuer's hands and body and without mechanical devices. The fracture site should be exposed before this is done. Circulation and nerve supply below the fracture should be assessed before and after alignment. Grasp the limb below the fracture site with both hands while an assistant supports the limb with one hand below and one hand above the site. Maintain gentle traction on the limb while straightening and, if necessary, rotating the limb into the most anatomically normal position possible.

Observe the fracture site to make sure the bone ends are not accidentally forced through the skin. After alignment has been completed, continue manual stabilization of the injured limb until the splint has been

applied. Please note that the purpose of alignment is *not* to reduce a fracture, but to correct the deformity enough so that a splint can be applied.

If resistance or severe pain occurs, stop attempts to align the limb, and splint it in the deformed position. The process of alignment is painful, but pain can be minimized by working smoothly and gently and by encouraging the patient to relax the muscles of the injured extremity.

Fractures of the ankle, lower leg, thigh, mid-forearm, mid-upper arm, hand, and finger usually can be aligned safely when necessary. Attempts usually are not made to align spinal fractures or fractures near or associated with the knee, wrist, elbow, and shoulder joints, all of which *should be splinted in the position in which they were found.*

Because dislocations frequently are locked in the displaced condition, the type of alignment done with fractures is not possible with dislocations, and they usually are splinted in the position in which they were found.

Remember that splinting is a *dynamic* and not a static process. Lifting, carrying, and transporting a splinted patient can cause shifting or loosening of the splint's attachments or, in the case of a traction splint, alter the traction mechanics. A splint *cannot* be applied and then forgotten, but must be checked periodically to make sure it is performing its duty and is not so tight that circulation and/or nerve supply to the extremity is compromised.

An injury that interrupts circulation to a limb may cause loss of the limb. An injury that damages a limb's nerve supply may cause permanent paralysis of the limb.

Signs of Loss of Circulation

1. Pulses distal to the extremity are absent.
2. The part distal to the injury turns white or blue.
3. The part distal to the injury feels cold.

4. The patient develops worsening pain in the part distal to the fracture rather than at the fracture site.
5. Ability to move parts distal to the injury is lost or impaired.

Signs of Loss of Nerve Supply

1. Reaction to touch or pain is lost or impaired distal to the injury.
2. Numbness or complete loss of sensation develops distal to the injury.
3. Ability to move parts distal to the injury is lost or impaired.

Because of the danger of tissue death or permanent disability, loss of circulation and/or nerve supply is an emergency, and the patient must be taken to a hospital as soon as possible. In the case of a fracture, if immediate medical help is not available, attempt to improve the circulation and/or nerve supply by correcting the fracture angle. Use the alignment process described above. When alignment is successful, the pulses return and limb color and temperature eventually improve. Improvement in sensation and motion may take longer.

Even though dislocations in general should not be aligned, if a dislocation interrupts the circulation or nerve supply to an injured limb, the rescuer should gently attempt to change the angle of deformity. If the attempt is successful, splint the dislocation in the new position.

Dislocations of the knee and ankle present a special problem because they frequently are accompanied by severe disruption of the joint and by damage to nerves and blood vessels. A dislocated ankle often is fractured as well. In these cases, attempts at realignment and rapid transportation to a hospital are important because, if the blood supply is not reestablished within a few hours, the part eventually may need to be amputated.

Check and *document* the circulation and nerve supply to the limb below an injury *during the first assessment*, immediately *before* and *after* alignment and splinting, and at *10- to 15-minute intervals* until the patient is transferred to the EMS system.

Increasing pain in an injured extremity may be an early indication of impaired circulation; this is an important sign that should be investigated and monitored closely. If there are signs of impaired circulation and nerve supply to an injured limb after it has been splinted, immediately inspect the splint to see if it is too tight. It may need to be loosened, the injury site may need to be re-exposed and/or, rarely, the splint may need to be removed and reapplied.

These precautions reflect the dynamic nature of musculoskeletal injuries which, even if properly splinted, may continue to swell, placing pressure on nerves and blood vessels.

Open fractures require special care because the overlying skin wound allows contamination of the fracture site. Be sure to institute universal precautions (Appendix F), which includes putting on rubber gloves—preferably sterile—at a minimum before caring for a patient with an open fracture. Before bandaging an open fracture, control bleeding by direct pressure and use sterile forceps to remove obvious foreign matter. However, do not probe the wound.

It takes several hours for infection to develop in an open fracture or other contaminated wound. If the patient will not receive definitive medical care within this time, it is preferable to clean the wound before bandaging and splinting the extremity. Cleaning is especially indicated for wounds that are very dirty. Cover the wound with a sterile compress, then wash the skin around the wound with a germicidal solution such as 10-percent povidone-iodine (Betadine or Hibiclens). Be sure to ask the patient about allergies to iodine and other chemicals. Then flush the wound with sterile physiological saline solution under pressure, using a sterile syringe and needle or Angiocath. Pouring 1-percent Betadine or other germicidal solutions directly on the ends of a broken bone or into an open wound is controversial, but is recommended by some medical personnel. To keep exposed bone ends moist, cover them with a sterile dressing saturated with sterile physiological saline, if available. After caring for the open wound, proceed with alignment and splinting as you would with a closed fracture.

Occasionally, exposed bone ends may retract into the wound during alignment and splinting. Do not

Table 8.1

Summary of Emergency Care of Musculoskeletal Injuries

1. Expose and inspect the injury site.
2. Stop bleeding and care for an open wound, if present.
3. Align a deformed fracture, if necessary.
4. Splint the injured part.
5. Assess and document circulation and nerve supply before and after alignment and splinting and at frequent intervals thereafter.
6. If circulation and/or nerve supply are impaired, attempt cautious alignment of the fracture or dislocation angle.
7. Treat sprains with support, cold packs, and by having the patient keep weight off the injured extremity.
8. Treat shock if necessary.

---

attempt to re-expose retracted bone ends or deliberately push bone ends into the wound. Remember that the purpose of traction splinting of an open fracture of the femur is to stabilize the fracture and reduce bleeding, *not* to pull the exposed bone ends back into the wound.

Shortly after reaching the hospital, the patient will be taken to surgery and the injury will be opened and cleaned. Therefore, do not give the patient anything by mouth. Tell the EMS personnel *exactly* what type of emergency care was given in the field and whether the bone ends were initially exposed and retracted into the wound during splinting.

The emergency care of sprains involves providing support with a cravat or elastic bandage (see Fig. 8.13e), applying cold packs (as described for closed soft-tissue injuries in Chapter 7), and advising the patient to avoid putting weight on an injured extremity and to see a physician if symptoms do not subside within 24 hours.

General Principles of Splinting

This section presents in detail a few commonly used examples of each type of splint. Splints used by nordic ski patrols and other rescue groups that have to carry equipment on their backs tend to be lighter and simpler than splints used by alpine ski patrols and vehicle-based groups. Suggestions are included for improvising splints from natural materials and familiar equipment. However, no attempt is made to describe every variety of splint ever invented.

Splints are of three general types: **fixation splints, traction splints,** and **spine immobilization devices**. All are designed to prevent motion at the injury site, and many prevent motion of the bones and joints above and below the site.

Either the splint or the patient should be well padded with foam or thick cloth to prevent pressure damage to superficial nerves and thin skin over bony projections. This is especially important at the knee and ankle. When metal splints are used, padding also prevents frostbite in cold weather and burns in hot weather. Ideally, splints should be made of a material that transmits X-rays so that complete films can be taken without removing the splint.

If possible, extremities should be splinted in the **position of function**. Thus, in the upper extremity, the shoulder is splinted with the arm next to the body, the elbow is bent to slightly less than a right angle, the wrist is bent slightly so that the hand is cocked upward, and the fingers are bent as if holding a ball. In the lower extremity, the hip should be splinted straight, the knee slightly flexed, and the ankle flexed to a right angle.

Fixation Splints

Fixation splints are simple devices that can be constructed from any rigid object of the proper size and shape. There are two types of fixation splints: **rigid** and **soft** (Fig. 8.4).

Fig. 8.4 *Types of Fixation Splints*

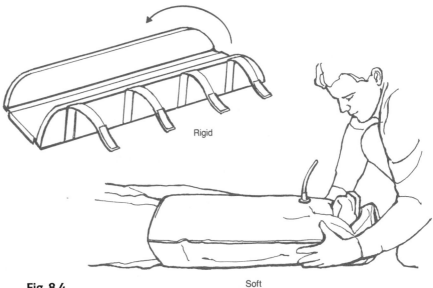

Rigid

Soft

Fig. 8.4

Rigid Fixation Splints

Common examples of rigid fixation splints are plywood **"quick splints"** and **cardboard splints** for injuries to the lower extremity, and **wire, ladder**, and **malleable metal splints** for the upper extremity.

Quick splints are made of plywood padded with foam and are designed for rapid application on a ski hill so that the chilled patient can be evacuated quickly to a warm first aid room. Open the splint flat next to the injured extremity (Fig. 8.5a), loosen the patient's boot, and grasp the booted foot using slight axial traction, while an assistant provides support with one hand distal and the other proximal to the injury site. The "pant leg pinch lift" (Fig. 8.5b) can be used instead to lift and support the extremity. Slide the splint underneath and gently lower the extremity onto the splint with the knee slightly flexed. Fold up the sides of the splint like a clamshell and secure them firmly against the extremity (Fig. 8.5c).

Cardboard splints are a favorite of ski patrols because they are effective, disposable, easy to apply, and inexpensive. They are especially useful when many patients with lower-extremity injuries are treated daily. A quick splint applied on the ski hill frequently will be replaced with a cardboard splint before the patient leaves the aid room. This allows the boot to be removed and circulation and nerve function to be assessed directly (Fig. 8.6). However, use judgment in deciding whether to subject the patient to a splint change. You may not want to change the splint if the patient has a very painful fracture, a bandaged open fracture, multiple injuries, or a fracture accompanied by shock.

Cardboard splints can be purchased or made from sturdy single-corrugation packing box cardboard. A convenient size is 15 inches by 42 inches. Cut the splint so that the corrugations run lengthwise. Cardboard splints are fitted individually to each patient, using the uninjured extremity as a guide. The splint should extend three-quarters of the way or more from knee to groin and be deep enough to contain the leg. If the splint is too long, part of one end can be cut off. Mark the bottom of the heel and cut the edges of the splint so that the end can be bent up at a right angle under the sole of the foot.

After removing the patient's boot, lift the injured extremity and slide the splint into position under it in the same manner as for the quick splint (Fig. 8.5b). Bend the end of the splint into position and anchor it with staples or tape. Protect the sides of the knee and ankle with padding, and place padding under the knee to keep it slightly flexed. Fold up the sides of the splint and secure them in position with adhesive tape.

Wire splints and ladder splints (Fig. 8.7) can be purchased in several sizes. The smaller sizes are compact enough to fit into a ski patrol first aid belt. Commercial ladder splints (3 inches by 31 inches) are available with widely spaced rungs that allow X-rays to be taken with the splint on.

Wire splints also can be constructed from 1/8-inch or 1/4-inch wire mesh. Practical sizes for homemade wire splints are 7 inches by 36 inches and 18 inches by 36 inches. The smaller splint can be rolled into a 2-inch by 7-inch cylinder. Fold 1-inch adhesive tape over all raw edges to avoid injury from the sharp ends of the wire.

Pad all wire and ladder splints and cut or bend them to fit the extremity. Lay the splints along the long axis of the extremity, bend them so that all joints are in the position of function, and secure them with self-adhering roller bandages or cravats. Depending on their size and strength, either one or two splints may be required to immobilize an extremity. The splints can be used singly or doubled on one side of an extremity, placed on opposite sides of the extremity singly or doubled, or applied like a "sugar tong." For example, two small wire splints

Fig. 8.5 *Quick Splint Application Technique*

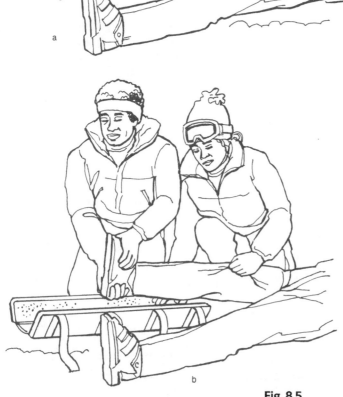

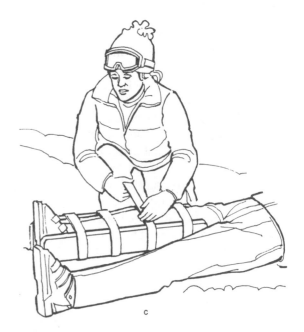

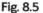

Fig. 8.5

can be doubled over to increase their strength and used one on each side to splint upper arm or forearm fractures. Two large wire splints can be used to immobilize a leg or an ankle, one on each side or two together posteriorly.

Malleable metal splints (Fig. 8.8) are made of soft sheet metal prepadded with thin sheets of foam glued to one or both sides. The SAM splint is one popular model. It measures 4¼ inches by 35½ inches and rolls into a 3-inch by 4¼-inch cylinder. It can be used singly or doubled, can be rounded sideways into a trough-like shape to better fit an extremity, or bent into a sugar tong shape. A malleable metal splint works as well or better than a wire or ladder splint and, if nothing better is available, also can be used as a rigid collar (extrication collar or c-collar). The material is soft enough to be cut, if necessary.

Soft Fixation Splints

Examples of soft fixation splints include **air splints, pneumatic anti-shock garments, vacuum splints**, the **sling and swathe**, and **improvised splints** made from folded parkas, blankets, or pillows.

Air splints (see Fig. 8.4) are compact and light. While air splints are probably the best fixation splint for most wilderness rescue groups and nordic ski patrols, their relatively high cost and poor durability make them less practical for alpine ski patrols that handle large numbers of injured patients.

Air splints are closed, shaped, airtight bags of plastic or coated nylon. They usually have a zipper running the length of the splint. Many different brands of air splints are available in sizes to fit the forearm, upper extremity, leg, or lower extremity. The manufacturer's directions for application should always be consulted. Generally, to apply, unzip the air splint, lay it flat, and slide it under the extremity in a manner similar to positioning a quick splint. Fold the splint around the extremity and close the zipper. Inflate the splint by mouth (Fig. 8.9), never with a pump. If you can indent an air splint slightly by pressing on it with a finger, it is properly inflated.

Air splints are comfortable, need no padding, and can apply firm pressure to a bleeding wound, an advantage when a wound is so large that direct pressure by hand is difficult.

Fig. 8.6 *A cardboard splint often replaces a quick splint in the first aid room.*

Fig. 8.7 *Wire and Ladder Fixation Splints*

Fig. 8.8 *Malleable Metal Splint*

However, they do have a few problems. An air splint may cause the limb to perspire, which in cold weather can increase heat loss and lead to frostbite. It is essential to monitor the splint and the circulation of the splinted extremity frequently because the pressure inside an air splint may vary with changes in temperature and elevation. When an air splint is brought into a warm room from the cold, the air in the splint expands, tightening the splint. A similar complication can occur during altitude changes when an air splint is used on a patient being transported in an unpressurized aircraft. The splint will tighten on altitude gain and loosen on altitude loss. Once an air splint has been used, it should be partially inflated if stored in the cold. Otherwise, the walls of the splint may be bound together when the moisture that condenses from the breath freezes.

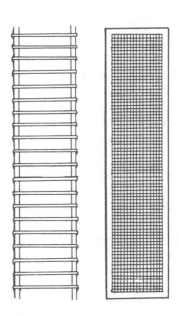

Fig. 8.7

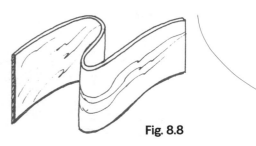

Fig. 8.8

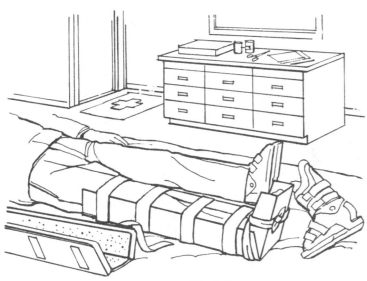

Fig. 8.6

Pneumatic antishock garments (PASGs) are pant-like garments originally designed to combat hypovolemic shock. They consist of three separate inflatable chambers, one for each leg and one for the abdomen. Each chamber is folded around its respective body part and fastened with Velcro straps. When all three are inflated, they provide good stability for fractures of the pelvis or upper femur. Special training, certification, and licensing are required to use these devices.

Vacuum splints also are closed, shaped, airtight bags. A vacuum splint is filled with many tiny plastic pellets. After the splint is put in place, the air inside is evacuated with a suction pump, which draws the plastic pellets close together to form a rigid encasement around the injured part. Vacuum splints are comfortable and work well although they are expensive and somewhat bulkier and heavier than air splints. Several types and shapes of large and small extremity splints and whole body splints (for spine injuries) are available.

A **sling and swathe** (Fig. 8.10a) immobilizes upper-extremity injuries by using the chest wall as a splint. Bend the patient's elbow to just under a 90-degree angle and lay a triangular bandage on the chest wall under the arm. The bandage's long edge should run along the opposite midclavicular line just medial to the fingertips, and the upper corner should pass over the opposite shoulder. The apex should be just beyond the elbow.

Bring the lower corner of the bandage anteriorly around the forearm and up and over the shoulder on the injured side. Tie the two ends together at the side of the neck. Bring the apex forward and pin it to the front of the sling. The tips of the fingers should be visible, and the forearm should be cradled in the sling with the weight of the forearm evenly distributed.

To make the swathe, fold a second triangular bandage to make a cravat about 3 inches wide. Wrap the cravat around the patient's chest and arm, and tie it snugly under the opposite armpit. The sling and swathe is used for shoulder dislocations and fractures of the clavicle and upper arm.

Alternatively, to avoid pressure on an injured shoulder or fractured clavicle, tie the sling as follows: bring the upper corner across the patient's chest, over the far (uninjured) shoulder, and around to the back (Fig. 8.10b). Bring the lower corner up and over the forearm and under the near armpit, where it is tied to the upper corner behind the patient's back. The swathe is tied around the patient's chest and forearm rather than arm.

Improvised fixation splints (Fig. 8.11) can be made out of boards and other rigid or semirigid materials of the proper size and shape. A splint

---

Fig. 8.9 *Air Splint*

Fig. 8.10 *Sling and Swathe*

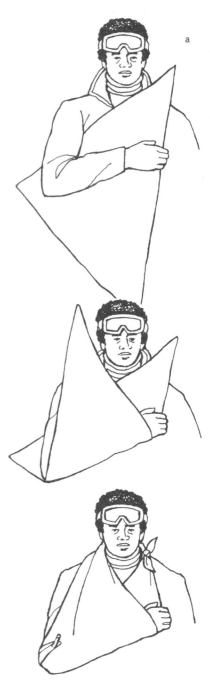

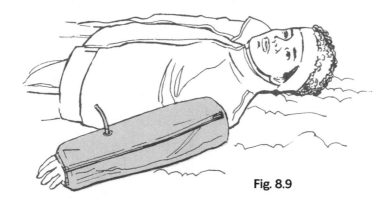

Fig. 8.9

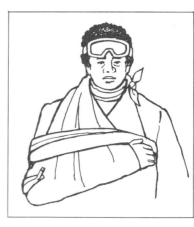

Fig. 8.10

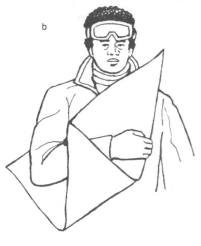

b

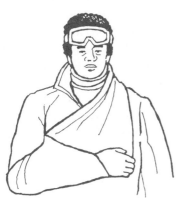

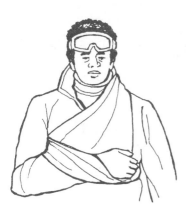

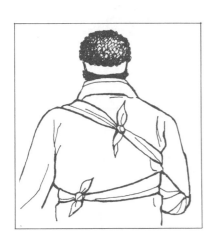

can be fashioned by rolling an inflatable mattress (such as the Therm-a-Rest) or a piece of Ensolite around the extremity, or by folding a blanket, parka or pillow. Semirigid and soft improvised splints can be reinforced with branches or ice axes if necessary. Padded pack straps and rolled newspapers and magazines make good splints for upper-extremity fractures.

Uninjured, nearby parts of the body can be used as splints. A fractured hip can be splinted by tying the injured lower extremity to the opposite extremity (pad between the knees and ankles), and the chest wall can be used to splint upper-extremity fractures. A substitute for a sling can be made from a long-sleeved shirt or jacket by fastening the sleeve to the side of the garment with safety pins.

Traction Splints

Traction splints are designed to counteract muscle spasm of the injured limb, which causes overriding of the broken bone ends, shortening of the limb, and laceration of the soft tissues with increased pain, bleeding, and the danger of shock. **Traction**

consists of a pull parallel to the long axis of the broken bone and opposite to the pull of the major muscles.

In emergency care, the classic indication for a traction splint is a fracture of the midshaft (middle one-half to three-fourths) of the femur. A traction splint also may be useful in oblique lower-leg fractures with shortening and overriding of the fragments. Traction should *not* be used for fractures at the upper and lower ends of the femur or for upper-extremity injuries.

If there is a question about applying traction, the following maneuvers can be useful in determining whether a traction splint is indicated. These maneuvers have been recommended by John Chandler, M.D. Place the heel of one hand on the patient's iliac crest with your fingers on the greater trochanter. If pressing on this hand with your other hand causes pain, the injury is in the hip area. If not, place the heel of one hand on the patient's pubic bone with your fingers pointing down the thigh, and the

Fig. 8.11 *Improvised Fixation Splints*

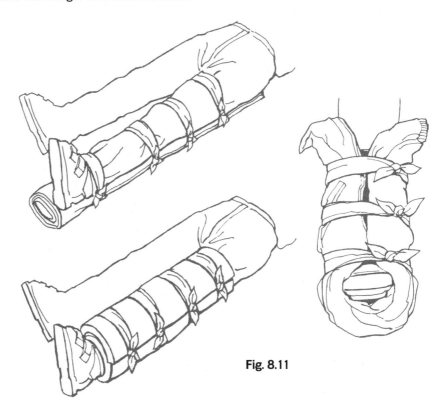

Fig. 8.11

heel of the other hand on the patient's patella with your fingers pointing up the thigh. If the suspected fracture is between the fingertips of the two hands, a traction splint is indicated.

The original traction splint was the **Thomas splint**, developed during World War I by Sir Hugh Owen Thomas. It was a revolutionary device that dramatically reduced mortality from fractured femurs during that war, probably because it reduced bleeding and prevented shock. The original splint had a full ring but was later modified by Keller and Blake to make the familiar half-ring splint (Fig. 8.12). For simplicity, in the following pages of this textbook the term "Thomas splint" will

be used generically to refer to Thomas types of half-ring splints, both commercial and improvised.

The basic Thomas splint is a rigid, longitudinal metal frame about 4 feet long, notched at the narrow end and attached at the wide end to a padded half-ring to which is fastened a strap with a buckle. The half-ring is angled

to fit comfortably behind the upper thigh against the ischial tuberosity and is hinged so it can be used for either the right or the left lower extremity. The strap is buckled in front of the thigh to keep the half-ring in place.

At least two rescuers are needed to apply a Thomas splint. If the splint is an adjustable model, it should be measured against the uninjured side and adjusted so that the end of the splint extends 12 inches beyond the foot or boot. Loosen the boot by unbuckling it and rebuckling it in a slightly looser mode. To stabilize the fracture manually, one rescuer grasps the toe of the patient's boot or foot with one hand and the patient's calf with the other, and exerts axial traction. If enough help is available, a second rescuer can support the patient's thigh with one hand above

Fig. 8.12 *Keller-Blake Half-ring Modification of Thomas Splint*

Fig. 8.13 *Application Technique for a Modified Thomas Splint*

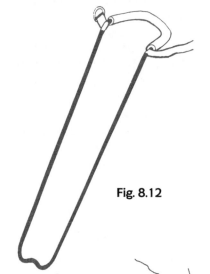

Fig. 8.12

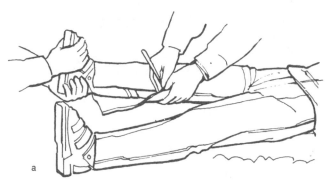

a

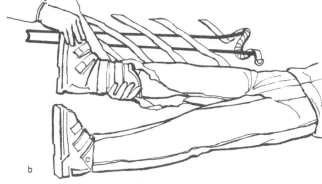

b

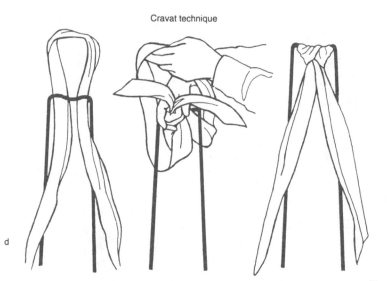

Nylon cord technique

Cravat technique

c

d

Fig. 8.13

and one below the fracture site. The first rescuer's hand position makes it easier to apply a traction hitch or cravat (described below) than if the boot were grasped with both hands. To expose the injury site, remove overlying clothing by cutting or ripping along a seam (Fig. 8.13a). Care for any wounds discovered as described previously under **Open Fractures**.

An angulated fracture must be aligned before the splint can be applied. This is done by two rescuers as described previously, one supporting and steadying the thigh and the other straightening the angulation while applying axial traction. Place the splint beside the injured extremity so that the long side will be on the outside of the extremity. Prepare four cravats (or Velcro support straps) and lay them on the splint, spaced so that two will lie above the knee and two below the knee (Fig. 8.13b). Tie the end of a 50-inch piece of $1/8$- or $1/4$-inch nylon line to the end of the splint with two half-hitches (Fig. 8.13c). Or, if you plan to use the Spanish windlass for traction, attach a cravat with a girth hitch (Fig. 8.13d). Meanwhile, the first rescuer continues axial traction on the boot and calf as the second rescuer puts an ankle hitch in place. This can be a sprained-ankle bandage made from a cravat (Fig. 8.13e), a hitch made from two cravats (Fig. 8.13j), or a commercial hitch made of nylon webbing (Fig. 8.14b). Note that many commercial hitches are too small to go around a ski boot.

To tie a sprained-ankle bandage (Fig. 8.13e), place the middle part of

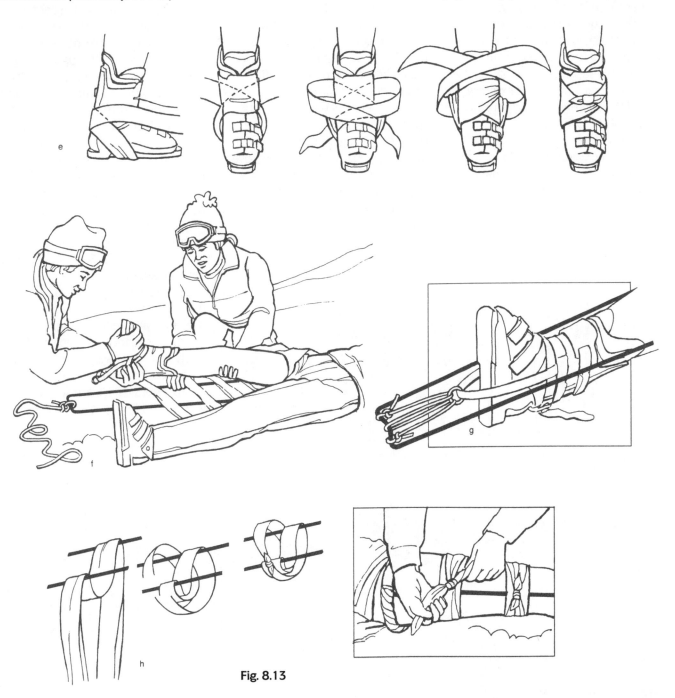

Fig. 8.13

a 2-inch cravat in the instep of the boot of the injured extremity, forming a stirrup. The ends are crossed behind the ankle, brought around in front of the ankle, and crossed again. Each end is run under the first part of the cravat on that side of the foot, then pulled medially around it. The two ends are tied together in front of the ankle with a square knot. The cravat should be free of wrinkles and snug but not tight.

After the ankle hitch is in place, the first rescuer continues to apply axial traction, and the second rescuer supports the injury site while both rescuers raise the extremity several inches off the ground. While supporting the injury site with one hand, the second rescuer slides the traction splint under the extremity until the half-ring is snugly in place against the ischial tuberosity (Fig. 8.13f).

Lay the distal end of the splint on a rock or piece of wood so that it is a few inches off the ground and will not allow the patient's heel to touch the ground when the splint is in place. Maintain axial traction while the extremity is lowered onto the splint. The second rescuer buckles the strap in front of the upper thigh to hold the half-ring in place and threads the end of the 50-inch nylon line through the stirrup of the ankle hitch, back over the end of the splint, back through the stirrup again, and back to the end of the splint, forming a pulley system with a 4-to-1 mechanical advantage (Fig. 8.13g).

As the second rescuer pulls the nylon line tight, the first rescuer gradually releases manual traction, transferring it to mechanical traction. The line is tightened until the pain is improved, then tied off to the end of the splint with two half-hitches. The loose ends of each of the four cravats lying across the splint are reversed, brought under and around the opposite sides of the splint, over and around the extremity, and tied together at the side of the splint, forming a series of cradle hitches (Fig. 8.13h). If Velcro straps are being used instead, they are put in place firmly around the limb.

Traction to the lower extremity is more comfortable when applied with the knee *slightly flexed*. Also, the knee joint is more rigid in this position, which allows the traction to be concentrated on the femur rather than on the knee joint. This can be achieved with a Thomas-type splint by putting padding on a strap placed under the knee.

A less-effective alternative to the pulley system described above is the venerable "Spanish windlass." In this method, a cravat or nylon cord is attached to the end of the splint with a girth hitch. The two loose ends are passed downward through the stirrup of the ankle bandage, run laterally around the bars of the splint, and tied together with a square knot. A short stick or dowel inserted between the two ends midway between the foot and the end of the splint is twisted to produce the desired amount of traction. The stick is then taped to the sides of the splint (Fig. 8.13i).

Commercially available modifications of the Thomas splint, such as the Hare splint (Fig. 8.14a), use Velcro straps instead of cradle hitches and a ratchet at the end of the splint for mechanical traction. Commercially available ankle hitches (Fig. 8.14b) are more comfortable and simpler to apply, but some are too small to fit over ski boots or heavy mountaineering boots. There are special conversion kits that give an ordinary

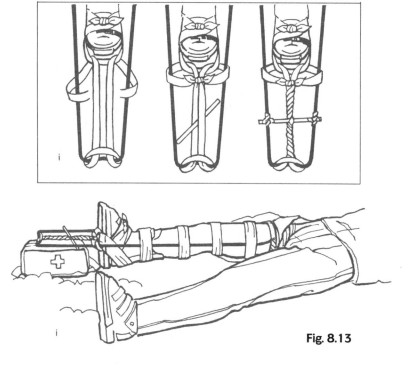

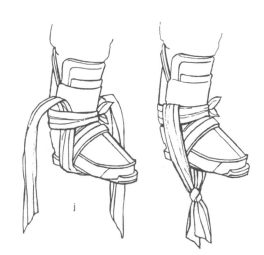

Fig. 8.13

Thomas splint some of the features of a Hare splint. Rescuers should not choose a splint that uses ratchet traction unless they are trained to use it properly. If applied too tightly, such devices are uncomfortable and can cause pressure damage to the buttock or even loss of pulses in the foot from pressure around the ankle.

In general, a traction harness applied over a boot is more comfortable than one applied over an unbooted foot. The boot protects against cold, provides additional support, and distributes the pressure from the harness over a larger area of the foot. When purchasing a traction splint for use on patients wearing boots, make sure the harness supplied with the splint is large enough to fit over most ski boots. In some cases a larger harness will have to be ordered separately; it should be the type labeled as "suitable for climbing, ski, or combat boots" and should be tried out before being used in the field.

In a pinch, improvise a traction hitch from one or two cravats (Figs. 8.13e, 8.13j). It is generally safe to apply traction to a booted foot for several hours; longer periods of time introduce the danger of pressure damage to the tissues of the foot. Question the patient periodically about his or her ability to wiggle the toes and any new numbness or pain in the toes or foot. If there is any question of pressure damage or compromise of circulation or nerve function, the traction should be released, manual traction substituted, the boot removed, the foot and ankle inspected, and traction reapplied to the unbooted foot, if necessary.

Several newer devices for traction are portable, lightweight, readily adjustable, and compact enough so that a splinted patient will usually fit into a helicopter. The Sager splint (Fig. 8.15) weighs less than 4½ pounds and breaks down to fit into a tapering package that measures 32 inches by 6 inches by 4 inches. It has a single longitudinal support that can be positioned either to the inside or the outside of the lower extremity. A new version of the Sager splint allows traction to be applied to both lower extremities at the same time. The Kendrick traction device is a similar splint that uses an aluminum pole to provide longitudinal support. It weighs about 20 ounces and breaks down to form a package about 10 by 5½ by 3 inches. Because of their simplicity, smaller size, and weight, these two splints are probably the

Fig. 8.14 *Commercial Traction Splint*

Fig. 8.15 *Sager Splint*

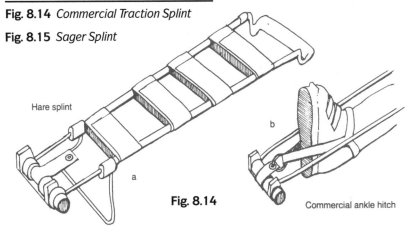

Hare splint

a

b

Fig. 8.14

Commercial ankle hitch

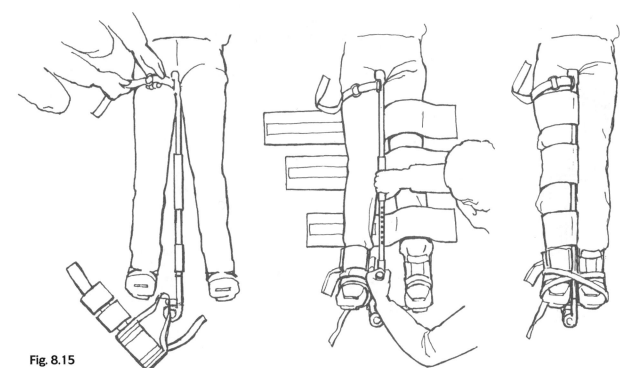

Fig. 8.15

best choices for backcountry rescue groups, whereas the Sager splint is replacing the Thomas types of splints in many urban EMS groups. Neither the Sager nor the Kendrick comes with a traction harness large enough to fit over a ski boot or large climbing boot, however, and the harnesses may have to be replaced or altered. Oversnow rescue groups may prefer to improvise traction splints from ski poles as described below.

The following is a summary of how to apply the Sager splint to the inside of the lower extremity. Also consult the manufacturer's directions.

1. Expose the fracture site and care for any wounds present. Remove the splint from its case, and attach the foam-covered, T-shaped groin piece to the top of the splint. Adjust the plastic buckle so that, when closed, it will be on the front of the thigh. Estimate the necessary splint length by holding the splint next to the lower extremity so that the wheel is just below the heel.

2. Slide the thigh strap under the extremity so that the groin

Fig. 8.16 *Improvised Traction Splint Using a Single Ski*

piece is snug against the crotch and the ischial tuberosity. Patients wearing tight under-clothing or jeans, especially men, may find this position uncomfortable unless the tight clothing is removed or cut open.

3. Close the buckle and tighten the thigh strap so that the groin piece is drawn sideways into the crotch.

4. Estimate the size of the ankle, and fold the number of (included) pads needed to provide padding around the ankle. Remove the patient's boot and sock, and apply the ankle harness tightly around the ankle above the malleoli. Check foot pulses before and afterward.

5. Shorten the loop of the ankle harness connected to the cable ring by pulling on the strap threaded through the square D-buckle.

6. Extend the splint by pressing down on the red thumb piece and sliding the inner part out until the desired amount of traction is noted on the cali-brated wheel. A rough guide is 10 percent of body weight up to a maximum of 22 to 25 pounds, with 10 to 15 pounds being average traction.

7. Fasten the splint to the extrem-ity by applying the three 6-

inch-wide straps. Place the longest as high on the thigh as possible. Pad the area between the metal bar and the extrem-ity. Apply the second longest strap around the knee and the shortest over the ankle har-ness and lower leg. Apply the figure-of-eight strap over and around the ankles to hold the extremities together.

Improvised Traction Splints

If standard traction equipment is not available, a Thomas-type traction splint can be improvised from a single ski or from two ski poles.

For the **single-ski technique** (Fig. 8.16), purchase or prepare in advance two canvas pockets—one to slip over each end of the ski. Each pocket should have a grommet on one side of the base. Cravats can substitute for the pockets. To construct the splint, slip the pockets in place, with the tail of the ski toward the patient's armpit, the tip turned out, and the grommets facing the patient.

One rescuer applies steady man-ual traction to the foot and calf until splinting is completed. Run a cravat around the patient's upper thigh and snug it up into the patient's groin. Tie the tails of the cravat through the grommet of the tail pocket. Apply an ankle bandage or hitch to the boot. Apply traction to the boot in the manner described above for the

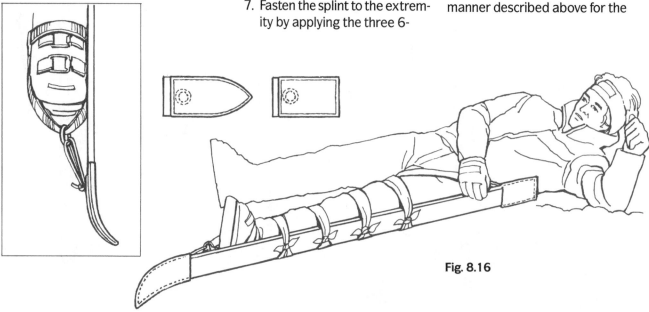

Fig. 8.16

Thomas half-ring splint, using either a nylon cord run in pulley-fashion through the grommet of the tip pocket and the stirrup of the ankle hitch, or a Spanish windlass with a cravat or cord.

Pad any areas where the lower extremity touches the ski. Wrap several wide cravats around the limb and ski from ankle to lower thigh. Support the tip of the ski to keep the patient's heel off the ground. After securing traction, stabilize the splint by wrapping cravats around the upper end of the ski and the trunk, and by tying the uninjured leg to the splint.

An acceptable type of Thomas splint can be made from two ski poles, provided they are long enough. The **two-ski-pole technique** (Fig. 8.17) makes a useful, improvised emergency traction splint for ski tourers and oversnow wilderness rescue groups. It requires a minimum of six cravats (five, if a commercial ankle hitch is available). Interlace or tie the pole straps together to form a half-ring no greater than one-half the thigh circumference. Join the baskets with a spreader such as an 8-inch length of ski pole that has two holes drilled in it the proper distance apart (prepared beforehand and carried in the first aid kit). Lay four cravats to use as cradle hitches across the two poles, apply an ankle bandage or ankle hitch to the boot, and attach a cravat or nylon cord to the spreader. Use manual axial traction in the same manner as described above for the Thomas splint. Slip the splint under the extremity so that the padded pole straps ride up under the buttock. Secure the splint at the groin by tying the handles of the poles together in front of the hip with a cravat. Set up a pulley device or Spanish windlass and apply traction. Finally, tighten the cradle hitches in place.

If no traction splint is available, traction can be applied to the lower extremity of a patient on a scoop stretcher (see **Spine Immobilization Devices**, below) by using the metal bar that forms the end of the stretcher as an anchor for a nylon cord pulley or Spanish windlass. However, the patient's torso first must be immobilized on the stretcher to keep the traction from pulling the patient toward the end of the stretcher. Use two cravats to immobilize the torso. Loop one around each thigh at the groin and tie them off to the side bar through a handhold.

Spine Immobilization Devices

Spine immobilization devices for neck and back injuries include the various types of long and short spine boards, modifications of the short board, such as vest-type devices, and collar-like devices applied around the neck.

When a person lies supine on a long spine board, the parts of the body *that contact the board* are the back of the head, the shoulders and upper back, the buttocks and sacrum, the calves, and the heels. The neck and lumbar spine do not contact the board and, depending on physical build, the thighs may or may not contact the board. Immobilization requires that immobilization straps be placed across the parts of the body that contact the board and that padding be placed beneath the parts that do not. So that the body is maintained in the neutral, in-line position, padding also may have to be placed beneath the head and, in small children (who have relatively large heads compared to the size of their bodies), beneath the trunk.

The spine can be thought of as composed of two long bones and three joints. The "bones" are the cervical and thoracolumbar segments of the spine; the joints are the joint between the first cervical vertebra and the skull, the joint between the seventh cervical and first thoracic vertebrae, and the joint between the fifth lumbar vertebra and the sacrum. The same principles that apply to immobilization of fractures of long bones also apply to the spine. Immobilizing the neck requires, at a minimum, immobilizing the joint above and below it; immobilizing the thoracolumbar spine requires immobilizing the joint above and below it. For practical purposes, however, immobilizing an injured back on a spine board requires that the shoulders, pelvis, thighs, and legs be immobilized. For an injured neck, the head also should be immobilized. Since these objectives can be accomplished only with a *long* spine board, short boards and their derivatives are used only temporarily for extrication and are "backed up" with a long spine board as soon as possible.

Long spine boards are also useful for fractures of the hip and pelvis, dislocations of the hip, and in multiple fractures where individual splinting of each fracture may be impractical. Many types of commercial long spine

Fig. 8.17 *Improvised Traction Splint Using Two Ski Poles*

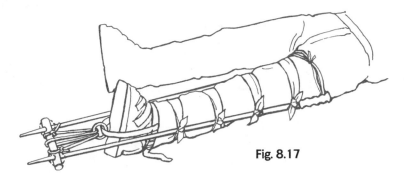

Fig. 8.17

boards are available, each of which has its enthusiastic proponents; however, homemade varieties are inexpensive and quite satisfactory. The spine board should *not* contain screws, nails, or other metallic objects, because a patient immobilized on a long spine board will need X-rays and frequently CT (computerized tomography) scans, MRI (magnetic resonance imaging) scans, and/or other special imaging after arrival at the hospital. Before choosing or constructing a long spine board, consider the type of terrain likely to be involved and the types and dimensions of transport devices or vehicles likely to be used (e.g., toboggans, litters, and helicopters).

A typical long spine board can be made from ¾-inch high-density marine or other high quality plyboard 72 inches by 17 inches. It is finished on both sides, sanded, and then varnished or painted. The eight handholes, which can double as strap holes, have rounded edges, measure 5 inches by 1¼ inches, and are 1¼ inches from the edge of the board. The strap holes, which are staggered between the handholes, measure ½ inch by 3 inches and are ¾ inches from the edge of the board. The runners, which are glued to the board, are 1-inch half-rounds with tapered ends to elevate the board so that the bearers can insert their hands under the board into the handholes. The ends of the runners and the board are tapered to allow the board to slide easily. For patient comfort, a sheet of Ensolite or similar material is glued to the top surface of the board.

The patient is secured to the board with a minimum of four adjustable straps of seat-belt-width nylon strapping, preferably fastened with adjustable Fastex buckles. A fifth strap or cravat helps to immobilize the patient's arms at the sides. Special one-piece, adjustable strap systems are available commercially. To immobilize the head and neck, place rolled towels or blankets on each side of the patient's head and tape in place. To keep the legs from shifting laterally, place a rolled towel on the outside of each leg and hold it in place with the leg strap. Commercial head immobilizers also are available. These, together with padding and extra cravats for additional immobilization, are kept in a stuff-sack stored with the board.

If the spine board is likely to be tipped into a head-up or head-down position (e.g., to ascend or descend a steep hill by toboggan), extra straps should be used to prevent axial shifting. Apply these over each of the patient's shoulders in a criss-cross fashion to prevent headward shifting, and around each groin to prevent footward shifting.

Also available are commercial boards that have multiple strap holes or that use an adjustable clamp system so the straps can be moved up and down the board to fit patients of various sizes. An adjustable system can be fashioned by using a strip of heavy-duty nylon webbing or 8-millimeter climbing rope fastened along each side of the board to form a series of 3-inch loops to which the straps are fastened with Velcro. To avoid using screws or bolts, drill a hole through the board every 3 inches, place a loop of the webbing or rope through the hole, and secure the loop with a knot. The straps are secured to the loops with plastic clamps.

The aluminum scoop stretcher (Fig. 8.18) is a recent variation of the long spine board that also is designed for extrication. Since it is not as rigid as a spine board, its use alone for immobilizing patients with neck or back injuries is not recommended. A rigid collar (described below) should be used with the scoop stretcher, and it should be backed up with a long spine board as soon as possible. The scoop stretcher is adjustable in length and breaks apart longitudinally into two halves that are slid under the patient from either side until they meet in the middle. This eliminates the manipulation needed to apply a short spine board or vest-type device (described below) or the need to lift or logroll the patient onto a long spine board. One version of the scoop stretcher folds in thirds so that it can be carried on a pack frame. Only two rescuers are needed to use a scoop stretcher, as opposed to three or four for a spine board.

Disadvantages of the scoop stretcher include the need to have access to both sides of the patient. Special care must be taken to strap the patient securely to the stretcher

Fig. 8.18 *Scoop Stretcher*

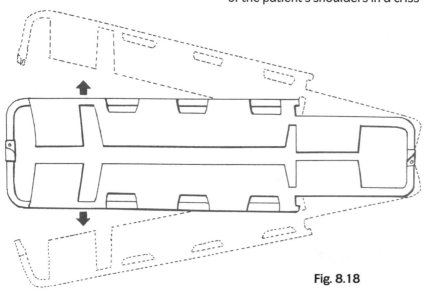

Fig. 8.18

so it can be safely tipped to the side if the patient vomits. Made of metal, the scoop stretcher interferes with X-rays and scans. It can be cold for the patient and for rescuers' hands unless padded, tends to split with tall, heavy patients, and has latches that can fill with snow and freeze.

Vacuum whole-body immobilizers based on the same principles as the vacuum splints (described previously under **Soft Fixation Splints**) also are available.

Long Spine Board
Application Technique (Fig. 8.19)

The patient is almost always strapped to a spine board in the supine position. This position provides the best immobilization and is easiest for monitoring the airway and vital signs and giving basic life support if needed. If not found supine, the patient should be turned by safe techniques (described in Chapter 13). If a head or neck injury is suspected, the patient's head and neck must be stabilized manually until the patient is fully immobilized on the long spine board. A rigid collar is applied also.

Lay the long spine board on the ground next to the patient (Fig. 8.19a). In the case of a child with a large head in relation to the size of the trunk, pad the board with a folded blanket under the patient's back and hips so that, when on the spine board, the head and neck will be in the neutral position. Tie the patient's ankles together with a cravat to keep the lower extremities from rotating outward during transfer and causing the lumbosacral spine to shift position. Transfer the patient to the board using the **four-person logroll** (Fig. 8.19b) or the **four-person direct ground lift** (Chapters 13 and 20). Assess and record sensation and motion below the injury immediately before and after the transfer and at regular intervals thereafter.

Secure the patient's trunk and lower extremities to the board, using at least four nylon straps as described above: one around the chest just below the armpits, one around the pelvis, one around the thighs, and

Fig. 8.19 *Long Spine Board Application Technique*

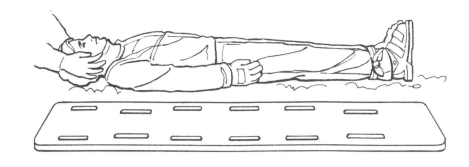

one around the ankles (Fig. 8.19c). If there is a pelvic fracture, place the pelvic straps around the patient's upper thighs and the thigh straps just above the knees. Immobilize the patient's upper extremities to his or her sides with the palms against the thighs, using a fifth strap or cravat. Place a rolled towel or other firm

a

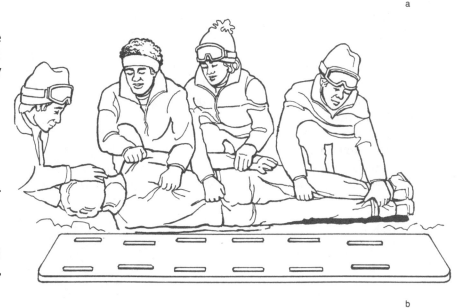

b

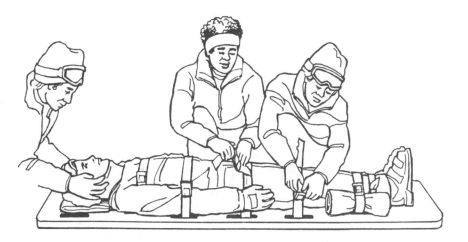

c

Fig. 8.19

padding under the leg strap against the outside of each leg to keep the legs from shifting laterally. Pad between the knees and beneath the small of the back and the back of the knees.

In the case of a neck injury, while maintaining manual head stabilization with the patient's head and neck in the neutral, in-line position, have another rescuer estimate the distance between the patient's head and the surface of the spine board, and insert enough padding into this space to maintain the neutral position. Secure the head (Fig. 8.19d) by placing a head support on either side of the head and running an immobilizing strap from the edge of the board, firmly around the head support on one side, across the forehead, around the head support on the other side, and to the other edge of the board. Run a second immobilizing strap in a similar manner from the edge of the board, across the head support, the rigid collar, the opposite head support, and to the other edge of the board. Adhesive tape, duct tape, roller bandage, or a Velcro strap or cravat can serve as immobilizing straps. The straps will be more stable if they are run completely around the bottom of the board as well; have an assistant lift the head off the board a few inches while you do this.

Do *not* place a strap across the chin. A chin strap cannot adequately secure the head because of the mobility of the jaw. Also, a patient who vomits with a chin strap in place may choke.

Head supports should be firm, lightweight, and noncompressible. Two large bath towels, firmly rolled and taped beforehand, are ideal. Fold each towel to one-quarter width lengthwise and roll it to form a cylinder 5 to 6 inches in diameter. Place one rolled towel on each side of the head. If smaller towels are used, two or more on each side of the head may be necessary.

Another good technique is to make a "horse collar" out of a rolled blanket folded into a U-shape. Do not use sandbags because, if the board is tipped on its side, their weight may make them sag and cause the neck to bend. Commercial head immobilizers also are quite satisfactory although more expensive. They should be used according to the manufacturer's directions.

Strap the patient to the board with enough properly tightened straps so the patient will not shift if the board is tipped onto its side.

Tipping may be necessary to aid in airway management and to avoid aspiration if the patient vomits. Back up the four basic straps with cravats or additional straps if necessary. As mentioned above, if axial shifting is a possibility, criss-cross straps over the shoulders and/or groin straps may be advisable (Fig. 8.19e). Attach each shoulder strap to the side of the board slightly below the top of the patient's shoulder, run it up and over the shoulder, cross it over the chest, and attach it to the opposite side of the board below the opposite armpit. The location of the buckles should be easily adjustable for the patient's comfort. Attach each groin strap to the side of the board at the level of the iliac crest and run it around the groin anteriorly, between the legs, and around the buttock, and attach it to the same side. Groin straps should not be used if a fractured pelvis is suspected.

Short Spine Boards and Vest-type Devices

Short spine boards were developed to evacuate patients with spine injuries from a sitting position in the front seat of a wrecked vehicle. They also can be used to immobilize the neck and back of a patient who must be extricated from an awkward position, for example, an injured climber on a narrow ledge or in a crevasse, a skier in a tree well, or a caver in a narrow cave passage. Short spine boards are quite functional. Most backcountry rescue groups and urban EMS units have, however, replaced them with vest-type devices, which are lighter, more compact, and easier to store and carry. Both short spine boards and vest-type devices are used *only for extrication*. The patient with the device in place should be immobilized on a long spine board as soon as possible.

Since a certain amount of manipulation is necessary to apply these

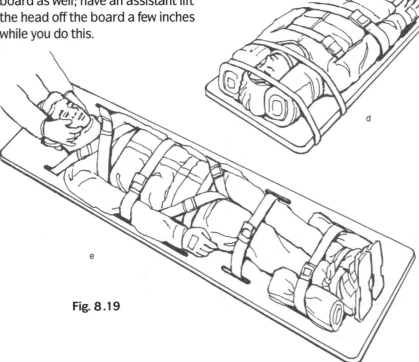

Fig. 8.19

short devices, each case should be individualized. In many cases, if a long spine board can be brought up quite near the patient, a multiple-rescuer lift or axial slide may cause less motion at the site of injury (Chapter 20). Many rescue groups use a vest-type device plus a semi-rigid litter such as the Thompson, Ferno-Washington, or SKED to both immobilize and transport patients with neck and back injuries. The SKED is designed to be used with the Oregon spine splint II (see below).

A short spine board (Fig. 8.20), which can be made from a piece of high-quality plyboard, should measure about half the length (36 inches) of a long spine board.

To position the short spine board, one rescuer stabilizes the patient's head and neck, while a second rescuer puts a rigid collar in place. Continue the manual stabilization until the patient is immobilized on the short board. Slide the short board behind the patient so that its bottom is level with the patient's hips. Secure the board to the patient's torso with cravats or straps. One strap goes around the chest under the armpits and a second strap goes around the abdomen below the costal arches. The patient's arms are placed at his

or her sides with the palms turned inward and secured with a third strap around the chest and upper arms. Place a rolled towel on each side of the patient's head, and secure the head to the board with one immobilizing strap (tape, Velcro strap, or a cravat) around the two towels and across the forehead, and a second one across the two towels and the rigid collar.

Next, carry the patient to a site where he or she can be fastened supine—with the short spine board in place—to a long spine board. The two-person seated carry (Chapter 20) is a suitable method to use.

Vest-type devices are made of sturdy nylon in the shape of a vest, strengthened with longitudinal slats, and provided with attached straps. This gives them fairly good longitudinal rigidity while allowing them to be rolled into a small cylinder for carrying. Two examples are the Kendrick extrication device (KED) and the Oregon spine splint II. Both are designed to be used with a rigid collar. The manufacturer's directions for applying these devices should be consulted in each case.

When moving a patient who has been fastened to a short spine board or who is wearing a vest-type device, move the *patient*, not the *device. Do not* use the board as a handle for moving or lifting the patient.

The KED (Fig. 8.21) was the first to be developed. It weighs about 7 pounds and rolls up into a package about 34 inches by 11 inches by 5 inches. Four 1-inch wide slats provide longitudinal stability.

To apply the KED, slide it behind the patient, wrap the sides around the patient's trunk, and secure them with the three horizontal chest straps. Wrap the groin straps around the patient's thighs at the groin. Immobilize the head using the side flaps on each side of the patient's head, and secure them with one strap across the forehead and one across the rigid collar.

The Oregon spine splint II is a similar device, but uses two 3½-inch-wide slats to provide longitudinal stability. It weighs about 9 pounds and rolls up into a package about 35 by 6 by 7 inches. This splint has four chest straps instead of three—two of which go over the shoulder and criss-cross the chest. This device may be preferred to the KED because it prevents axial shifting better and the groin straps are positioned so the patient can be laid from a sitting to a supine position on a long spine board without loosening them.

A spine board can be improvised from a long, sturdy board, a door, or two skis fastened rigidly side-by-side with crosspieces such as thick tree branches.

Rigid Collars

These devices, also called **cervical collars**, **c-collars**, and **extrication collars**, are widely used in the EMS system to immobilize the neck in patients with suspected neck injuries (Fig. 8.22). They are used not only for extrication but are an essential part of vest-type devices. Many protocols specify that *all* patients immobilized on a long spine board have a rigid collar applied as well, because any trauma capable of causing a

Fig. 8.20 *Short Spine Board*

Fig. 8.21 *Kendrick Extrication Device (KED)*

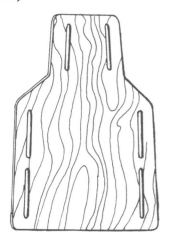

Fig. 8.20

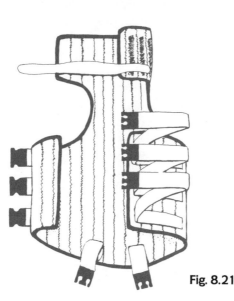

Fig. 8.21

back injury also may have caused a neck injury. However, there is *no* currently available rigid collar that satisfactorily prevents all excessive flexion, extension, rotation, and lateral bending of an injured neck. Therefore, although the collar will add some stability, *do not rely upon the collar alone to stabilize a neck injury*. Also, do not use the collar alone, except perhaps in the rare case when a patient with a possible neck injury must be removed from danger too rapidly to allow full spine board application. Application of a rigid collar always must be accompanied by manual stabilization followed by immobilization of the patient on a spine board.

There is another important reason why a patient with a neck injury should have a rigid collar in place even though immobilized on a long spine board: the rigid collar is the only available device that will *resist axial loading* of the cervical spine. Axial loading, an important cause of further injury, is inevitable in a patient who is being transported by toboggan or motor vehicle, because changes in speed and the pull of gravity when going up- or downhill cause compression of the head on the neck.

The collar also provides the important function of *calling attention to the possible presence of a neck injury*.

It is easier to apply a collar if the rescuer puts his or her hands on the sides of the patient's head to stabilize the neck, rather than lower down with the fingers under or behind the jaw. Applying a collar can be very difficult if the patient is wearing several layers of garments with high necks.

There are many good commercial collars available, both single piece and two piece. Many brands come in multiple sizes. Always follow the manufacturer's instructions for size selection, application, and care of the collar. The best collar is one that is familiar to the rescuer, fits the patient, and produces a minimum of head and neck motion during application. The collar should limit neck motion well but at the same time allow the patient's mouth to be opened if vomiting occurs. Two-piece collars are somewhat easier to apply than one-piece collars. Rigid collars should be stored in a warm place, since they tend to stiffen in the cold. *Soft collars have no place in the emergency care of an injured neck.*

A rigid collar can be improvised from a blanket tightly rolled into a 4- to 6-inch diameter. The blanket should be centered at the back of the neck, with the ends brought over the shoulders, crossed over the chest in an X, and brought under the opposite armpits (Fig. 8.23). The SAM splint, mentioned earlier, can be molded into a rigid collar, and suitable collars can be made from tightly rolled towels or garments made into a sausage shape by being wrapped round and round with a rubberized bandage.

Fig. 8.22 *Rigid Collar*

Fig. 8.23 *Improvised Rigid Collar Using a Blanket*

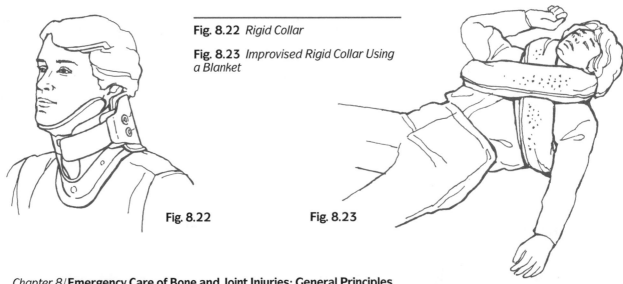

Fig. 8.22   Fig. 8.23

Scenario #8 (Fig. 8.24)

The following scenario illustrates the care of two types of injuries to bones.

You have just received a transmission from the hill chief asking you to check out a jump that some skiers have made on an ungroomed run just below the summit. As you approach, you see a group of teenaged boys gathered at the top of a narrow run leading to a heaped-up mound of snow. One boy is preparing to push off from the top of the run. To your experienced eye, the landing area below the mound looks too close to a small rock pile. Before you can get within shouting distance, the skier is on the run and heading swiftly for the jump. His form doesn't look good to you, and as he sails off the top of the mound, his balance is off. When he lands, he bounces off a large rock, falls, and starts to scream. One of his companions waiting below starts side-stepping up to him. You arrive at his side, kick out of your bindings, and stick your skis in the snow in the form of an X. You quickly approach the skier, who is lying on his back, moaning softly, with his left thigh bent back at an abnormal angle.

You: "I'm Ben Schussen of the High Range Ski Patrol. Can I help you?"

Skier: "Oh! Oh! Oh! Please, my leg."

You: (Removing one of his gloves, you assess his radial pulse. It is strong, regular, and about 100 beats per minute. His breathing appears easy and quiet but faster than normal, about 20 per minute.) "I saw you land. Did you hurt yourself anywhere else besides your thigh?"

Skier: (moaning) "My back hurts between my shoulder blades."

You: (after radioing for a toboggan, backboard, traction splint, oxygen, suction, and some help) "Did you hit your head?"

Skier: "No."

You: "Did you hit your neck?"

Skier: "No."

You: "Try to lie still until we get some help and can get you down the hill. What's your name?"

Skier: "Dan Jerass."

You: "Where are you from?"

Skier: "Denver."

You: "Do you know your age and what day it is?"

Skier: "I'm 17 and it's Saturday, March third."

Fig. 8.24 *Scenario #8*

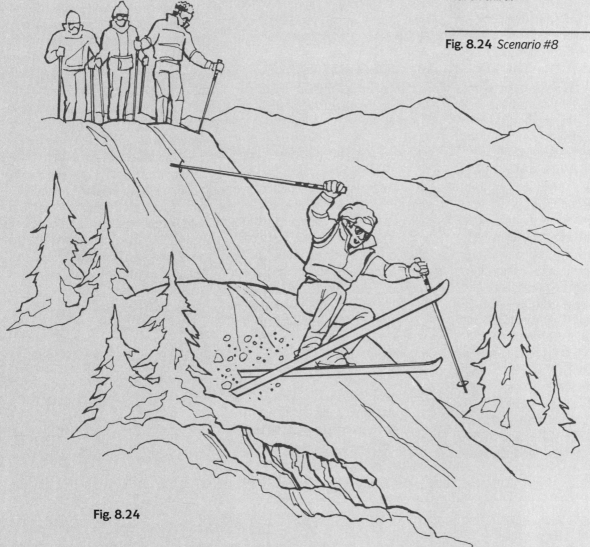

Fig. 8.24

You are satisfied that the patient's airway is normal, his breathing is adequate, and his circulation normal. It is time to examine the areas of complaint.

You: "I'm going to examine your thigh. I'll let you know everything I'll do before I do it."

You gently palpate the patient's left thigh starting at the groin. He winces when you reach the midthigh and you believe there is a bulge there. You compare it with the same part of the right thigh and see that there definitely is a difference. You continue down the thigh and palpate the knee and leg. There are no obvious abnormalities. You then assess the right lower extremity; it appears normal.

You: "Can you feel your left foot?"

Skier: "Yes."

You: "Can you wiggle your toes?"

Skier: "Yes."

You: "Next, I'm going to run my hand behind your neck and back. Let me know if I hit a tender spot. Try not to move."

You gently palpate each spinous process in turn from the base of the skull to the lower sacrum. There is definite tenderness over two of the midthoracic spinous processes.

So far there is no sign of the other patrollers and the toboggan. You start the secondary survey, assessing his scalp, face, eyes, ears, nose, and mouth. There is no sign of any wounds, bleeding, tenderness or swelling. The pupils are equal and respond to light. There is no bleeding or discharge from the nose and ears. Your flashlight is not working, but you do not see any obvious abnormalities in his mouth. Moving down to his neck, you find no wounds, bleeding, tenderness, or swelling. The trachea is in the midline.

By the time you have assessed his chest, abdomen and pelvis, you catch sight of your friend Joe headed

this way with the toboggan, accompanied by two other patrollers. You quickly assess the patient's upper extremities as Joe arrives with the toboggan and anchors it with his skis below the patient.

You direct your three fellow patrollers to assist you. Mike places one hand on each side of the patient's head and stabilizes the head and neck manually. Pete affixes a Stifneck hard collar around the patient's neck. Joe takes the Sager splint out of the toboggan pack and removes the splint from its container. Meanwhile, you have unbuckled the patient's left boot and rebuckled it slightly looser. While Joe supports the patient's thigh with one hand on each side of the injury, you grasp the toe of the patient's boot with one hand and his calf with the other.

You: "Dan, we are going to put this traction splint on your leg. It will feel much better as soon as we get it on. First, I have to straighten your leg a little. I'll be as gentle as I can, but it will hurt for a short time."

You gently straighten the angulated thigh with the aid of slight axial traction. Meanwhile, Joe has assembled the splint and slipped the groin piece between the patient's legs and up against his left ischial tuberosity while Pete supports the patient's leg and thigh. He next secures the upper end of the splint by tightening the groin strap, then secures a special ankle harness—large enough to go around the ski boot—to the patient's ankle and attaches it to the end of the splint. He extends the end of the splint slowly until the gauge reads 15 pounds. You tie the two ankles together.

You: "Does that feel better?"

Patient: "Yes."

The patient's thigh and leg are secured to the splint with the three 6-inch straps. Meanwhile, Pete brings the long spine board over and lays it on the snow beside the patient.

You assess his pulse and breathing again. The pulse is strong and about 100 beats per minute; his respirations are slower at 18 per minute.

You: "Dan, because you may have hurt your back, we are going to transport you down the hill on this special board. I'm going to straighten your arms and then the four of us will lift you carefully onto the board."

Patient: "Okay."

Carefully, the patient's arms are arranged by his side and his wrists tied together in front of him. Four patrollers are needed to lift the patient 6 inches off the snow and slide the long board under him without any twisting or bending of his spine. Quickly, the patient is strapped to the board with one strap across his chest just under his axillae, one across his pelvis, one across his lower thighs, and one across his legs. His arms are secured to his sides with a fifth strap. Towel rolls are placed on the outside of each leg beneath the leg strap, and padding is placed under the small of his back and beneath his head. His head is immobilized with two towel rolls and two straps of adhesive tape. One strap of tape is placed around the top of the board, over the towel rolls, and across his forehead. The other goes across the towel rolls and the hard collar. The board with the patient on it is lifted into the toboggan with its head toward the front of the toboggan. In a few minutes, Dan is on his way to the warm patrol room.

Chapter 9

Mechanisms and Patterns of Injury

Accident, n. An inevitable
occurrence due to the action
of immutable natural laws.

—*Ambrose Bierce*
  The Devil's Dictionary

Injuries in the outdoors are not random examples of the workings of capricious Fate, nor are they the deliberate actions of malevolent gods. The production of injuries is governed by certain laws of physics, anatomy, and physiology. Knowledge of these laws enables us to

1. *understand* how injuries occur and why some injuries are more common than others;
2. *predict* the types and severity of injuries likely to have resulted from an accident based on observation of the accident scene; and
3. *anticipate* the development of life-threatening complications.

The ease with which human body parts are injured depends on their tissue characteristics, the mechanics of their construction, their location, and the manner and frequency of their use.

An elastic tissue such as the skin will deform when a force is applied to it. As the force increases, the threshold of injury eventually will be exceeded, and the skin will be torn or contused. Because skin is soft and elastic, it can be easily deformed without injury, but, conversely, it is more susceptible than harder tissues to cuts and punctures. On the other hand, the hardness and inelasticity of bone make it more resistant to cuts and punctures but less resistant to fracture from deforming forces. Solid organs, such as the spleen and liver, are more susceptible to rupture than are hollow organs, such as the stomach or bladder. However, when hollow organs are distended with fluid, they may be more easily injured than solid organs. Flexible organs that are rigidly anchored, such as the aorta, are more susceptible to injury from displacing forces than are loosely attached, flexible organs that can move within body cavities, such as the intestines.

Organs that are protected by parts of the skeletal system, such as the brain, spinal cord, and the organs of the chest and pelvic cavities, are less prone to injury from equivalent forces than less-protected organs, such as those of the abdominal cavity. The activities of daily life injure the extremities more often than the trunk. The extremities are prone to injury because they frequently are in motion, are located more peripherally, have less protection, and often are used to protect the trunk from injury, e.g., extending the arms to break a fall. The shoulder joint, which has a shallow cup and a wide range of motion, is more often injured than the hip joint, which has a deep cup and a narrow range of motion.

Most injuries are associated with motion—either motion of the human body itself or motion of another object that impacts the body. Therefore, the student should be familiar with the physical laws of motion and with the laws of kinetic energy in particular.

The term **force** is used for any action that changes the state of rest or motion of a body to which it is applied. In physics, a **body** is *any* mass of matter that is distinct from other masses of matter. (In the following pages of this chapter, the term "body," when used alone, will refer to any mass of matter; when the "human body" is meant, it will be so stated). **Energy** is the capacity for doing work. It can be either **potential energy,** which is derived from the position of a body in a gravity field with respect to its own parts or to another body, or **kinetic energy,** which is energy created by motion.

The terms **trauma** and **injury** frequently are used interchangeably. Both refer to damage to the human body by an external force. However, in this chapter, "trauma" refers to the end effect of a force applied to the human body, and "injury" refers to the actual type and extent of human body damage produced by the force or forces.

Newton's First Law of Motion states that a body at rest will tend to remain at rest and a body in motion will tend to remain in motion unless acted upon by an outside force. For example, a moving skier will continue to move in a straight line unless he or she applies energy through the leg muscles to produce a turning motion (Fig. 9.1a) or collides with an obstacle such as a tree (Fig. 9.1b).

The Law of Conservation of Energy states that energy can neither be created nor destroyed but may be changed from any form to any other form. For example, the energy of a moving object that strikes the human body does not just disappear. It **dissipates** as it deforms and injures the tissues. The amount of injury is roughly proportional to the amount of energy that has to be dissipated.

The most important aspect of kinetic energy is its *relationship to velocity,* or speed. The speed of a moving object is much more important than its mass, or weight; since while the amount of kinetic energy produced goes up in *direct* proportion to the increase in mass, it goes up in proportion to the *square* of the speed as the speed increases. For example, if the speed of the object *doubles,* the amount of kinetic energy produced increases *four* times.

Another important type of kinetic energy is the energy of a falling body. Because of the force of gravity, a falling body, regardless of mass, increases its speed by 32 feet per second every second (980.6 centimeters per second per second)—as measured at sea level at 45 degrees latitude—regardless of its mass. This means that a free-falling climber will build up kinetic energy very rapidly. However, the speed of a falling body does not increase infinitely. Because of the resistance of the atmosphere against the body, a final speed of fall is reached, called the **terminal velocity,** when the air resistance equals the pull of gravity.

This varies with the shape of the body, the position in which it is falling, and the density of the air.

Kinetic energy causes injury because it is applied to the human body in the form of a force. Forces have both magnitude (strength) and direction. They act on the human body to move it from a resting position, speed it up (**accelerate**), slow it down or stop it (**decelerate**), and/or change the direction of its motion.

The amount of kinetic energy of a body in motion is equal to one-half the product of the mass of the body times the velocity squared. Thus, when E_k = kinetic energy, M = mass, and V = velocity, then $E_k = M/2 \times V^2$. For example, a 100-pound (45-kilogram) skier traveling at 15 miles per hour (24 kilometers per hour) has a kinetic energy of approximately 1,000 Joules (one Joule = one Kg/m²/second²). A skier who weighs 50 percent more (150 pounds or 70 kilograms) and is traveling at the same speed has a kinetic energy that is 50 percent greater (1,500 Joules). However, a 100-pound skier traveling *twice* as fast (30 miles per hour/48 kilometers per hour) has *four times* (not twice) the kinetic energy (4,000 Joules). If such a skier hits a tree, a large part of the kinetic energy is dissipated by crushing or tearing the skier's body. Thus, hitting a tree at 30 miles per hour can theoretically cause four times as much damage as hitting a tree at 15 miles per hour. (However, remember that the skier can be just as dead after a 15-mile-per-hour collision as after a 30-mile-per-hour collision.)

Types of Trauma

Changes in speed or direction can lead to the following types of trauma: **penetration, compression** ("blunt trauma"), **flexion** (bending), **rotational,** and **distraction** (stretching). Flexion trauma is further divided into **hyperflexion** and **hyperextension**. Pure examples of injuries caused by one force and one type of trauma are unusual; most serious injuries involve more than one force and more than one type of trauma.

The specific injury depends on the magnitude and direction of the force or forces, the type of trauma, and the human body part involved. The type of surface that impacts the human body and the rate of deceleration or acceleration also are important. Landing in deep powder snow after a fall is less dangerous than landing on ice or concrete. Because the rate of deceleration is slower, it is less dangerous to be in a car that runs into a soft snowbank or a stand of small trees than to be in a car that hits a brick wall or a large tree at the same speed.

The effects of trauma can be modified by controlling velocity (i.e., avoiding higher speeds), wearing protective devices such as helmets and seat belts, and slowing the rate of deceleration by trying to tuck and roll when falling forward rather than landing head on and skidding.

Penetration and **compression traumata** are caused by similar forces. The difference is that, in penetration trauma, the size, shape, and sharpness of the wounding object and its speed and/or direction (or the speed and direction of the moving human

Fig. 9.1 *A moving skier will travel in a straight line unless he or she applies energy to turn or collides with an object.*

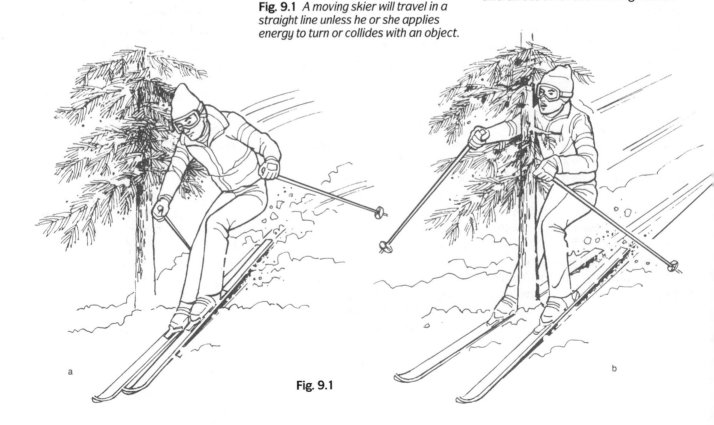

a

b

Fig. 9.1

body that impacts it) are such that the force per unit area is great enough to drive the object through the skin. This may cause a laceration or puncture wound plus damage to deeper tissues. Penetration trauma can be caused by bullets, knives, ice axes, ski pole tips, arrows, and other sharp objects moving at moderate to high speeds. It also can be caused by a moving human body striking a sharp, rough object such as a rock, or a sharp, narrow object such as a broken tree limb (Fig. 9.1b).

In compression (blunt) trauma, the wounding object tends to be larger in diameter and less sharp, or the force is weaker and/or the direction different, so that the skin is not broken (Fig. 9.2). However, compression trauma frequently damages tissues beneath the skin, causing a closed wound, such as a contusion or hematoma, as well as damage to internal organs.

The types of trauma and the various actions of forces can be further illustrated using several common accident patterns. An example of **deceleration** is a full-impact collision between a skier and a tree. On striking the tree, the skier's body comes to an abrupt halt, and its kinetic energy is dissipated through the production of various types of trauma to the skier (Fig. 9.3) and damage to the tree. The specific types of trauma depend on the skier's speed, the skier's body position as it strikes the tree, the angle of impact, the rate of deceleration, the skier's physical condition, the number and strength of layers of clothing worn, and whether the skier is wearing a helmet.

The body parts that directly impact the tree trunk are subject to compression trauma, which squeezes the soft tissues, rupturing blood vessels and producing contusions and hematomas. Compression trauma also can break underlying bones, such as the skull and ribs, and bruise or rupture internal organs. A glancing blow or impact with a sharp part of the tree, such as a broken branch, can produce a shearing type of penetration trauma (produced by one object moving parallel to another object), such as a laceration or abrasion. Full impact with a sharp part of a tree can produce a puncture type of penetration trauma, such as an open chest or abdominal wound.

If the skier strikes the tree at an angle that impacts the midtorso and bends the upper and lower parts of the body like a horseshoe around the tree, the **hyperflexion** type of **bending trauma** can result (Fig. 9.3a). This type of trauma can cause wedge-shaped vertebral compression fractures with the narrow side anteriorly (Fig. 9.3b) or fracture-dislocations of the spine as well as the types of compression and penetrating trauma described above.

The hyperflexion type of bending trauma also can result in a wedge-shaped compression fracture of one or more thoracic or lumbar vertebrae when the body is forced into forward flexion by a decelerating force. This can occur when a climber falls, lands hard on the feet, and pitches forward.

Stronger forces of this type can cause a fracture-dislocation of the spine.

If the skier strikes the tree with the midthigh, hyperflexion trauma can produce a fracture of the middle part of the femoral shaft (Fig. 9.3c). Striking a tree with a bent knee can bring the thigh and leg to a sudden halt (deceleration type of compression trauma) while the pelvis and the rest of the body continue to move forward. This situation, which also is common in automobile accidents when an occupant's knee strikes the dashboard, can cause a patellar fracture (Fig. 9.3e), femur fracture, or fracture-dislocation of the hip joint (Fig. 9.3d) as the force is transmitted up the femur and pops the head of the femur out through the rear of the acetabulum.

If this skier's other foot is wedged under a log for a half hour or longer before it is freed, the resulting tissue damage is a slowly developing type of compression trauma called a **crushing injury** (Fig. 9.3a). A crushing injury involves both direct tissue injury and secondary injury when pressure on the blood vessels causes interference with circulation. Crushing injuries are common in victims of building collapses, mine tunnel collapses, and natural disasters such as earthquakes and hurricanes.

Fig. 9.2 *Compression trauma is produced when a collision with a blunt object stops motion abruptly.*

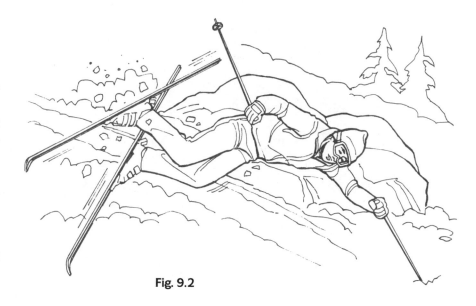

Fig. 9.2

Because many organs are somewhat free to move inside body cavities, they can be injured by **secondary collisions.** When the human body suddenly stops moving (decelerates), internal organs continue to move forward until they collide with the body wall or until their movement is stopped by the tightening of their attachments. At times the attachments will tear, causing severe bleeding. Secondary collisions can injure the brain within the cranial cavity, the heart and aorta within the chest cavity, and the liver, spleen, and intestines within the abdominal cavity.

An example of **acceleration** is when the speed of an automobile suddenly increases when it is struck from the rear by a faster-moving vehicle. Unless an occupant's seat is equipped with a properly positioned headrest, the occupant's neck can be subjected to the **hyperextension** type of **bending trauma.** This type of trauma can cause the type of distraction (stretching) and compression injuries to ligaments and tendons

called a "whiplash," and can even fracture the cervical spine. If a body part strikes or is struck violently and bends suddenly, it tends to develop compression injuries on the side that was struck and distraction injuries on the opposite side.

Catching a pole basket in a tree while wearing the pole strap around the wrist can dislocate a shoulder due to a decelerating force that causes a mixed type of injury. Because of **hyperextension** and **distraction** trauma, the shoulder joint is rotated externally, hyperabducted, and pulled apart by the resulting forces (Fig. 9.4).

Rotational trauma is well known to ski patrollers, who are familiar with the twisting type of deceleration fall that can cause a knee sprain or a spiral fracture of the tibia (Fig. 9.5).

An example of the injury caused by an accelerating force that produces **distraction trauma** alone occurs when a person with long hair

is scalped after the hair is caught in moving machinery such as a surface ski lift.

Frequently, multiple injuries occur, partly because of the continued dissipation of forces over time. The climber who suffers a hard fall may fracture both feet on landing (Fig. 9.6), plus the pelvis and spine as the deceleration force is transmitted headward. Then, as energy continues to dissipate, the climber may pitch forward and land on outstretched hands, fracturing one or both wrists, forearms, or clavicles, and/or dislocating one or both shoulders.

The amount of damage is proportional to the amount of energy involved. For example, if ski bindings do not release, an easy fall may produce a simple fracture of the tibia (Fig. 9.7), while a fall at high speed may cause a comminuted fracture of the tibia (Fig. 9.8). A high-velocity rifle bullet causes much more internal damage and a larger exit wound than a low-velocity pistol bullet of the same caliber.

Fig. 9.3 *Types of Injuries Produced by a Collision*

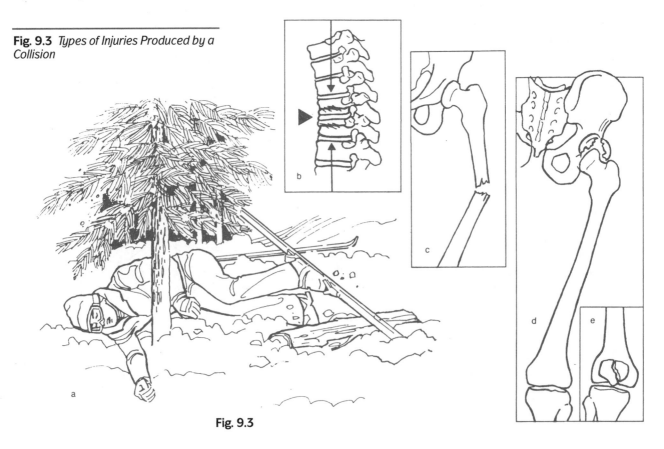

Fig. 9.3

Injuries can be either **direct** or **indirect**. In a direct injury, the trauma occurs at the place where the force meets the body. An example is the contusion produced by compression trauma when a skier falls and hits a rock. In an indirect injury, the force meets the body in such a way that energy is transmitted to another part of the body where the trauma is concentrated and the injury occurs. An example is the dislocated shoulder or fractured clavicle caused by falling forward on an outstretched hand. An important complication of indirect injuries is the development of a **fulcrum point**—the hinge-like point about which a lever turns—which allows an extremity or equipment item such as a ski to function as a lever. This fulcrum can focus forces and multiply them many times.

One of the most valuable benefits derived from the skills of analyzing and understanding mechanisms of injury is the ability to predict potential **internal injuries**. This ability is most important in compression trauma, where visible signs of injury on the body surface may be minimal, and

the signs and symptoms of serious internal injury may not have had time to develop. Although understanding the significance of the mechanism of injury does not replace good assessment skills, it is an additional tool especially important in predicting the possibility of spinal cord injuries and internal injuries to the head, chest, abdomen, and pelvis.

A decelerating force causing compression trauma to the head frequently produces a double injury to the brain: the first injury occurs when the brain strikes the inside of the skull on the side of impact; the second occurs when the brain bounces back and strikes the inside of the skull on the opposite side. This combination is called a **contrecoup** injury.

In addition to causing a compression injury of the chest wall with contusions and multiple broken ribs, a decelerating force may shear off the movable aortic arch from the more fixed thoracic aorta. This type of chest injury also can injure the heart by squeezing it between the sternum and the spine. Such a cardiac contusion can cause the pumping function of the heart to fail or can tear the

heart muscle and cause bleeding into the sac around the heart (pericardial tamponade, see Chapter 14).

In the abdomen and pelvis, compression trauma can fracture the pelvic bones, and the sharp ends of the bones can lacerate the bladder (Fig. 9.9) and pelvic blood vessels. Deceleration and shearing forces also can rupture abdominal organs—particularly the pancreas, spleen, liver, and kidneys—producing serious intra-abdominal bleeding.

Injuries tend to occur in predictable types and combinations. Injuries caused by automobile accidents tend to group according to the vehicle's velocity, the seat the injured person was occupying, whether the seat belt was fastened, whether the impact was direct or rotational, and whether it came from the front, rear, or side.

Most non-vehicular outdoor injuries are related to the type of terrain and the mode of transportation. Skiing is more dangerous than walking and snowshoeing, because the increasing

---

Fig. 9.4 *A ski pole basket that catches on a tree can cause hyperextension and stretching trauma.*

Fig. 9.5 *A twisting fall can produce rotational trauma.*

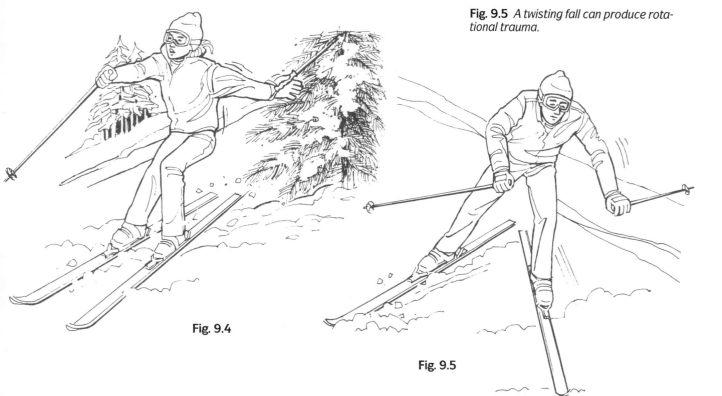

Fig. 9.4

Fig. 9.5

velocity inherent to the sport gives the skier less time to make decisions and can lead to high-speed collisions and falls involving higher kinetic energy. Ski-related accidents will be discussed in detail in Chapter 21 because of the volume of data, the unusual characteristics of these injuries, the hazards of ski equipment, and the existence of a well-organized and trained rescue system.

Hikers who slip or fall are subject to decelerating forces that can cause compression and penetration trauma, producing lacerations, abrasions, contusions, sprains, and fractures. Less frequently, falling trees and limbs cause injuries. Mountain hiking and technical mountaineering introduce the possibility of falls from heights with serious, multiple injuries. As a rule of thumb, a fall from three times or more a person's height will cause critical

injury, depending to some extent on the softness and compressibility of the landing surface.

Water sports introduce a different type of terrain and mode of transportation. The kinetic effect of rapidly moving water must be experienced to be appreciated; it can pin canoeists and kayakers against rocks, fallen trees, and other obstacles. Compression and penetration trauma can be caused by collisions with sharp prows of watercraft or with rocks and other stationary objects. Underwater obstacles that entrap extremities can cause fractures due to bending trauma (as well as pin the victim underwater and cause drowning). Compression and bending trauma to the head and neck can result from diving into too-shallow water.

Careful inspection of the accident scene and mental reconstruction of the sequence of events reveal a good deal about the type, location, and severity of possible injuries. In determining the mechanism of injury, the rescuer should ask himself or herself the fol-

lowing questions.
1. Considering the estimated speed of travel, the distance of the fall, or the speed of the striking object, what is the probable amount of kinetic energy involved? Were the forces produced strong enough to cause fractures and serious internal injuries, or weak enough so that less serious injuries should be expected?
2. What are the characteristics of the ground or any other surface the patient impacted? Is the surface smooth or rough, hard or soft, compressible or rigid?
3. What forces were involved? On what part of the patient's body and in what direction did they act? Were they accelerating or decelerating? What was the patient's body position at impact?
4. Based on the above, your assessment of the patient, and your knowledge of the patterns of injury discussed earlier in this chapter, what types of trauma were or could have been involved (compres-

Fig. 9.6 *Injuries caused by Landing on the Feet After a Hard Fall*

Fig. 9.7 *Tibia Fracture*

Fig. 9.8 *Comminuted Tibia Fracture*

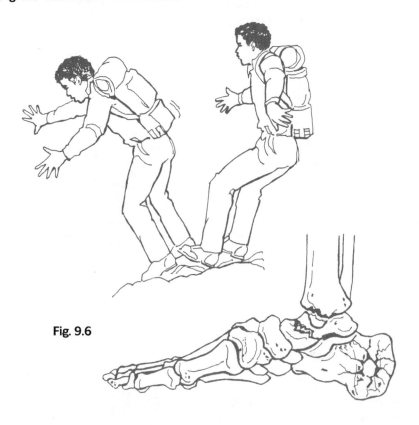

Fig. 9.6

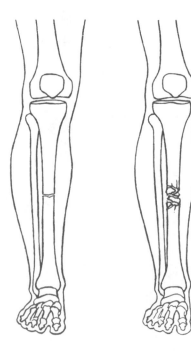

Fig. 9.7   Fig. 9.8

sion, penetration, bending [hyperflexion, hyperextension], rotation, or distraction)?

5. Based on the types of trauma, what *visible* injuries would you expect to see? Do you see them?

6. Based on the types of trauma and your knowledge of surface anatomy and the location of underlying organs, what types of *internal* injuries might have occurred? Is there any pain, tenderness, ecchymosis, swelling, or other signs or symptoms that indicate the presence of these injuries?

7. Are there any signs of developing shock in the absence of obvious external bleeding? If not, could it be too soon for signs and symptoms to have developed?

8. Based on your analysis of the mechanism of injury, is there any likelihood of a spine injury?

In motor vehicle (especially automobile) accidents, the location and amount of damage to the vehicle gives an indication of the amount of kinetic energy involved and provides clues about the type and location of body impact. A broken windshield, especially with a "star" pattern, suggests that one or more occupants might have struck the windshield with the head. A broken steering wheel or bent steering column indicates the possibility of a fractured sternum, crushed chest, flail chest, or injuries to the heart and lungs. A bent dashboard raises the possibility of a deceleration injury to a lower extremity. A vehicle hit from the side indicates the possibility of lateral chest, abdominal, and other injuries.

Determining the **mechanism of injury** is part of the first impression registered as the rescuer arrives at the accident scene. It is also part of the primary survey after dealing with emergency problems, and the secondary survey as you search for additional injuries. By acquiring experience and a feel for types of injuries likely to have been produced, you can ensure that few injuries will be missed.

When first seen, patients may be free of symptoms and have a normal or unimpressive assessment despite having suffered a serious injury that is potentially fatal or permanently disabling. Early recognition of internal bleeding may depend on the rescuer's alertness and careful patient monitoring based on an understanding of the mechanism of injury and its significance. When the mechanism of injury suggests a possible spinal cord injury, the patient must be immobilized on a spine board even if pain is minimal and paralysis or loss of sensation is absent. Neck fractures and internal injuries of the head, chest, abdomen, and/or pelvis are notorious for initially appearing to be minor.

Based on a combination of the calculated **kinetic** energy produced, the amount of protection, and the human body area involved, anticipate **multiple, serious injuries** if the following has occurred:

1. The patient has fallen from a height of two-and-one-half to three times his or her own height (or less if horizontal motion was involved as with a moving chair lift).

2. The patient was in a vehicle that crashed going 25 miles per hour (40 kilometers per hour) or faster, particularly if no seat belt was worn and especially if another occupant of the same vehicle was killed.

3. The patient was hit by an auto going 25 miles per hour (40 kilometers per hour) or faster.

4. The patient was involved in a motorcycle, all-terrain vehicle, or snowmobile accident, especially if no helmet was worn.

5. The patient was ejected from a vehicle or was in a vehicle that rolled over during a crash.

6. The patient was a passenger in a car whose front end or front axle was displaced rearward 20 inches or more.

7. The patient collided at high speed with another skier or an immobile object such as a tree or ski lift tower.

8. The patient has a gunshot wound of the head, neck, or trunk.

9. The patient is in shock or respiratory distress following trauma and no external bleeding is detected (this is especially true of compression trauma to the chest, abdomen, or pelvis).

10. The patient is unconscious due to a head injury.

All such patients should be cared for as though they had actual or potential spinal cord injuries and internal injuries involving the head, chest, abdomen, and pelvis.

Fig. 9.9 *Fractured pelvic bones can lacerate the bladder.*

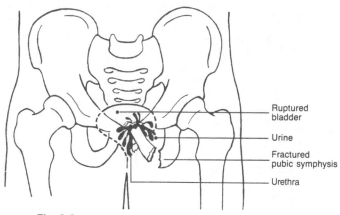

Ruptured bladder

Urine

Fractured pubic symphysis

Urethra

Fig. 9.9

Chapter 10

Specific Injuries to the Upper Extremity

Sticks and stones will break
my bones, but words will never
hurt me.

—Traditional nursery rhyme

The care of soft-tissue injuries in general is discussed in Chapter 7, and the principles of the care of bone and joint injuries are discussed in Chapter 8. This chapter describes the care of **specific sprains, fractures**, and **dislocations** of the upper extremity. Before reading this chapter, please review Chapters 7 and 8 and be familiar with the appropriate sections on anatomy, physiology, and surface anatomy in Chapters 2 and 3.

In the outdoors, upper-extremity injuries usually result from a fall on a shoulder or outstretched hand, although skiers can suffer these injuries during collisions as well. Fractures, dislocations, and soft-tissue injuries such as lacerations, contusions, and sprains can occur. The extent and type of injury depend on the age of the patient; the characteristics of equipment, if any; the type, direction, and magnitude of the forces involved; the position of the upper extremity at the time of impact; and the characteristics of the ground, snow, or other surface. A fall on an outstretched arm can sprain the shoulder, elbow, wrist, or hand; dislocate the shoulder, elbow, wrist, or fingers; or fracture the clavicle, humerus, forearm bones, or bones of the hand.

When the arm is in the **adducted** position, the head of the humerus moves upward against the arch formed by the lateral end of the clavicle and the acromion of the scapula. A patient who falls with an arm in this position (Fig. 10.1) is more likely to sprain the shoulder joint or the acromioclavicular joint or fracture the upper humerus than to injure other parts of the shoulder girdle.

If the patient falls with the arm **partly abducted** (Fig. 10.2a), force is transmitted directly to the clavicle, which is likely to be fractured (Fig. 10.2b). If the arm is **fully abducted** and **externally rotated** (a common position when holding a ski pole or ice ax), the force of the fall is transmitted to the joint capsule. In young people with strong bones, this frequently produces an anterior dislocation of the shoulder (Fig. 10.3a). In elderly people, whose bones are more fragile than the tendons and ligaments of the shoulder capsule, a fracture of the upper end of the humerus is more common than a shoulder dislocation (Fig. 10.3b).

In many types of upper-extremity injuries, pain increased by motion causes the patient to self-splint the injured extremity in a characteristic manner. The patient internally rotates the upper arm, flexes the elbow, and holds the extremity against or near the chest wall while supporting the forearm with the opposite hand (Fig. 10.4).

Rings, bracelets, and any other jewelry must be removed from an injured upper extremity as soon as possible, before swelling occurs and before the extremity is splinted.

Fig. 10.1 *A fall with the arm adducted can cause a sprain.*

Fig. 10.2 *A fall with the arm partly abducted concentrates force on the clavicle.*

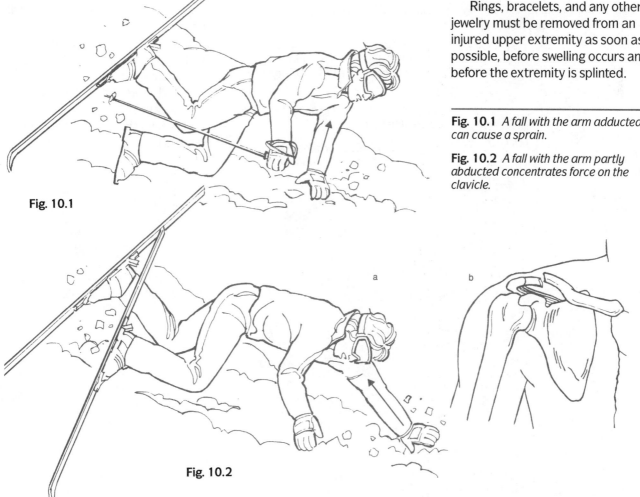

Fig. 10.1

Fig. 10.2

Sprains

Shoulder Sprains

Shoulder sprains usually are caused by a fall on an outstretched hand as described above. Climbers can sprain a shoulder if they slip while one hand is anchored above the head. The joint is tender, painful, and may be slightly swollen, but the contour is basically normal when compared with the opposite shoulder. Shoulder motion increases the pain.

Emergency care consists of applying cold packs as described in Chapter 7 and, in severe cases, a sling and swathe.

AC Separations

Acromioclavicular (AC) separations are third-degree sprains of the acromioclavicular joint, usually caused by a hard fall on the shoulder that forces the distal shoulder footward. Comparison with the smooth slope of the opposite, normal shoulder reveals an obvious, tender, shelf-like deformity at the point of the injured shoulder (Fig. 10.5).

Emergency care consists of preventing swelling with cold packs and limiting joint motion by supporting the arm with a sling and swathe.

Elbow Sprains

Elbow sprains have the same causes as shoulder sprains, but are rare and *should be x-rayed* since they may be confused with non-displaced fractures or partial dislocations. They are most common in children. The elbow is slightly swollen, tender, and painful; pain is increased by use.

Emergency care consists of applying cold packs and splinting with a sling and swathe. If in doubt, use a fixation splint as you would with a fracture above the elbow (see below).

Wrist Sprains

Wrist sprains are less common than wrist fractures. The injured wrist is swollen, tender, and painful to use.

Emergency care consists of applying cold packs and, for a severe sprain, splinting with a rigid, all-purpose

forearm and hand splint (also used for hand and finger sprains and forearm, wrist, and hand fractures). This is a board, wire, ladder, or malleable metal splint applied to the anterior (volar) surface of the forearm and hand, and which extends at least to the elbow and holds the hand in the **position of function** (Fig. 10.6). The fingers should be curled around a roll of gauze held in the palm as if holding a ball. Then the entire extremity and splint should be wrapped with a self-adhering roller bandage and the forearm supported by a sling. The fingertips should be left visible so that circulation can be assessed easily. Wrist injuries should be x-rayed because sprains are difficult to tell from fractures of the small wrist bones.

Hand and Finger Sprains

Hand and finger sprains also are common. The most common upper-extremity injury in skiers is the "skier's thumb," also called "gamekeeper's thumb." This is a sprain of the medial ligament of the joint at the base of the thumb (first metacarpophalangeal [MCP] joint) caused when the skier tries to break a fall with an outstretched hand while holding a ski pole. Because of the position of the hand around the ski pole grip, the thumb is bent backward on impact

---

Fig. 10.3 *Anterior Dislocation of the Shoulder and Fracture of the Upper Humerus*

Fig. 10.4 *Self-splinting an Upper-extremity Injury*

Fig. 10.5 *An AC separation causes a shelf-like deformity of the shoulder.*

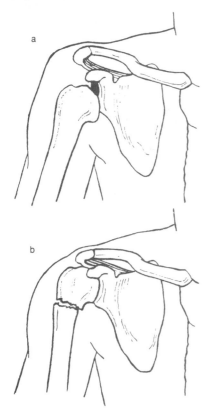

Fig. 10.3

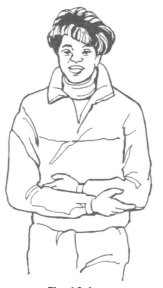

Fig. 10.4

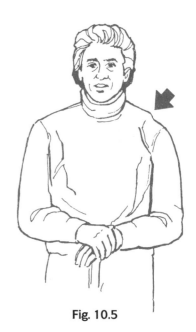

Fig. 10.5

with the snow. Twenty to 30 percent of these sprains are accompanied by a small fracture at the base of the first phalanx, and some involve a ligament tear that is severe enough to require surgery; therefore, all patients with skier's thumb should be seen by an orthopedic surgeon.

Do not manipulate an injured thumb since excessive motion at the MCP joint may displace a previously non-displaced fracture. The injury can be splinted with an all-purpose forearm and hand splint (Fig. 10.6) or taped so that it is held in adduction (Fig. 10.7).

Sprains of the other fingers and the small joints of the palm are less common. Mild sprains may not require splinting; severe sprains can be splinted with a bulky hand bandage (Fig. 7.13, Chapter 7) or with an all-purpose forearm and hand splint (Fig. 10.6).

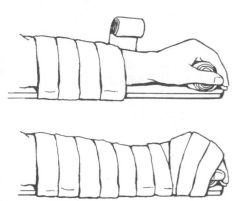

Fig. 10.6

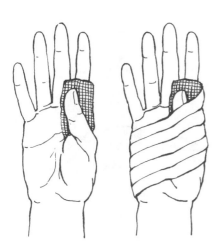

Fig. 10.7

Fractures

Clavicle Fractures

The clavicle is one of the most frequently fractured bones in the body. The patient complains of pain in the shoulder area and attempts to self-splint the injury as described above. Assessment of the clavicle reveals a tender swelling and often a deformity when compared to the opposite side (Fig. 10.8a). The injured shoulder is frequently lower than the normal shoulder.

Emergency care consists of splinting with a sling and swathe (Fig. 10.8b and Chapter 8, Fig. 8.10b). However, to avoid pressure on the injured clavicle, the lower end of the sling is run around the forearm, *under the armpit* on the injured side, and around the patient's back, where it is tied to the upper end of the sling behind the uninjured shoulder.

Scapula Fractures

A strong force is required to fracture the scapula, which lies against the side of the upper back and is protected by large overlying muscles. The mechanism of injury usually is a direct blow, as in landing on the back after a hard fall. Therefore, anticipate and search for other injuries, particularly of the spine, adjacent chest wall, and lungs. Examination reveals tender-

ness, swelling, and ecchymosis over the scapula, with pain on attempted use of the upper extremity.

Although an isolated scapular fracture can be immobilized with a sling and swathe, the mechanism of injury usually requires immobilizing the patient's entire body on a long spine board.

Upper-arm Fractures

The humerus usually is fractured in one of three places: just below its head, at its midshaft, or just above the elbow.

Fractures below the head of the humerus are more common in elderly people and may be confused with shoulder dislocations or severe sprains. Examination reveals swelling, tenderness, and ecchymosis of the arm just below the shoulder joint, with pain on attempting to use the upper extremity.

Emergency care consists of splinting with a sling and swathe. In a fracture below the head of the humerus, the bone ends are rarely displaced or

---

Fig. 10.6 *Splint a wrist sprain with an all-purpose forearm and hand splint.*

Fig. 10.7 *A sprained thumb can be taped in adduction.*

Fig. 10.8 *Use a sling and swathe when there is a deformity over the clavicle.*

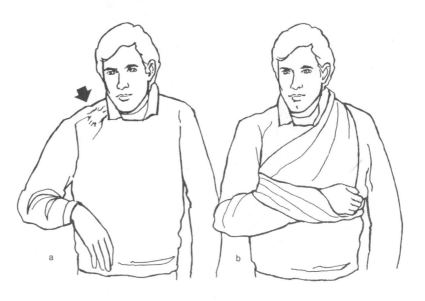

Fig. 10.8

angulated and, as in most other fractures near a joint, alignment should *not* be attempted.

Midshaft fractures of the humerus tend to occur in younger adults. These fractures usually are characterized by marked swelling, angulation, and instability. The radial nerve may be injured where it winds around the back of the humerus, causing wrist drop. Assessment discloses swelling, tenderness, ecchymosis, and loss of use of the extremity. If angulation is severe, the fracture cannot be splinted without alignment.

To align the fracture, support it with a hand just above the fracture site, grasp the two condyles of the humerus with the other hand, and straighten the fracture while exerting gentle, axial traction (Fig. 10.9). After alignment, apply a padded rigid splint to the outside of the upper arm, and incorporate the splint into a sling and swathe. Occasionally, a second rigid splint must be placed on the inside of the upper arm to provide adequate stability (Fig. 10.10). As with any fracture, if pain, resistance, numbness, or loss of the radial pulse occurs during alignment, stop the process and splint the injury in the angulated position using a sling and swathe plus a pillow or folded parka placed between the upper arm and the chest wall (Fig. 10.11).

Fractures above the elbow (Fig. 10.12) are common and may be difficult to distinguish from elbow dislocations. These fractures frequently are accompanied by nerve and blood vessel injury from the jagged bone fragments. Assessment usually reveals marked swelling and deformity of the elbow area, with tenderness, pain, and ecchymosis. The point of the elbow often is displaced backward.

Be sure to assess circulation and nerve supply below the fracture site.

Emergency care consists of splinting the injury in the position found. A good method is to use two rigid splints, one on either side of the extremity, which are attached to the mid or upper part of the upper arm above and the midforearm below so that they form the base of a triangle whose apex is the elbow (Fig. 10.13). An alternative method is to use a SAM splint or ladder splint folded into the shape of a sugar tong.

Loop a cravat around the neck and tie it to the wrist to support the weight of the extremity. It is preferable not to use a full sling because the cradling effect of the sling on the proximal forearm decreases the straightening effect of the pull of gravity on the upper arm and may aggravate the injury by increasing the deformity at the fracture site.

If there are signs of impaired circulation such as a cold, pale hand; pain in the hand and forearm; or an

Fig. 10.9 *Alignment of an Upper-extremity injury.*

Fig. 10.10 *A rigid splint provides upper arm stability.*

Fig. 10.11 *A pillow sling and swathe will support an angulated humerus fracture.*

Fig. 10.12 *Fracture above the Elbow*

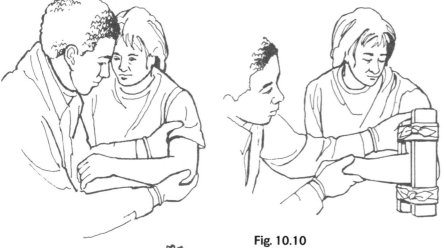

Fig. 10.9

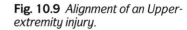

Fig. 10.10

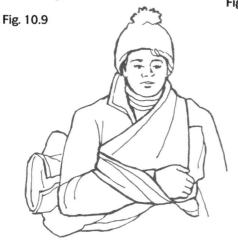

Fig. 10.11

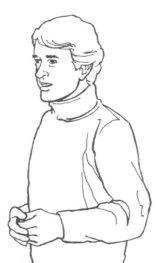

Fig. 10.12

absent or weak radial pulse, the situation is an emergency and the patient must be transported to a hospital as soon as possible. If transportation will take more than 30 minutes, attempt to improve circulation by gently aligning the fracture. Exert axial traction by grasping the upper forearm with both hands and pulling gently downward while an assistant steadies the upper arm above the fracture. Splint the extremity in the position that produces the strongest pulse. If the first attempt is unsuccessful or causes resistance or severe pain, make no further attempts at alignment, and splint the arm in the most comfortable position.

Forearm and Wrist Fractures

Forearm and wrist fractures are common, especially in children and

---

Fig. 10.13 *Two padded board splints will stabilize a fracture above the elbow.*

Fig. 10.14 *Silver-fork Deformity*

Fig. 10.15 *Self-splinting of an Anterior Dislocation*

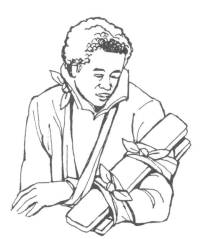

Fig. 10.13

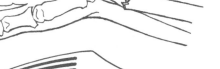

Fig. 10.14

the elderly. Assessment reveals swelling, tenderness, ecchymosis, pain on motion, and usually some deformity. The common **Colles' fracture** at the end of the radius produces a characteristic deformity, called a "silver-fork deformity" because of its resemblance to an upside-down fork (Fig. 10.14).

Emergency care consists of splinting the injury with an all-purpose forearm and hand splint that also must support the hand firmly and hold it in the position of function (Fig. 10.6). Support the forearm with a sling.

Hand Fractures

Fractures of the hand are important injuries because a functional hand is so necessary for normal living. The hand contains a large number of bones, muscles, nerves, and blood vessels, all of which are crowded together with little padding or protection. Hand and wrist injuries, other than superficial lacerations, should be seen by a physician. Fractures of the bones of the hand usually produce an obvious deformity along with swelling, tenderness, ecchymosis, and loss of function.

Emergency care consists of immobilizing the entire hand with an all-purpose forearm and hand splint (Fig. 10.6) and supporting the extremity with a sling.

Dislocations
Shoulder Dislocations

The shoulder is the most commonly dislocated joint in skiers and probably in outdoor enthusiasts in general.

The injury usually is caused by a fall on an externally rotated, outstretched hand, causing the head of the humerus to lever out of its socket using the acromion as a fulcrum. Some individuals have recurrent shoulder dislocations, with each one stretching the joint capsule further, making it easier to dislocate the next time. The dislocated head of the humerus frequently can be felt in the armpit.

The most common type of shoulder dislocation is an **anterior dislocation**. In this type of dislocation, the patient attempts to splint the upper extremity by holding the upper arm *slightly* away from the chest, with the elbow bent and the forearm supported by the opposite hand (Fig. 10.15). In the rare case of a **posterior** or **inferior dislocation**, the patient will hold the arm in front of the body away from the chest or over the head.

When the shoulder is assessed, it looks and feels more square than a normal smooth, round shoulder. There is tenderness over the shoulder and the patient resists attempts to move it because of pain. Be sure to assess circulation and nerve supply below the dislocation. Because the axillary nerve is located close to the shoulder joint and is commonly injured in shoulder dislocations, its function should

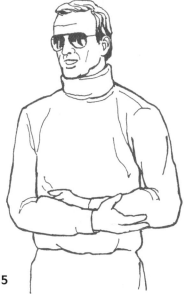

Fig. 10.15

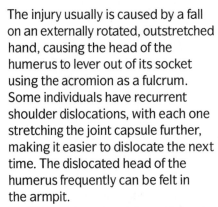

be assessed specifically. Test for pain and touch directly over the lateral part of the patient's deltoid muscle, then place your hand on the deltoid and ask the patient to tighten the muscle and try to abduct the arm. Even though the patient will not move the shoulder because of pain, if the axillary nerve is intact you will be able to feel the deltoid muscle contract.

Emergency care consists of splinting the injury in position with a sling and swathe. A pillow, rolled blanket, or parka usually is needed as padding between the upper arm and the chest, since the arm cannot be brought against the chest without pain (Fig. 10.16a). If the patient is holding the extremity at shoulder level or over the head and is unable to lower it because of pain, an alternative is to splint the injury by tying the hand to the top of the head. The patient usually is more comfortable when transported sitting rather than lying down. During transportation by toboggan, another patroller may have to sit behind and support the patient (Fig. 10.16b).

Elbow Dislocations

Elbow dislocations are serious injuries because of the possibility of nerve injury and circulatory impairment. The patient should be taken to a hospital as soon as possible. The radius and ulna usually are displaced posteriorly, producing a marked deformity with the point of the elbow more posterior than normal. This may resemble the deformity seen in a fracture above the elbow. The elbow joint usually is locked in slight flexion. Examination reveals marked swelling, tenderness, deformity, and pain on attempted motion. It is important to check the radial pulse and movement and sensation in the forearm and hand.

Emergency care consists of splinting the injury in the position found (Fig. 10.13), as described above in **Upper-arm Fractures**. Evidence of impaired circulation and/or nerve injury justifies an attempt to realign the elbow using gentle axial traction as described in the same section. Circulation is more likely to be improved by increasing the angle of elbow flexion rather than decreasing it.

Wrist Dislocations

Wrist dislocations are uncommon and may be accompanied by a frac-

ture. Examination reveals marked swelling and deformity, with pain on attempted motion of the joint.

Emergency care consists of immobilizing the injury in the position found, using an all-purpose forearm and hand splint (Fig. 10.6) and supporting the extremity with a sling.

Finger Dislocations

Finger dislocations are common injuries. Assessment shows a grossly deformed finger joint locked in position, with pain on attempted motion. Swelling can be minimal or marked.

Emergency care consists of immobilizing the injury in the position found with an all-purpose forearm and hand splint.

Fig. 10.16 *Care of a Dislocated Shoulder*

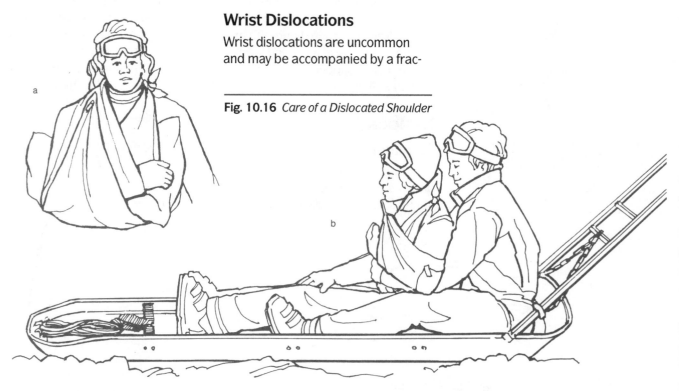

Fig. 10.16

Scenario #9 (Fig. 10.17)

The following scenario illustrates the management of a typical upper-extremity injury.

You and a group of friends are taking a four-day fishing and backpacking trip through the Moose Flop Wilderness Area. This involves a 20-mile approach by trail to a mountain range that forms the backbone of the area, followed by 3 miles of scrambling and boulder hopping to get across a pass, then 4 miles of travel to a campground where you have left a van. The weather forecast is favorable.

The first two days go well. The steaks and heavy fresh food are eaten the first night so that the packs are noticeably lighter the next day. You start to feel the altitude as you make camp the second night at timberline in a beautiful meadow below a small lake. Lucky gets his harmonica out that night and you sing old western songs around a small campfire.

The next morning, after burying the remains of the campfire, you set out, scrambling across boulders at the lake edge until you reach the inlet, then up steep grassy slopes to a small saddle. As you are descending through a large boulder field on the other side of the saddle, you hear a cry behind you. Turning, you see that Lucky has fallen between two large boulders. His pack is over his head and all you can see are his legs. You and the other two reach him at about the same time.

You: "Are you okay, Lucky?"

Lucky: "I can't move my shoulder. Help me get this damn pack off." (You and the other hikers carefully remove the pack and set it aside. Lucky is twisted so that he is lying on his side with his feet on one of the boulders. He is holding his left arm with his right.)

You: "Where does it hurt?"

Lucky: "My shoulder."

You: "Anywhere else?"

Lucky: "No."

You: "Did you hit your head or hurt your neck or back?"

Lucky: "No."

You: "Can you get up by yourself?"

Lucky: "I need some help." (You and the others gently help him to a sitting position on a small boulder, being careful to avoid moving his left upper extremity.)

You: "I'll check your arm for you." (You hold his left wrist and assess his radial pulse. It is strong and regular. You carefully palpate the left clavicle, shoulder joint, arm, elbow, and forearm. There is a large, tender bulge in the center of the clavicle.)

"Can you feel this?" (You scrape the back of his hand with your fingernail.)

Lucky: "Yes."

You: "Can you wiggle your fingers?" (Lucky does so.) "Make a fist and then spread your fingers." (Lucky does so.) "Does your arm or hand feel numb or tingly?"

Lucky: "No."

You: "Looks like you got your collarbone."

Fig. 10.17 *Scenario #9*

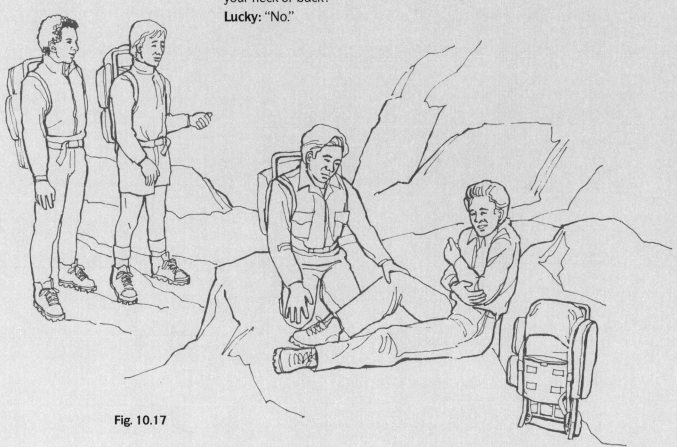

Fig. 10.17

Lucky: "I was afraid of that. I put my hand out to catch myself when I slipped, but I hit too hard."

You: "Well, we can get a sling and swathe on your arm and take your pack. Do you feel up to walking out? It's 4 miles to the van from here. The trail starts about a quarter mile from where we are."

Lucky: "I don't know, I'll have to see."

You: "We can give it a try. If it doesn't work we can send out for help. Have you ever ridden a horse?"

Lucky: "Sure."

You: "Before I put on the sling, I need to check a few other things." (You open Lucky's shirt, pull his undershirt out of the way, and expose the clavicle. There is an ecchymosis over the lump at its midpoint, but no open wound. You note that the chest shows no open wounds, ecchymosis, or swellings. You palpate each rib in turn. Lucky winces when you hit the left fourth rib.) "Does that hurt?"

Lucky: "Yes."

You: "Take a deep breath." (Lucky does so and winces again.) "You may have gotten that rib when you hit."

Lucky: "I didn't notice it until you touched it. I guess the collarbone was hurting too much."

You reach in your pack and pull out your first aid kit. Fortunately, you have two triangular bandages. You make a sling with one, supporting Lucky's left forearm but putting all the weight on his right shoulder. You fold the other into a cravat and bind his left arm to his chest.

You: "How does that feel?"

Lucky: "Better."

You then assess his head, neck, abdomen, lower extremities, and back, and ask him about previous illnesses and injuries, medications taken, allergies, and any additional problems. The answers are all negative. Lucky's pack is emptied and its contents distributed into the other three packs. With the aid of a walking stick donated by one of his companions and some steadying over rough spots, Lucky slowly and carefully makes his way through the rest of the boulder field to an area of rolling tundra that leads to the trail at the tree line. The pace picks up as soon as he reaches the trail, and it looks like he will be able to self-evacuate.

You: "Lucky, you've got to quit doing things like this, or the next time we'll leave you at home."

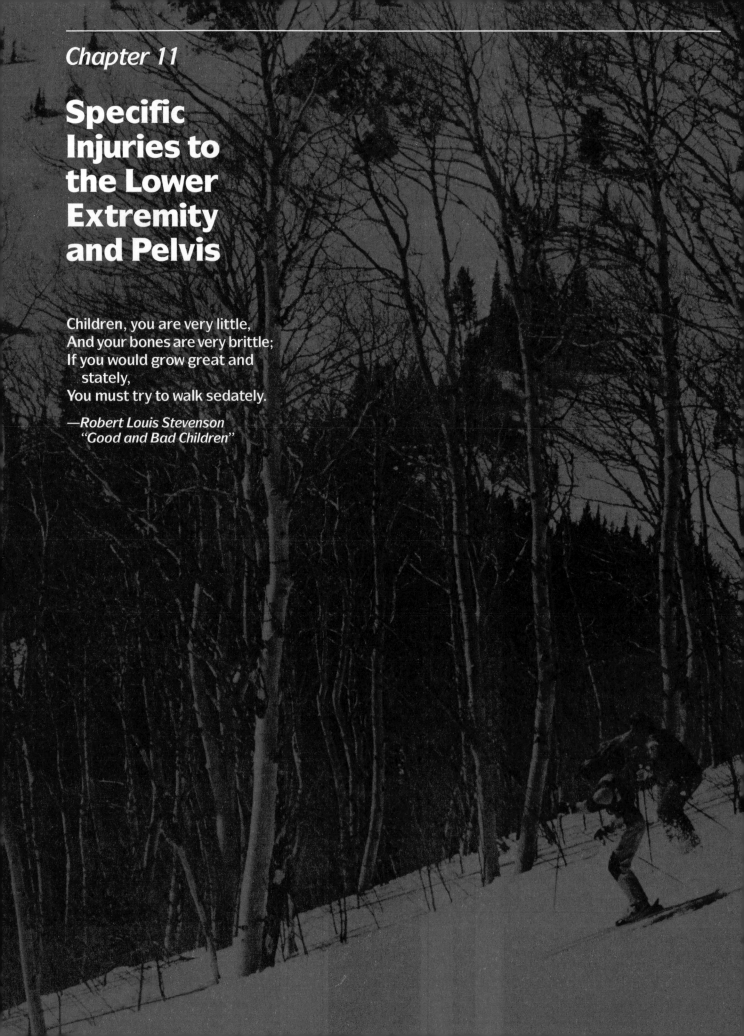

Chapter 11

Specific Injuries to the Lower Extremity and Pelvis

Children, you are very little,
And your bones are very brittle;
If you would grow great and
    stately,
You must try to walk sedately.

—*Robert Louis Stevenson*
    "Good and Bad Children"

Injuries to the lower extremity and pelvis are not rare in outdoor enthusiasts, particularly skiers. Knee and ankle injuries are probably the most common lower-extremity injuries, with knee sprains being the most commonly reported skiing injury. Lacerations, contusions, and other soft-tissue injuries occur in the lower extremity as they do in other areas of the body. As with the upper extremity, injuries to the lower extremity and pelvis are caused mainly by falls, collisions, and direct blows. The extent and type of injury depend on the age of the patient; the type, direction, and magnitude of the forces involved; the position of the lower extremity at the time of injury; the condition of the snow or other ground surface; and whether skis or other equipment that introduce a lever arm are involved.

When the hip is abducted, a direct blow to the side of the hip or to the knee can drive the head of the femur directly into the acetabulum, shattering it (Fig. 11.1). With the hip in other positions, forces transmitted along the femur can fracture the pelvis at other places; these fractures usually involve the weaker, thinner ischial and pubic bones (Fig. 11.2). If the hip is flexed, these forces can cause a posterior dislocation of the hip joint with or without a fracture of the lip of the joint. A blow to the side of the iliac crest can fracture the crest or other parts of the pelvis, depending on how the force is transmitted. An antero-posterior blow to the pelvis also will tend to fracture the weaker parts of the ischial and pubic bones Fig. 11.3).

Hip fractures (actually fractures of the upper end of the femur) usually are caused by falls in which compression, distraction, rotational, and shearing forces are generated. Fractures of the shaft of the femur usually are caused by direct blows; a classic example is when a motorcyclist is thrown upward and forward, striking the handlebars of the motorcycle with both thighs and fracturing both femurs (Fig. 11.4). Skiers can fracture a femur in a hard fall against a rock (Fig. 11.5) or occasionally in a slow twisting fall with the rotational force exerted on the femur rather than the knee or lower leg. Climbers occasionally will fracture a femur in a long, hard fall.

The causes of knee-joint injuries and leg fractures are discussed in detail below and in Chapter 21.

The ankle usually is injured in one of three ways. The first method is when the foot is forced into abduction and external rotation, e.g., by falling when the foot is fixed by a ski binding (Fig. 11.6) or trapped between rocks while hiking or kayaking. Such a fall can tear the medial ligament of the ankle, fracture the tip of the medial malleolus, or fracture the fibula just above the lateral malleolus. The second situation occurs when the foot is forced into adduction and

---

Fig. 11.1 *A blow to the lower extremity with the hip abducted may transmit force directly to the acetabulum.*

Fig. 11.2 *When the hip is adducted, force is transmitted to other parts of the pelvis.*

Fig. 11.3 *Effect of an Antero-posterior Blow to the Pelvis*

Fig. 11.4 *This type of motorcycle accident can fracture both femurs.*

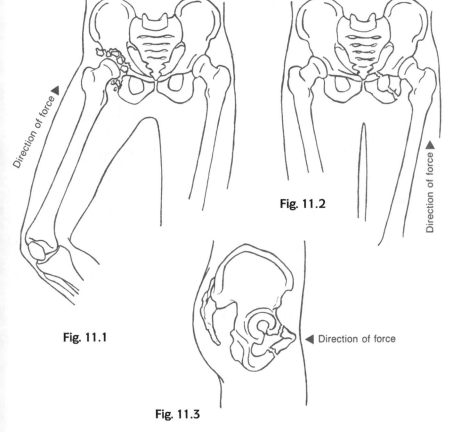

Direction of force

Fig. 11.2

Direction of force

Fig. 11.1

Direction of force

Fig. 11.3

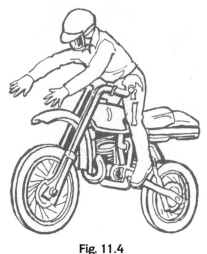

Fig. 11.4

internal rotation, e.g., when a person trips—the mechanism that produces the most common type of ankle sprain (Fig. 11.7). The lateral ligament may be stretched or torn, and the tip of the medial malleolus may be fractured. The third situation involves axial compression of the type that occurs when landing on the feet after a hard fall. This can crush the lower end of the tibia, fracture the large bones of the foot (the talus and calcaneus), and damage ligaments and soft tissues (Fig. 11.8).

Before reading the material on specific sprains, fractures, and dislocations of the lower extremities and pelvis, please review Chapters 7 and 8 and the appropriate sections on anatomy, physiology, and surface anatomy in Chapters 2 and 3.

Sprains

Knee Sprains

Knee sprains are common among people who participate in most outdoor sports and recreational activities, particularly skiers. Because of

the knee's importance, the rescuer should be thoroughly familiar with its anatomy (Fig. 11.9) and function, discussed briefly in Chapter 2.

The knee is a **modified hinge joint**. Although its motion is mainly in the single plane of flexion-extension, some degree of rotation of the tibia on the femur can occur during full flexion and full extension.

The bones of the knee joint are the **femur** proximally, the **tibia** distally, and the **patella** anteriorly (Fig. 11.9 a and b). The **fibula** is only indirectly involved in the knee joint.

The riding surfaces of the knee are the convex **condyles** of the femur, which are semicircular and covered

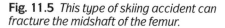

Fig. 11.5 *This type of skiing accident can fracture the midshaft of the femur.*

Fig. 11.6 *Results of a Fall with the Foot Abducted and Externally Rotated*

Fig. 11.7 *Results of a Fall with the Foot Adducted and Internally Rotated*

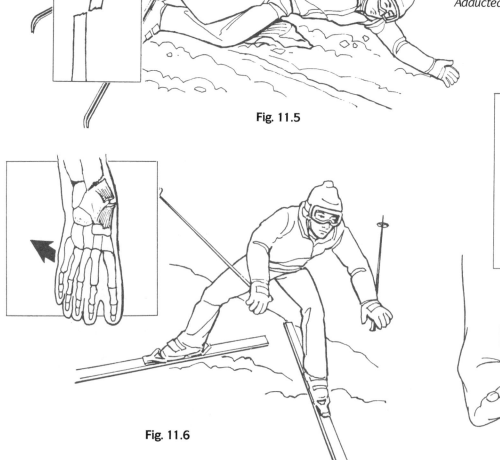

Fig. 11.5

Fig. 11.6

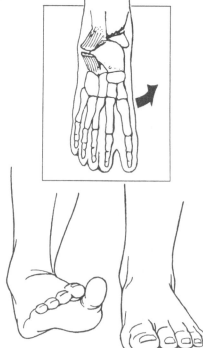

Fig. 11.7

with cartilage, and the concave **tibial plateau**, also covered with cartilage, on which the femoral condyles sit. The C-shaped **medial** and **lateral cartilages** (menisci) sit atop the tibial plateau, deepen its concavities, cushion the joint, and align the femur as it sits on the tibia. The **patella** is in front of the knee joint in the groove between the femoral condyles.

The knee joint is enclosed by a fibrous joint capsule (Fig. 11.9c), lined by a synovial membrane that secretes lubricating synovial fluid. The medial and lateral parts of the knee joint capsule are thickened and strengthened, forming the **medial** and **lateral ligaments** of the knee (Fig. 11.9d), also called collateral ligaments. The front and back of the capsule are loose, permitting flexion and extension of the joint.

There are two other important ligaments of the knee joint: the **anterior** and **posterior cruciate ligaments** (Fig. 11.9 d and e). These originate in the groove between the femoral condyles, cross each other in an X, and insert into the tibial plateau. The anterior cruciate ligament inserts in front of the posterior cruciate ligament. Because the concavities of the tibial plateau are shallow, the knee joint would be easy to dislocate if not for these four powerful ligaments and the muscles and tendons around the knee. The lateral

and medial ligaments are probably the most important in preventing medial and lateral dislocation of the knee; the anterior cruciate in preventing forward dislocation; and the posterior cruciate in preventing backward dislocation. Hyperextension is prevented by both cruciates, mainly the anterior cruciate, and also by the posterior part of the joint capsule.

The major muscles associated with the knee joint are the **quadriceps femoris** ("quad") anteriorly, which extends the knee (Fig. 11.10a), and the **medial** and **lateral hamstrings**, which flex the knee (11.10b). The patella is actually a "sesamoid" bone—a bone that forms within a muscle tendon. The quadriceps tendon attaches to the top of the patella, surrounds it, and finally attaches to the tibia at the **tibial tubercle** (Fig. 11.9a).

When the knee is in *slight flexion*, most ligaments and tendons are tight and the joint is in its strongest position. When the knee joint is stabilized in this way, a rotational force of the type frequently exerted during skiing is more likely to cause a binding release than a knee injury. This is one of the reasons beginning skiers are told to "bend ze knees."

Fig. **11.8** *Injuries Caused by Landing on the Feet After a Hard Fall*

Fig. **11.9** *Anatomy of the Knee*

The medial cartilage (meniscus), which is partly fixed by its attachment to the medial ligament, is torn more often than the lateral cartilage, which can move to some extent within the joint.

Prolonged flexion of the knee at close to a 90-degree angle, as in "sitting back" while skiing bumps, puts a severe strain on the patella. If done frequently, this eventually injures the cartilage that lines the posterior surface of the patella, producing a painful condition called chondromalacia

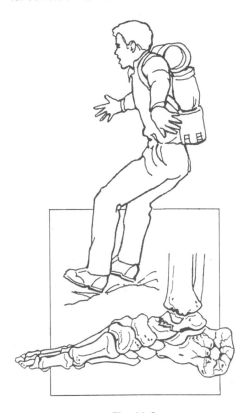

Fig. 11.8

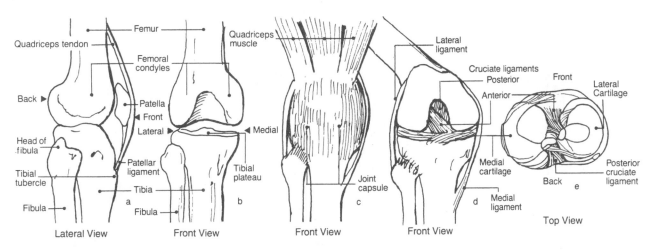

Fig. 11.9

of the patella. Chondromalacia can cause pain in the knee when ascending or (especially) descending stairs or hills. The knee also is less stable in the 90-degree flexed position, and the partly relaxed anterior cruciate seems to be more prone to injury.

The patella provides an advantage in completing knee extension when the knee is *partly* extended, since the patella lies on the lower end of the femur just above the condyles, holds the quadriceps tendon away from the joint, and lengthens the lever arm (Fig. 11.11a). However, in *full flexion*, the mechanical advan-tage of the patellar system is lost because the patella moves down-ward, sinks between the femoral condyles, and allows the quadriceps tendon to move closer to the joint (Fig. 11.11b). Modern ski boots with a built-in forward lean put consider-able stress on the patella. Skiers are advised to loosen their boots and stand up straight when they are not skiing.

Knee sprains continue to make up 20 to 25 percent of all reported ski-ing injuries in both alpine and nordic skiers. Sprains of the medial ligament are the most common, occurring with about 10 times the frequency of sprains of the lateral ligament. The anterior cruciate ligament is the next most commonly injured ligament. Minor anterior cruciate injuries are more common in women and novice skiers; severe anterior cruciate inju-ries are more common in advanced skiers of either sex.

Even experienced physicians have trouble specifically diagnosing knee injuries because serious liga-ment tears may not appear to be that severe when first seen. Physical examination of an injured knee is easier and provides more information if it can be done before the knee swells and becomes very painful. Success-ful treatment of many knee injuries depends on prompt diagnosis, which may require examining the interior of the joint with an arthroscope, and surgery within a week or two. There-fore, every patient with a knee injury should be advised to see a physician promptly—preferably an orthopedic surgeon—especially if knee symp-toms do not clear up within 24 hours.

Fig. 11.10 *Major Muscles Associated with the Knee Joint*

Fig. 11.11 *Mechanics of the Patellar System*

Fig. 11.12 *Immobilization of a Knee Sprain with a Suitable Fixation Splint*

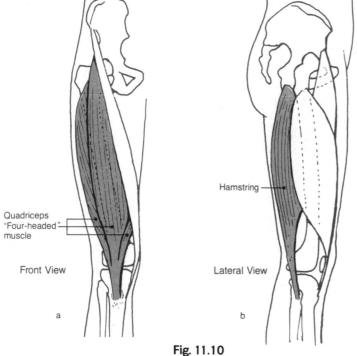

Quadriceps "Four-headed" muscle

Front View

a

Hamstring

Lateral View

b

Fig. 11.10

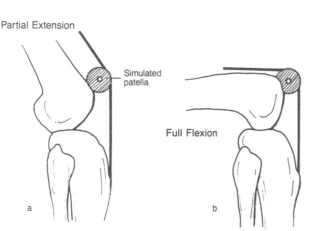

Partial Extension

Simulated patella

Full Flexion

a

b

Fig. 11.11

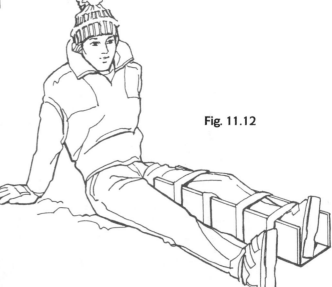

Fig. 11.12

The examiner frequently can form a good idea of which ligament or ligaments have been injured by noting the circumstances of the injury and the areas of tenderness. Severe anterior cruciate ligament injuries can occur without a fall, but frequently the patient hears or feels a pop in the knee at the time of injury.

When assessing an injured knee, first ask the patient to describe the events immediately preceding the injury, including the exact way in which he or she fell. Try to reconstruct the probable mechanisms involved. Then, look for swelling and gently feel for tenderness of the medial and lateral ligaments, the ligaments attached to the patella, the posterior part of the joint capsule, and the hamstring tendons.

Emergency care of a knee sprain consists of applying cold packs and immobilizing the knee with a suitable fixation splint (Fig. 11.12). It is best to let a physician decide when the patient can remove the splint and bear weight on the injured extremity.

because of the low tops of nordic ski boots. As the use of higher nordic boots and higher, stiffer telemark boots increases, the number of ankle sprains in nordic skiers probably will decrease.

Depending on the mechanism of injury and the particular ligaments injured, assessment may reveal tenderness, swelling, and ecchymosis over the top of the foot and/or around one or both malleoli. Emergency care of *mild* sprains consists of applying cold packs and supporting the ankle with a cravat ankle bandage (Fig. 11.13a) or a figure-of-eight made from an elastic bandage (Fig. 11.13b). The patient should avoid bearing full weight on the injured ankle but, if necessary, can be allowed to walk with the aid of a cane or crutches. *Severe* ankle sprains are hard to tell from fractures and should be treated with a fixation splint designed for the lower leg. All patients with severe ankle sprains, or mild sprains that do not improve within a day or two, should see a physician.

Under wilderness conditions, a patient with a mild to moderate ankle sprain may have to self-evacuate. An adhesive-tape boot may stabilize the sprain enough to allow the patient to walk or ski out (Fig. 11.14 and Appendix C).

Fractures

Pelvic Fractures

A pelvic fracture should be suspected when the mechanism of injury and the magnitude of the forces involved could produce such a fracture. Most pelvic fractures are caused by compression trauma to the side or front of the pelvis, or by forces transmitted to the pelvis from one or both femurs, as in landing on the feet after a hard fall.

Pelvic fractures frequently are accompanied by other serious injuries, such as spine and lower-extremity fractures. The major hazard of a pelvic fracture is damage to blood vessels and pelvic organs from sharp bone fragments. Internal bleeding from large pelvic blood vessels may be difficult to detect initially but should be

---

Fig. 11.13 *Two Types of Support for a Sprained Ankle*

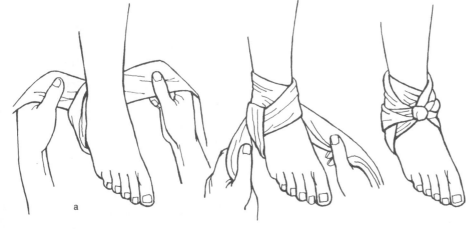

Ankle Sprains

An ankle sprain, another common injury, is a hazard for outdoor travelers walking on uneven ground and for alpine and nordic skiers. Although modern hiking and alpine skiing boots tend to protect the ankle, ankle sprains still are common in nordic skiers

Fig. 11.13

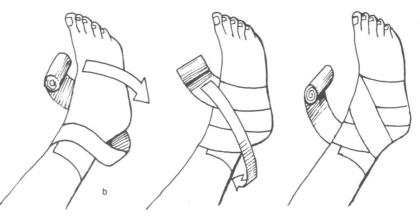

anticipated in all pelvic fractures. Monitor the vital signs closely to detect early signs of continued bleeding and impending shock. Pelvic fractures also can injure the bladder, urethra, and rectum, and the uterus of a pregnant woman.

The patient with a fractured pelvis will be lying down and complaining of lower-abdominal or pelvic pain that usually is increased by movement. Because the pelvis is a continuous bony ring, pressure on one part of the pelvis is transmitted to any injured area, causing pain in that area. During assessment, place one hand on each iliac crest and press gently inward with a rotary motion toward the midline with both hands. If this does not cause pain, press gently backward on each iliac crest in turn with one hand. If the pelvis is fractured, one or both of these maneuvers should cause pain.

Emergency care of a patient with a pelvic fracture consists of immobilization on a long spine board and treatment for shock, if needed. Carefully raise the patient using a three-or four-person direct ground lift (see Chapters 13 and 21), slide the board under the patient, and secure him or her in place with straps, padding, and rolled towels as described in Chapter 8. Do *not* put straps across the pelvis. The patient may prefer to lie with the knees and hips bent and should be allowed to do so. A pneumatic antishock garment (PASG) is useful to control severe bleeding, if personnel trained and licensed in its use are present. Blood in the urine indicates injury to the bladder or urethra. Anyone with a suspected pelvic fracture should be transported to a hospital without delay.

Hip Fractures

The term "hip fracture" usually refers to a fracture of the upper part of the femur. This injury, while common in elderly persons after a minor fall, is less common under outdoor conditions except with severe trauma.

A patient with a fractured hip usually complains of severe pain and inability to move the involved extremity. In some cases, a patient with a hip fracture may complain of moderate pain that is increased by walking or passive manipulation of the hip joint. Some patients complain of mild pain and are able to walk despite the fracture. The involved lower extremity almost always is externally rotated and usually is shortened as well. The upper thigh below the groin or around the greater trochanter usually is tender when palpated.

Emergency care consists of immobilizing the patient on a long spine board as described in the section on pelvic fractures. Do not run straps across the site of injury and do not attempt to flex the hips or knees. If the hip is flexed, do not attempt to straighten it. Instead, stabilize the hip in position with folded parkas and padding as needed. If the patient must be moved before a long spine board is available, you may be able to splint the injury against the normal lower extremity by putting padding between the extremities and tying the thighs and legs firmly together with cravats.

Femoral Shaft Fractures

The term "femoral shaft fracture" is used for a fracture of the middle one-half to three-fifths of the femur. Assessment will disclose an externally rotated and shortened limb, with a large, tender bulge in the thigh. If that patient is seen early, this bulge—which represents hematoma and edema—may not have had time to develop yet. The patient usually experiences severe pain and is unable to move the extremity. The fracture may be angulated.

A femoral shaft fracture is best treated by traction splinting (technique described in Chapter 8), which counteracts the spasm and pull of the large, powerful thigh muscles, controls overriding of the bone ends and further shortening of the limb, prevents further damage from the sharp bone fragments, reduces pain by immobilizing the fracture site, and minimizes blood loss into the thigh.

Fig. 11.14 *Adhesive Tape Boot*

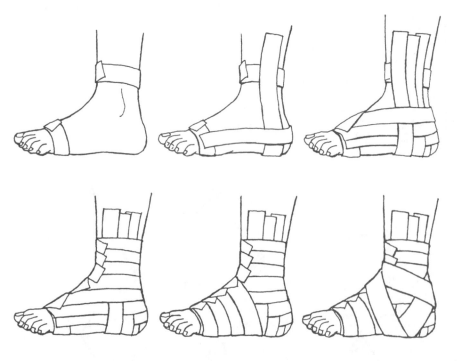

Fig. 11.14

The purpose of traction splinting is *not* to pull the bones apart or to reduce the fracture, although a deformity, if present, must be aligned enough to permit the application of the splint. Bleeding into the thigh is decreased because the traction stretches and tightens the musculofascial "envelope" surrounding the fracture, keeping it in a cylindrical shape rather than allowing it to assume a spherical shape. This tamponades the bleeding by increasing the pressure inside the envelope. (A fixation splint stabilizes the fracture without tightening the envelope, thereby allowing continued bleeding into the loose envelope before enough pressure builds up to tamponade the bleeding.)

Because the patient may lose up to 1.6 quarts (1,500 milliliters) of blood into the fracture site, mild to moderate shock should be anticipated, with a pulse rate of over 100 beats per minute. The blood pressure may be normal as long as the patient is lying down (see Table 6.1, Chapter 6). Nerves and blood vessels may be damaged as well. The circulation and nerve supply to the part below the injury must be assessed during the primary survey, before and after splinting, and at frequent intervals thereafter. If circulation and nerve supply are impaired, there may be improvement after splinting.

In general, a traction splint should not be removed except in a hospital. However, in ski patrol operations, special circumstances may arise in which a traction splint applied to a fractured femur might legitimately be removed in the aid room and traction reapplied. It is advisable to establish local protocols with the aid of medical advice. Such special circumstances might include the following:

1. When a makeshift splint has been applied for a transport from a wilderness accident or off-ski-area rescue, or any other instance where the splint is clearly not doing an adequate job.
2. When a patient is unable to wiggle the toes or feel the foot, and it is desirable to remove the boot so that pulses and nerve function can be assessed directly. (Even here, however, a strong case can be made for immediate transport of the patient to a hospital as being a better way to spend your time, depending on the distance to the nearest hospital.)
3. When helicopter transport is necessary and the splint is too big to fit in the helicopter.
4. When splint removal is necessary to apply the PASG in a patient with shock.
5. When a patient is in great pain where adjusting traction does not help.

If the traction splint is removed or the traction loosened, **manual stabilization** of the injured extremity must be maintained until the new splint is in place and traction reapplied.

A **subtrochanteric** fracture resembles a classic midshaft fracture of the femur but cannot be splinted with a traction splint. This type of femoral fracture involves the upper part of the femur below the trochanters. The pull of the iliopsoas muscle holds the proximal fragment in a flexed position; attempts to straighten the hip cause severe pain.

Emergency care consists of placing the patient on a long spine board with the limb stabilized in position with rolled parkas or pillows. The patient may prefer to sit up during transportation.

Above-knee Femur Fractures

A fracture of the femur above the knee (**supracondylar fracture**) is a serious injury (Fig. 11.15). The pull of the thigh muscles tips the lower fragment so that its jagged upper end lies against the nerves and blood vessels running down the back of the thigh, and they may be injured.

Assessment reveals a large, tender swelling in the lower thigh just above the knee, with pain and inability to move the knee. Circulation and nerve supply to the extremity below the injury should be assessed during the primary survey, before and after splinting or alignment (if this becomes necessary because circulation and nerve supply are impaired), and at regular intervals thereafter.

Emergency care consists of immobilizing the fracture with a lower-extremity fixation splint that extends to just below the groin (Fig. 11.16), as described in Chapter 8. Do not use a traction splint.

The patient must be taken to a hospital as soon as possible if there are signs of interrupted nerve supply, such as weakness in ankle, foot, or toe movement or loss of sensation below the fracture. Other indications of the need for immediate transport

Fig. 11.15 *Supracondylar Fracture*

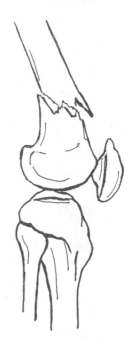

Fig. 11.15

are signs of impaired circulation, such as a cold, pale foot, pain in the foot and leg, or absence or weakness of the posterior tibial and dorsalis pedis pulses.

If transportation will take more than 30 minutes, try to improve matters by gentle alignment of the fracture. Do this with the patient's knee bent. Grasp the leg just below the knee while an assistant steadies the pelvis. Exert axial traction to reduce the angle of the fracture site slightly (Fig. 11.17). If alignment produces a return of pulses and capillary refill, decrease in pain, or improvement in color, splint the extremity in the position that produces the strongest pulses. If the first attempt is unsuccessful or causes resistance or severe pain, make no further attempts and splint the injury in the most comfortable position.

Lower-leg Fractures

A lower-leg fracture involving the tibia and/or fibula can occur at any place from the knee to the ankle joint. Boot-top and spiral fractures are common in skiers. The extremity distal to the fracture usually is angulated or rotated. Occasionally, it may be ro-

tated as much as 180 degrees. The patient will complain of severe pain and resist movement of the leg. Assessment shows swelling, tenderness, and ecchymosis at the fracture site.

Emergency care of a patient with a lower-leg fracture consists of applying a fixation splint designed for the lower leg as described in Chapter 8. To apply the splint, the fracture must be aligned so that the foot is in its proper relationship to the leg. Grasp the foot firmly with both hands while an assistant supports the leg with one hand above and one hand below the fracture site. With the aid of gentle axial traction, the injured extremity usually can be straightened and rotated into position so that it will fit into the splint. The sooner alignment is done after the injury, the easier it is to perform. Assess circulation and nerve function in the distal extremity during the primary survey, before and after alignment and splinting, and at frequent intervals thereafter.

Ankle Fractures

An ankle fracture actually is a fracture of the lower end of the tibia and/or fibula, although the bones of the foot occasionally may be involved. The ankle joint has two "shear pins,"

Fig. 11.16 *Fixation Splint for a Fracture Above the Knee*

Fig. 11.17 *Technique of Gentle Alignment of a Fracture to Improve Circulation*

the lateral and medial malleoli, which usually break first when a rotational force is applied to the ankle joint, thus preventing a more extensive fracture of the shafts of the bones. Ankle fractures are caused by twisting falls and falls from heights; such fractures are now less common in skiers because of improved boot designs.

An ankle fracture may be hard to tell from a severe sprain. Assessment reveals swelling, tenderness, and ecchymosis of the tissues around the ankle joint. The patient may or may not be able to move the joint. If a malleolus is fractured, gentle pressure over its tip will evoke tenderness.

Emergency care consists of applying a fixation splint designed for the lower leg, as described in Chapter 8. An improvised splint made of a folded pillow or a tightly rolled blanket or parka also is satisfactory (Fig. 8.10).

Foot Fractures

Fatigue ("stress") fractures of the metatarsals can occur in long-distance runners, joggers, and hikers who carry heavy packs for long distances. The foot also may be fractured in a fall or when struck by a rock or other falling object.

Assessment reveals tenderness, swelling, ecchymosis, and occasionally deformity at the fracture site. In the case of a fatigue fracture, the only symptom may be pain that is increased by walking or running.

Patients with foot fractures should stay off their feet. If there is

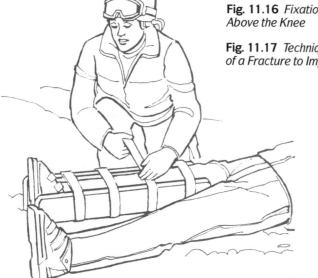

Fig. 11.16

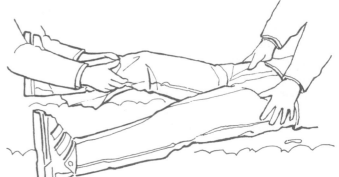

Fig. 11.17

little swelling, the patient's boot or shoe can be used to protect and splint the injury. Severe fractures should be splinted with a pillow or a rolled, folded blanket or parka (Fig.8.10).

Dislocations

Hip Dislocations

Because the hip socket is deep, the hip is rarely dislocated without fracturing the socket. The most common type of hip "dislocation" is a **posterior fracture-dislocation** (Fig. 11.18a). This injury can occur in auto accidents when an occupant's knee strikes the dashboard and the force is transmitted along the shaft of the femur to the posterior lip of the socket. A skier can suffer the same type of fracture-dislocation if a ski binding inadvertently releases during rapid skiing. This may allow the boot to jam deeply into the snow, bringing the lower

extremity to a sudden halt while the skier's momentum carries the rest of the body forward. The posterior lip of the hip joint is torn away as the hip is dislocated posteriorly. A severe fall from a height also can dislocate a hip.

In a posterior dislocation, the lower extremity is internally rotated and the knee is bent (Fig. 11.18a and Chapter 8, Fig. 8.3). In the rare anterior dislocation (Fig. 11.18b and Chapter 8, Fig. 8.3), the hip is slightly flexed and externally rotated, and usually cannot be straightened. Attempted motion produces severe pain, and there is tenderness over the upper thigh just below the groin. The sciatic nerve, which runs behind the hip joint, may be injured when the hip is dislocated, causing paralysis of the foot, foot drop, and numbness in the lower leg and sole of the foot. An additional hazard is inter-

ruption of circulation to the head of the femur, which receives most of its blood supply through vessels in a ligament attached directly to the head. If this ligament is stretched, circulation will be slowed; if torn, it is likely that the head of the femur will atrophy and eventually have to be replaced by an artificial joint.

Emergency care of a patient with a dislocated hip consists of immobilization on a long spine board. The involved lower extremity is maintained in the position found with pillows, wadded jackets, straps, and cravats. Ability to preserve circulation to the head of the femur and prevent serious long-term disability diminishes each minute the head of the femur remains out of the socket. Therefore, treat this situation as an emergency and transport the patient to a hospital without delay.

Knee Dislocations

A knee dislocation is a rare but very serious injury. The blood vessels and nerves that run behind the knee frequently are damaged, impairing the circulation and nerve supply to the

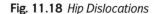

Fig. 11.18 *Hip Dislocations*

Fig. 11.19 *Knee Dislocation*

Fig. 11.20 *Axial traction improves circulation when the knee is dislocated.*

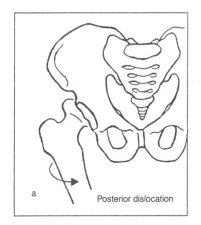
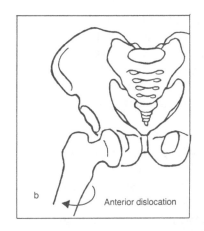

a — Posterior dislocation

b — Anterior dislocation

Fig. 11.18

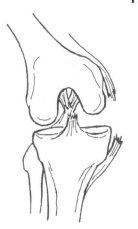

Fig. 11.19

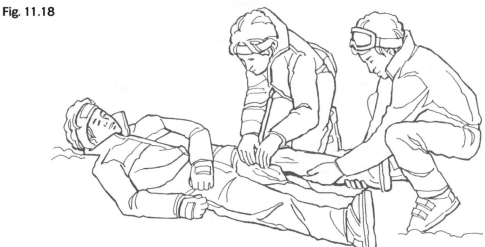

Fig. 11.20

lower leg. This injury is another true emergency and the patient must be taken to a hospital as soon as possible.

A knee dislocation (Fig. 11.19) involves complete disruption of all or most of its ligaments. Severe trauma, usually a fall or hard collision, is necessary to produce this degree of injury. The patient experiences severe pain, swelling, and gross deformity of the knee, and is unable to move the knee.

Immediately expose the injury, remove the boot, and assess circulation and nerve supply to the foot and leg. If distal pulses are good, splint the dislocation in the position found. A clamshell type of lower-extremity fixation splint, such as the quick splint, is a good choice (Fig. 11.16). The knee also can be splinted like a dislocated elbow, with a padded board splint or two doubled SAM splints on each side of the extremity, and attached to the thigh just below the hip and to the ankle so that a triangle is formed with the knee at its apex (Fig. 10.13).

If pulses are weak or absent and transport to a hospital will take more than 30 minutes, an attempt to restore circulation by axial manual traction is justified. Grasp the patient's ankle with one hand and the patient's calf with the other hand, while an assistant steadies the lower thigh. Then, exert gentle traction while flexing the knee slightly (Fig. 11.20). Test the pulses in the foot with the knee in the new position. If the maneuver is successful, splint the limb in the position that produces the strongest pulses. If the attempt is unsuccessful or if severe pain or resistance is encountered, splint the limb in the most comfortable position and take the patient to a hospital as soon as possible.

Patella Dislocations

A dislocated patella is a bizarre injury that can occur during athletic activities. The patella usually dislocates laterally and locks the knee in the flexed position, producing a marked deformity. It occasionally moves back into place when the knee is extended. The mechanism of injury usually is a twisting fall or maneuver such as a poorly executed kick turn, rather than a hard blow to the patella, which is more likely to produce a fracture. Emergency care consists of splinting the injury using the same technique as for a dislocated knee.

Ankle Dislocations

An ankle dislocation is hard to distinguish from an ankle fracture and usually is associated with fractures of both malleoli. Assessment reveals tenderness, swelling, and deformity of the ankle joint, with pain on motion. A severe injury can produce a flail (excessively mobile) ankle. The deformity usually will have to be aligned to allow splinting. Remove the boot and assess the circulation and nerve supply below the injury by feeling for the dorsalis pedis pulse (the posterior tibial pulse usually will not be detectable due to local swelling), testing sensation over the foot, and having the patient move the toes. Repeat the assessment after alignment and at regular intervals thereafter.

Use gentle axial traction to achieve alignment, with one hand grasping the toes and the other the heel of the foot while an assistant steadies the lower leg. Splint the ankle with a lower-leg fixation splint as with a fractured ankle. If attempts at alignment are unsuccessful or produce increased pain or resistance, splint the ankle in the position found with a folded pillow or rolled blanket splint. Take the patient to a hospital immediately.

If circulation and nerve function are impaired, an attempt to realign the injury in the position that gives the strongest pulse is justified.

Scenario #10 (Fig. 11.21)

The following scenario illustrates the management of a typical lower-extremity injury.

It is after 4 p.m. and the upper lift has closed. The last skier has just gotten awkwardly off the lift and skied down the cat track. You hope he doesn't plan to ski Mad Dog, but that's not your problem—your sweep assignment is Autobahn. You get into your bindings and push off, making slow, wide turns and looking at the remaining skiers far ahead. One of them falls, sending up a huge cloud of snow.

As you come nearer, the skier is still down. As far as you can tell, he has not moved. Several other skiers have stopped and are looking uphill at their companion. One of his skis is off, the other still on. You ski to a stop just below the skier.

You: "Hello, I'm Ben Schussen of the High Range Ski Patrol. Can I help you?"

Skier: "Yes. I think I did a job on my leg."

You take off your skis and approach. You take the patient's wrist and feel his pulse. It is strong, regular, and about 80 beats per minute. You notice that the left foot (the one with the ski still attached) seems to be rotated out to an abnormal degree. Keying the radio transmission key, you call the sweep chief at the summit and ask her to bring down a toboggan.

You: "What's your name?"

Skier: "Will Clyde."

You: (pointing to the leg with the ski on) "That leg?" (The skier nods.) "Lets get that ski off."

(You carefully release the heel piece of the binding without moving the leg or foot, then remove the ski. Then you carefully unbuckle the boot.) "I'm going to stick your skis up in the snow to warn other skiers that we are down here." (You form an X uphill from the skier.)

You: "Can you feel your toes?"

Skier: "Yes."

You: "Can you wiggle them?"

Skier: "Yes."

You: "Did you hurt yourself anywhere else?"

Skier: "No."

You: "Did you hit your head, or hurt your neck or back?"

Skier: "No."

You: "I'm going to examine your leg. Where exactly does it hurt?" (The skier points to a place just above the top of the boot.) "Do you remember how you fell?"

Skier: "I caught an edge, one ski went one way, and this ski went another. It didn't release, and I twisted my leg when I fell."

You: "Did you feel a pop?"

Skier: "No."

You palpate the leg and find a swollen, tender area just above the top of the boot.

Fig. 11.21 *Scenario #10*

Skier: "Ouch!"

At this point, the toboggan arrives, pulled by veteran patroller Bea Friendly.

You: "Bea, this is Will Clyde. He has a hurt left leg."

Bea parks the toboggan below the patient, anchors it with her skis, and unpacks it. She removes the quick splint, opens it, and lays it on the snow by the skier's injured left lower extremity.

You: "We're going to have to expose your injury to make sure there is no open wound. We'll use a seam ripper so that you can have the ski pants re-sewn and no one will know the difference." (The skier nods assent.)

You open your first aid belt, take out a seam ripper, and expertly open the seam of the left pant leg to the knee. Then you open the seam of the left long-john leg to the knee. There is no sign of blood and no open wound. There is a swelling of the midleg without any ecchymosis as yet.

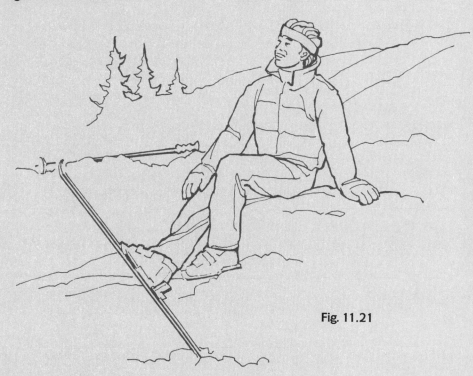

Fig. 11.21

You: "Bea, I'll put some slight traction on the foot if you will steady the thigh."

Bea uses the "pant leg pinch lift" to steady the thigh and raise it slightly while you grasp the toe and heel of the boot. Using axial traction, you straighten and rotate the leg slightly so that it is back in anatomical position. The skier grimaces and you notice some pallor and sweat on his forehead.

Bea reaches over with one hand and slides the opened quick splint beneath the skier's extremity. Then, as you lower the skier's extremity into the splint, she folds up the sides and closes the Velcro straps.

You: "We'll lift you into the toboggan and then give you a ride down the hill."

Chapter 12

Injuries to the Head, Eye, Face, and Throat

For, as the substance of the brain, like that of the other solids of our body, is nearly incompressible, the quantity of blood within the head must be the same, or very nearly the same, at all times, whether in health or disease, in life or after death.

—*Alexander Monro*
Observations of the Structure and Functions of the Nervous System

Before reading this chapter, please review the section on the anatomy and physiology of the skeletal and nervous systems in Chapter 2.

Head injuries are a major cause of death and disability; in half of all trauma deaths, head injury is a major factor. In the urban setting, head injuries are most frequently caused by motor vehicle accidents. In the outdoors they also can be caused by snowmobiles and all-terrain vehicles, as well as by falls and collisions while hiking, climbing, and skiing. These injuries can be prevented to some extent by wearing helmets when climbing, ski racing, riding mountain bikes, and driving off-road vehicles.

The importance of a head injury depends on the amount of **brain injury**. The degree of recovery obtained by a head-injury patient depends on the sum of the damage occurring at the time of the accident and the secondary damage caused by complications following the accident.

As with fractures, head injuries can be either **open** or **closed** (Fig. 12.1). In an open injury, the scalp is incised or lacerated, the skull fractured, and the brain exposed. A head injury is considered open if spinal fluid is draining from a head wound, even if the brain itself cannot be seen. The brain can be injured both by the initial trauma and by infection that may develop later. In a closed injury, brain damage is caused by shearing forces and compression trauma, both from the original impact and the subsequent contrecoup effect. While rescuers have no control over this initial damage, they may have considerable control over secondary damage.

The main cause of secondary injury to the brain is hypoxia, or decreased tissue oxygen level. This can be caused by interference with the brain's blood supply because of shock in a patient with multiple injuries, restriction of blood supply as a result of increased pressure inside the rigid skull caused by swelling or bleeding, or by airway obstruction. The longer the hypoxia lasts, the greater the damage. The rescuer can prevent or improve hypoxia to some extent by maintaining an open airway, giving oxygen, and preventing shock by stopping external hemorrhage; however, in most cases little can be done outside of a hospital.

A head injury by itself *rarely causes shock*. If shock develops and severe bleeding from the scalp is not present, the patient probably has additional injuries to the chest, abdomen, pelvis, or spinal cord. *Any patient with a head injury should be assumed to have a cervical spine injury*.

Field emergency care for patients with head injuries is limited to little more than providing airway and ventilation support. Therefore, the most important emergency care is *transportation of the patient to a hospital without delay*. Any head injury that causes loss of consciousness, even for a moment, is of concern. Most patients with significant head injuries are already unresponsive (unconscious) when discovered and remain so during emergency care. *Changes in responsiveness are important, especially if the patient is initially* alert but gradually becomes more lethargic, confused, and sleepy. In every patient with a head injury, frequently assess and record the level of responsiveness (by the AVPU Scale or Glasgow Coma Scale, Chapter 3), the state of the pupils, and the ability to perceive touch and pain or to move the extremities in response to pain. It is especially important to note a decreasing level of unconsciousness, progressive enlargement of a pupil, and a decrease in the ability to move one side of the body. Send the recorded information with the patient to the hospital.

As swelling and/or bleeding progress in a head injury, the inability of the rigid skull to enlarge causes the pressure inside it to rise. This development, called increased **intracranial pressure (ICP)**, produces local signs and symptoms, due to pressure on vital centers, and general signs and symptoms, due to restriction of blood circulation in the brain, resulting in hypoxia. The local signs and symptoms include changes in the pupils, a rise in blood pressure, slowing of the pulse, slowing and irregularity of breathing, incontinence, and weakness or paralysis of one or more extremities. The general ones include

Fig. 12.1 *Some Types of Head Injuries*

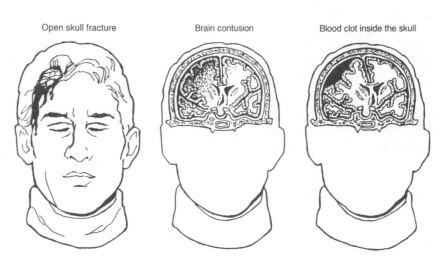

Open skull fracture   Brain contusion   Blood clot inside the skull

Fig. 12.1

headache, nausea, vomiting, and a progressive decrease in the level of responsiveness. Lack of oxygen in the brain causes enlargement of brain blood vessels as the body attempts to get more oxygen-containing blood to the brain cells; however, blood vessel enlargement tends to increase the swelling inside the brain. This raises the ICP even higher and starts a "vicious circle." One technique available to rescuers that can help reverse this process is to *hyperventilate the patient with 100-percent oxygen*. This is done with the bag-valve-mask at 24 to 30 breaths per minute. The increased breathing rate and depth not only provides more oxygen but removes the carbon dioxide at a faster rate. Higher oxygen and lower carbon dioxide both cause the blood vessels to narrow, which decreases brain swelling.

At this point, please review the **Assessment of the Unresponsive Patient** presented in Chapter 4. The steps of this assessment are summarized in Table 12.1. Remember that a head-injury patient may have lost consciousness for reasons other than the head injury itself. For example, a patient who suffers a sudden stroke or seizure may lose consciousness, fall to the ground, and suffer a head injury because of the fall.

The rescuer must always anticipate and prevent problems, because an unresponsive patient cannot tell the examiner how he or she feels and may be unable to perform actions such as coughing that are carried out routinely by responsive individuals. The emergency care of a patient unresponsive due to a head injury is much the same as the emergency care of a patient unresponsive for any reason.

Table 12.2 lists several possible causes of unresponsiveness.

Table 12.1

Summary of Assessment of an Unresponsive Patient

1. First impression
   Is there any danger to the rescuer or patient? Is there a need for extrication? Is there need for additional help? What has most likely occurred? What is the probable mechanism of injury? Institute universal precautions—wear disposable rubber gloves at a minimum.
2. Primary survey
   a. Level of responsiveness: Ask, "Are you okay?" If the patient does not respond, call for help.
   b. Airway: Open, usually with the jaw-thrust technique. Maintain manual stabilization of the head and neck in a trauma patient.
   c. Breathing: Assess and assist or provide ventilation (mouth-to-mask, bag-valve-mask) and/or care for airway obstruction as needed.
   d. Circulation: Assess and give CPR as needed.
   e. Control severe bleeding.
   f. If the patient has labored breathing and/or a fast, weak pulse not explained by injuries already discovered, assess the neck and chest, followed by the abdomen, pelvis, and extremities. Care for significant injuries as discovered.
   g. Assess the head. Monitor repeatedly and record the level of responsiveness (AVPU, Glasgow Coma scales), state of pupils, and movement of the extremities in response to pain.
   h. Stabilize the patient's body temperature.
   i. Transport the patient as soon as possible. *Do not delay transport of a seriously ill or injured patient in order to conduct a secondary survey in the field.*
3. Secondary survey
   a. Record and monitor vital signs. Take temperature with a low-reading thermometer if hypothermia-producing conditions exist (estimate temperature in the field [see Chapter 18], measure temperature after reaching patrol room or other shelter).
   b. Assess skin color, moisture, and temperature.
   c. Obtain the patient's medical history from companions to determine:
      (1) Events leading up to present state
      (2) Pre-existing illness or injury
      (3) Allergies
      (4) Medicines or drugs
      (5) Anything else we should know?
   d. Conduct a general body examination from head to toe. Look for wounds, other injuries, ability to move normally, reaction to pain and touch. Conduct the examination in the following order:
      (1) Head
      (2) Neck
      (3) Chest
      (4) Abdomen and pelvis
      (5) Lower extremities
      (6) Upper extremities
      (7) Back
   e. Look for medical-alert bracelets and wallet cards.

Table 12.2

Some Causes of Unresponsiveness

1. Head injury
   a. Damage to both cerebral hemispheres or to the reticular activating system of the brainstem. Damage may be temporary (e.g., concussion) or more severe (e.g., contusion or hemorrhage).
   b. Hemorrhage
      (1) Subdural or epidural
      (2) Into the brain substance itself, especially the cerebral cortex or brainstem
2. Stroke
   a. Brain hemorrhage
   b. Clot in a cerebral artery
3. Infection
   a. Brain abscess
   b. Meningitis
   c. Encephalitis
   d. Toxic effect on the brain from severe, generalized body infection such as pneumonia or septicemia (bloodstream infection)
4. Brain tumor
5. Metabolic abnormalities
   a. Hypothermia, hyperthermia
   b. Hypoglycemia
   c. Hypoxia, including acute mountain sickness
   d. Poisoning, including illegal drugs
   e. Starvation, severe dehydration
   f. Acidosis or alkalosis
   g. Low thyroid state
   h. Kidney or liver failure
   i. Hypercarbia (excess carbon dioxide)
6. Seizure
7. Shock

General Care of the Unresponsive Patient

When providing emergency care, always institute universal precautions against blood-borne pathogens (see Appendix F), which means putting on disposable rubber gloves, at a minimum.

Arrange for transport without delay. Then treat problems uncovered during the primary survey. The most immediate danger to an unresponsive person is obstruction of the upper airway, most commonly caused by the tongue, although mucus, vomitus, or foreign matter such as food or snow are other possible causes.

Use the jaw-thrust technique (Fig. 12.2) to open the airway of *every* unresponsive trauma patient and every patient in whom the onset of unresponsiveness was unobserved. The cervical spine could have been injured by the initial trauma or by a fall if the patient lost consciousness while sitting or standing.

Remove any foreign material using the finger-sweep method, suction, or, if necessary, the Heimlich maneuver or modifications of it (see Chapter 4 and Appendix B). Insert an oral airway to keep the airway open (see Chapter 5), unless the patient has a

gag reflex. If necessary, provide ventilation by mouth-to-mask or bag-valve-mask, and if pulses are absent, perform CPR. A patient unresponsive due to a head injury should be hyperventilated by bag-valve-mask at 24 to 30 breaths per minute. Be sure to allow the patient sufficient time to *exhale* between breaths.

If the patient is unconscious for a reason other than trauma, the semiprone (coma or NATO) position (Fig. 12.3) is useful in maintaining the airway and promoting drainage of vomitus and other secretions from the mouth and nose; this position is especially important if the patient cannot be watched constantly.

Assess the scalp for wounds and bleeding. Since shock may cause unresponsiveness by itself and can worsen brain injury from other causes, look for external bleeding from other parts of the body. If the signs of shock are present without any obvious external bleeding, assess carefully for signs of internal bleeding (see Chapter 6). Stop external bleeding by direct pressure, as described in Chapter 6 and in **Scalp Lacerations** below. An open skull fracture is extremely serious because of the danger of meningitis or brain infection. Protect any open scalp wound with sterile compresses.

Give unresponsive patients oxygen in high concentration and high flow rate to ensure that each unit of

Fig. 12.2 *Use of Jaw-thrust Technique to Open and Maintain the Airway*

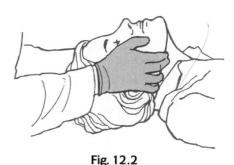

Fig. 12.2

blood will carry the greatest possible amount of oxygen to the sensitive brain tissues.

Since any patient unresponsive due to trauma is assumed to have a neck or back injury, apply a rigid collar and maintain manual stabilization of the head and neck until the patient is completely immobilized on a long spine board. Vomiting is common in unresponsive patients, particularly those with head injuries, and is a common cause of airway blockage. Anticipate vomiting and watch for it constantly. It should be managed with suction equipment, if available, and in the non-trauma patient by rolling the patient into the semiprone (NATO) position. A trauma patient already immobilized on a long spine board can be tipped on the side if vomiting occurs. If not yet on a spine board, the trauma patient must be logrolled. If only one rescuer is available, the patient's head and neck must be stabilized manually as well as possible when the patient is turned to one side to vomit. There is no completely safe way for a single rescuer to do this, but the alternative may be suffocation from airway blockage due to aspirated vomit. *Aspirated vomit is a disaster to be avoided at all costs.*

Figure 12.4 illustrates a reasonably satisfactory one-rescuer logroll. Quickly kneel at the patient's side, far enough away so that you can roll the patient toward you. Bend the patient's far elbow and place the far hand behind the head. Straighten the patient's near arm and place it at the patient's side with the palm against the thigh. Cross the patient's far ankle over the near ankle. With one hand behind the patient's far shoulder and the other behind the patient's far hip, roll the patient quickly onto the side toward you, being careful that the patient does not vomit on you. A minimum of bending or rotation of the spine may occur with this maneuver, but it is preferable to having the patient vomit and aspirate.

Note any bleeding or drainage of clear fluid from the ears, nose, and mouth. Test pinkish fluid by letting a drop fall on a paper towel or white cloth (see **Skull Fractures**).

Keep the patient lying down. If the patient is on a spine board, elevate the *head* of the board about 6 inches to raise the patient's head and trunk slightly higher than the rest of the body. This position retards swelling of the brain to some extent. However, if the patient is in shock, it may be preferable to leave the board level or to raise the *foot* of the board 6 inches. If transporting the patient by toboggan, position the patient in the toboggan so the head will be uphill or downhill as desired, depending on the major problem(s).

Do *not* use a pillow, because it would cause flexion of the patient's neck and might interfere with the airway or aggravate a neck injury. Keep the patient warm but not hot. Remove hard contact lenses, if present (see Chapter 4 for technique), and keep the patient's eyelids closed to prevent the corneas from drying out.

Unconscious patients may convulse. Because convulsions cannot be stopped, emergency care consists of protecting the patient from inadvertent self-injury by removing obstacles and using padding, if available (see Chapter 17). Breathing that stops temporarily during a convulsion usually will start again in one to two minutes. The only treatment required is to maintain an open airway.

Treat any additional injuries uncovered during the secondary survey.

Fig. 12.3 *The NATO Position*

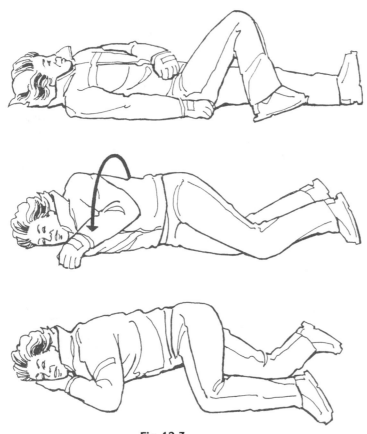

Fig. 12.3

Table 12.3

Summary of General Care of Unresponsiveness

1. Use universal precautions.
2. Conduct the primary survey. Treat life-threatening conditions. Support or provide ventilation, relieve respiratory obstruction, give CPR, and control severe bleeding as necessary.
3. Arrange for transport to a hospital without delay.
4. Guard and monitor the airway. Use the semiprone position in a non-trauma patient.
5. Insert an oral airway unless the patient has a gag reflex.
6. Give oxygen in high concentration and high flow rate. Assist inadequate ventilations with a mouth-to-mask or bag-valve-mask. In head injuries, consider hyperventilation by bag-valve-mask at 24 to 30 breaths per minute.
7. Keep the patient's head slightly higher than the feet unless shock is present.
8. Dress wounds.
9. Watch for vomiting. Use suction if available. Turn the patient to the side to avoid aspiration of vomitus.
10. Keep the patient warm but not too warm.
11. Keep the patient's eyelids closed to prevent the eyes from drying.
12. Watch for convulsions.
13. Care for all unresponsive trauma patients as though they had neck and back injuries.

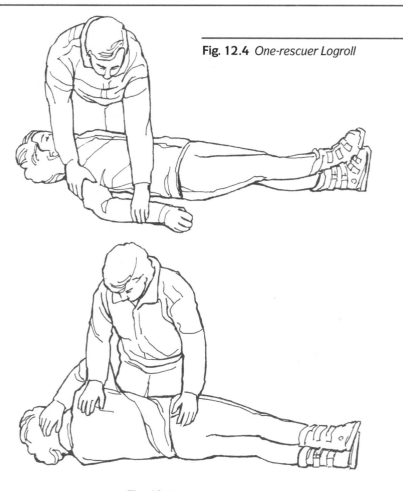

Fig. 12.4 *One-rescuer Logroll*

Fig. 12.4

Specific Types of Head Injuries

Scalp Lacerations

Because of the scalp's generous blood supply, a scalp laceration usually bleeds freely and can cause considerable blood loss. Assess the wound to see whether the skull or brain is exposed and whether there is an indentation that suggests a depressed skull fracture.

Control bleeding by careful direct pressure. If the patient has a depressed skull fracture, exert pressure *around the edges* of the injury rather than on top of it.

Open skull fractures are extremely serious and may not be obvious. Take care to avoid introducing dirt or loose hair into the wound. Do *not* irrigate scalp wounds or trim the patient's hair near the wound, since contaminants may be washed into an open fracture and hair clippings may get into the wound. However, a dirty scalp avulsion should be cleaned, if necessary, by irrigating it with either sterile physiological saline solution or clean water to which one-half teaspoon of table salt has been added per quart. Be careful not to wash anything into the wound.

After cleaning, replace the tissue, then bandage the wound by covering it with a sterile compress held in place by a triangular bandage or stocking cap as described in Chapter 7. Infection in simple scalp wounds is unusual because of the scalp's excellent blood supply.

Concussions

A patient who has lost responsiveness, even momentarily, or has other symptoms of temporary brain dysfunction after a blow to the head is said to have a concussion. Symptoms can include "seeing stars," confusion, loss of memory, dizziness, severe headache, nausea, vomiting, weakness, and double vision or other visual changes. Some patients are unable to remember events that occurred just before the injury. These symptoms usually are temporary and will subside without residual damage. They probably occur because the brain has been jarred, causing a temporary "short circuit" of its electrical connections.

A concussion is significant because its symptoms are similar to early symptoms of brain hemorrhage and other serious illness or injury. In every patient who has symptoms of a brain concussion, the rescuer should monitor and record at regular intervals the vital signs, especially the level of responsiveness, state of the pupils, ability to move, and response to touch and pain. In a remote setting where the patient cannot be transferred to a hospital immediately, monitoring should continue at least every two hours during the following night.

Any person who loses responsiveness, even momentarily, should be examined by a physician.

Brain Contusions

Brain contusions involve bruising of brain tissue and swelling of the brain. Because the brain lies within a "tight, bony box," only a small amount of swelling can occur without causing an increase in pressure inside the skull. The signs and symptoms of a brain contusion are similar to those of a concussion but are more severe. They include loss of responsiveness longer than five minutes, repeated loss of responsiveness, weakness, paralysis or loss of sensation—especially of one side of the body—changes in the pupils, and convulsions.

A contusion is a serious injury and the patient should be taken to a hospital without delay. During transport, closely monitor the patient's airway, level of responsiveness, pupils, and other vital signs, and give care for unresponsiveness, as outlined above, if it develops.

Bleeding Inside the Skull

Bleeding inside the skull can be caused by a head injury or by the spontaneous rupture of a blood vessel. Blood vessel ruptures can be caused by high blood pressure, blood vessel damage in arteriosclerosis, or breakage of a berry-like weak spot on a vessel, called an **aneurysm**.

Bleeding can occur within the brain itself or into the spaces between the coverings of the brain (**meninges**). The signs and symptoms are caused by direct pressure on the brain, hypoxia secondary to increased intracranial pressure, and destruction of brain tissue. The neurologic status of the patient may deteriorate rapidly.

Monitor the patient closely and record findings at regular intervals. Transport the patient to a hospital without delay, caring for unresponsiveness if it develops.

Skull Fractures

Because a considerable force is required to fracture the skull, some degree of brain damage almost always accompanies a skull fracture. An unstable cervical spine injury should be assumed as well. The seriousness of the injury is related to the brain damage and not the skull damage.

Skull fractures can be open or closed. A frequent cause of open skull fractures is a penetrating injury from a sharp or high-velocity object such as an ice pick or bullet. The signs and symptoms of a skull fracture are mainly those of the underlying brain damage as described in **Brain Contusions** above. In addition, the patient may have a scalp wound that exposes the skull or brain tissue. Cerebrospinal fluid, which is watery and colorless or pink, may exude from the wound or drip from the nose or ear; there may be bleeding from the nose, ear, or mouth. Bleeding from a skull fracture also may be present under the skin as

ecchymosis, usually in the skin around the eyes ("raccoon eyes") or at the tip of the mastoid process behind the ear (Battle's sign). However, these signs of bleeding usually do not appear until several hours after the injury occurs.

Cerebrospinal fluid coming from the nose or ear may be overlooked if it is mixed with blood. If the discharge is allowed to drop onto a paper towel or piece of cloth, a target-like figure is produced, with dark red in the center, surrounded by a dark pink area with a light pink rim.

The emergency care of a patient with a skull fracture is similar to that of a patient with a brain contusion or hemorrhage (see above). Local wound care is discussed in the section on **Scalp Lacerations** above. Do not remove an impaled object; instead immobilize it in place with a stabilizing dressing. Give general care for unresponsiveness as required.

Patients with head injuries may be alert and may not appear to be seriously injured when first seen. However, because of slow bleeding or progressive swelling inside the skull, they may develop increased intracranial pressure many hours or days after the injury. Development of any of the following signs and symptoms in a head-injured patient means that the patient should be taken to the hospital without delay.

1. Decreasing level of responsiveness or difficulty in awakening the patient.
2. Recurring nausea or vomiting.
3. Unexplained visual changes, including double vision, blurring, blindness, "spots" or "stars."
4. Increasingly severe headaches.
5. Change in personality, memory, ability to concentrate or ability to think.
6. Weakness, paralysis, or loss of sensation, especially of one side of the body.
7. Seizures.

Eye Injuries

Eye injuries have special significance because of the associated risk of blindness. An understanding of eye injuries and their emergency care requires a brief overview of the anatomy (Fig. 12.5) and physiology of the eye.

The eyeball is a hollow globe about 1 inch in diameter that lies in the eye socket of the skull. The optic nerve connects the eyeball with the brain through an opening in the back of the socket. The posterior five-sixths of the globe is formed by a dense tissue, the **sclera**, and the anterior one-sixth is formed by the transparent **cornea**. In front, the visible part of the sclera is white and is called the "white of the eye." It is covered by a transparent tissue, the **conjunctiva**, that contains small visible blood vessels. When this tissue is inflamed (**conjunctivitis**), the blood vessels enlarge, turning the conjunctiva pink or red.

The eyeball is divided into two compartments, or chambers, by the transparent **lens** and its supporting ligaments. The posterior chamber is filled with a jellylike fluid, the **vitreous humor**; the anterior chamber is filled with a watery fluid, the **aqueous humor**. The pressure of these two fluids maintains the globular shape of the eyeball. A laceration that allows fluid to leak out will cause the eyeball to collapse.

Fig. 12.5 *Anatomy of the Eye*

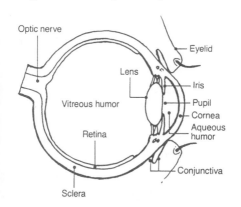

Fig. 12.5

Between the cornea and the lens lies a circular sheet of muscle, the **iris**, with a central hole, the **pupil**. The iris adjusts the size of the pupil to regulate the amount of light entering the eye. The outer surface of the iris is covered with pigmented cells that account for the color of the eye. The inner surface of the sclera is covered with a thin sheet of tissue, the **retina**, containing light-sensitive cells.

The eye can be compared to a simple camera. The cornea acts as a transparent lens cover, the lens of the eye corresponds to a camera lens, the iris to the camera diaphragm, and the retina to the film. The lens of the eye is elastic and can change shape to focus an image on the retina. In people over 45 years of age, this elasticity often is lost and must be compensated for by eyeglasses, usually bifocals or trifocals.

The cornea is protected by the **upper** and **lower eyelids** and is kept from drying out by **tears** produced by **tear glands** that lie above the outer part of each eye. The tears flow down across the cornea and drain at the inner corner of the eye through the **tear ducts** into the nasal cavity.

When evaluating an eye injury, the rescuer should ask the patient to describe in detail exactly what happened, then ask specifically whether vision is normal, whether there is a red haze, flashing lights, or other abnormal visual phenomena, and whether there is double vision. Look for skin wounds, bleeding, swelling, or ecchymosis of the eyelid, and for abnormal prominence of one eye compared with the other. Inspect the conjunctiva for injuries or abnormal redness from bleeding or dilated blood vessels. Examine the pupils for size and symmetry, test them with a flashlight for reaction to light, and compare them to each other to detect differences in size and shape. An irregular or non-reactive pupil following

trauma may mean a serious eye injury. Unless there is an obvious injury to one or both eyes, ask the patient to follow the movement of your finger with the eyes. Observe whether the patient's eyes move together and are able to follow the finger as it is moved up, down, and from side to side. Test vision in each eye separately by having the patient cover one eye and read ordinary print from a magazine or newspaper; then do the same with the other eye. Record exactly what you find on the eye assessment.

The technique of removing contact lenses is described in Chapter 4. Do not remove a contact lens from an injured eye.

Eye motion can aggravate an injured eye. Because the eyes normally move together as a unit, the only way to keep an injured eye quiet is to *cover both eyes*. Because eye injuries are a serious matter (except for irritation from small, easily removed foreign bodies), a patient with an eye injury must be taken to a hospital emergency department or to a physician (preferably an ophthalmologist) as soon as possible. Transport the patient in the supine position.

Foreign Bodies

The conjunctiva is designed to protect the eye and is well supplied with nerves. Any object that touches the eyelashes or conjunctiva causes an instantaneous blink reflex, which is the body's attempt to keep the object out of the eye. A foreign body that penetrates these defenses and lodges on the conjunctiva causes severe pain and irritation. The eye produces copious tears in an attempt to flush out the object, and the eyelids go into spasm.

Warn the patient never to rub or press on an eye containing a foreign body, because this can grind the object into the delicate eye tissues.

Small foreign bodies, such as cinders, frequently lodge under the upper eyelid. These can be removed using the moistened corner of a clean handkerchief after rolling the lid back (Fig. 12.6). Place a matchstick horizontally against the center of the eyelid, and lift the lid up over the stick by pulling on the eyelashes while the patient looks downward.

It is safe for a well-coordinated layperson to remove small, loose foreign bodies from the inner eyelid or conjunctiva, but only a physician should remove a large or embedded foreign body or an object lying on the cornea. Impaled foreign bodies should be stabilized in place by sterile compresses that have been moistened with sterile physiological saline solution. Cover the injured eye with an inverted paper cup and patch the normal eye.

Fig. 12.6 *Removal of a Foreign Body from the Inside Surface of the Upper Eyelid*

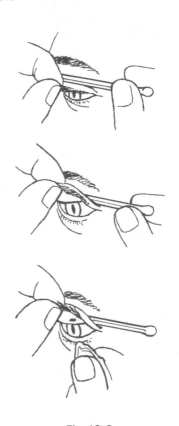

Fig. 12.6

Eye Lacerations

Lacerations of the eyelid require delicate suturing to preserve normal function and appearance. Bleeding from a lacerated eye*lid* can be controlled by gentle direct manual pressure. However, do not press on a lacerated eye*ball*.

The emergency care of patients with eyeball lacerations and penetrating injuries consists of protecting the injured eye with a sterile dressing covered by an inverted paper cup and patching the opposite (normal) eye. Do not replace an exposed or displaced eyeball; instead, cover it with a sterile dressing moistened with sterile physiological saline solution or, if this is unavailable, with clean water, preferably with one-half teaspoon of table salt added per quart. Protect the eye with an inverted paper cup. It is important to prevent the eyeball from drying out.

Eye Contusions

Blunt trauma to the eye can injure its structures and fracture the bones of the orbit. Bleeding into the eyeball may occur; at times blood may be seen in the anterior chamber. Normal eye motion may be impaired.

Emergency care consists of protecting the eye with an inverted paper cup or metal eye shield and patching the normal eye.

Eye Burns

Eye burns can be caused by heat and caustic chemicals. Sunburn of the eye (snowblindness) is discussed in Chapter 18.

Thermal burns usually involve a burn of the face that injures the eyelids, which close reflexively to protect the eyes. Eyelid burns are serious injuries that require expert care, and the patient should be transported immediately to a hospital. Both eyes should be covered. To keep the cornea of the injured eye from drying out, cover that eye with a sterile compress moistened with sterile physiological saline solution (or clean water to which one-half teaspoonful of table salt has been added per quart).

Chemical burns are also serious injuries that may cause extensive destruction of delicate eye tissues. Major offenders are acids and alkalis; alkalis cause the worst injuries. Because these injuries progress rapidly, every second counts.

The sole emergency care is immediate and prolonged flushing of the eye with copious amounts of clean water. This can be accomplished by pouring water into the eye, holding the patient's head under a running faucet, or immersing the patient's face in a bucket of water with instructions to blink rapidly. The eyelids may be in spasm and may have to be held open forcibly during flushing. Flushing is continued for at least five minutes; alkali burns should be flushed for 20 minutes. While flushing, prevent the water from running from the injured eye into the uninjured eye. After flushing, patch both eyes and take the patient to a hospital without delay.

Eye Changes With Head Injuries

Head injuries that damage the orbits or eyeballs or interfere with nerve or muscle function can cause eye changes. These changes should alert the rescuer to the possibility of a head injury and should be monitored to detect deterioration in the patient's condition. Such changes include the following:

1. Differences in the size and/or shape of the pupils (see Chapter 3, Fig. 3.19), due either to direct eye trauma or to increased intracranial pressure affecting the cranial nerve that controls the pupil.
2. Complaints of double vision.
3. Failure of the eyes to move together or to point in the same direction.

4. Bleeding into the eyeball or orbit, which can produce visible blood in the anterior chamber or "raccoon eyes" (see above).
5. Increased or decreased protrusion of one or both eyes.

Injuries to the Face and Throat

Facial and throat injuries can be caused by the same mechanisms that injure the head and are accompanied by the same risk of cervical spine injury. Soft-tissue injuries, bleeding, and/or facial bone fractures may occur. The greatest danger is upper-airway blockage because of bleeding, swelling, deformities, loose teeth, dentures, or direct injury to the larynx or trachea. Vomitus, blood, mucus, and other materials obstructing the mouth and pharynx may have to be suctioned. In addition, patients with facial injuries may not be normally responsive and may have the airway problems commonly associated with altered responsiveness. Lacerations and other open injuries of the face are important from a cosmetic standpoint because they may heal with unsightly scars.

Assessment of a face or throat injury is similar to that of a head injury (see Table 12.1). Patency of the airway must be reassessed at regular intervals.

Emergency care of soft-tissue injuries of the face and neck is similar to that of any soft-tissue injury (see Chapter 7). Always examine the inside of the mouth for bleeding, broken teeth, vomitus, and foreign material.

Control bleeding by direct pressure; however, pressure should not be excessive if you suspect an underlying fracture. It may be necessary to apply pressure simultaneously from both inside and outside the cheek to control bleeding from cheek lacerations. Patients who are bleeding from the mouth or nose should be positioned on one side or sitting up and leaning forward to prevent them from swallowing blood and to allow gravity drainage to help keep the airway clear.

Bandage open wounds. Because infected wounds heal with severe scarring, dirty wounds and wounds that will not receive medical care within a few hours should be cleaned (see Chapter 7).

Cover exposed important structures such as the brain and eye with sterile compresses moistened with sterile physiological saline solution or the cleanest possible water (preferably boiled and then cooled) to which one-half teaspoonful of salt has been added per quart.

Control swelling with cold applications.

Preserve amputated pieces of ear or nose tissue and send them along to the hospital with the patient (see Chapter 7 for technique).

Clean an avulsed flap of skin by irrigating it with sterile saline solution (or clean water to which one-half teaspoonful of salt has been added per quart). Replace the flap over the wound before bandaging.

Nose Injuries

The inside of the nose is lined by a thin mucous membrane containing fragile blood vessels. The anterior part of the thin bone dividing the two halves of the nasal cavity (nasal septum) is the most common area to bleed.

Bleeding can be caused by disease of or damage to the vessels or by interference with the normal blood-clotting mechanisms; however, most nosebleeds occur without obvious cause. In other cases, nosebleeds can be caused by facial or head injuries, the effects of high blood pressure or altitude, or by blowing the nose hard. People with allergies or head colds frequently have nosebleeds.

Most spontaneous nosebleeds will stop of their own accord; those caused by disease or injury may be harder to stop. The patient usually is alarmed by the sight of so much blood and may become nauseated from swallowing blood. Instruct the patient to sit up and lean slightly forward so the blood will drain out of the nose rather than down the throat (Fig. 12.7).

Stopping or Slowing a Spontaneous Nosebleed
(Fig. 12.8)

1. Have the patient blow the nose gently to clear out any clots.
2. Press the upper nostril against the septum for five minutes (Fig. 12.8a).
3. If the previous steps are ineffective, place a pencil-sized roll of gauze between the upper lip and the teeth, and press inward on it for several minutes to shut off the artery to the septum (Fig. 12.8b).
4. Then place a wad of Vaseline gauze in the bleeding nostril and press the side of the nostril against the septum (Fig. 12.8c).
5. Finally, place an ice bag over the nose (Fig. 12.8d).

Fig. 12.7 *A patient with a nosebleed should sit up and lean forward.*

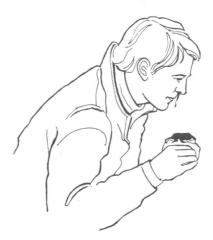

Fig. 12.7

Facial Fractures

Facial fractures may be accompanied by difficulty in talking and swallowing; facial deformity, asymmetry, and swelling; bite irregularity; and bleeding. The major risk is airway obstruction, which may worsen as swelling and bleeding progress.

Emergency Care of a Patient with a Facial Fracture

1. Open and maintain the upper airway, clearing it of secretions, if necessary.
2. Stabilize the cervical spine manually and with a rigid collar.
3. Use suction if necessary.
4. Insert an oral airway if the patient is unresponsive and without a gag reflex. The patient may have to be turned onto one side so that copious secretions or bleeding can drain away. The patient, if responsive, may insist on sitting up and leaning forward in order to breathe and drain secretions.

5. Give oxygen in high concentration and flow rate.
6. Stop external bleeding with direct pressure.
7. Consider immobilizing the patient on a long spine board.

Oral-Dental Injuries

Lacerations inside the mouth can occur with or without injury to teeth. If bleeding occurs following the fracture or avulsion of a tooth, use sterile gauze to wipe out blood and clots, then place several gauze squares over the bleeding area. Ask the patient to bite down gently on the gauze. If this does not control the bleeding, direct finger pressure may be required. Do not let the patient rinse the mouth, since this may worsen bleeding. Send extra gauze pads along with the patient during transportation.

Facial blows may chip or fracture teeth. If a sensitive dental nerve is

---

Fig. 12.8 *Methods for Stopping a Nosebleed*

Fig. 12.9 *Method of Handling an Avulsed Tooth*

exposed, it should be covered with gauze to protect it from cold air. If teeth are displaced or avulsed, the patient should see an oral surgeon immediately. If an avulsed tooth can be found, it should be handled by the crown only (Fig. 12.9a). Do not touch, rub, or vigorously clean the tooth, although it can be gently cleaned by holding it under running water or a stream of sterile saline poured from an IV bottle. Replace the tooth in the socket, if possible (Fig. 12.9b). Otherwise, send the tooth along with the patient in a container of milk, saline solution, water, or, if the patient is alert and dependable, inside the patient's cheek. If at all possible, the tooth should be re-implanted by an oral surgeon within 30 minutes; the success rate falls off rapidly if replacement takes longer.

Immobilize a fractured lower jaw by gently lifting the mandible into proper position against the upper teeth. Secure it with a cravat tied snugly under the jaw and around the head so that it can be slid off quickly if the patient retches (Fig. 12.10). A dislocated jaw usually is locked open and requires no splinting; it should be relocated only by a physician.

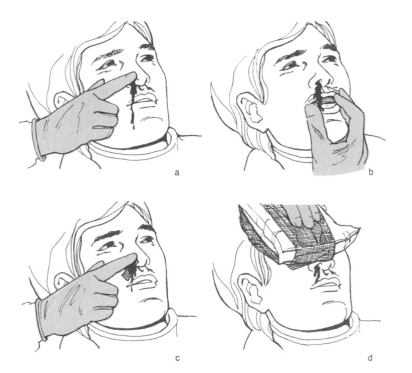

Fig. 12.8

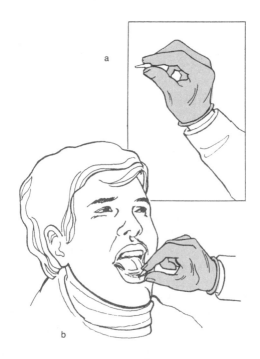

Fig. 12.9

Throat Injuries

Injuries to the soft tissues of the neck and direct injury to the larynx or trachea can cause bleeding, swelling, and upper-airway obstruction. Injury to the air-containing structures of the neck can cause subcutaneous emphysema with a characteristic crackling sensation when the examiner touches the area with a finger. Injuries to the larynx usually cause voice loss. Since an associated cervical spine injury frequently accompanies a throat injury, immobilize the head and neck manually and with a rigid collar.

Bleeding or swelling from a throat injury may cause or worsen airway obstruction. Because this type of airway obstruction frequently cannot be managed without an endotracheal tube or a tracheostomy, the patient must be transported to a hospital without delay. Give oxygen in high concentration but *do not use a bag-valve-mask unless absolutely necessary to assist breathing*, because the positive pressure may force air into the damaged tissues, worsening the obstruction. For the same reason, instruct the patient to breathe slowly and quietly.

Fig. 12.10 *Immobilization of a Fractured Lower Jaw*

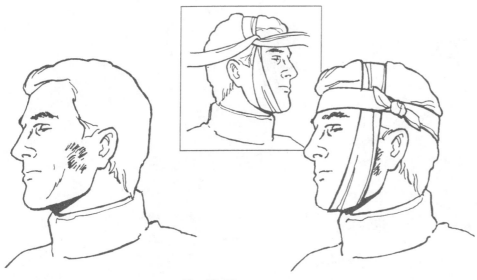

Fig. 12.10

Scenario #11 (Fig. 12.11)

The following scenario illustrates how to provide emergency care for a patient with a head and face injury. Although some of the techniques described are beyond the scope of this book, they are included to provide a comprehensive view of the proper management of this type of injury in the nonurban environment.

You are the sub-district ranger in charge of an area of Grandstone National Park that adjoins a national forest where snowmobiling is popular in the winter. The park has a mutual aid agreement with the county to help out with medical emergencies. The nearest doctor is 50 miles away, the nearest hospital 100 miles away.

You are relaxing after your second cup of coffee one Sunday morning in February when the phone rings. It is the manager of a motel in a town several miles away, a community where hundreds of snowmobilers congregate each weekend during the snowy months. A snowmobiler has lost control of his machine and crashed into a tree several miles north of town. One of his friends drove out to get help, while several others stayed with the injured snowmobiler, who is described as unresponsive and having difficulty breathing. One of the friends has had first responder training, but the group has no first aid equipment.

You reach for your radio and alert Scott, the other ranger in the compound, then run outside. Parked next to the ambulance is a large snowmobile trailer with two snowmobiles and a toboggan on it. You back the ambulance up and hitch the trailer to it.

Scott arrives and the two of you drive up the road to town, where several of the local snowmobile search and rescue people have assembled. It takes only a few minutes to orient all personnel, unload the toboggan and a snowmobile, and transfer the trauma bag, monitor-defibrillator, portable suction unit, oxygen backpack, and a long spine board from the ambulance to the toboggan. Shortly afterward, you are heading up the unplowed road north of town, the friend of the injured snowmobiler leading the way.

Twenty minutes later you arrive at the accident scene. An expensive racing snowmobile is lying on its side, the windshield and front end smashed. Nearby, the patient is lying supine on a space blanket in the snow with a friend stabilizing his head and neck and keeping his airway open with the jaw-thrust technique. The patient's helmet is off, and he is breathing

Fig. 12.11 *Scenario #11*

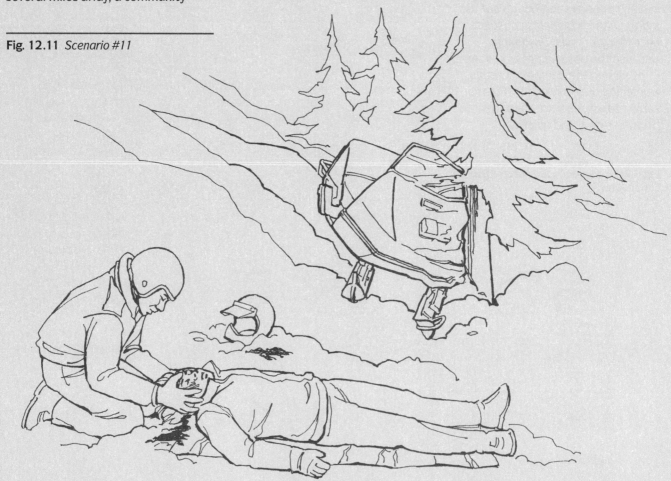

Fig. 12.11

deeply and noisily. There is blood on the snow near his head, his face is bruised and covered with blood, and his eyes swollen partly shut. He is not moving. You lift the trauma bag and suction machine from the trailer and approach the patient.

You: (putting on a pair of rubber gloves from the kit) "Hi, I'm Ranger Brian Weeks and this is Ranger Scott Manley. What's the situation?" (You set up the suction machine and attach a Yankauer tip to the tubing.)

Friend: "Thanks for coming. I'm Duane Crotchroquette and this is Will Clyde. He's in a bad way. He's unresponsive, and I'm having trouble keeping his airway clear because of the blood and mucous."

You: "Let's try some suction. You keep his airway open, and keep his head and neck stabilized."

You grasp the patient's wrist and feel the radial pulse. It is strong and slow. You don't take time to count it but take out a tongue blade and a small flashlight and gently open the patient's mouth. Several teeth are missing and several more turned at an abnormal angle, obviously loose. There is so much blood in the mouth you cannot see anything. Blood is coming from both nostrils.

You insert an oral airway, then turn on the machine and use the suction tip to remove blood and mucous from the mouth and nose, sucking in 15-second spurts and removing your finger from the side port whenever you move the tip. A lot of material ends up in the jar, and the patient's respirations become easier and less noisy. You turn off the machine for a minute. Scott has gotten the patient's arm out of his sleeve and is taking the blood pressure. You remove the oxygen backpack from the sled, attach a non-rebreather mask and tube to the outlet nipple, and turn the flow valve to 12 liters per minute. You position the mask on the patient's face.

You: "Have you assessed the patient? What have you found?"

Friend: "You know about his airway. His breathing is slow, deep, and regular—10 to 12 respirations per minute. His carotid pulse is strong, and I got 60 beats per minute about five minutes ago. He isn't responding to my voice. I've been too busy to check his response to pain. He isn't moving spontaneously at all."

Scott: "His blood pressure is 160 over 90."

You: "Did you see the accident happen?"

Friend: "No. I was on the other side of the hill. When he didn't show up, I turned around and went back, and found him like this but face down in the snow. I turned him as carefully as I could so I wouldn't hurt his neck, and he started breathing right away on his own. The way the machine looks, he was booking when he went over that ridge and hit the tree. Looks like he went through the windshield."

You: "Scott, take over with the suction. I'm going to check a few things."

You grasp the patient's wrist and assess the pulse. It is strong, regular, and 56 beats per minute. Respirations are deep, regular, and 16 per minute. Capillary refill in a finger is normal.

Starting at the patient's head, you carefully assess the scalp. There are no obvious wounds and no bleeding there. On the face, there is a large blue swelling over the left forehead and a large laceration above the left eye, which is oozing blood. You take a sterile compress out of the trauma bag and place it on the laceration. Moving down, you note that the area around the left eye is quite swollen and blue; the area around the right eye is swollen but not blue. The left eye is swollen shut; the right eye almost so. There is a lot of swelling around the nose, which is obviously flattened and bent to the right side, with blood flowing slowly from each nostril. The skin

over each maxilla is swollen and blue. There is blood around the mouth and a large swelling at the midpoint of the left jaw. The lower teeth are clearly not matched to the upper, so you suspect the jaw is broken.

Moving back to the eyes, you open each one with some difficulty, shining a flashlight into each eye in turn. The left pupil is larger than the right and does not react as well to light. Turning to the ears, you find some pinkish fluid draining out of the left ear. To assess his level of responsiveness, you shout into his ear, "Will, are you okay?" He doesn't respond.

You reach for your radio and contact the Park Communication Center at Mastodon Hot Springs. You explain the situation and arrange for a Life-Flight helicopter to meet you at the helipad in town as soon as possible. Next, you reach into the trauma bag and take out the bag-valve-mask. You remove the non-rebreather mask from the patient's face, hook up the oxygen line to the bag-valve-mask, and start assisting the patient's respirations at 30 breaths per minute (one breath every two seconds).

Scott takes over for you as you proceed downward to assess the patient's neck. The skin is pale, cool, and moist. There are no swellings, wounds, or deformities, and the neck seems lined up normally with the shoulders. The trachea is in the midline. Running your fingers down the spinous processes, there is no step-off deformity and no swelling.

At this point, you remove a "short-neck" size Stifneck collar from the trauma pack, snap it into shape, and apply it to the patient's neck.

You zip open the patient's heavy snowmobile suit, open the patient's shirt, and pull up his undershirt to palpate each rib in turn. You find no swellings, wounds, or crepitation. Placing a hand on each side of the lower chest, you note that expansion of the chest on each side is equal. You pull a stethoscope out of your pocket and listen to the breath sounds on each side of the chest; they are normal.

You then open the lower part of the snowmobile suit to assess the abdomen. There are no obvious wounds, bleeding, bruises, or swellings. You push the two iliac crests together with a rotary motion and then push each crest backward. There is no crepitation and the patient does not wince.

You move on to the lower extremities. Not taking time to cut the suit legs away or remove the boots, you palpate each extremity through the clothing. There are no swellings or deformities and the extremities are the same length. You pinch the skin of each lower leg hard. He withdraws the left leg; the right does not move.

Moving to the upper extremities, you again find no swellings or deformities through the clothing. You pinch the skin of the midpoint of each inner arm hard. He withdraws the left arm; the right does not move.

You pause to think. Scott is doing a good job with the bag-valve-mask, and Duane is doing a good job of stabilizing the patient's head and neck. You suction the patient's nose and mouth again. His airway is open and his pulse is good although somewhat slow for the severity of his injuries. You retake the blood pressure; it is 170 over 100 and the pulse is 48. Capillary refill is normal. The patient is responsive to pain, but is moving only the left side of the body. He has a badly injured face, with probable facial bone fractures, a probable fractured jaw, and evidence of a skull fracture. There are no other obvious severe injuries, in particular to the chest, abdomen, or pelvis. The rising BP, slowing pulse, large left pupil, and right-sided weakness make you concerned about a progressive brain injury with increasing intracranial pressure, probably a hematoma or contusion of the left side of the brain. He needs a neurosurgeon as soon as possible.

Friend: "You know, this guy broke his leg last year at High Range Ski Area. That's why he took up snowmobiling this year. Maybe he should have stayed with skiing."

You: "If you're not careful, you can get hurt doing anything."

With the assistance of other members of the rescue team, the patient is lifted onto the long spine board and strapped into place, then lifted into the sled. An IV of lactated Ringer's solution is started with a large bore needle in his right arm. You start slowly back to town, trying to avoid a bumpy ride. You and Scott are riding in the toboggan with the patient, managing the ventilation and suction. You know that the helicopter will be there to meet you when you arrive.

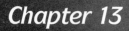

Chapter 13

Injuries to the Neck and Back

And sadly reflecting,
That a lover forsaken
A new love may get,
But a neck when once broken
Can never be set.

—*William Walsh*
   "The Despairing Lover"

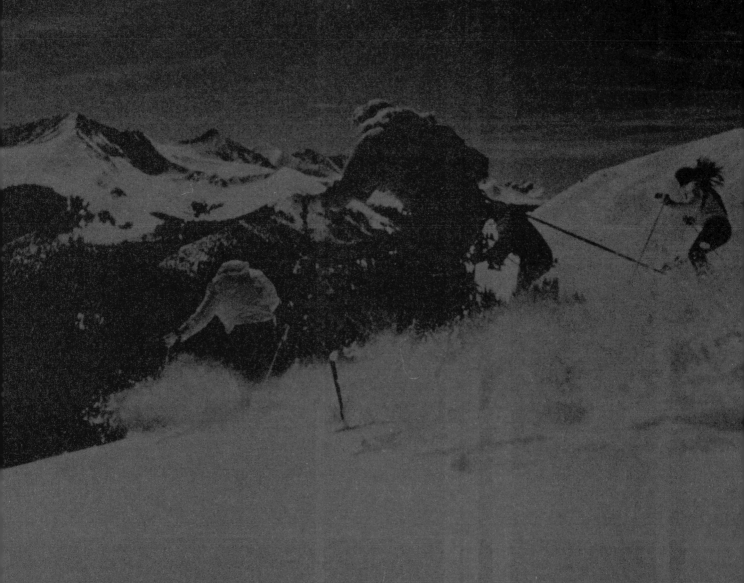

Neck and back injuries are significant because major, often permanent disability may result if the spinal cord is involved. In urban settings, these injuries most commonly are caused by motor vehicle accidents, falls, and contact sports such as football. In outdoor pursuits, they can be caused by collisions and hard falls while skiing; snowmobile and all-terrain vehicle accidents; direct blows from falling objects such as rocks; cave-ins; surfing accidents; and dives into shallow water. Injuries to the soft tissues of the neck and back have been discussed in previous chapters. This chapter covers injuries to the major parts of the skeletal and nervous systems found in the neck and back: the **spine** and **spinal cord**.

As discussed in Chapter 2, the spinal cord lies in a long tunnel, the spinal canal, formed by the successive arches of the vertebrae. The cord extends from the base of the brain to the level of the second lumbar vertebra. Although the cord is somewhat protected by this arrangement, the close relationship between the spine and the cord means that severe injuries to the spine are likely to involve the cord as well.

Disabling spinal cord damage is more common with neck injuries than with upper and lower back injuries. The neck is more vulnerable to injury than the back because it has a wide range of motion, is located in an exposed position at the top of the body where it is not protected by other body parts, and functions like a large ball on a chain because of the weight of the 20-pound head at its free end. These relationships place the cervical spine at more risk from trauma than other areas of the spine. Dangerous mechanisms of injury include the following:

1. Axial compression forces generated by collisions, falling objects, and dives into shallow water.

2. Hyperextension, hyperflexion, rotation, and excessive lateral bending from acceleration and deceleration forces in high speed accidents, especially when the trunk is partly immobilized and the head is free to move.

The thoracic and lumbosacral parts of the spine are stronger and less mobile than the cervical spine and are protected more by the bones and soft tissues of the chest, abdomen, and pelvis. However, they still can be injured by forces causing axial compression and by acceleration, deceleration, rotational, and bending forces that drive one part in a direction different from the rest. Common causes of injury to the thoracic and lumbosacral spine are falls where the spine is axially compressed or hyperflexed, seat-belt injuries where the body is jack-knifed over the belt, and pedestrian-motor vehicle accidents.

A spinal cord injury is a *medical emergency*. Although the rescuer has no control over the amount of cord injury caused by the initial trauma, he or she has considerable control over subsequent injury to the cord due to shock, hypoxia, and improper moving and immobilization techniques. The major goals of emergency care are to *prevent further injury* and *to transport the patient without delay to a hospital*.

The amount of disability caused by a spinal cord injury depends on both the **extent** and the **location** of the injury. The spinal cord is similar to a telephone cable running from the main office through town giving off wires to individual telephones. If the cable is completely cut, more phones are out of service than if it is partially cut. If the cable is cut close to the telephone office, more phones go dead than if it is cut far from the telephone office. A major spinal cord injury or one that is close to the brain damages more nerve fibers and

nerve cells than a minor cord injury or one that is farther from the brain. Thus, if the cord is severed in the lumbar or low thoracic area, the legs will be paralyzed; in the high thoracic area, the legs and chest muscles will be paralyzed; in the midcervical area, the legs, chest muscles, and arms; and in the upper cervical area, the legs, chest muscles, arms, and diaphragm. Paralysis of both legs is called **paraplegia**; paralysis of both arms and both legs, **quadriplegia**; paralysis of the arm and the leg on the same side, **hemiplegia**.

When the patient is first seen, the examiner usually can tell only that the patient has a neck or back injury. It may be impossible, at least initially, to tell whether the spine or spinal cord is injured or, more important, *whether the spinal cord is in danger of being injured*. Nevertheless, *all* neck and back injuries must be treated as though they could be spinal cord injuries, since the consequences of missing an actual or potential spine injury or spinal cord injury are so serious. Fortunately, most neck and back injuries are minor, heal well, and produce no long-term disability. In the field, however, it may not be possible to distinguish minor neck and back injuries from major ones.

Before reading further in this chapter, please review the anatomy and physiology of the spine and spinal cord in Chapter 2.

Classification of Neck and Back Injuries

(Fig. 13.1)

1. Soft-tissue injury *alone* (skin, muscles, tendons, and/or ligaments), without bony spine or spinal cord injury (Fig. 13.1a).
2. Spine injury *without* spinal cord injury (Fig. 13.1b).

3. Spine injury with *incomplete* spinal cord injury (Fig. 13.1c).
4. Spine injury with *complete* spinal cord injury (Fig. 13.1d).

Neck and back injuries also can be classified as **stable** or **unstable**. In a stable injury, there usually is little or no dislocation of the joints between the vertebrae, and the injured area does not contain sharp bone fragments located where they menace the spinal cord. Impaction of fractured bones, tightening of injured ligaments, and muscle spasm splint the injury so that movement causes little or no change in the relationships of the injured parts to each other. The patient may be able to move the body at the injured area to some extent without increasing pain.

In an unstable injury, the body does not splint the injury site enough to prevent further motion, and spinal cord damage may be caused or increased due to worsening of the deformity or laceration by sharp bone fragments. Even normal motion that could be performed safely by an uninjured person may cause further displacement at the injury site with cord injury and the risk of permanent paralysis.

Table 13.1

Mechanisms of Injury That May Indicate Neck and Back Injuries

1. Any significant injury above the clavicle, especially to the head.
2. Any injured patient with impaired responsiveness.
3. Any injury involving high kinetic energy and sudden acceleration or deceleration, especially if there is axial compression, distraction, rotation, or severe bending of the spine.
   a. Any person involved in an accident while driving or riding in an automobile, motorcycle, snowmobile, all-terrain vehicle, trail bike, motorbike, etc. Be especially suspicious if the person was involved in a rollover, ejected from a vehicle, involved in a crash while traveling 25 miles per hour (40 kilometers per hour) or faster, or if another occupant of the same vehicle was killed.
   b. Any skier who collides with a stationary object or other skier.
   c. Any skier who hits hard during a jump or high-speed fall.
   d. Any person who falls from more than two-and-one-half to three times the person's height, or less if from a moving vehicle or chair lift.
   e. Any person hit by a rock, tree, or other falling object.
   f. Any pedestrian or bicyclist struck by a motor vehicle.
4. Any injury from surfing or shallow-water diving.

There is no way that a neck or back injury can be classified as stable or unstable in the field. The patient may or may not have any of the signs and symptoms of spine or spinal cord injury (Table 13.2). Therefore, if a **mechanism of injury** exists that might cause a spine or spinal cord injury (Table 13.1), or if the mechanism of injury is unclear but the patient has other significant injuries that indicate a dangerous mechanism of injury or a high amount of kinetic energy, care must be given for a possible unstable neck or back injury even though the patient has *no* positive signs or symptoms. "After considering the mechanism of injury, the patient's other injuries, and doing the assessment, if you have any reasonable doubt always consider the spine unstable and immobilize it," —Alex Butman, co-author of *Pre-Hospital Trauma Life Support*, second edition (Emergency Training Division, Educational Directions, Inc., Akron, Ohio, 1990).

Fig. 13.1 *Types of Neck and Back Injuries*

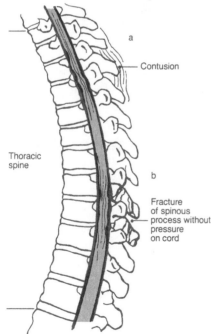

Thoracic spine

a — Contusion

b — Fracture of spinous process without pressure on cord

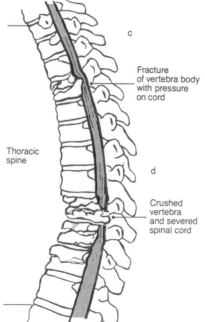

Thoracic spine

c — Fracture of vertebra body with pressure on cord

d — Crushed vertebra and severed spinal cord

Fig. 13.1

Signs and Symptoms of Neck and Back Injuries

1. When the **soft tissues** alone are injured, there may be pain, tenderness, local swelling, ecchymosis, and/or open wounds, but deformity and evidence of neurologic injury usually are absent.
2. When the **spine**, but not the spinal cord, is also injured, pain, tenderness, and swelling usually are worse than with a soft-tissue injury alone. Signs and symptoms of spine injury include the following:
   (a) **Pain at the injury site**. Spontaneous motion at the injury site may cause or increase pain, but *never ask a person with neck or back pain or a suspicious mechanism of injury to move the body at the injured site*. Except possibly in the rare emergency, never move such a patient except by techniques designed to safely place the person on a spine board with a minimum of spine motion.
   (b) **Localized tenderness**. Gently press the spinous processes of all the vertebrae; tenderness of one or more suggests injury at that site. If the patient is being examined in the supine instead of the lateral or prone position, slide your hand under the patient's back from the side so your fingers touch the spinous processes. Do not allow the patient's trunk or neck to turn or rotate during this examination.
   (c) **Deformity or unusual positions** of the spine may or may not be present. Common types of deformities are an abnormal prominence of one spinous process or a "step-off" deformity separating one area of the spine from another.
   (d) **Self-splinting or guarding** of the head, neck, or back.
3. In addition to the signs and symptoms listed above for soft-tissue and spine injuries, patients with **spinal cord** injuries may have signs and symptoms that involve *one* or *both* (usually both) sides of the body **at** and **below** the injury site. Signs and symptoms of spinal cord injury include the following:
   (a) Varying degrees of **loss of sensation** to touch and pain.
   (b) **Abnormal sensations** such as tingling or unusual types of pain such as radiating or "shooting" pains.
   (c) **Muscle weakness** or complete **paralysis**.
   (d) Signs and symptoms of **vascular shock** of the neurogenic type (see Chapter 6).
   (e) **Difficulty breathing** due to paralysis of the chest muscles, or the chest muscles plus the diaphragm.
   (f) **Incontinence** (involuntary urination or bowel movements).
   (g) In males, a prolonged erection of the penis called **priapism**.

Spinal cord injuries may be **partial** or **complete**. With a partial injury, the patient suffers some but not complete paralysis and loss of sensation at and below the injury site. Repeated monitoring is necessary to detect possible progression. The presence or absence of progression should be documented because it is important information for the emergency department physician.

When the injury is complete, the patient suffers complete paralysis and loss of sensation below the injury site. Although the outlook for recovery or improvement is much worse than for a partial cord injury, prompt surgery and other measures may relieve pressure on the cord, permitting some recovery over time.

Table 13.2

Summary of Signs and Symptoms of Spine and Spinal Cord Injuries

1. Spine
   a. Pain at the injury site
   b. Localized tenderness
   c. Possible deformity or unusual position
   d. Associated soft-tissue injuries
   e. Patient self-splinting or guarding
2. Spinal cord
   a. Any or all of the above are usually but not always present
   b. Numbness
   c. Abnormal sensations
   d. Weakness or paralysis
   c. Neurogenic shock
   d. Difficulty breathing
   e. Incontinence
   f. Priapism

Assessment of a Patient with a Neck or Back Injury

Form your first impression as you approach the accident site, considering the mechanism of injury to determine whether the accident would be expected to produce a neck or back injury (Table 13.1). Institute universal precautions (see Appendix F).

Ask the patient or witnesses what happened. Ideally, at this point, if you suspect a neck injury you should stabilize the head and neck manually, applying a rigid collar as soon as the primary survey is completed and the neck assessed. In practice, however, the ABC's (Airway, Breathing, and Circulation) are more important, and lack of help and other urgent problems may force delay of specific manual stabilization to the head and neck. If so, tell the patient not to move, and try to immobilize the head and neck in place with a pack, parka, branches, piled snow, etc.

Perform the primary survey and treat urgent problems. Assess the patient in the supine position. If the patient is found prone or semiprone, carry out the initial assessment in that position until additional help arrives, unless an emergency logroll is necessary because of airway obstruction, severe bleeding, or similar urgent problems. Labored breathing in the absence of airway obstruction is particularly important because it suggests either a concurrent throat or chest injury, or a cord injury with paralysis of the respiratory muscles. If there is time, assess the back before turning a patient into the supine position. The technique of turning is described below in **Emergency Care of a Patient with a Neck or Back Injury**.

If the neck is bent or twisted, whether or not there is an airway problem, bring the head and neck into the neutral, in-line position with the trunk. Not only is assessment, care, and monitoring of the patient much easier, but breathing is easier, and rigid collars, head immobilizers, and vest-type devices are designed to be applied to the patient in this position. Therefore, gently move the patient's head and neck into the in-line position unless there is a deformity or the motion produces muscle

Table 13.3

Summary of Assessment of a Patient with a Neck or Back Injury

1. First impression. Determine the mechanism of injury. If positive mechanism, manually stabilize the head and neck as early as possible. Institute universal precautions (see Appendix F).
2. Primary survey. Treat urgent problems. Logroll the non-supine patient to the supine position as soon as possible, or if required by an emergency.
   a. Airway. Perform the jaw-thrust technique, if necessary.
   b. Breathing. Significance of respiratory distress. Move the head and neck into a neutral, in-line position if necessary to improve breathing.
   c. Circulation. Consider the possibility and significance of shock. Assess pulse, blood pressure, skin color, and moisture.
   d. Assess the level of responsiveness.
   e. Assess the ability to move and response to pain and touch.
   f. Assess the neck, move the head and neck into a neutral, in-line position, and apply a rigid collar.
   g. Ask, "Where do you hurt?"
   h. Assess the back.
3. Secondary survey. Assess the vital signs, take the history, and assess the remainder of body.

spasm, pain, resistance, airway difficulty, or abnormal neurologic signs and/or symptoms, such as numbness, tingling, or sudden weakness. In that case, immobilize the head and neck as found with blankets, towels, etc.

If a patient with the neck bent or twisted has upper airway obstruction that does not respond to the jaw-thrust technique, gently move the head and neck toward the in-line position in a series of steps, stopping after each step to see whether the jaw-thrust technique will open the airway. The head and neck should be immobilized in the position that produces the easiest breathing.

After caring for any urgent problems, ask the patient to indicate the location and type of any pain, and assess painful areas. If the patient complains of pain in the neck or back, ask whether there are (or have been at any time since the injury) numbness, weakness, and/or abnormal sensations below the site of pain. Ask the patient to wiggle the toes

and squeeze your hands. Assess the patient's four extremities for ability to perceive pain and touch. If the patient is prone or semiprone, assess the back for wounds, swellings, tenderness, or deformity. If the patient is supine, *without moving the patient*, run your hand under the back and neck, feeling for any deformity or tenderness of the spinous processes. (Be careful not to cut yourself if there are broken glass fragments or sharp stones on the ground.)

During the secondary survey, note the rate and strength of the pulse, the capillary refill time, and the color, temperature, and moisture of the skin. Reassess the level of responsiveness and, if possible, measure the patient's blood pressure. Abnormal findings may suggest the presence of such conditions as neurogenic shock due to spinal cord injury or hypovolemic shock due to loss of blood from other injuries. Question the patient or witnesses for information about events leading up to the present problem; the patient's medical history; medicines taken; allergies; and "anything else important we should know." Proceed with a careful assessment of the head, neck, chest, abdomen, pelvis and extremities. If you detect abnormalities during the assessment that lead you to suspect a neck or back injury, do not allow the patient to move. The patient should be moved only by trained rescuers using proper techniques.

The steps of the assessment that require direct interaction with the patient obviously cannot be performed on an unresponsive patient. This is irrelevant in cases of unresponsiveness due to trauma, since all such patients should be treated as though they have neck and back injuries.

Emergency Care of a Patient with a Neck or Back Injury

Definitive emergency care of a patient with a neck or back injury, or with a mechanism of injury that might produce such an injury, is *immobilization on a long spine board* so that head, neck, back, pelvis, and lower extremity movement is prevented. During the initial assessment, try to foresee the extrication and immobilization techniques that will be required so that hand position, spine board orientation, and rescuer location will be suitable. The patient must be transferred to the board using *proper techniques* so that there is *minimal* bending or rotation of the head, neck, and back during transfer. When the board cannot be brought all the way in to a patient in an unusual position (e.g., in a tree well), use the extrication techniques described in Chapter 20.

The immobilization of a patient on a spine board is basically the same whether the patient has a neck

injury, a back injury, or both. Patients with neck injuries alone require immobilization of the entire body on a long spine board, since any body movement carries the risk of producing movement of the neck. Patients with back injuries alone theoretically might not require head and neck immobilization but in practice are usually suspected of having a neck injury as well because of the mechanisms involved. In both cases, a rigid collar is applied and the patient's head and neck are stabilized manually until the patient is immobilized on the long spine board.

As mentioned previously, a patient with a neck and/or back injury is best assessed and immobilized in the supine position. This simplifies maintenance of the airway, monitoring of vital signs, transfer to the spine board, and management of vomiting by suction. In rare cases, a patient with a marked deformity of the back may be found in a position that justifies immobilization in other than the supine position. The multiple-rescuer direct ground lift is probably the best technique to use to avoid producing motion at the site of injury while transferring such a patient to a spine board. This lift is described below in **Patient Found in the Supine Position** and also in Chapter 20.

A patient found in a *non-supine* position usually is rolled as a unit into the supine position as soon as possible. This maneuver, called logrolling (Fig. 13.2), also can be used to roll a supine patient onto one side so that a spine board can be slid underneath. Unless logrolling is urgent, assess the back while the patient is still non-supine. Although logrolling should be performed carefully, it should take no longer than 30 seconds to complete.

At least three (but preferably four) rescuers are required for the logrolling maneuver. To avoid unnecessary movement of the patient, logrolling should be delayed until the patient

can be logrolled directly onto a long spine board, unless a non-supine patient has to be logrolled into the supine position because of airway complications or other problems.

Patient Found in the Prone or Semiprone Position

Before logrolling the patient, open the airway with the jaw-thrust technique, assess breathing, and control any obvious severe bleeding. If breathing is absent or if the jaw-thrust technique fails to adequately open the airway, the patient must be logrolled *immediately* into the supine position. If no help is available, this is done by the one-person technique described in Chapter 4 (Fig. 4.5).

If breathing and circulation are adequate, assess the presence of motion and perception of pain and touch in all four extremities *before* logrolling the patient.

To perform the logroll, first tie the patient's legs together with a cravat if there is time. The first rescuer kneels by the patient's head, facing the patient, and is responsible for stabilizing the patient's head and neck throughout the maneuver and until the patient is immobilized on the board. This is done with one hand on each side of the patient's head, as illustrated in Figure 13.2a. The head and neck usually will be rotated to the side and not in line with the rest of the body. A rigid collar *cannot* be applied at this point.

The patient should be rolled *away* from the side the head is facing so that, as the torso is turned, the head and neck will move as little as possible. The direction of roll is *toward* the rescuers at the patient's side. The first rescuer gently restores the head and neck to the neutral, in-line position during the logroll. If resistance or marked pain occur during turning, stop and maintain the head and neck in the position just before the one

Fig. 13.2 *Technique of Logrolling a Patient from the Prone to the Supine Position*

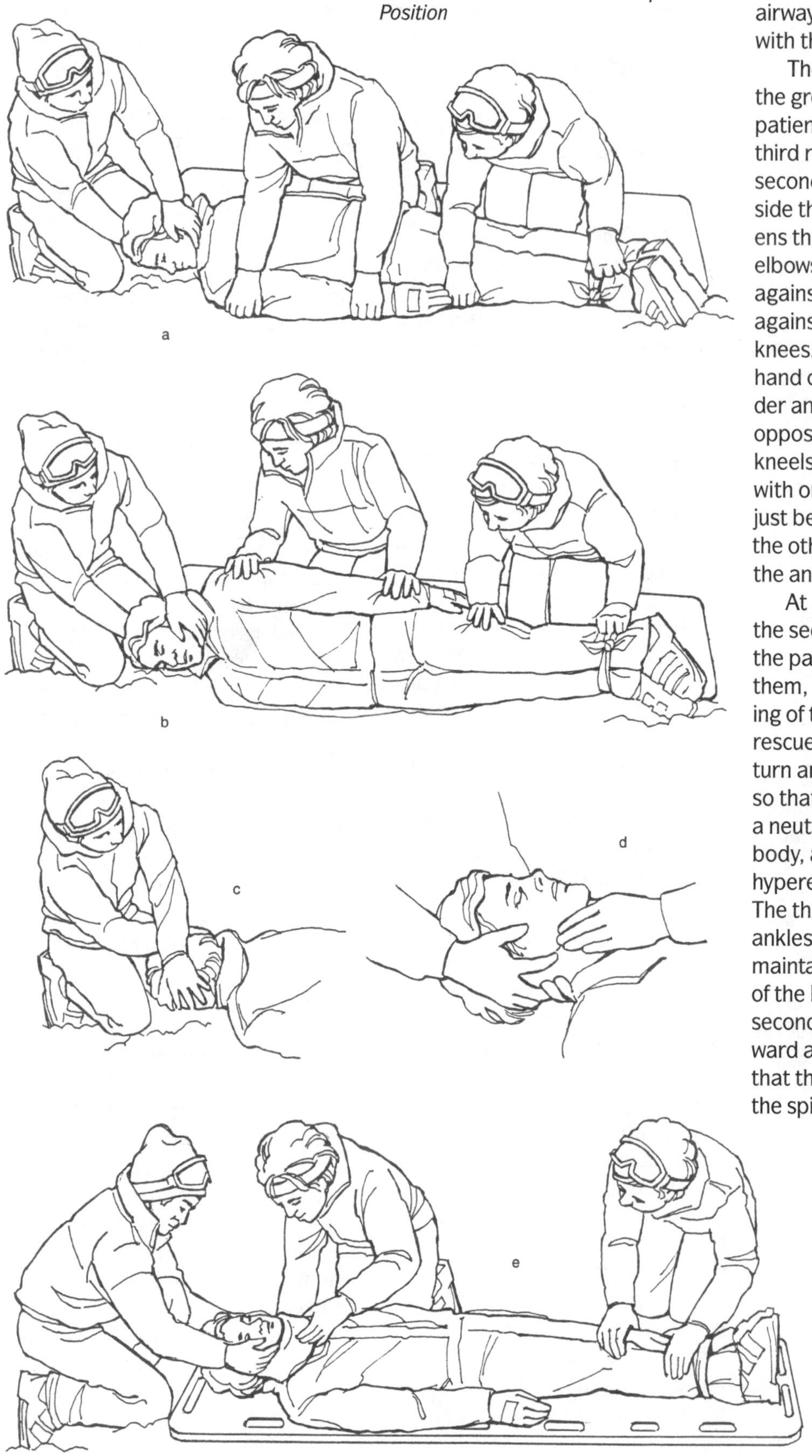

a

b

c

d

e

Fig. 13.2

causing pain or resistance. The first rescuer can maintain the patient's airway by thrusting the jaw forward with the fingers.

The long spine board is placed on the ground 4 to 5 inches from the patient's side with the second and third rescuers kneeling on it. The second rescuer, who is kneeling beside the patient's midchest, straightens the patient's arms, locking the elbows and holding the arms tightly against the body and the palms against the thighs with his or her knees. This rescuer then places one hand on the patient's opposite shoulder and the other hand over the opposite wrist. The third rescuer kneels beside the patient's knees, with one hand on the opposite hip just below the patient's far hand and the other grasping both pant cuffs the ankles.

At a signal from the first rescuer, the second and third rescuers roll the patient's body slowly toward them, avoiding any twisting or bending of the back (fig. 13.2b). The first rescuer watches the patient's chest turn and rotates the patient's head so that the head and neck come into a neutral, in-line position with the body, and the neck is not flexed, hyperextended, or bent sideways. The third reser lifts the patient's ankles slightly off the ground and maintains them in line with the rest of the body as the patient turns. The second and third rescuers move backward as the patient's body turns so that the patient ends up supine on the spine board.

By the time the patient's body has rolled 90 degrees onto the side, the first rescuer may find that he or she is being forced off balance. This can be prevented by starting the loggroll with the hands crossed (Fig. 13.2c). As the patient turns, the hands uncross.

If enough help is available, another suitable technique is for the log-rolling to stop at the 90-degree position with the patient on the side (Fig. 13.2b). At this point, an additional rescuer can stabilize the head and neck with one hand behind the patient's neck and occiput and the other cupped under the patient's chin in a manner similar to that used for helmet removal (see below and also Fig. 13.2d). This allows the first rescuer to regain a more comfortable position before taking over again.

After the patient reaches the supine position, airway and breathing are reassessed, a rigid collar is put in place around the neck, and the first rescuer continues manual stabilization of the head and neck in the neutral, in-line position until the patient has been immobilized on the long spine board (Fig. 13.2e).

If a fourth rescuer is available, the technique is the same except that the second rescuer kneels by the patient's shoulders, holding the patient's arms tightly against the body with his or her knees and placing one hand on the patient's opposite shoulder and the other and over the opposite forearm. The third rescuer kneels beside the patient's buttocks, with one hand on the opposite iliac crest and the other on the near midthigh. The fourth rescuer kneels beside the patient's knees, with one hand on the opposite knee and the other hand grasping both pant legs at the ankles (fig. 13.3). At a signal, the patient is turned as described above, except by three rescuers at the side instead of two. The fourth rescuer lifts the patient's ankles lightly off the ground during the roll so that they remain in line with the rest of the body as the patient turns.

Assess all four extremities for motion and sensation after logrolling the patient.

Patient Found in the Supine Position (or Logrolled from the Prone Position)

If the patient is found in the supine position, the primary and secondary surveys are performed in the usual fashion, with temporary halts as necessary to deal with any urgent problems discovered. The head and neck should be stabilized manually in the neutral in-line position while this is done. If a second rescuer is available, this is done by standard techniques; if not, the patient is cautioned not to move the head or neck, which are stabilized with a pack, parka, fanny pack, or other gear, or with natural substances such as snow.

If needed, the airway is opened and maintained with the jaw-thrust technique. If the neck is bent or twisted, whether or not there is an airway problem, the head and neck should be brought into the neutral, in-line position with the trunk as mentioned previously. After the head and neck are in line, apply a rigid collar. Continue manual stabilization of the head and neck until the patient is immobilized on a long spine board.

Helmets, if worn by injured climbers, ski racers, and snowmobilers, usually should be removed since they may prevent access for assessment and control of bleeding, interfere with stabilization of the head and neck, and obstruct breathing or interfere with resuscitation, suction of secretions, and application of a rigid collar. To avoid twisting or bending the neck, two rescuers are needed (Fig. 13.4).

One rescuer stabilizes the patient's head and neck with one hand behind the patient's occiput and the other cupped under the patient's chin. The second rescuer releases the helmet chin strap and removes the helmet.

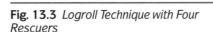
Fig. 13.3 *Logroll Technique with Four Rescuers*

Fig. 13.4 *Helmet Removal*

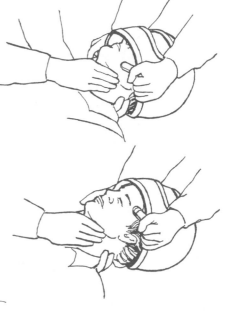
Fig. 13.4

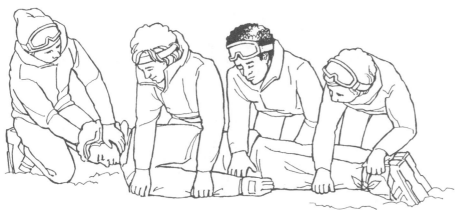
Fig. 13.3

To put a long spine board in place under the patient, the **multiple-person direct ground lift** (also discussed in Chapter 20) or **logroll** can be used. The direct ground lift, which produces less motion of the head, neck, and back, is preferred. Assess and record the patient's ability to move and his or her perception of pain and touch *before* and *after* any of these maneuvers.

1. **Direct ground lift** (Fig. 13.5). This method requires at least four but preferably six rescuers. The rescuer at the patient's head is the leader, who maintains manual stabilization of the head and neck during the procedure and calls out the commands. A rigid collar should be in place. The patient should be supine in the neutral, anatomic position, and if not, should be logrolled and aligned into this position.

   When only four rescuers are available, the first rescuer stabilizes the head and neck; the second rescuer places one hand under the patient's shoulders and the other under the patient's midback; the third rescuer places one hand under the patient's lower back and the other under the patient's upper thighs or buttocks; and the fourth rescuer places one hand under the patient's lower thighs and the other under the patient's calves (Fig. 13.5a). If six rescuers are available, one stabilizes the head and neck, two interlace their hands from each side to support and stabilize the patient's shoulders and upper back, two interlace their hands from each side to stabilize the patient's hips and lower back, and the sixth rescuer supports the patient's legs (Fig. 13.5b). On command, the rescuers simultaneously lift the patient a previously specified distance—usually 6 to 12 inches. Care is taken to maintain the head, shoulders, and hips in line with each other and at right angles to the spine, and that minimal rotation of the neck or back occurs. At this point a long spine board is slid under the patient, and on command the patient is lowered onto it.

   In some cases, the spine board cannot be brought up close enough to the patient, and the patient *must be carried* a short distance. The rescuers simultaneously stand on command, walk in unison to the spine board, and lower the patient onto it.

2. **Logroll** (Fig. 13.6)

   a. The first rescuer stabilizes the patient's head and neck in the neutral, in-line position throughout the procedure and until the patient is immobilized on the long spine board. A rigid collar should be in place. The board is placed at the patient's *far* side and lined up so that the patient will end up on it in the proper position.

   b. The second and third rescuers kneel at the side of the patient to which he or she will be rolled (Fig. 13.6a).

   c. The patient's legs are placed side-by-side in line with the body, the feet are tied together, and the arms are extended at the sides with the palms against the upper thighs and the elbows locked.

   d. The second rescuer kneels at the patient's midchest, placing the hand nearest the patient's head behind the patient's far shoulder and the other hand on the patient's far wrist.

Fig. 13.5 *Direct Ground Lift for a Patient with a Suspected Spine Injury*

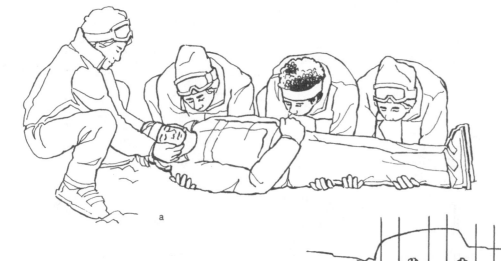

Fig. 13.5

e. The third rescuer kneels at the patient's knees, placing the hand nearest the patient's head on the patient's far thigh just below the patient's hand. The other hand grasps both pant cuffs at the patient's ankles.

f. At a signal from the first rescuer, the patient's body is rolled 90 degrees onto the side, facing the two rescuers. During this, the third rescuer keeps the patient's ankles slightly off the ground enough to keep the legs in line with the body during the roll, and the first rescuer watches the chest turn and rotates the head and neck in line with the chest (Fig. 13.6b).

g. While the patient's body is on its side, an assistant (or the second or third rescuer if no one else is available) pulls the board toward the patient so that its side is touching the patient's back, and tips it toward the patient at a 30- to 45-degree angle (Fig. 13.6c). The patient is then rolled back onto the board and the board lowered onto the ground.

h. If a fourth rescuer is available, the procedure is the same except that the second rescuer kneels at the patient's shoulders, placing the hand nearest the patient's head behind the patient's far shoulder and the other hand on the patient's near elbow. The third rescuer kneels at the patient's pelvis, placing the hand nearest the patient's head on the patient's far iliac crest and the other hand on the patient's near

Fig. 13.6 *Logroll Technique for Placing a Spine Board Under a Patient*

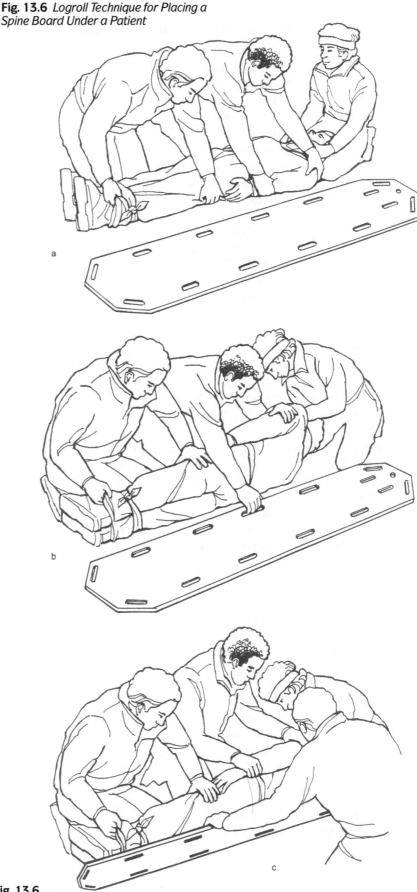

Fig. 13.6

Table 13.4

Summary of Long Spine Board Immobilization Technique

1. Lay the board on the ground next to the patient.
2. Apply a rigid collar, with the patient's head and neck stabilized in the neutral, in-line position. Continue manual stabilization of the head and neck until the patient is completely immobilized on the spine board.
3. Tie the patient's ankles together.
4. In the case of a child with a large head, pad the board with a folded blanket under the torso area.
5. Assess and record sensation and motion below the injury immediately before—and after—transferring the patient to the spine board.
6. Transfer the patient to the board using the direct ground lift or logroll.
7. Secure the patient to the board with a minimum of four adjustable straps. Seat-belt-width straps with adjustable Fastex buckles or Velcro closures are suitable. Place the straps as follows:
   a. One around the chest just below the armpits.
   b. One around the pelvis.
   c. One around the midthighs.
   d. One around the legs.
8. Using a fifth strap, immobilize the patient's upper extremities with the palms against the thighs.
9. Place a rolled towel against the outside of each leg. Include the towels in the leg strap to keep the legs from shifting laterally.
10. Pad between the knees, under the backs of the knees, and under the small of the back. While doing this, avoid any unnecessary movement of the patient.
11. Add additional straps or cravats as necessary to provide adequate immobilization. To prevent axial shifting when going up or down a steep hill, add over-the-shoulder straps and groin straps.
12. Pad between the back of the head and the board to maintain the head and neck in a neutral, in-line position.
13. Immobilize the head and neck with a commercial head immobilizer or with a rolled towel on each side, using straps across the forehead and across the rigid collar.

accidently apply traction to the head and neck while centering the patient. The technique of immobilizing a 13.8) is described in Chapter 8 and summarized in Table 13.4

Difficult Extrications

When a patient is found **sitting** or in a difficult-to-extricate position, a special extrication device such as a short spine board or vest-type device may be preferable. The immobilization technique is described in Chapter 8. These short devices are always used with a rigid collar and are designed for use *only* during extrication. The patient should be immobilized on a long spine board or strapped into a rigid litter as soon as possible. Always leave the short device in place when the patient is transferred to the second device. Because the short device does not immobilize the spine completely, never lift an unsupported patient by the short device alone.

Use judgment in deciding whether to use a short extrication device. Using the direct ground lift and a short transfer to place the patient

Fig. 13.7 *Logrolling a Patient on a Spine Board with Four Rescuers*

midthigh. The fourth rescuer kneels at the patient's knees, with one hand on the opposite knee and the other hand grasping both pants' cuffs at the patient's ankles (Fig. 13.7).

Once the patient has been placed on the spine board, he or she may have to be **centered**. Do this by pulling the patient headward or footward in the direction of the long axis of the body rather than pushing the patient sideways. Be careful that you do not

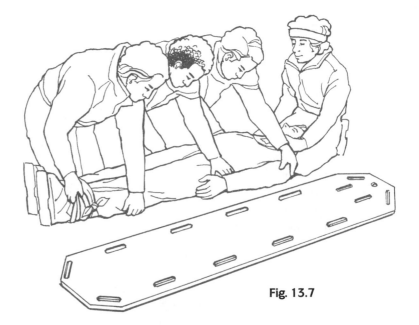

Fig. 13.7

directly on a long spine board may cause less spine motion than applying a short device.

Frequently, a patient with a neck or back injury is found **standing** or even **walking** around. The patient may be complaining of pain in the neck or back, or the mechanism of injury may cause the rescuer to strongly suspect a neck or back injury. In such cases, having the patient lie down or sit may cause dangerous movement of the spine. Therefore, it is preferable to apply the board with the patient *standing* in order to minimize spine motion. At least four rescuers are needed for this technique (Fig. 13.9), as recommended by the authors of *Prehospital Trauma Life Support*.

1. The first rescuer stands behind the patient and stabilizes the patient's head and neck manually.
2. The second rescuer inserts the board from the side, between the patient and the first rescuer (Fig 13.9a). The board is held vertical and placed so that the patient is centered on it. The second and third rescuers stand facing the patient, one on either side. Each inserts the hand nearest the patient under the patient's armpit and grasps

the nearest handhold on the board above the armpit (Fig. 13.9b).
3. The second and third rescuers each grasp a handhold near the top of the board with their free hand.
4. A fourth rescuer stabilizes the foot of the board so that it cannot slip. The second and third rescuers lower the patient and the board toward the ground, stopping halfway down, if necessary, to allow repositioning so that their arms will clear those of the first rescuer when the board is fully lowered. The first rescuer continues manual stabilization of the head and neck of the patient. This rescuer will need to rotate the hands slightly against the patient's head as the board is lowered and kneel as the board reaches the ground (Fig. 13.9c).
5. After the patient and board reach the ground, a rigid collar is applied, the patient is centered on the board by axial sliding and is strapped to the board by standard techniques.

If the patient is **partly or totally unresponsive**, provide the appropriate care (see Chapter 12). If available, give oxygen in high concentration

and flow rate. Anticipate and watch for vomiting. Since a patient immobilized on a long spine board is helpless to guard his or her own airway, you must have suction equipment available and manage vomiting by tipping the spine board on its side and using suction.

If the patient has **associated fractures**, you must decide whether to splint these before or after immobilizing the patient on the spine board. In general, fractures that can be splinted without moving the patient, and major ones, such as open fractures and fractures of the femur, should be splinted beforehand, since a patient with a spine injury is stable as long as he or she is stationary. Splint minor fractures, stable fractures, and relatively painless fractures after the patient is on the spine board, as long as the patient can be boarded without disturbing these fractures. In the multiple-trauma patient where rapid transport is desired, it is almost always preferable to immobilize the patient on a long spine board and treat fractures temporarily by immobilizing the involved body parts to the board rather than take the time to treat each fracture separately. An exception to this is a fracture of the shaft of the femur, which usually requires traction splinting in order to tamponade bleeding and prevent shock.

A patient with a **cervical** or **high thoracic spinal cord injury** may have paralysis of the chest wall and the abdominal muscles, and may be *breathing with the diaphragm alone*. The motor supply of the diaphragm comes from the two **phrenic nerves**, which exit the spinal cord at the level of the third, fourth, and fifth cervical vertebrae and run down through the neck and mediastinum to each side

Fig. 13.8 *Immobilizing a Patient on a Long Spine Board*

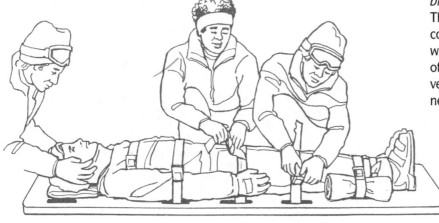

Fig. 13.8

of the diaphragm. Their pathways can be interrupted by injury to the chest, neck, or highest part of the cervical spinal cord.

When the chest wall and abdominal muscles are paralyzed, the patient's respirations will be rapid and shallow and the chest wall will not move, but the abdomen will move in and out with each breath as the diaphragm moves up and down. If both the chest wall muscles and diaphragm are paralyzed, the patient will be unable to breath. If only half of the diaphragm is paralyzed (as in injury to a single phrenic nerve), the patient will still be breathing, but the breathing will be ineffective. Therefore, in a patient with a neck or back injury, monitor the patient's respirations, give the patient oxygen in high concentration and flow rate, and if respirations appear too slow or too shallow or the patient becomes cyanotic, agitated, or develops altered responsiveness, assist breathing by using a bag-valve-mask or pocket mask so that oxygen can be given at the same time.

The neurogenic type of **vascular shock** may occur in a patient with a high thoracic or cervical cord injury because of injury to the autonomic nerve pathways that control blood vessel tone and speed the heart rate. As a consequence, the blood vessels in the abdomen and lower extremities relax, allowing blood to pool in them; the heart does not speed up, and the blood pressure drops. In this type of shock the heart rate is slow instead of fast, the skin may be warm and pink below the level of injury instead of cool and gray, and since the nerve supply to the sweat glands has been interrupted, the skin usually will be dry instead of clammy. If there are accompanying injuries, hypovolemic shock due to blood loss may be present as well.

Emergency care consists of controlling bleeding, splinting extremity fractures, especially of the femur, and elevating the foot of the long spine board about 12 inches so that the patient is in the head-down position. However, since this position usually makes it more difficult for the patient to breathe, use of a pneumatic antishock garment (PASG) may be preferable, if one is available and there are rescuers present who are trained and licensed in its use.

When a patient has suffered **multiple injuries**, a head or chest injury may indicate elevating the patient's head and chest, but the presence of shock may indicate a head-down position. The rescuer always should care for the condition that appears to be the most life-threatening first, even though some treatment requirements conflict with others.

A patient with a serious injury of any kind may be unable to urinate, but if the injury is to the spinal cord, involuntary urination (**incontinence**) also is common. Male patients with serious spinal cord injuries may develop a prolonged type of erection of the penis called priapism.

Fig. 13.9 *Backboarding Technique for a Standing Patient*

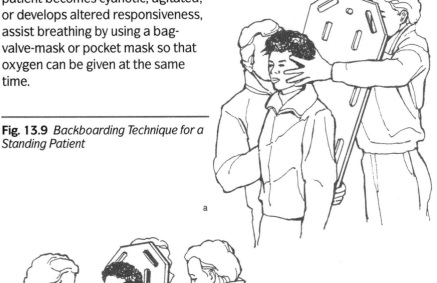

a

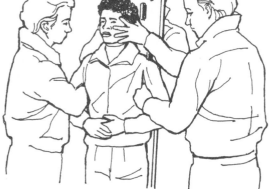

b

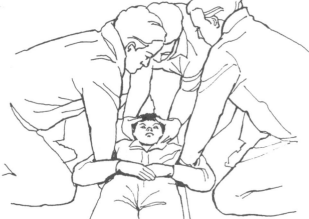

c

Fig. 13.9

Table 13.5

Summary of Emergency Care of a Patient with a Neck or Back Injury

1. Maintain the airway and stabilization of the head and neck.
2. Move the head and neck gently into the neutral, in-line position as necessary.
3. Give additional basic life support as needed. Assist ventilation if necessary.
4. Assess sensation and movement in all four extremities before and after logrolling, lifting, and placing the patient on the long spine board.
5. If the patient is found prone or semiprone, logroll the patient into the supine position when appropriate.
6. Remove the patient's helmet, if present.
7. Assess the neck and apply a rigid collar.
8. Care for unresponsiveness, if present.
9. Care for any bleeding and/or open wounds and fractures.
10. Place the patient on a long spine board using the direct ground lift, logroll, or interim short extrication device as appropriate. Immobilize the patient on the board.
11. Watch for vomiting and treat it by turning the board on its side and using suction.
12. Give oxygen in high concentration and flow rate.
13. Monitor and record ABC's, vital signs, level of responsiveness, ability to move, and perception of pain and touch in all four extremities at regular intervals.
14. Anticipate and care for shock if it develops.
15. Transport patient to hospital without delay.

Scenario #12 (Fig. 13.10)

The following scenario illustrates the care of a patient with a possible neck and back injury, among other problems.

You have just stepped off Number 2 lift at High Range Ski Area and are tightening your boots when you intercept a transmission from the base. There is a report of a skier having fallen off Number 5 lift just beyond Tower 30. Realizing that this is about 200 yards below and to the north of where you are at the moment, you note the time on your watch (11:15 a.m.) and call to the patroller at the top of Number 2: "Joe, I'll check it out. Get the backboard, oxygen, and suction loaded on the toboggan and I'll call you as soon as I get down there. Tell the base that I'm answering the call but will need more help."

In 60 seconds you are at the scene. The patient is spread-eagled face down in the snow, surrounded by a crowd of curious onlookers. You quickly get out of your bindings and hurry to him, meanwhile noting that the patient is not moving and that there is no blood on the snow. You cannot tell whether he is breathing because of his heavy clothing. Quickly, you scoop the snow away around his nose and mouth—being careful not to cause movement of his head and neck—and create a large breathing space.

You: (shouting in his ear) "Sir, are you okay? Don't move!" (You carefully perform the jaw-thrust technique as he stirs with a faint groan, and you are relieved to see that he is breathing. Keeping the airway open with one hand, you key your lapel microphone.) "Schussen to Midway, copy." (Midway replies.) "Need the toboggan, spine board, oxygen, suction, and lots of help, just north of Tower 30 on Number 5 lift."

You relax the jaw-thrust and note that his respirations remain strong and about 20 per minute. You perform a finger sweep and find no snow in his mouth. His carotid pulse, which is strong and regular, is 100 beats per minute. "Things are under control at this point," you think to yourself, stabilizing the head and neck with both hands. At this point, an excited skier approaches you.

Skier: "Ski Patrol, how's my brother?"

You: "Okay so far. Were you with him?"

Skier: "Yes."

You: "I'm Ben Schussen of the High Range Ski Patrol. Pardon me for not shaking hands. What is his name?"

Skier: "Barry Careless. I'm his brother Les."

You: "What happened?"

Skier: "We were sitting in the chair together when he started to act strange. He grabbed me, mumbled something, almost pulled me off, then the next thing I knew he went head-first out of the chair and landed face-down in the snow. I came down as soon as I could get off the lift. Is he going to be okay?"

You: "It's too early to tell just what is going on. Right now, he's breathing well and has a good pulse. I'm stabi-

Fig. 13.10 *Scenario #12*

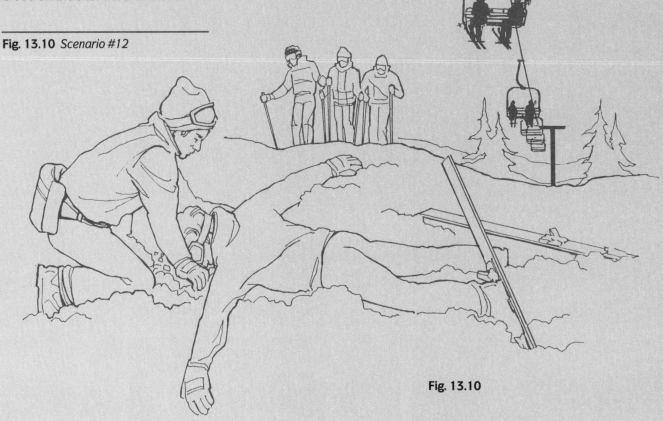

Fig. 13.10

lizing his head and neck in case he has a neck injury. We have some help coming. In a minute, we'll turn him over, get him on a backboard, and get him to a doctor. Do you have any idea what went wrong with him? Was he partying last night? Did he skip breakfast?"

Skier: "He was up pretty late last night drinking with some buddies, and had a thumper this morning. He didn't feel like eating breakfast—wanted to go skiing. He thought the cold air would help his headache. He fell down several times on the first run and didn't seem to be in his usual form."

You: "Was he feeling okay before he went out last night?"

Skier: "Yes, he looked okay to me."

You: "Is there anything medically wrong with him?"

Skier: "He's a diabetic."

You: "Does he take good care of his diabetes?"

Skier: "Most of the time. He tries to eat right and takes his insulin every day, but occasionally he gets fed up with it and really pigs out, like last night.

You: "Did he take his insulin this morning?"

Skier: "I don't know."

You: "Does he take any other medicine besides insulin?"

Skier: "No."

You: "Does he have any allergies?"

Skier: "No."

You: "Is there anything else we need to know about his health in order to help him?"

Skier: "That's about it. He's always been healthy and active."

At this point, several other patrollers arrive with the toboggan. You ask one of them to call the base and the hill chief to arrange for an ambulance from town, then you ask another to assess the patient's neck and back. After putting on a pair of rubber gloves, she runs her fingers beneath the patient's jacket, along the spinous processes of the cervical, thoracic, and lumbar vertebrae. There are no prominences, step-off deformities, swelling, obvious tenderness, or obvious open wounds. Next, she pinches the nail of each index finger hard between her index finger and thumb. The patient withdraws both upper extremities equally. She presses her knuckles firmly against the tibia of each leg. The patient withdraws both lower extremities equally.

One of the patrollers brings the long spine board, oxygen, and portable suction unit from the toboggan. You then assemble three patrollers, and the four of you carefully logroll the patient into the supine position on the long spine board. A rigid collar is placed around his neck. He has to be pulled 6 inches headward once and 6 inches feetward before he is centered on the board. Oxygen is started by non-rebreather mask at 12 liters per minute.

The patient now has his eyes open and is starting to stir. You again ask him if he is okay, and he says, weakly, "No." He is able to tell you that he has pain in his face—where the skin over the cheekbones and around the eyes is red and noticeably swollen—his neck, and his anterior chest. Despite this, his breathing remains regular, deep, and 16 to 20 respirations per minute. His pulse is strong and steady at 90 beats per minute.

You ask him if he took his insulin this morning, and he says he did. After asking him whether he feels nauseated and receiving a negative reply, you ask one of the other patrollers, John, to take a tube of Instant Glucose out of your first aid belt and squeeze some of it into the patient's mouth for him to swallow.

John quickly assesses the patient's head and face while you continue manual stabilization of the head and neck. The pupils are equal and respond to light. The swollen area over the cheekbone is tender but there are no open wounds. The teeth are symmetrical and there are no lumps or tender areas over the sides of the jaw. John quickly performs the remainder of the body survey. There are no obvious open wounds, bleeding, deformities, or swellings, and no tenderness except over the midsternum. Both sides of the chest expand equally during breathing. The patient is able to squeeze both of the patroller's hands and says he can wiggle his toes and feel his feet. He is able to feel a gentle pinch on all four extremities. The patient's body is then strapped securely onto the spine board, and his head and neck are immobilized.

You retrieve a notebook and pencil from your fanny pack and start making notes. It is 11:30 a.m. (Can all this have happened in only 15 minutes?)

As the board and patient are being lifted into the toboggan, he starts to gag. Quickly, the four of you lower the board to the snow, snatch the oxygen mask from the patient's face, and tip the board on its side, while one patroller hands you the V-Vac suction unit. The patient vomits about a cupful of thin, yellow material onto the snow. You play the suction tip in and around his mouth and nose, wishing that you had thought to put on some rubber gloves too when you had time. When he has stopped vomiting, the boarded patient is lifted into the toboggan, covered with a sleeping bag, and strapped into place. The oxygen backpack is beside him. Before the toboggan starts to move, you give him another dose of Instant Glucose.

You: "I'll take the V-Vac and ski beside him. If he vomits again we'll have to stop right away and tip the toboggan on its side. Remember, slow and easy."

You think: he must have passed out from low blood sugar and was limp when he hit the snow. The adrenalin surge due to the low blood sugar itself, plus the injury, raised the blood sugar enough to wake him up. He lucked out: he did a 20-foot whole-body plant face-first into 3 feet of snow, but the most obvious injury seems to be soft-tissue damage to the face. Even if he has a cervical spine fracture, there probably is no cord damage."

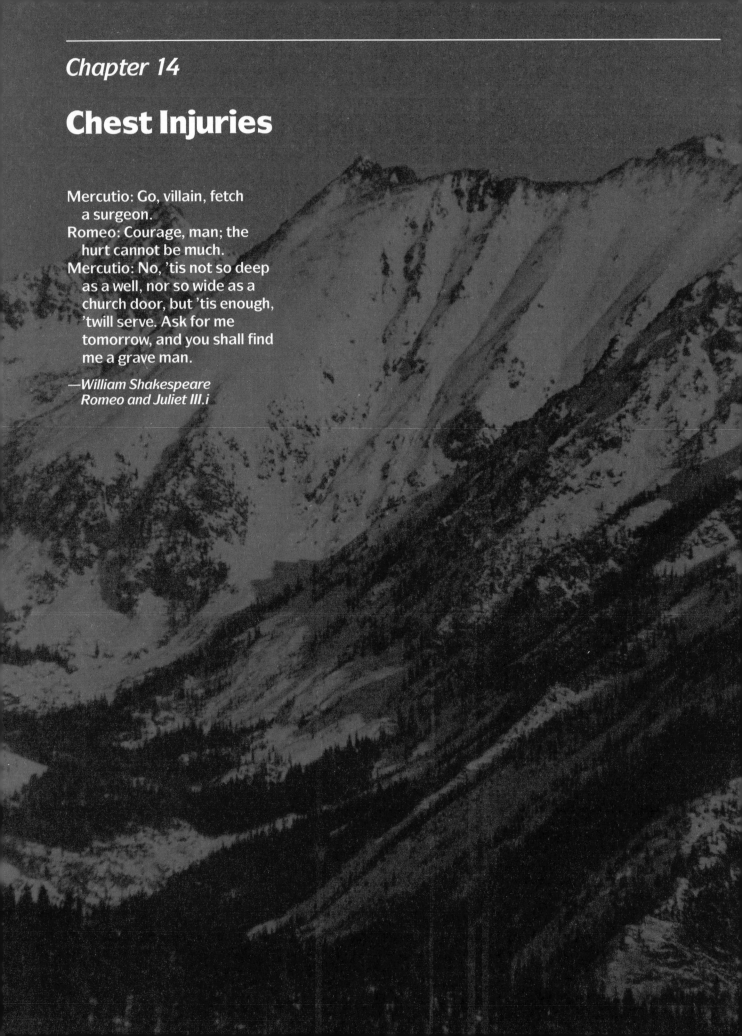

Chapter 14

Chapter 14

Chest Injuries

Mercutio: Go, villain, fetch
   a surgeon.
Romeo: Courage, man; the
   hurt cannot be much.
Mercutio: No, 'tis not so deep
   as a well, nor so wide as a
   church door, but 'tis enough,
   'twill serve. Ask for me
   tomorrow, and you shall find
   me a grave man.

*—William Shakespeare
Romeo and Juliet III.i*

Chest injuries are a significant cause of death and disability. In the urban environment, these are most commonly caused by motor vehicle and industrial accidents and lethal weapons such as guns and knives. In the outdoors they can be caused by collisions and falls while skiing; falls while climbing; direct blows from rockfall; snowmobile and all-terrain vehicle accidents; hunting accidents; and so on.

Before reading this chapter, please review the sections on anatomy and physiology of the respiratory and circulatory systems in Chapter 2. Remember that normal functioning of the circulatory system requires the following:

1. The heart must beat with a normal rate, rhythm, and strength of contraction so that the blood moves effectively through the vessels.
2. There must be adequate blood volume for the heart to pump.
3. The blood vessels must be able to perform their function of containing and moving the blood.

Normal functioning of the respiratory system requires the following:

1. There must be enough oxygen in the air.
2. The upper and lower airways must be open.
3. The pleural space must be intact with negative pressure.
4. The chest wall must move as a unit.
5. The intercostal muscles and the diaphragm must contract in synchrony and at the proper rate.
6. The control pathways of the nervous system must be intact.

The chest is most commonly injured by either compression or penetrating trauma. Depending on the type, magnitude, and direction of the forces involved, injury can occur to the structures of the chest wall only—skin, subcutaneous tissues, muscles, tendons, ligaments, and ribs. Injury may involve important deeper structures as well, including the heart, pleura, lungs, diaphragm, great vessels, trachea, and nerves.

Chest wounds can be either **open** or **closed**. Open chest wounds are caused by objects that penetrate the chest wall, either because they are sharp (e.g., ice axes, ski pole tips, tree branches, knives) or because of their high velocity (e.g., bullets). Air enters the pleural space through the wound, causing loss of the normal negative pressure and collapse of the lung. Structures inside the chest can be lacerated and punctured as well as contused, causing bleeding and loss of function.

Closed chest wounds are caused by compression ("blunt") trauma, such as when a skier collides with a fixed object such as a tree. The skin may be broken or unbroken; the chest wall and organs within the chest can be contused, torn, or sheared from their attachments. Single or multiple ribs can break, and their sharp ends can lacerate blood vessels, the lungs, and other organs, causing bleeding and lung collapse. Fractures of multiple ribs can change the integrity and rigidity of the chest wall, causing interference with the normal ability of the chest cage to expand and contract as a unit during breathing.

The seriousness of a closed chest injury is determined by the underlying injuries to the **lungs, heart,** and/or **blood vessels** and the resulting interference with respiratory and circulatory system function, although these injuries may be initially overshadowed by more obvious chest wall damage. In a contused area of the lung, damage to bronchi and blood or edema fluid within alveoli prevent air from entering the alveoli. Blood vessel damage may prevent blood from reaching the alveoli.

Chest injuries, other than simple chest wall contusions and uncomplicated fractures of one or two ribs, are potentially serious and should be treated as emergencies. In addition to **pain, swelling, tenderness,** and/or **ecchymosis** at the injury site, the presence of one or more of the following signs and symptoms usually means that a serious chest injury has occurred.

Signs and Symptoms of a Serious Chest Injury

1. An **open wound**, especially if bloody air bubbles or a whistling sound is noted as the patient breathes, indicating that air is moving in and out of the chest cavity through the wound.
2. **Respiratory distress**, which can include difficult or labored breathing (dyspnea), increase in the breathing rate (tachypnea), and increase in the breathing depth (hyperpnea). Dyspnea also includes the patient's awareness of the need to make extra efforts to get enough oxygen. If breathing is painful, breaths tend to be rapid and shallow.
3. **Cough** developing after the injury. This may be mild or severe.
4. **Coughing up blood** (hemoptysis).
5. **Failure** of one or both sides of the chest—or part of one side—to **expand normally** during breathing. This can be due to direct chest wall injury, to collapse of the underlying lung with over-expansion of the opposite lung, or to the patient's attempts to self-splint the injured side because of pain.

6. **Deviation of the trachea** to one side. This is seldom seen but is an important sign of a tension pneumothorax (see below), where the trachea is deviated to the side opposite the injury. It is not seen in a simple pneumothorax.

7. **Subcutaneous emphysema**. This may be found under the skin of the neck or chest (see below).

8. **Cyanosis**, a bluish discoloration of the skin, fingernails, and lips that means the blood is not adequately oxygenated.

9. Signs and symptoms of a **myocardial contusion** (see below). These include a fast or irregular heartbeat, a weak pulse, and low blood pressure.

10. Signs and symptoms of **shock** (see Chapter 6).

Specific Chest Injuries

Rib Fractures

Rib fractures are common injuries usually caused by falls and collisions. Fractures can be single or multiple and can involve one or more ribs. The broken ends of the ribs can be non-displaced or displaced (Fig. 14.1). The most commonly fractured ribs are the fifth through tenth, since the upper four ribs are protected by the shoulder girdle and the last two are small and their front ends are free.

Simple forward falls usually do not break ribs because people tend to break a fall with their hands. However, falling to the side and striking the ground with the arm against the body may cause lateral rib fractures. Multiple ribs can be broken in hard falls, in long pendulum swings during climbs, in high-speed collisions while skiing, and in motor vehicle accidents.

Several adjacent ribs fractured in more than one place can produce a

loose section of chest wall that moves *in* instead of out when the patient *inhales*, and *out* instead of in when the patient *exhales*. This abnormal motion is called **paradoxical motion of the chest wall**, the condition is called a **flail chest**, and the loose section is called a **flail segment** (Fig. 14.2).

The sharp, displaced end of a fractured rib can tear a hole in the lung (Fig. 14.3), producing a **pneumothorax** (Fig. 14.4) as air leaks into the pleural space and causes the lung to collapse. If a blood vessel is lacerated, significant bleeding can occur as well, producing a **hemothorax**.

Fractured ribs are very painful. Pain is increased by anything that causes them to move at the fractured site, such as twisting, breathing, coughing, straining, or sneezing. Advise the patient to stabilize the painful area with a hand before coughing. The proper treatment for a fractured bone is splinting, which limits motion of the bone on both sides of the fracture site. Because the patient must breathe, the chest wall cannot be splinted so tightly that rib motion is prevented completely. Fortunately, a fractured rib will heal even without complete immobilization.

The pain of a broken rib usually is well-localized, so that the patient often can point to the painful spot with one finger. Breathing typically is shallower and more rapid because of the pain. The patient usually prefers to sit up

Fig. 14.1 *Types of Rib Fractures*

Fig. 14.2 *Paradoxical Motion of the Chest Wall*

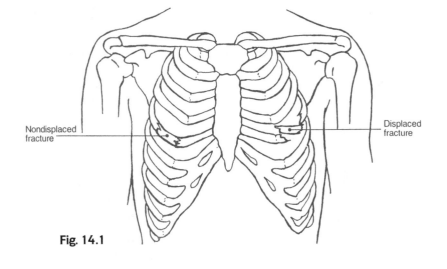

Nondisplaced fracture

Displaced fracture

Fig. 14.1

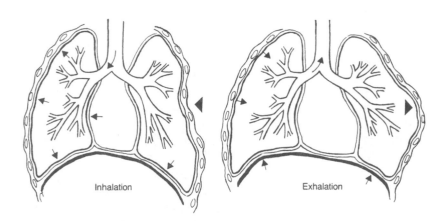

Inhalation

Exhalation

Fig. 14.2

and tries to splint the chest by leaning to the injured side. Signs that the patient has a lung injury in addition to a rib fracture include respiratory distress, cyanosis, severe cough, coughing up blood, subcutaneous emphysema, and deviation of the trachea.

A flail chest is a serious injury because there frequently is a crushing injury of the underlying lung in addition to disruption of the normal breathing mechanics on the injured side. The patient has severe respiratory distress and may be cyanotic. Assessment of the chest usually discloses the paradoxical motion of the flail segment described above. In an adult, however, the chest muscles may be strong enough to splint the flail segment at first, so that paradoxical motion does not develop until the muscles tire.

Penetrating Injuries

Penetrating injuries occur when an object such as a knife or bullet penetrates the chest wall. The object may stop in the chest wall but usually enters the chest cavity where it can injure any organ within the chest. Abdominal organs also may be injured in a penetrating injury of the lower chest. If you know chest and abdominal anatomy, the penetrating object's direction of motion and the location of the wound can give clues as to which organs may be injured. The organs of most concern are the heart, lungs, large blood vessels, and upper abdominal organs such as the liver and spleen. A penetrating injury can cause air and/or blood to leak into the pleural space. Massive bleeding with shock can occur; the bleeding may not be obvious because it is internal.

If the entrance wound is small, the wound may seal itself; if large, a **sucking chest wound** usually develops. This wound is an open hole in the chest wall that establishes a connection between the pleural space and the outside air. The lung on that side collapses and, during breathing,

air moves in and out of the hole in the chest rather than in and out of the lung through the normal airway (Fig. 14.5).

A patient with a penetrating chest injury complains of pain, is short of breath, usually prefers to sit up rather than lie down, and may be cyanotic. The patient may cough up blood, the affected side of the chest may not move as well as the normal side, and the signs and symptoms of hypovolemic shock may be present. Assessment discloses the entrance wound and, in the case of a gunshot wound, usually an exit wound as well. The trachea may be deviated, usually to the injured side. There may be an impaled object in the wound and external bleeding may be significant. If the wound is open, a peculiar sucking noise may be heard as the air moves in and out of the hole.

Fig. 14.3 *The sharp, displaced end of a rib can lacerate the lung.*

Fig. 14.4 *Pneumothorax*

Fig. 14.5 *Sucking Chest Wound*

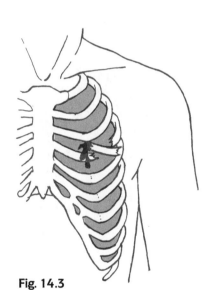

Fig. 14.3

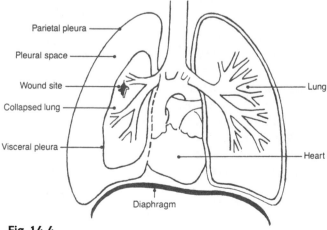

Fig. 14.4

Parietal pleura
Pleural space
Wound site
Collapsed lung
Visceral pleura
Lung
Heart
Diaphragm

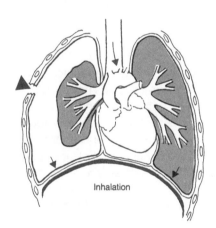

Inhalation

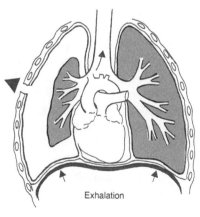

Exhalation

Fig. 14.5

Massive Compression Injuries

Massive compression trauma of the type seen in cave-ins and explosions can cause severe injury. Multiple rib fractures and crushing injuries to the lungs, heart, great vessels, and other intrathoracic organs can occur. The accompanying sudden, rapid increase in intrathoracic pressure can produce swelling of the upper body, distension of the neck veins, and bulging of the eyes. The patient usually is cyanotic, severely short of breath, and goes into shock rapidly.

Injuries to the Back of the Chest

Trauma to the back of the chest can injure the posterior chest wall, thoracic spine, scapulae, back muscles, and underlying organs such as the lungs, pancreas, and kidneys. Any injured person who complains of pain in the back of the chest should be logrolled onto one side for a careful assessment of this area.

Pneumothorax

The term pneumothorax means air in the pleural space. The normal pleural space is a closed sac whose negative pressure is essential for normal breathing. If an abnormal passage connects the pleural space with the outside air, the pressure in the pleural space becomes equal to that of the outside air. Loss of the pressure differential causes the elastic lung to collapse and fail to expand with air when the chest cage expands. Such an abnormal passage can be either in the chest wall, where it connects the pleural space directly with the outside air, or within the lung, where it connects the pleural space with the outside air via the bronchi and trachea.

Even though a small abnormal passage usually seals itself off, the air in the pleural space takes many days to be absorbed. Larger passages require surgery because they do not seal by themselves.

Pneumothorax can occur spontaneously or be caused by an injury. A bleb (blister-like abnormality of the lung surface) or congenital lung cyst can rupture without warning, or the lung can be lacerated by an object that penetrates the chest wall from without or by the sharp ends of a broken rib from within.

The signs and symptoms are those of the condition that caused the pneumothorax and always include pain and respiratory distress. Decreased motion of the affected side of the chest may occur during breathing, and breath sounds (heard with a stethoscope or the naked ear against the chest) will be decreased or absent on the injured side.

Spontaneous pneumothorax usually occurs in young people who have blebs or congenital cysts on the lung surfaces, but may also occur in older people with emphysema. This condition should be suspected in a patient—especially a young, healthy person—who develops sudden chest pain and respiratory distress in the absence of a chest injury.

Tension Pneumothorax

Tension pneumothorax is a serious complication of a pneumothorax that occurs when a defect simulating a one-way valve develops at the injury site (Fig. 14.6). Each time the patient inhales, the valve opens and air is pumped into the pleural space. When the patient exhales, the valve closes and the air cannot escape. The pressure within the pleural space becomes higher and higher, eventually compressing the lung into a ball a few inches in diameter. The mediastinum is forced toward the other side of the chest, interfering with the function of both the heart and the opposite, normal lung. When pressure in the pleural space exceeds pressure in the venae cavae or the mediastinal shift causes them to kink, blood can no longer flow back to the heart, and the patient rapidly goes into cardiogenic shock and dies.

Tension pneumothorax can occur with spontaneous pneumothorax and with both open and closed chest injuries. It occasionally occurs after a sucking chest wound has been sealed with an occlusive bandage.

Signs and symptoms are due to the effects of increased pressure inside the chest, failing lung function, and failing circulation. They include severe, rapidly worsening respiratory distress; engorgement of the neck veins; a weak, rapid pulse; falling blood pressure; bulging of the chest wall tissues between the ribs and above

---

Fig. 14.6 *Tension Pneumothorax*

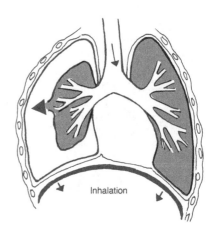

Inhalation

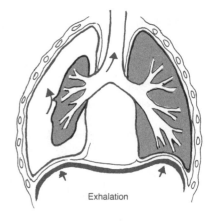

Exhalation

Fig. 14.6

the clavicle on the involved side; deviation of the trachea to the opposite side; and cyanosis.

The condition progresses rapidly, and death can occur within a few minutes. To relieve a tension pneumothorax, a physician or paramedic decompresses the chest by piercing it with a large needle or a special tube.

If a patient whose sucking chest wound has been treated with an occlusive dressing suddenly gets worse, the rescuer should suspect development of a tension pneumothorax due to a valve-like effect of the dressing.

Hemothorax

Hemothorax, or blood in the pleural space, is caused by bleeding from vessels in the lung or chest wall that have been damaged by a closed or open chest injury. Hemothorax frequently is accompanied by air in the pleural space (hemopneumothorax). The pressure of the blood partly collapses the lung.

The signs and symptoms are similar to those of pneumothorax, except that significant blood loss into the pleural space may cause hypovolemic shock. In the field, hemothorax and pneumothorax are difficult to tell apart; a patient with a pneumothorax whose condition is worsening is probably developing a hemopneumothorax or a tension pneumothorax if unrelated conditions can be ruled out.

Subcutaneous Emphysema

Injury to air-containing parts of the respiratory tract in the neck and chest can allow air to escape and spread as small bubbles through the subcutaneous tissues. When the involved area is assessed, the examiner feels a unique crackling sensation.

The signs and symptoms are mainly those of the underlying injury, frequently a compression injury to the chest wall with damage to the underlying lung from a fractured rib or a laceration of the trachea or large bronchi.

Myocardial Contusion

Compression trauma to the chest may injure the heart as well as the lungs, most frequently causing a heart muscle bruise called a myocardial contusion.

The signs and symptoms include low blood pressure and a fast and/or weak heartbeat. Muscle irritability due to injury may produce abnormal electrical discharges causing the heartbeat to be irregular as well. Large contusions may injure enough heart muscle to cause heart failure or cardiogenic shock. However, in the early stages, the pulse and blood pressure may still be normal. Always suspect a myocardial contusion in any patient who has sustained trauma to the mid-anterior chest.

Pericardial Tamponade

Pericardial tamponade is the accumulation of fluid in the pericardium, a fibrous sac surrounding the heart that ordinarily contains only a small amount of fluid. Penetrating injuries to the chest occasionally lacerate the heart, causing bleeding into the pericardium. Pressure buildup from the accumulation of blood or other fluid interferes with the heart's ability to relax and refill with blood between heartbeats. Less blood is ejected with each heartbeat. As a result, blood pressure falls and cardiogenic shock may occur.

The signs and symptoms of pericardial tamponade include a weak, fast pulse, falling blood pressure, and progressively decreasing pulse pressure (the difference between the systolic and diastolic pressures). Because of back pressure on the veins, the neck veins engorge and the face swells.

Injury to the Great Vessels

Compression trauma to the chest can damage the great vessels: the aorta, venae cavae, or their larger branches. Vessel walls may be lacerated, or entire vessels can be fractured or sheared. Such injuries usually are rapidly fatal because of massive internal bleeding from these large vessels.

Assessment of a Patient with a Chest Injury

1. Ask the patient or witnesses what happened. Determine the mechanism of injury, and consider whether it would be expected to produce a serious chest injury. Institute universal precautions (see Appendix F).
2. Perform the primary survey. Open and maintain the airway, assess the pulse, and search for severe bleeding.
3. Give basic life support and control bleeding as needed.
4. If a chest injury is suspected or the pulse is fast, weak and/or irregular, or the breathing is labored, move rapidly to expose and assess the neck and chest. Ask the patient about chest pain, pain on breathing or coughing, shortness of breath, and coughing of blood. Look for neck vein engorgement, cyanosis, subcutaneous emphysema, deviation of the trachea, equality of chest expansion, open wounds—especially sucking chest wounds—impaled objects, and the presence of a flail segment. Care for any injuries found.
5. Ask, "Where else do you hurt?" Assess any additional painful areas the patient

indicates, and care for any injuries discovered.

6. Perform the secondary survey.
   a. Assess the blood pressure, pulse pressure, pulse, respiratory rate, capillary refill, and skin temperature, color, and moisture.
   b. Obtain the details of the present problem, the patient's medical history, medicines taken, and allergies. Ask, "Is there anything else we should know?"
   c. Assess the remainder of the body: head, abdomen, pelvis, extremities, and back.
7. Monitor and *record* the vital signs at 15-minute intervals.

Table 14.1

Summary of Assessment of a Patient with a Chest Injury

1. Ask, "What happened?" Determine the mechanism of injury. Institute universal precautions (see Appendix F).
2. Perform the primary survey: airway, breathing, circulation, bleeding.
3. Provide basic life support techniques as required. Give rescue breathing, CPR, and control bleeding.
4. If you suspect chest injury, or pulse or breathing are abnormal, assess the neck and chest.
5. Care for any injuries found.
6. Ask, "Where does it hurt?"
7. Assess any additional painful areas and care for any injuries found.
8. Perform the secondary survey: assess vital signs, obtain medical history, and assess remainder of body.
9. Record and monitor vital signs at regular intervals.

Fig. 14.7 *Emergency Care of an Open Chest Wound*

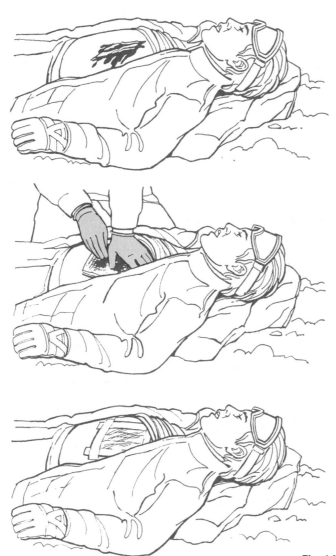

Fig. 14.7

Emergency Care of a Patient with a Chest Injury

1. Monitor the airway and keep it open.
2. If breathing is inadequate, support ventilation with a mouth-to-pocket mask or, preferably, a bag-valve-mask.
3. If available, give oxygen in high concentration and flow rate.
4. Allow the patient to assume a comfortable position. The patient usually will want to sit up, which often makes breathing easier.
5. Control external bleeding by direct pressure.
6. Cover an open chest wound with an airtight occlusive dressing large enough to prevent the dressing from being sucked into the wound (Fig. 14.7). The dressing should consist of a sterile compress covered by an airtight layer of aluminum foil, plastic wrap, a plastic bag, or Vaseline gauze. If airtight material is not available, substitute with multiple layers of standard dressing material.

Tape the edges of the dressing securely to the skin of the chest wall to ensure an airtight seal. Tape the dressing on three sides, then instruct the patient to exhale forcefully just before the fourth side is taped so that the minimum possible amount of air remains in the pleural space.

On rare occasions, symptoms of tension pneumothorax will develop after an open chest wound is taped, because the dressing itself causes a one-way valve effect. If this occurs, remove the tape on one side of the dressing. If pressure has developed inside the chest, you will hear air whistle out and the symptoms usually will be relieved. If this does not work, gently pull the sides of the wound apart to see if air whistles out. Try leaving the dressing taped on only three sides, since this may form a beneficial one-way valve effect so that air will be expelled from the opening during exhalation but will not enter the opening during inhalation because the dressing is sucked up against the wound. Continue to monitor the patient for signs and symp-

oms of recurrence of pressure buildup inside the chest.

7. Stabilize a flail chest to reduce the paradoxical motion of the flail segment, thus decreasing pain and improving the mechanics of chest wall motion during breathing. Stabilize the segment in the *inward* position by splinting it with a pillow, large thick compress, or wadded parka fixed against it with tape or a self-adhering roller bandage. Or, have the patient lie with the segment against a hard surface such as the side rail or base of the litter or toboggan. If the flail segment is anterior, the patient may be able to hold a pillow or wadded parka against it. Since the patient cannot expand the lung normally because of the abnormal chest wall mechanics, the rescuer should help it expand by supporting ventilation with positive pressure from the bag-valve-mask.

8. Stabilize an impaled foreign body (Fig. 14.8) in place. A long object, such as a ski pole, can be cut off short with a pipe-cutter.

9. Observe the patient closely to detect any changes in condi-

tion. Obtain vital signs initially and at 15-minute intervals thereafter.

10. If necessary, treat the patient for shock (see Chapter 6).

11. Splint simple rib fractures for comfort and to permit the patient to ambulate. Have the patient sit up and place the hand that is on the injured side on top of the head (Fig. 14.9). Place several cravats, elastic bandages, or padded trouser belts around the injured area. Ask the patient to take a deep breath, exhale deeply, and hold the breath while the material is tightened around the chest and fastened in place. If increased pain or respiratory distress occurs, remove the material immediately.

If evacuation will be prolonged or the patient must self-evacuate on foot, splint the chest with adhesive tape to control pain better (Fig. 14.10). Tape the rib cage in the unexpanded position by applying tape to the injured area while the patient holds his or her breath after an exhalation as described above. If a razor is available, shave hair off the area before taping. After each exhalation, apply a long strip of 2-inch-wide adhesive tape

Fig. 14.8 *An impaled foreign body should be stabilized in place.*

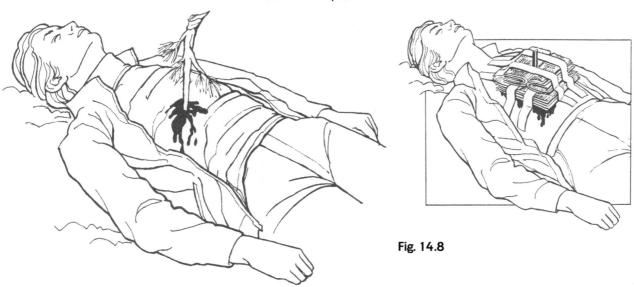

Fig. 14.8

from the midline in front to the midline in back. Six to eight strips are required; they should overlap each other like shingles on a roof. The nipple should be protected with gauze before tape is laid over it.

Splinting of the chest as described above should be regarded as a temporary measure for pain control only; if prolonged it may interfere with lung function.

12. Chest injuries—other than simple chest wall contusions and uncomplicated fractures of one or two ribs—are potentially serious and should be treated as emergencies. Every effort should be made to notify EMS and transport the patient promptly to a hospital. The medical facility should be notified in advance, if possible.

Fig. 14.9 *Emergency Care of a Simple Rib Fracture*

Fig. 14.10 *Adhesive Tape Splint for a Rib Fracture to Permit Self-evacuation*

Table 14.2

Summary of Emergency Care of a Patient with a Chest Injury

1. Open and maintain the upper airway. Institute universal precautions (see Appendix F).
2. Support ventilation, if needed.
3. Give oxygen in high concentration.
4. Allow the patient to find a position of comfort (usually sitting up).
5. Control external bleeding by direct pressure.
6. Cover a sucking chest wound with an airtight dressing.
7. Stabilize a flail chest and support ventilation with the bag-valve-mask.
8. Stabilize an impaled object in place.
9. Monitor vital signs.
10. Treat shock if it develops.
11. Splint simple rib fractures.
12. In any significant chest injury, transport the patient to a hospital without delay.

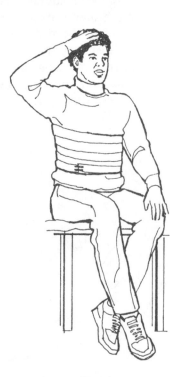

Fig. 14.9

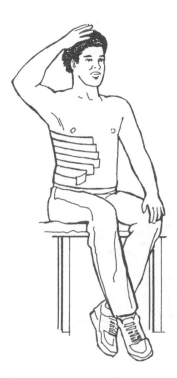

Fig. 14.10

Scenario #13 (Fig. 14.11)

The following scenario illustrates management of a patient with an open chest wound.

You and three companions are all students at State University, located 100 miles from Grandstone National Park. You have a four-day spring break and have decided to use the time to explore the country just north of the Park boundary. The snowpack has been light, but there was a foot of snow two days ago, and this is the first time all winter that the snow has been good and the avalanche danger acceptable.

The plan is to leave your vehicles at a parking area off the main road and take a trail 5 miles north into a range of 10,000-foot peaks where there should be some good powder telemarking. You will establish a base camp and spend two-and-a-half days exploring the high country before heading back after lunch on Sunday. All four of you have your Ortovox transceivers, and Lucky has brought Bandit, an avalanche-trained 2-year-old German shepherd with a good nose. You discover that some other skiers have broken trail ahead of you—this means easier trail skiing and more time for the powder.

The party is 2 miles up the trail and going strong through a narrow draw between two meadows. Bandit is out in front. You round a bend and see a huge male bison about 30 yards away. He is standing sideways on the trail; you hear him snort as he swings his head around to look at you. "Bandit, noooooooooo!" cries Lucky, but it is too late. Bandit is heading full tilt for the bison, barking aggressively. The big animal lowers his head and raises his tail as he turns toward the dog. The party members have all halted and are nervously side-stepping off the trail—there are steep banks on each side and no place to go to avoid a charge. You recall that male bisons weigh a ton and can run at 25 miles per hour.

"Bandit, COME!" shouts Lucky. The dog is dancing around in front of the bison, barking furiously. The bison takes a step forward and hooks his head up sharply. The tip of a horn catches Bandit and tosses him high up on the bank. He lies there yelping loudly. With a snort, the bison heads for Joe, the nearest skier, who is yelling and frantically side-stepping up the bank. The other three stand frozen and watch in horror as the big animal hooks a horn below Joe's armpit and tosses him straight up. Joe lands screaming in the snow, half-way up the snowbank.

Fig. 14.11 *Scenario #13*

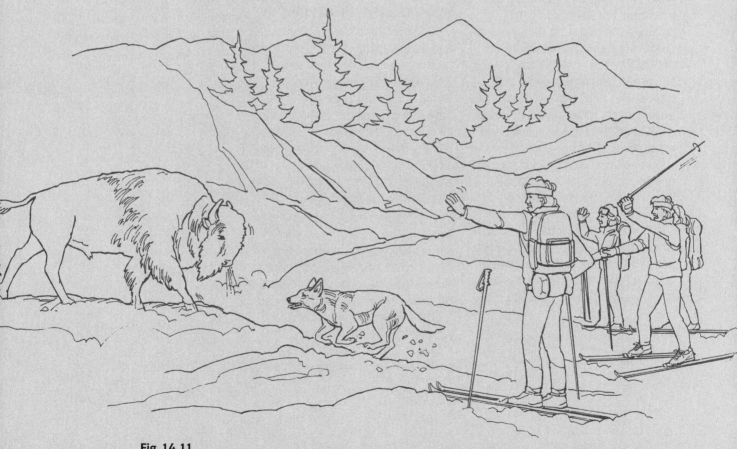

Fig. 14.11

The bison stops, snorts, then turns and walks slowly away up the trail.

Joe is lying on his side. He is moaning with pain—the moans interrupted by gasps for breath. As soon as the bison is out of sight, you take off your skis and approach Joe. His parka is torn below his left armpit, and there is blood on his clothing and on the snow.

You: (grasping his wrist and feeling his pulse) "Joe, are you okay?"

Joe: "He got me in the chest. I can't breathe."

Joe's pulse is strong, regular, and 110 beats per minute. His breathing rate is about 40 respirations per minute and obviously labored. His skin is pale with a cyanotic cast; there is cold sweat on his forehead.

You: "Joe, did he get you anywhere else? Did you hit your head or hurt your neck or back when you landed?"

Joe: (weakly) "No."

By now you know that Joe's airway, breathing, and circulation are functional but stressed. He has clearly suffered a serious injury to his chest. Asking your companions to get the first aid kit out of your pack, you unzip Joe's windbreaker, unbutton his shirt, and expose his chest by pulling up his undershirt. Both sides of his chest are moving equally with respirations. There is an open wound the size of a 50-cent piece in the right anterolateral chest. The clothing is blood-soaked and there is blood coming out of the wound. You hear a sucking noise as he inhales, and when he exhales you can see bloody bubbles in the wound as air comes out of it. You think, "So this is what a sucking chest wound looks like."

Opening the first aid kit, you take out a pair of rubber gloves, a roll of 2-inch adhesive tape, and a plastic baggie full of sterile compresses of various sizes. "Mike, look in the top flap pocket of my pack and get out one of those clean, empty plastic bags." You put on the gloves, open three of the sterile 3 x 3's, and stack them over the wound. "Lucky, tear me off four strips of the tape, about 6 inches long." You place a clean Ziploc bag over the top compress and tape three edges to the skin, which you have wiped dry of blood with a cravat. You ask Joe to exhale and tape down the fourth edge.

You: "Can you breathe better, Joe?"

Joe: "Yes, a little. I need to sit up!"

You: "Let me check your neck and back first—won't take a minute. Does this hurt anywhere?" (You quickly run your fingers from the base of Joe's skull down to his coccyx, pressing on each spinous process in turn).

Joe: "No."

You: "I'll help you sit up" (doing so).

Joe now appears less anxious, and his breathing rate has dropped to 30 per minute. You look at the wound; the blood has not soaked through the compresses yet. "We have to move Joe out of this bowling alley in case the bull comes back," you say. The three of you carry Joe slowly and carefully 60 yards out of the gulley and into the woods, laying him down on an Ensolite pad.

You: "Mike, you're the best skier. Take your pack and head back to the cars as fast as you can. Here are my keys. Drive to the Alpine Motel in town—the man who runs it is head of the local rescue unit. Get a snowmobile and a toboggan so we can get Joe back to town. Call the Life-Flight helicopter to meet us there. Lucky and I will stay here with Joe."

Lucky has retrieved his dog, who now seems its usual self. Bandit has a superficial laceration of the skin of his side where the big horn caught him, but the skin was so loose that no deeper injuries appear to have resulted.

Joe is starting to shiver, so you pull his shirt and parka around him and help him into his pile jacket. As Mike disappears down the trail, Lucky starts to collect wood for a fire and you start the secondary survey. Joe has always been healthy, is on no medications, and has no allergies. His capillary refill is greater than 2 seconds, which is not surprising in the cold. There are no abnormalities of his head, face, pupils, ears, nose, mouth, or neck. The trachea is in the midline. There are no abdominal wounds and no tenderness on palpation. There are no deformities, swellings, or tenderness over the extremities. He is able to wiggle his toes and squeeze both your hands. You set about making Joe comfortable while waiting for help.

You: "Lucky, you should train that dog not to chase anything bigger than a cat."

Chapter 15

Injuries to the Abdomen, Pelvis, and Genitalia

Certainly, it is by their signs and symptoms, that internal diseases are revealed to the physician. But daily observation shows, that there is no uniform and invariable relationship between the extent and intensity of the disease, and its external signs. The prominence, the number, and the combination, of these, depend upon many circumstances beside the disease with which they are connected.

—Elisha Bartlett
Philosophy of Medical Science

Injuries to the Abdomen

Before reading this chapter, please review the sections on the abdomen, pelvis, and the digestive and urinary systems in Chapters 2 and 3.

Abdominal injuries can be either **open** or **closed**. Open injuries are caused by sharp or high-velocity objects that create an opening between the peritoneal cavity and the outside. Abdominal organs along the path of these penetrating injuries can be punctured or lacerated. Closed injuries, which usually are caused by compression trauma, include contusions and other injuries of the abdominal wall in addition to contusions, lacerations, ruptures, or shear injuries of underlying internal organs.

The results of an abdominal injury depend to some extent on whether the involved organs are **hollow** or **solid**. Hollow organs, such as the stomach, intestines, and gallbladder, contain liquid or semisolid material such as partly or fully digested food; enzymes; hydrochloric acid; bacteria; and emulsifying agents. When these hollow organs rupture, their highly irritating and infectious contents spill into the peritoneal cavity, producing a painful, inflammatory reaction called **peritonitis**.

Solid organs such as the liver, spleen, and kidneys have a rich blood supply; damage to these organs usually causes severe bleeding. Blood in the peritoneal cavity irritates the peritoneum although less so than stomach or bowel contents. The signs and symptoms of mild peritonitis usually are present, although they may be overshadowed by those of hypovolemic shock. One solid organ, the pancreas, is rich in potent digestive enzymes; injury to it can cause severe chemical peritonitis and hypovolemic shock.

Signs and Symptoms of Peritonitis

During the hour or more after organ rupture occurs, localized pain and tenderness at the injury site spread to involve the rest of the abdomen. The abdomen usually becomes rigid and distended, the pulse faster and weaker, and normal bowel sounds—as heard by listening with a stethoscope or ear placed against the abdomen—disappear as the intestines become paralyzed by the inflammation and infection. Failure of normal peristalsis and muscle tone causes the intestines to enlarge and fill with fluid. Signs and symptoms of hypovolemic shock can develop due to bleeding and loss of fluid from the circulation. The patient appears progressively sicker and frequently vomits. Abdominal pain is increased by moving, straightening the knees, or taking a deep breath, so the patient may prefer to lie quietly on the back or side with the knees flexed. Injury to upper abdominal organs such as the liver and spleen may cause pain in the shoulder due to irritation of the diaphragm.

It is important to note that the patient may not be able to locate the pain precisely, other than to say that it is in one of the four abdominal quadrants. Intra-abdominal pain is occasionally referred to an uninolved part of the abdomen, or even to the back, chest, or shoulder.

Abdominal trauma also may injure the aorta, inferior vena cava, or large arteries and veins, resulting in severe or fatal hemorrhage.

Abdominal injuries may be obvious, such as a large, open wound with protruding bowel, or quite subtle, such as a blow to the flank that initially causes little pain but has damaged the liver or spleen. Suspect serious internal injuries in any patient who has a penetrating abdominal wound or who has suffered compression trauma to the abdomen in an accident involving high kinetic energy and acceleration or deceleration. Examples include motor vehicle accidents, gunshot or knife wounds, hard falls, and collisions.

Injuries to the Pelvis and Genitourinary System

Kidney Injuries

The kidneys lie against the posterior abdominal wall on either side of the spine, where they are partly protected by the ribs. Because a kidney injury usually is associated with fractures of the overlying ribs or adjacent vertebrae, suspect an accompanying kidney injury when such injuries are discovered.

The patient usually develops tenderness, swelling, and ecchymosis in the costovertebral angle or the flank. Injured kidneys may bleed severely, resulting in hypovolemic shock. Usually, but not always, there is blood in the urine.

Bladder Injuries

The bladder is a hollow organ that serves as a reservoir for the urine. A full bladder is more easily injured than an empty one; therefore, the bladder should be emptied before any type of contact sport or other strenuous activity and emptied frequently during prolonged vehicle rides.

Pelvic fractures frequently lacerate the bladder or tear the urethra (Fig. 15.1). The assessment of injuries to the lower abdomen and genital area should always include a search for pelvic fractures (see below), an inspection of the opening of the urethra for bleeding, and inspection of a specimen of voided urine for the presence of blood. The rescuer should anticipate the development of hypo-volemic shock if there is evidence of a fractured pelvis or bleeding into the urinary system.

The Male Genitalia

Injuries to the male genitalia are extremely painful and generally cause the patient considerable anxiety and concern. Any type of soft-tissue injury can occur and bleeding may be severe. Amputation of the penis causes considerable bleeding because of its blood-filled sinuses. The amputated part should be preserved as described in Chapter 7 and sent to the hospital along with the patient.

The foreskin of the penis occasionally gets caught in a trouser zipper, causing a very painful injury. If the zipper is stuck, cut it out of the trousers to make transport more comfortable.

A testicle contusion is very painful and should be treated by application of a cold pack and temporary stabilization of the groin area with clothing or an athletic-supporter type of garment made of triangular bandages.

The urethra can be bruised by a fall when the patient lands in a straddle position, or lacerated by sharp fragments from a pelvic fracture. A patient with an injured urethra is usually unable to void.

The Female Genitalia

The internal organs of the female reproductive system are seldom injured because they are well protected by the pelvis. Since they are located in the center of the pelvis away from its walls, they are rarely lacerated by sharp fragments of a fractured pelvis. However, the uterus of a pregnant woman is susceptible to injury from compression trauma to the abdomen or pelvis. Such injury can cause severe internal or external bleeding or precipitate a miscarriage or premature labor.

Soft-tissue injuries to the external female genitalia, particularly straddle injuries, are very painful. Bleeding may be profuse but is usually controllable by local pressure. Anchor dressings with a diaper-like arrangement made from triangular bandages (Fig. 15.2), or use tight-fitting underpants. *Never* insert dressings or packs into the vagina.

Assessment of a Patient with an Abdominal or Pelvic Injury

1. Ask the patient to describe the circumstances of the accident. Note the mechanism of injury and consider whether it might be expected to produce a significant abdominal or pelvic injury. Institute universal precautions (Appendix F).
2. Perform the primary survey and give basic life support, as needed. Follow up a rapid pulse, weak pulse, and/or labored breathing by assessing the neck and chest. Care for any urgent problems discovered.
3. Ask the patient where it hurts. If there is abdominal or pelvic pain, determine the characteristics of the pain, including time of onset, location at onset, severity, change in position or severity with time, radiation (including to the shoulder), character (dull, aching, sharp, burning, stabbing, crampy, constant, intermittent), and relationship to position or motion (including breathing and coughing).
4. Assess the abdomen and pelvis while the patient lies supine with the knees bent and the assessed area exposed.

Fig. 15.1 *The sharp fragments of a fractured pelvis can lacerate the bladder.*

Fig. 15.2 *Diaper-like Bandage for a Wound of the Perineum*

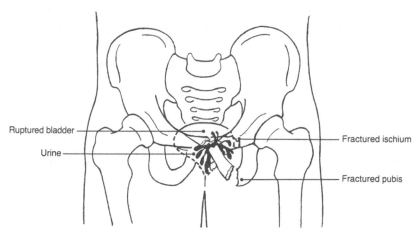

Ruptured bladder

Urine

Fractured ischium

Fractured pubis

Fig. 15.1

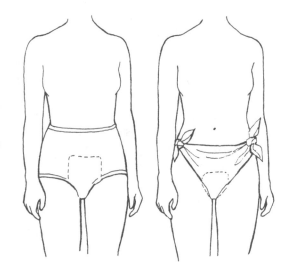

Fig. 15.2

Inspect and palpate for open wounds, bleeding, bruises, swelling, tenderness, muscle rigidity, and abdominal distention, noting the skin color, moisture, and temperature. Inspect any obvious wounds for protruding fat or intestines. If there is a wound made by a bullet or long, sharp object, search for an exit wound. Stabilize impaled objects in place. Gently press the iliac crests together with a rotary motion. If this maneuver causes pain, abnormal motion, or crepitus, the pelvis is fractured. If it is negative, push the iliac crests and pubis firmly backward to see if this causes pain. If there has been an injury to the suprapubic area or if a pelvic fracture is suspected, inspect the urethral opening for blood.

The surface location of tenderness, wounds, swelling, or bruises is significant because internal organs known to lie underneath may have been injured as well.

Table 15.1

Summary of Assessment of a Patient with an Abdominal or Pelvic Injury

1. Ask, "What happened?" Determine the mechanism of injury. Institute universal precautions (see Appendix F).
2. Perform the primary survey. Give basic life support as needed. Follow up an abnormal pulse or breathing by assessing the neck and chest.
3. Ask, "Where do you hurt?" Ask the patient to describe the location and character of the abdominal pain. Assess the abdomen and pelvis. Give any urgent care required.
4. Anticipate vomiting and inspect vomitus.
5. Perform the secondary survey. Assess and record vital signs; obtain the medical history.
6. Assess the remaining body areas. Expose and assess the perineal area if you suspect genital injury, with concern for privacy and with a witness present.
7. Inspect voided urine for the presence of blood.
8. At regular intervals, monitor and record the vital signs and any change in the character and location of the pain.
9. Assess for additional (internal) injuries if the level of shock is not explained by the seriousness of the injuries already found.

If there has been an injury to the genitalia, expose the perineal area for assessment. This should be done with regard for the patient's privacy and with a witness of the same sex as the patient present.

5. Nausea and vomiting usually will develop and should be anticipated. Keep a receptacle handy and help the patient turn the head to one side to avoid aspiration. Suction the mouth and nose if necessary. Inspect the vomitus for blood, bile, undigested food, etc.

6. Proceeding to the secondary survey, check and record the vital signs. Note the character and rate of breathing, the

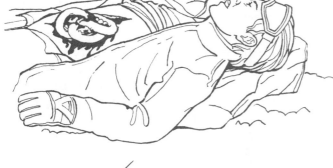

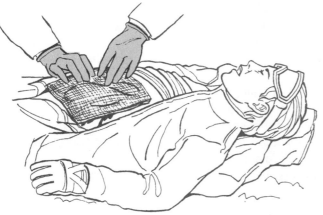

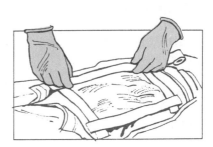

Fig. 15.3 *Care of an Open Abdominal Wound with Protruding Bowel*

Fig. 15.3

patient's position, and whether the patient resists moving or changing position. Obtain the patient's medical history, find out what medicines are taken, if there are allergies, and ask, "Is there anything else we should know?"

7. Assess the remainder of the body, particularly the back if the mechanism of injury makes you suspect a kidney injury.

8. Collect any voided urine and inspect it for the presence of blood.

9. Reassess and record the vital signs, change in location and character of pain, and any other new events at regular intervals. If the signs and symptoms of shock are present or develop, decide whether the injuries you have found are serious enough to explain the level of shock. If not, continue to reassess the patient for evidence of internal bleeding.

Emergency Care of a Patient with an Abdominal or Pelvic Injury

1. Keep the patient warm and lying down in the most comfortable position, usually on the back or side with the knees flexed.

2. Do not give the patient anything by mouth. Watch for vomiting and monitor the upper airway if it occurs, using suction if necessary. Monitor breathing and assist ventilation as needed.

3. Control external bleeding by direct pressure.

4. Consider any visible abdominal wound as an *open* abdominal injury, even if the abdominal wall has not been completely

penetrated. The rescuer has no way of knowing whether underlying organs have been injured, although the gradual development of the signs and symptoms of peritonitis may lead you to a suspect that they have. Apply a dry, sterile dressing to the wound and monitor the patient for signs of internal bleeding, shock (Chapter 6), or peritonitis (see above).

5. If abdominal organs are protruding from an open wound, cover them with an **occlusive dressing** (Fig. 15.3) consisting of a universal dressing or several layers of sterile compresses moistened with sterile physiological saline or the cleanest water available to which one-half teaspoonful of salt has been added per quart. Cover this with a layer of clean (preferably sterile) airtight material, such as Vaseline gauze, foil, plastic wrap, or a plastic bag, to keep the organs from drying out.

6. Stabilize impaled objects in place using large, bulky dressings held firmly with tape or self-adhering roller bandages.

7. Regularly monitor and record the vital signs, particularly the pulse, respirations, and blood pressure. Record any changes in the amount, type, or location of pain. Also record the amount of abdominal distention, occurrence of vomiting, and the amount and description of urine passed.

8. Anticipate and treat shock (see Chapter 6). Stabilize the patient's temperature, elevate the legs, and provide oxygen at high concentration and flow rate.

9. The pneumatic antishock garment (PASG) is effective in treating intra-abdominal and pelvic bleeding and stabilizing a fractured pelvis. The PASG should be used for these indications if personnel trained and licensed in its use are available.

Table 15.2

Summary of Emergency Care of a Patient with an Abdominal or Pelvic Injury

1. Keep the patient warm and recumbent in the position of greatest comfort.
2. Control external bleeding by direct pressure.
3. Give the patient nothing by mouth.
4. Maintain the airway. Manage vomiting, using suction if necessary. Assist ventilation as needed.
5. Bandage wounds.
6. Protect eviscerated organs with a sterile, moist occlusive dressing.
7. Stabilize an impaled object in place.
8. Monitor and record vital signs; change in location or character of pain; amount of distention; vomiting and description of vomitus; amount and description of urine; and any other changes.
9. Anticipate and treat shock.
10. Use the PASG if possible to treat intra-abdominal or pelvic bleeding and stabilize a fractured pelvis.
11. Immobilize the patient with a fractured pelvis on a long spine board.
12. Transport the patient to a hospital.

---

10. If you suspect a fractured pelvis, immobilize the patient on a long spine board. In some cases, the patient is more comfortable with the knees bent.

11. Transport the patient to a hospital as soon as possible. Allow the patient to lie down in the most comfortable position. Remember that a pelvic fracture is a true emergency because of the danger of serious internal bleeding.

Scenario #14 (Fig. 15.4)

The following scenario represents the assessment and emergency care of a patient with an abdominal injury.

It is a cold, blustery day in early March. The sky is overcast with a light snow falling. You have just finished your lunch and have dropped by the patrol room when the telephone rings. It is your friend, Sheriff Brown. There has been an accident at Silver Falls, a popular ice-climbing area about 2 miles inside the Big Bear Wilderness just beyond High Range Ski Area. He needs some experienced ski mountaineers to help the county search and rescue team.

According to a phone message from the victim's companion, the victim was putting on his crampons at the bottom of the main icefall when he slipped on the ice and slid down the frozen stream below the fall, over a series of small staircase areas of ice for about 100 feet. He had abdominal pain and was unable to stand, so the companion wrapped him in spare clothing and, realizing that he needed medical attention, skied out to the road where there was a public campground with a phone. The companion notified the sheriff, then skied back to the falls to do what he could for his friend. Emergency care and an oversnow evacuation will be needed since the weather is too bad for a helicopter evacuation.

You mentally go over the things you need to know as you question the sheriff. There was no sign of bleeding at the accident site. The victim was conscious and coherent, although having considerable abdominal pain. The companion saw him slide at full speed into a large log at the side of the frozen stream and believes he hit the log belly first. The companion also believes his friend may have an ice-ax wound of the abdomen. The victim had grabbed his ice ax as he slipped, but could not self-arrest on the glare ice.

You check the roster. Fortunately, there are four other patrollers on duty besides yourself who are trained ski mountaineers. There are enough off-duty people available to keep the mountain covered. You clear your plans with the area operator, radio the assistant hill chief to take over your duties, then call the other four patrollers to assemble at the base. You call the summit and ask the duty patroller to send down the four-handle fiberglass Akja. While waiting, you open the off-area locker and take out five off-area rescue packs, an off-area first aid kit, and two 150-foot coils of climbing rope. You then retrieve a long spine board and an oxygen backpack from the gear closet. You put a liter bag of sterile physiological saline inside your undershirt against your chest.

By this time, the four other patrollers have arrived. Fortunately, you all have your telemarking equipment in your vehicles, one of which is a large pickup truck. Within a few minutes, the equipment is loaded and, after calling the sheriff's office to notify them of your departure, you leave for the trailhead about 10 miles away.

Fig. 15.4 *Scenario #14*

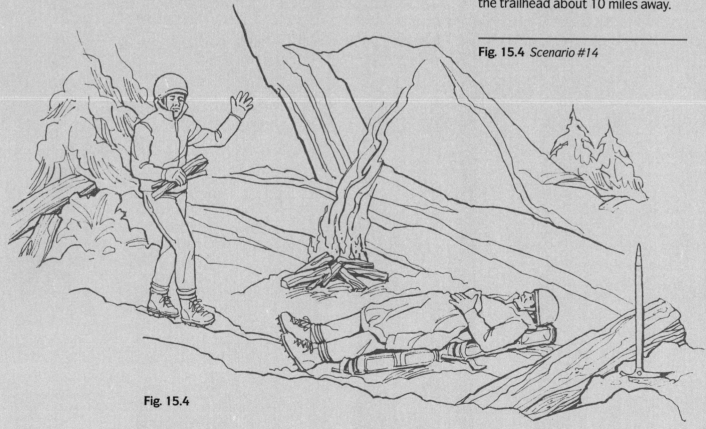

Fig. 15.4

When you arrive, half a dozen members of the local search and rescue (SAR) unit are assembling their equipment. Your party puts on climbing skins and gets into its bindings. Together with several members of the SAR unit, the patrollers set off up the trail with the Akja, three skiers pulling on a length of rope attached to its front end and one between the rear handles. You and one of the search and rescue team unit members ski on ahead with the off-area first aid kit and oxygen. It is about 18°F and still overcast and snowing lightly, but the wind has died down.

It takes you 45 minutes to ski 2 miles up the narrow trail and ¼ mile through deep snow to the accident site. You can see the bright flames and smoke of a fire as you approach. The victim is lying on two daypacks covered with a parka, a few feet from the fire. An ice ax is standing in the snow nearby. There is blood on the pick, but no obvious blood on the snow. The companion comes to meet you. You recognize him as an acquaintance you have climbed with in the past. He took the Winter Emergency Care course with the patrol candidates two years ago. You glance at your watch: it is 2 p.m.

You: "Bill, how does it look?"

Bill: "I've checked him over as well as I can. We don't have any first aid equipment along. He took a long slide down the ice of the creek and hit that log. He has a wound in his abdomen—probably landed on the pick of his ice ax. He's bleeding some but not much. His pulse is strong, but he is in a lot of pain."

You: "What time did this happen?"

Bill: "About 11 a.m."

You: "What's his name?"

Bill: "Howard Angle, we call him 'Hi.' "

You: "Howard, I'm Ben Schussen from the High Range Ski Patrol (grasping his wrist and feeling his pulse). "Can we help you?" (The pulse is strong, regular and 110 beats per minute.)

Patient: "Yes, I've met you before" (He speaks carefully—it obviously hurts to talk.) "Thanks for coming."

You count his respirations; they are 24 per minute and shallow. You then scan his body from head to toe, noting that there is no obvious blood on the clothing.

You: "Exactly what happened?"

Patient: "Slipped and took a fast ride down the ice. Hit that log pretty hard, landed on my ax. Terrible pain in my gut."

You: "Did you hit the log with your abdomen?"

Patient: "Yes."

You: "Do you have any pain anywhere else? How about your neck and back?"

Patient: "No."

You: "Did you hit your chest? You're having trouble breathing."

Patient: "My gut hurts when I breathe."

You: "Did you hit your head?"

Patient: "No."

You: "Are you cold?"

Patient: "Not bad. The fire helps."

You: "Sorry to have to ask you so many questions, but we need to know what happened."

You have now established that his airway is open, he is ventilating well, his pulse is strong, and he is alert and able to give a coherent history. It is time to examine the area of chief concern: the abdomen.

You: "I'll have to open your clothes to get a look at your abdomen" (putting on a pair of rubber gloves).

There is a small tear penetrating all the way through his parka, down sweater, pile jacket and expedition polypropylene undershirt. It matches up with an open wound the size of a 25-cent piece in the mid-abdomen, just to the right side of the umbilicus. There is a small amount of blood around the wound and along the track through the clothing. The wound looks free of dirt and bark, which is expected under the circumstances. Some shiny, yellow material covered with blood—probably fat—is protruding from the wound.

You open the first aid kit and take out a flashlight, tongue blade, several large, sterile compresses, some 2-inch tape, a large package of sterile Vaseline gauze, the V-Vac suction unit, and a set of IV tubing. You remove the IV bag of physiological saline from inside your undershirt. You carefully inspect and palpate the abdomen, avoiding the area immediately around the wound. The abdomen is distended and generally tender. There are no other open wounds, swellings, or ecchymosis. You press the iliac crests toward each other, and then backward. None of these maneuvers causes any additional pain.

At this point, the patient starts to retch. You help him turn on his side and he vomits into the snow. You grab the V-Vac and suction his mouth. When he seems to have finished, you change to a new pair of rubber gloves, open two large compresses, and place them over the wound. Attaching the IV tubing to the bag, you let enough sterile saline flow into the compresses to wet them all the way through, then put a large piece of sterile Vaseline gauze over the top. You cover this with a large dry dressing and tape its edges to the skin of the abdomen.

You: "Howard, you have an ice ax wound in your abdomen. The toboggan will be here in a few minutes and we're going to load you into it and take you back to the trailhead. First, I need to ask you a few questions and make sure nothing else is wrong, if you don't mind. Are you still warm enough?"

Patient: "I'm okay."

You: "Do you have anything medically wrong with you we should know about? Any previous chronic illnesses?"

Meanwhile, you start a rapid head-to-toe assessment, beginning with the head. There are no open or closed wounds of the scalp or face, the pupils are equal and respond to light, there is no bleeding or drainage from the ears or nose, and no injuries inside the mouth.

Patient: "No."

You: "Are you taking any medicines for anything? Any allergies?"

You proceed to the neck. The jugular veins are not distended, there are no open or closed wounds, no tenderness, and no medical-alert tags. The trachea is in the midline.

Patient: "No."

You: "Anything else about you at all that we should know?"

You proceed with an assessment of the chest. There are no obvious open or closed wounds or tenderness. Both sides of the chest expand equally.

Patient: "No."

You: "When did you eat last?"

Patient: "I had breakfast about 6 a.m. and a candy bar just before this happened."

You palpate the lower and then the upper extremities through the patient's clothing. There are no areas of tenderness or deformity.

You: "Can you feel your toes? Can you wiggle your toes?" (The answer is yes to these questions.) "Squeeze both my hands with your hands." (The patient does so. You note that both his hands are warm.) "Do your hands and arms feel numb or tingly at all?"

Patient: "No."

You next run your hand down the patient's neck and back, feeling for any tenderness, swelling, or deformity of the spinous processes. There is none.

By this time, your companions have finally arrived with the Akja, maneuvered it beside the patient, and opened the tarp and sleeping bag. The patient is raised carefully using a four-person lift, laid in the Akja with his knees bent for comfort, and covered up. His head is exposed so he can be watched. Oxygen is started at 6 liters per minute, by nasal cannula in case he vomits again.

One patroller takes the front handles, another the rear. You ski immediately behind the rear patroller, carrying the suction unit. Four skiers are carrying the climbing rope attached to the front of the Akja in case they are needed to pull, and two are in a belay position holding the other rope attached to the back. Fortunately, it is mostly downhill to the road. You have radioed ahead so that an ambulance will meet you at the trailhead—about a half-hour away with luck and strong legs.

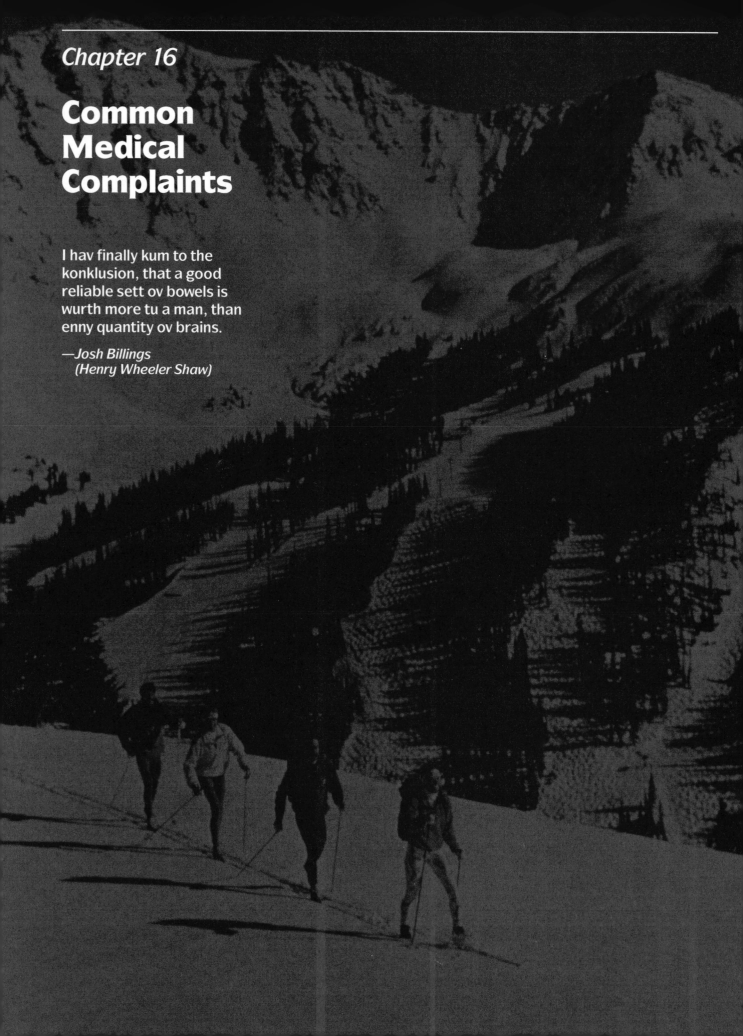

Chapter 16

Common Medical Complaints

I hav finally kum to the konklusion, that a good reliable sett ov bowels is wurth more tu a man, than enny quantity ov brains.

—*Josh Billings*
  (Henry Wheeler Shaw)

With the exception of a short section on medical assessment in Chapter 4, the preceding chapters of this textbook have emphasized the effects of injury on the body and the assessment and care of the injured patient. This strong emphasis on trauma is deliberate. Each year in the United States, one person in three suffers a nonfatal injury. Trauma is the leading cause of death and disability in children and young adults, killing more Americans under the age of 35 than all diseases combined. Nevertheless, nontraumatic illness also is a major public health problem, particularly in older Americans.

Fifteen years ago, it was accurate to say that advances in medical care had controlled or eliminated the major infectious diseases, leaving cancer and degenerative diseases of the circulatory and respiratory systems as the principal causes of death. However, since the early 1980s, the infectious disease AIDS has become the most common cause of death in men aged 20 to 40 in major metropolitan areas. By the end of this century, AIDS is predicted to be the major cause of death in young to middle-aged men throughout the entire United States and will be an increasingly common cause of death in women. Childhood diseases such as measles are making a comeback despite the availability of potent vaccines, because children are not being vaccinated.

Antibiotics have controlled acute infections that at one time killed millions, such as pneumococcal lobar pneumonia and scarlet fever; however, older people and those with defective immune systems continue to die of infections caused by organisms that are poorly controlled by available antibiotics.

The human body has limited ways to respond to a wide variety of illnesses. This chapter discusses signs and symptoms that are common to many illnesses. It is important that the rescuer know the possible causes of each "common medical complaint," its significance, and its emergency care. The emergency care of a complaint frequently is the same regardless of the underlying disease. Chapter 17 discusses medical illnesses as entities and their care, based on the specific illness rather than the signs and symptoms. This chapter examines specific medical illnesses such as heart disease and diabetes with emphasis on their causes, signs and symptoms, and emergency care.

In medical care, the ending "itis" added to an anatomical term implies infection or inflammation of the anatomical part. For example, appendicitis is an infection of the appendix, and bronchitis is an infection of the bronchi.

Common Respiratory Complaints

Respiratory Distress

Respiratory distress, frequently called "shortness of breath" or **dyspnea,** means breathing that is labored or difficult for the patient, i.e., abnormally rapid, deep, shallow, or slow. Combinations frequently occur, such as rapid breathing that is shallow, or slow breathing that is deep. In particular, respiratory distress refers to the patient's *awareness* of the need for making an extra effort to obtain enough air. It is important to determine whether the cause of the respiratory distress is located in the upper or the lower respiratory tract or elsewhere in the body.

Respiratory distress can have a number of causes, including the following:

1. Difficulty moving air in and out through the passages of the respiratory tract. This usually is due to partial obstruction because of swelling, secretions or, occasionally, a foreign body.
2. Unusual lung stiffness, as with blood, pus, or edema in the alveoli and the spaces between them.
3. Compression of the lung from the outside by air or fluid in the pleural cavity.
4. Interference with respiratory mechanics, as in chest wall injury.
5. Changes in the amount of oxygen or carbon dioxide in the blood or in its acidity or alkalinity (pH).
6. Working muscle demand for more oxygen.
7. Psychological problems such as anxiety that are interpreted by the brain as a need for greater respiratory efforts.

Common medical illnesses that produce respiratory distress include respiratory infections, pulmonary edema from heart failure or high altitude illness, emphysema, asthma, a foreign body in the airway, lung cancer, a blood clot in the lung (pulmonary embolism), fluid in the pleural space (pleural effusion), blood in the pleural space (hemothorax), air in the pleural space (pneumothorax), acidosis from uremia or uncontrolled diabetes, and anxiety. A cause of "normal" respiratory distress is increased muscular activity as seen in strenuous exercise.

Coughing

The term cough refers to a short, harsh sound produced by air suddenly rushing out through the larynx. Coughing helps to rid the body of mobile material, such as pus, that is irritating a part of the respiratory tract.

The act of coughing consists of a short inhalation followed immediately by closing of the **glottis**, the part of the larynx around the vocal cords. Next, the chest wall muscles contract, increasing pressure within the chest. The glottis then opens suddenly and the air rushes out, carrying the offending material with it. Coughing continues until the material is either expelled completely or is moved to a less sensitive part of the airway. The most sensitive areas are the trachea and the larynx, but irritation of the smaller air passages, the lungs, and the pleura also can cause coughing. Nonmobile irritants, such as infection of the lining of the bronchi, also cause coughing, but since the irritant cannot be removed by coughing alone, the cough may be particularly irritating and prolonged.

Coughing can result from irritation caused by infection, allergy, injury, excessive dryness or wetness of the airway lining, a mucous plug, or a foreign body. Illnesses that produce coughing are the same as those that cause respiratory distress.

Wheezes, Rhonchi, and Stridor

Wheezes are high-pitched sounds produced by air traveling through small air passages in the lungs narrowed by swelling or spasm. They typically occur on expiration but may also occur on inspiration. Rhonchi are coarser, usually lower-pitched sounds produced by air moving in and out through larger air passages partly blocked by mucus or other secretions. Stridor is a high-pitched, crowing sound on inhalation produced by air moving through a narrowed part of the upper respiratory tract. These sounds often can be heard with the unaided ear.

Wheezes are characteristic of conditions involving the smaller air passages, such as asthma, emphysema, pulmonary edema, and certain infections (bronchiolitis and bronchitis). Rhonchi typically are heard in patients with diseases of the larger air passages, such as bronchitis and tracheitis. Stridor is heard in patients with irritation, infection, or a growth that causes

swelling or obstruction of part of the upper airway, usually the larynx. A common cause of stridor in infants is croup.

Pain

Pain coming from the respiratory tract usually is felt in the throat, neck, beneath the sternum, or on one side of the chest. Throat pain ("sore throat") is due to an infection of the tonsils or posterior pharynx and is most noticeable during swallowing. Neck pain can be seen in infections of the larynx (laryngitis). Pain beneath the sternum is common with infection or irritation of the trachea or large bronchi. The patient usually describes this pain as a dull ache increased by cough. Pain on one side of the chest may be seen in infection or irritation of the pleura (pleuritis or pleurisy) and pneumonia. Frequently it is a sharp, knife-like pain increased by deep breathing or coughing.

Common Medical Causes of Respiratory Complaints

Respiratory Infections

Respiratory infections may involve the upper respiratory tract, the lower respiratory tract, or both. The most common **upper respiratory tract infection** (URI) is the **common cold**, a viral infection characterized by a stuffy, runny nose, sneezing, and a scratchy throat. Fever usually is absent or low-grade. In some cases the infection will move downward to involve the larynx and bronchi. Hay fever, an allergic condition of the nose and sinuses, can cause similar symptoms. Patients with a URI may complain of shortness of breath when they actually mean nasal stuffiness caused by swelling of the nasal passages.

Influenza, or "flu," is a more severe type of respiratory infection. The symptoms are the same as those

of the common cold, plus a high fever, generalized aching, sore throat, and severe cough.

A **sore throat** may occur by itself or may be part of a general URI. It is a commonly seen illness due to infection of the tonsils, posterior pharynx, or soft palate by a virus or bacterium. Severe sore throats with chills, fever, swelling, pus and/or white spots on the tonsils or throat, and/or tender lymph nodes under the back of the jaw usually are caused by a bacterium (streptococcus).

Earache occasionally may occur by itself but usually is part of a URI when infection in the posterior pharynx moves up the eustachian tube to the middle ear. The eustachian tube keeps pressure equal on both sides of the eardrum by serving as a connection between the middle ear and the throat. Swallowing will open the tube, which is how you "pop" your ears when they feel full during rapid ascents and descents. Blockage of this tube by swelling during a sore throat also interferes with the normal drainage of secretions out of the middle ear.

Infections of the **epiglottis** and **larynx** occasionally cause enough swelling to obstruct the upper respiratory tract, especially in children whose respiratory passages are smaller than those of adults. Stridor, hoarseness, and coughing are typical of these infections; the patient is anxious and frequently prefers to sit up and lean forward with the mouth open. An upper respiratory infection with stridor and respiratory distress is a medical emergency.

Pneumonia, pleurisy, and bronchitis are **lower respiratory tract infections. Pneumonia** is an infection of the lung caused by a virus or bacterium. The infection causes stiffening (consolidation) of the involved part of the lung as the alveoli and the spaces between them become filled with blood and pus (Fig. 16.1b). Patients with pneumonia have respiratory distress because of this stiffness and also because of the lowered level of oxygen in the arterial blood. The areas of lung consolidation can be seen heard with the stethoscope and seen on X-rays.

Pleurisy (pleuritis) is an infection of the pleura, the thin membrane that lines the pleural space. The layer of pleura that covers the lung moves across the layer of pleura that lines the inside of the chest cage as the lung expands and contracts during normal breathing. The small amount

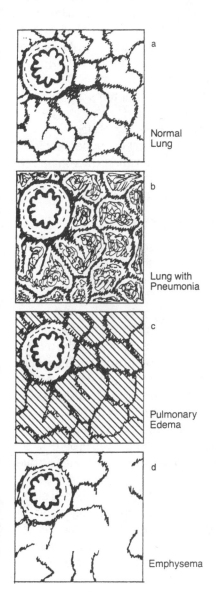

Fig. 16.1

of fluid in the normal pleural space lubricates this motion. Inflammation or irritation of the pleura roughens it and thickens the pleural fluid, so that breathing and coughing become painful.

In **bronchitis**, the main infection is in the bronchi rather than the alveoli. Rhonchi and wheezes may be heard by stethoscope, but there are no or few signs of consolidation by stethoscope or X-ray.

Although pneumonia, pleurisy, and bronchitis are separate diseases, there frequently is some overlap since the infected parts of the respiratory tract are closely associated. Patients with pneumonia usually have some bronchitis as well, and patients with severe bronchitis also may have small patches of pneumonia (bronchopneumonia). Pneumonia involving parts of the lung close to the pleura often is accompanied by pleurisy.

All three conditions usually are accompanied by fever. In both pneumonia and bronchitis, the patient usually has a severe cough that produces greenish or yellowish sputum. Pain beneath the sternum may be seen in either pneumonia or bronchitis; pain on the side or back of the chest usually means pneumonia or pleurisy. Blood in the sputum of a patient with a lower respiratory tract infection usually means pneumonia.

Pulmonary Edema

In pulmonary edema, the fluid portion of the blood leaves the capillaries and collects in the alveoli (Fig. 16.1c). This is due to either:

1. Increased capillary pressure caused by back pressure from a failing heart or to high pressure shunts that develop at high altitude; or
2. Alveolar and capillary wall damage caused by infection, the hypoxia of high altitude, or inhalation of toxic material such as smoke or chemical fumes.

Stiffening of the lung and interference with oxygen uptake result. Bubbly sounds, wheezes, and rattles often can be heard with the unaided ear. The patient is short of breath, coughs frequently, may be cyanotic, and finds it easier to breathe in a sitting position. In severe cases, frothy, pink sputum is produced because the capillaries are so damaged that they allow leakage of red cells as well as plasma.

Emphysema

Emphysema is a chronic, degenerative lung disease caused by cigarette smoking or breathing polluted air. It is a serious problem in modern society. The mechanism is progressive lung damage from years of exposure to pulmonary irritants and repeated infections. This causes scarring, obstruction of the alveoli, and narrowing and chronic inflammation of the bronchi. The walls between the alveoli break down, creating fewer, larger alveoli (Fig. 16.1d). As the patient's lungs become larger and less efficient, the chest enlarges, creating a characteristic barrel-chested appearance (Fig. 16.2).

Fig. 16.1 *Microscopic Appearance of Various Lung Conditions*

Fig. 16.2 *An Emphysema Patient with an Enlarged Chest*

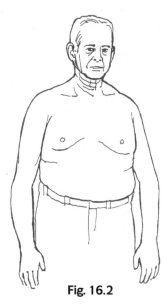

Fig. 16.2

Breath sounds heard with a stethoscope typically are quieter than normal. Exhalation is prolonged because it takes longer to exhale through the narrowed bronchi. Eventually, the lungs become so inefficient that the oxygen level in the blood drops and the carbon dioxide level rises. Respiratory distress is caused by the increased work required to breathe and the altered blood levels of carbon dioxide and oxygen. Coughing, wheezing, and rhonchi are commonly noted. Patients with severe emphysema cannot exert themselves enough to walk even a few steps without supplemental oxygen from a portable tank. Because of their disability, these patients are unlikely to engage in active outdoor sports.

Asthma

Asthma is a condition in which periodic episodes of bronchial narrowing occur, causing attacks of coughing, wheezing, and shortness of breath. Some asthmatics suffer attacks when they inhale substances they are allergic to, such as pollen. In others, attacks are precipitated by emotional stress or irritation from infection, air pollution, cold air, or exercise.

During an asthma attack, the patient is short of breath, prefers to sit upright, and wheezes audibly. Respiratory distress is caused by the increased work required to move air in and out of the narrowed bronchi.

Pulmonary Embolism

Pulmonary embolism occurs when blood clots that form in the veins of other parts of the body are carried by the venous blood flow into the lungs, where they are trapped eventually as the branches of the pulmonary arteries become smaller and smaller. Blockage of a pulmonary artery branch reduces or shuts off blood flow through the segment of the lung it supplies, in some cases producing an **infarct**, an area where the segment dies and the alveoli and their walls become filled with blood and edema fluid.

Symptoms of pulmonary infarct include respiratory distress, spitting up blood, and chest pain that worsens upon coughing and deep breathing. Large emboli may block such large vessels that blood flow through the lung is interfered with enough to cause cardiogenic shock.

Pulmonary emboli most commonly originate from clots in the deep veins of the legs and pelvis. Clots in a lower extremity may be asymptomatic or may produce leg swelling and tenderness of the calf. Bending the foot upward at the ankle frequently produces pain in the calf ("Homan's sign," Fig. 16.3).

Pulmonary emboli usually develop in people who are forced to be inactive because of illness or during recovery from surgery. They also can develop after severe injury, especially fractures of the pelvis or extremities. The blood thickening that results from increased production of red blood cells during acclimatization to high altitude predisposes expeditionary climbers to clotting, especially if confined to a tent or snow cave by long periods of bad weather. Pulmonary embolism is a serious medical emergency, and there is no effective field emergency care.

Fig. 16.3 *Test for a deep blood clot in the leg by bending the foot toward the head.*

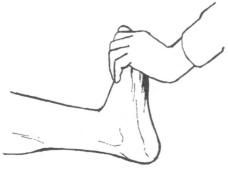

Fig. 16.3

Airway Obstruction

Most of the important causes of **upper airway obstruction** are related to trauma or unconsciousness and have been discussed in Chapters 4, 12, and 13. Medical conditions such as malignant disease and infections of the larynx and epiglottis also can cause upper airway obstruction. The accidental inhalation of food, such as a peanut, or a small foreign body, such a bead, is an important cause of upper (and lower) airway obstruction in infants and small children.

Lower airway obstruction is most commonly chronic and is caused by malignant disease. Acute lower airway obstruction occasionally is seen in emergency care due to blockage of bronchi by inhaled vomitus or a foreign body.

Signs and symptoms of airway obstruction include respiratory distress, coughing, wheezing, and cyanosis. In addition, upper respiratory obstruction may be accompanied by hoarseness, inability to talk, and a crowing type of stridor.

Malignant Disease

Malignant disease of the upper or lower respiratory tract, especially cancer of the lung, is a common cause of death and disability. Lung cancer has long been the most common cancer in men and has recently replaced breast cancer as the most common cancer in women. The recent decrease in smoking in some Western countries is predicted to decrease the incidence of this cancer.

Replacement of normal lung tissue by cancer causes progressive respiratory distress and coughing due to irritation and obstruction of the respiratory tract and decreased blood oxygen. Other common signs and symptoms of respiratory tract cancer include blood in the sputum, weakness, weight loss, and chronic hoarseness.

Hyperventilation

Hyperventilation is a common and benign form of respiratory distress that involves a progressive and predictable series of events leading to frightening signs and symptoms in the affected individual and considerable alarm in family and friends. The respiratory distress of a patient who hyperventilates is rarely caused by actual respiratory system disease.

The episode usually starts with an increase in the rate and depth of breathing caused by altitude, nausea, an emotional reaction such as anxiety or fright, or chest pain from gas in the digestive tract. These breathing changes cause excessive loss of carbon dioxide from the blood. Because carbon dioxide is acidic, its loss makes the blood more alkaline. This alkalinity (alkalosis) interferes with the normal function of muscles and nerves, causing coldness, numbness, and tingling of the hands, feet, and mouth, as well as a feeling of lightheadedness and increased shortness of breath.

Such symptoms alarm the patient, who may fear that a stroke, heart attack, or other catastrophe is occurring, and cause him or her to breathe even harder. As the alkalinity of the blood increases further, the patient's hands and feet turn blue and go into flexor spasms (Fig. 16.4). If untreated, this series of events ultimately leads to unconsciousness, which returns the breathing to normal and allows the patient to recover.

Benign hyperventilation almost always occurs in children, teenagers, and young adults. Hyperventilation in older people must be distinguished from respiratory distress caused by a stroke, pulmonary embolus, heart attack, or other serious illness.

Assessment of a Patient with a Respiratory Complaint

1. First impression. The patient appears to have an illness rather than an injury. Institute universal precautions (see Appendix F).
2. Introduce yourself. Ask, "Can I help you? What's the trouble?"
3. Perform the primary survey, giving basic life support and otherwise caring for any urgent problems discovered. Note deviations of the pulse and breathing rate from normal, whether breathing is labored, whether the patient is sitting upright to make breathing easier, and whether the patient is too short of breath to talk normally. Note the presence of cough, hoarseness, and obvious audible, abnormal breathing sounds such as wheezing and stridor.
4. Ask the patient to describe the problem and to elaborate on any respiratory complaints, particularly the time and manner of onset, duration, whether the complaint is getting better or worse, and whether it is accompanied by pain or fever. Patients with severe respiratory distress frequently have trouble conversing.
5. Assess the vital signs. Obtain information about the patient's medical history, especially whether there has been any chronic heart or lung condition such as coronary artery disease,

congestive heart failure, asthma, and emphysema. Determine whether the patient has any allergies and is taking any medicines. Do not forget to ask, "Is there anything else we should know about your health?"
6. Start the body assessment with the head and neck. Assess the skin, particularly for color (cyanosis), temperature, and moisture. Inspect the nose for drainage of mucous or blood, and the mouth and throat for redness, swelling, and white patches. Feel for tender swellings under the sides of the jaw. Listen for stridor. Look for a medical-alert tag.
7. Assess the chest, noting the type of respiratory distress present, if any. Observe whether the sides of the chest are moving together, and if pain is present, whether the patient is self-splinting the chest. Listen for wheezes and rhonchi.
8. Proceed with assessment of the remaining parts of the body.

Emergency Care of a Patient with a Respiratory Complaint

1. Allow the patient to assume the most comfortable position.
2. Give oxygen, if available, to patients with moderate to severe respiratory distress, especially if cyanotic.
3. If ventilations appear to be ineffective, i.e., too fast, too slow, and/or too shallow, assist ventilation with mouth-to-pocket mask or bag-valve-mask. For further discussion of ineffective ventilations, see Chapter 19.
4. Assist an asthmatic to take his or her own medications.

Fig. 16.4 *A patient who hyperventilates may develop flexor spasms in the hands.*

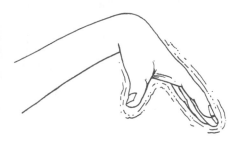

Fig. 16.4

5. The traditional management of hyperventilation has been to have the patient breathe in and out of a paper bag. This theoretically would tend to correct the alkalosis as the patient rebreathes the exhaled carbon dioxide. However, since pure hyperventilation is difficult to distinguish from more serious diseases, it is best to try to calm the patient and give oxygen at high concentration and flow rate.

6. Relief of specific symptoms:
   a. For nasal congestion, the patient can take nonprescription decongestants such as Sudafed, Actifed, or Dimetapp. Patients with high blood pressure should use these with caution.
   b. For cough, the patient can take a nonprescription cough suppressant. Combinations of cough suppressants with decongestants also are available.
   c. For discomfort, the patient can take nonprescription analgesics such as aspirin, acetaminophen, or ibuprofen.

7. The patient should see a physician if he or she has any of the following:
   a. Suspected pneumonia or severe bronchitis.
   b. Earache.
   c. Yellow or green sputum, or blood in the sputum.
   d. Stridor.
   e. A severe sore throat, especially with white spots on the tonsils, or enlarged, tender lymph nodes under the back of the jaw.
   f. Fever higher than 101°F (38.3°C), especially with chills.
   g. Fever of any degree associated with respiratory distress.
   h. Evidence of heart disease, such as a positive medical history, abnormal heart rate or rhythm, suspicious chest pain (see below), or swelling of the ankles.
   i. Any respiratory distress of uncertain cause or that does not respond to rest or other simple measures.

Chest Pain

Chest pain is a common complaint in modern society. Because of the association of chest pain with heart disease, any type of unexplained chest pain is very alarming to the patient. There are five general causes of chest pain:

1. Minor chest wall injury.
2. Heart disease.
3. Respiratory system disease.
4. Gastrointestinal system disease.
5. Stress and anxiety.

Chest wall pain usually occurs at weak points in the chest cage, such as the joints between the ribs and sternum, or the costochondral junctions where the bony part of the rib is connected to its cartilage. Minor compression trauma and lifting a heavy weight or other activities can buckle or sprain these areas and also bruise ribs and intercostal muscles. Symptoms include pain on breathing or using the upper extremities. The painful area usually is tender when pressed on.

Most pain due to heart disease is associated with **coronary artery disease**, discussed in detail in Chapter 17. The pain is of two major types:

1. Pain of short duration, called **angina pectoris**. This is due to a temporary mismatch between the need of the heart for blood and the ability of the diseased coronary arteries to supply it.
2. A more severe pain due to **myocardial infarction**. In this condition, there is actual death of a portion of the heart muscle (myocardium), usually caused by sudden blockage of a coronary artery by a clot.

Angina pectoris most commonly occurs during physical exertion or emotional stress. The characteristic pain is felt beneath the sternum, frequently radiating to the neck, jaw, one or both shoulders (usually the left), the left arm, and occasionally the upper abdomen (Fig. 16.5). At times, it may be felt only in the throat, jaw, or back between the shoulder blades. The patient describes the pain as squeezing, crushing, vise-like, burning, and occasionally as aching but almost never as sharp or sticking. It rarely lasts longer than 15 minutes, is relieved by rest, and responds to a nitroglycerin tablet under the tongue within three to five minutes. Most patients with angina will have been diagnosed previously and will be carrying nitroglycerin or other heart medication.

The pain of myocardial infarction resembles that of angina pectoris but

Fig. 16.5 *Most Common Locations of Anginal Pain (shaded area)*

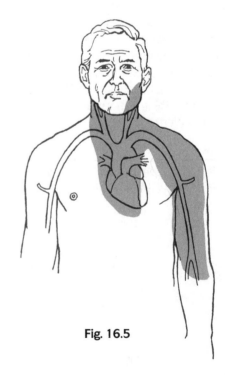

Fig. 16.5

is more severe and lasts longer. It is unrelated to exertion and is not relieved by nitroglycerin. Frequently, the skin is cold, clammy, and pale. The patient usually is anxious and short of breath and prefers to sit up or lie with the chest elevated. In rare cases the patient may want to walk around.

Pain due to **respiratory disease** has been described above in **Common Respiratory Complaints**. It includes sore throat, substernal irritation due to bronchitis and tracheitis, and lateral chest pain on coughing or deep breathing due to pleuritis or pneumonia. It rarely should be confused with pain due to heart disease.

Pain caused by **gastrointestinal disease** is commonly mistaken for pain due to heart disease (see below under **Gastrointestinal Complaints**). It may originate in the esophagus, stomach, gallbladder, intestines, or pancreas, and frequently is associated with indigestion (see below). Pain from inflammation of the esophagus or from a hiatus hernia (a condition where part of the stomach herniates into the chest) may resemble the pain of coronary artery disease since it frequently is burning in nature and substernal in location. It occasionally radiates to the neck or left shoulder; however, it often is relieved by antacids such as Tums or Maalox.

Pain due to stomach irritation usually is described as burning and is epigastric in location, also being relieved by antacids. Pain from an inflamed gallbladder usually is a pressure or aching in the right upper quadrant but may be substernal. It may radiate through to the right shoulder blade. Pain from an inflamed pancreas is deep in the epigastrium and is a severe, boring, burning pain that may radiate into the lower substernal area and through to the back. Pain due to gas accumulation or irritation of the intestines (usually the

colon) frequently is confused with heart disease by the uninitiated, although it usually is aching, sharp, or sticking in nature and located under the ribs on the left side of the anterior chest (occasionally under the right side). Many of these patients are anxious and stressed, which is not helped by having pain "over the heart."

Although pain from many types of gastrointestinal disease is characteristically relieved by antacids, pain from heart disease may occasionally be relieved as well, at least temporarily. All patients with **substernal pain**—especially pain that radiates to the neck, jaw, left shoulder, left arm, or both arms—should be cared for as heart disease patients.

Pain due to **stress** and **anxiety** usually is caused by sustained contractions of the muscles of the chest wall, esophagus, stomach, or intestines. It often is described as a chronic ache, beneath the sternum if the esophagus is involved, or in the lower left or right anterior chest if the stomach or intestines are involved. It often is constant, may last for days, is worse if the patient's anxiety level is increased, and may be accompanied by various symptoms of indigestion, such as heartburn, bloating, frequent belching, increased passage of intestinal gas (flatus) and changes in bowel habits.

Assessment and Emergency Care of a Patient with Chest Pain

1. First impression. The patient appears to have an illness rather than an injury. Institute universal precautions (see Appendix F).
2. Ask the patient what is happening. Perform the primary survey, with particular attention to whether the patient looks relatively healthy or seems seriously ill as evidenced by an abnormal pulse, abnormal

breathing pattern, cyanosis, altered mental status, hot skin, or cold, clammy skin.
3. Question the patient as to the exact location of the pain, type (sharp, sticking, aching, crushing, squeezing, vice-like, burning), how long the pain has been present, whether it has changed in type or location, and whether it is related to such activities as breathing, coughing, exertion, eating, belching, moving the bowels, passing flatus, using the arms, or turning over in bed.

Also ask about chills, fever, cough, production of sputum, shortness of breath, sore throat, and earache.
4. Assess the vital signs, especially the temperature, pulse, breathing rate, and blood pressure. Assess the skin color, temperature, and moisture. Obtain the patient's medical history, including whether similar pain has occurred before, whether there has been a recent injury to the chest or unusual physical activity involving the chest muscles, whether there has been a recent respiratory infection, and whether there is a history of heart disease. A history of lung or digestive system disease, especially gallbladder disease, "nervous stomach," hiatus hernia, and irritable bowel disease, may be important also.
5. Assess the neck and chest, looking for tender lymph nodes, deviation of the trachea, areas of tenderness or slight swelling on or between the ribs, audible rhonchi or wheezes, and a difference in chest expansion between the two sides.

6. Assess the abdomen, looking for tenderness, rigidity, swelling, distension, and audible bowel sounds.
7. Assess the head. Using a tongue blade (or spoon handle) and a flashlight, inspect the mouth, tonsils, and throat.
8. Perform the rest of the secondary survey.
9. If you suspect a serious cause for the chest pain, such as pneumonia, severe bronchitis, a gallbladder attack, pancreatitis, or a heart attack, arrange to transport the patient to a hospital as soon as possible. Give oxygen at high concentration and flow rate, if available. Allow the patient to assume the position of greatest comfort, and keep the patient warm, since shivering adds to the work of the respiratory and circulatory systems. The following types of chest pain should always be considered serious:
   a. Chest pain with fever, especially pain that is made worse by deep breathing or coughing.
   b. Chest pain with shortness of breath, weakness, cyanosis, and/or cold sweating.
   c. Substernal chest pain described as crushing, squeezing, or heavy.
   d. Chest pain that radiates to the neck, jaw, left shoulder, left arm, or both shoulders.
10. If the cause is clearly minor, such as mild chest wall pain, gastrointestinal tract pain, or stress and anxiety, advise the patient to do the following:
    a. For chest wall pain, use mild analgesics such as aspirin, acetaminophen, or ibuprofen; apply local heat; and avoid pain-producing activities.
    b. For pain that appears to originate in the stomach, try antacids such as Tums or Maalox.
    c. For pain associated with stress and anxiety, avoid irritating, gas-producing foods such as cabbage and similar vegetables, tomatoes, dried beans, onions, popcorn, raw fruit, melons, and fried and spicy foods.
11. If in doubt about the cause of chest pain, always assume that it is potentially serious and call an ambulance or take the patient to a hospital without delay (see 9 above).

Gastrointestinal Complaints

Indigestion

Indigestion is a sign that the stomach is not functioning normally. Symptoms include heartburn, pain, nausea, and vomiting.

Heartburn is a burning feeling in the epigastric area that radiates to the substernal region and throat. It is due to regurgitation of acid stomach contents into the lower esophagus. The **pain** associated with indigestion can be a burning pain, dull discomfort, cramp, or feeling of fullness or pressure. It usually is felt in the epigastric area and frequently is accompanied by epigastric tenderness.

The symptoms **nausea** and **vomiting** are discussed below.

The symptoms of indigestion are due to a mild to severe stomach inflammation frequently associated with excessive acid production, and usually are brought on by such things as stress, a viral infection, excessive alcohol intake, or a meal that is too large, too rich, or too spicy. It also can be an early symptom of an ulcer or stomach cancer. Persistent indigestion should be investigated by a physician.

Nausea and Vomiting

Nausea and vomiting are common symptoms that reflect the stomach's tendency to react to any noxious stimulus by emptying its contents. These stimuli can act directly on the stomach or indirectly through nerve pathways. Direct stimuli include infection; food poisoning; irritating drugs or chemicals such as aspirin, arthritis drugs (ibuprofen, etc.), or alcohol; abdominal trauma; or an ulcer or tumor of the stomach. Indirect stimuli include effects of high altitude; severe headache; motion sickness; stress ("nervous stomach"); psychosomatic illness; or a severe injury or illness of any type.

Vomiting may be mild or severe, acute or chronic. The major effects of severe vomiting include the following:
1. Inability to eat and loss of fluids and electrolytes, leading to starvation, dehydration, metabolic abnormalities, and occasionally even shock.
2. Aspiration of vomitus, causing airway obstruction and severe lung infection.
3. Bleeding due to tears in the stomach or esophagus.

In the outdoor setting, vomiting usually is caused by gastroenteritis, food poisoning, or the effects of altitude, and eventually subsides. However, if vomiting is prolonged, the patient must be evacuated to a hospital.

Vomiting of blood almost always indicates a serious condition. Although it can be caused by swallowing blood from a nosebleed, it usually is caused by bleeding from disease of the stomach or esophagus. The most common causes are inflammation of the stomach, a stomach or duodenal ulcer, a tear in the esophagus caused by severe vomiting, or esophageal varices (large, fragile veins in the lower esophagus that accompany cirrhosis and other chronic liver diseases).

Vomited blood can be bright red or, if partly digested, can resemble coffee grounds. A patient who is vomiting blood should be taken to the hospital as soon as possible.

Diarrhea

Diarrhea is the passage of soft or liquid stools with abnormally high frequency. In severe cases there may be pus or blood in the stools. Prolonged, severe diarrhea can lead to dehydration, starvation, and occasionally even shock because food and liquid are lost through the frequent stools. Diarrhea may be accompanied by nausea and vomiting.

Since diarrheal diseases frequently are caused by contaminated food or water, the causes of diarrhea differ in different parts of the world due to variables such as climate and state of sanitation. In the urban areas of developed countries, the most common cause of mild to moderate diarrhea is a viral infection of the bowel. Severe bacteria-caused bowel infections, such as cholera and dysentery, are rare. A protozoan, *Giardia lamblia,* carried by beavers and many other wild animals, is a common cause of diarrhea in persons who drink untreated surface water in the backcountry. Chronic, mild diarrhea may be caused by chronic emotional stress. *Staphylococci* ("staph"), a common cause of minor skin infections, grow easily in bland, creamy foods left at room temperature for a few hours. They produce a toxin that causes violent vomiting, diarrhea, and cramps. This toxin is not destroyed by reheating the contaminated food.

Severe diarrhea is common in undeveloped countries. It usually is caused by bacteria or amoebae introduced into food by dirty hands or flies or into groundwater through contamination by human feces. Diarrhea can be prevented by scrupulous attention to personal cleanliness, by washing hands before eating and preparing food, by protecting food from spoilage and contamination by flies, and by proper treatment of drinking water. In undeveloped countries, avoid raw or partly cooked meat or seafood, salads, cooked food that has cooled before being served, and raw fruit or vegetables (unless they can be peeled). Bottled drinks are usually safe, but ice, which can be contaminated, should not be added to them. Do not drink or wash your teeth with water that has not been boiled or disinfected.

Diarrhea and vomiting frequently occur together. When vomiting prevents the fluid and minerals lost by diarrhea from being replaced orally, dehydration, starvation, and shock are even more likely to occur. Hospitalization with intravenous fluid therapy is frequently required.

Blood in the Stools

Bright red blood in the stools usually means either bleeding from the rectum or lower colon or bleeding higher in the gastrointestinal tract with rapid passage of blood through the bowel.

The most common cause is bleeding from hemorrhoids or a fissure (crack or small ulcer) of the anus. The color of blood in the stools depends on how long it has been in the bowel. Maroon or reddish-black blood (frequently called "tarry stools") usually comes from higher up, most commonly from a bleeding ulcer of the stomach or duodenum, but at times from a bleeding polyp or cancer of the colon. The darker color is caused by partial digestion of the blood. Bismuth preparations such as Pepto-Bismol and vitamin-mineral supplements containing iron also can turn the stool black. Eating large amounts of beets can turn the stool (and urine) red. Some types of colon inflammation (colitis) can cause either bright red or dark blood in the stools.

Dark-colored or reddish-black blood in the stool almost always signifies a serious condition; the patient should see a physician as soon as possible. Bright red blood accompanied by pain in the anal area on moving the bowels is almost always caused by bleeding from hemorrhoids, a fissure, or an abrasion from a hard stool.

Colic

Colic is intermittent, severe abdominal pain caused by obstruction of a hollow, tubular organ such as the gallbladder, bowel, or ureter. The pain is caused by the strong contractions of the muscles of the organ as they try to force the organ contents past the obstruction. Pain resembling colic also can occur with severe gastroenteritis because of irritation and spasm of the bowel muscles.

Common causes of colic or colic-like pain are stones in the gallbladder or bile ducts, severe gastroenteritis, stones in the ureter, and intestinal obstruction cause by adhesions, a twisted bowel, or a tumor. Gallbladder or bile duct colic usually is felt in the right upper abdominal quadrant and in the back near the lower angle of the scapula; ureteral colic is felt in the flank; and intestinal colic around the navel.

Colic frequently is a symptom of serious disease and, in any case, is so painful that medical assistance is required.

Constipation

Constipation is the passage of hard, dry stools at less-than-normal intervals. It can be caused by insufficient physical activity, partial dehydration, chronic anxiety, or lack of bulk in the diet.

Constipation must be distinguished from the infrequent passage of stools of normal consistency, a situation that is normal in many people. Excessive bowel consciousness is a common human preoccupation, encouraged by laxative peddlers. The elderly, who may be inactive and subsist on a bulk-poor diet, are more likely to be afflicted with constipation than younger, more active people.

Persistent constipation or other changes in bowel habits without apparent cause should be investigated; they may be early symptoms of bowel cancer. In some cases of constipation, hard stool accumulates in the rectum, cannot be passed normally, and must be dug out of the rectum with a lubricated, gloved finger. This condition, called "fecal impaction," may cause intestinal obstruction if not cared for promptly.

Difficulty in Swallowing

Difficulty in swallowing (dysphagia) may be caused either by abnormal function of the esophageal muscles that move food and liquids from the mouth and pharynx toward the stomach, or by obstruction of the esophagus by scar tissue, tumor, or a swallowed foreign body.

Dysphagia may be acute, chronic, or intermittent. The most common cause is a temporary spasm of the esophageal muscles. The most serious cause is cancer of the esophagus, which usually causes slowly progressive dysphagia with difficulty swallowing solids at first, followed by difficulty swallowing both solids and liquids. All patients with dysphagia should be investigated by a physician.

Jaundice

Jaundice is a yellow discoloration of the skin, mucous membranes, and the whites of the eyes caused by an abnormal accumulation of **bilirubin** in the blood. Bilirubin, an end product of normal red blood cell breakdown, is excreted by the liver. It will accumulate if red cell breakdown is above normal or if the normal excretion pathways are diseased or blocked.

The most common causes are liver disease (such as hepatitis) and obstruction of the bile ducts by a gallstone or tumor. Jaundice is the sign of a serious condition, and the patient should see a physician promptly.

The Acute Abdomen

Acute abdomen is a collective term for a number of painful abdominal conditions that may require surgery or at least consultation with a surgeon. The longer the pain lasts, the more likely surgery will be required.

The signs and symptoms are either those of **inflammation of the peritoneum** (peritonitis, discussed in Chapter 15), of **colic**, or both. The pain usually is localized at first to the site of the diseased (or injured) organ, gradually spreading to involve nearby areas and then the entire abdomen. Signs and symptoms include fever, abdominal pain (which may be steady or crampy), tenderness, rigidity of the abdominal muscles, abdominal distention, loss of appetite, nausea, and vomiting. Diarrhea, if present, usually is mild. The patient may breathe rapidly and shallowly and lie quietly because it hurts to move or breathe. Later, signs of hypovolemic or vascular shock may develop.

An acute abdomen is caused by disease of the peritoneum or the organs within the abdominal cavity. Similar signs and symptoms can occur following blunt or penetrating abdominal trauma. A knowledge of the location of the major abdominal organs can give the examiner a clue as to the responsible organ (Fig. 16.6). Common causes include the following:

1. Acute appendicitis.
2. Mesenteric adenitis (inflammation of intra-abdominal lymph nodes in a patient with a respiratory infection).
3. Rupture of a peptic ulcer.
4. Acute inflammation of the gallbladder.
5. Diverticulitis (inflammation of a small, finger-like pouch on the side of the colon).
6. Pancreatitis.
7. Intestinal obstruction, due to adhesions from previous surgery, a tumor, or a twisted bowel.
8. Bowel infarction due to disease of bowel blood vessels.
9. Acute gastroenteritis without diarrhea.
10. Severe kidney infection.
11. Infection of an ovary or a fallopian tube.
12. Rupture of a pregnancy developing outside the uterus (ectopic pregnancy).
13. Peritonitis, either primary, or secondary to a ruptured abdominal organ (perforated peptic ulcer, ruptured appendix, ruptured gallbladder, ruptured diverticulitis, etc.).
14. Ruptured aneurysm (weak place on the aorta or other large blood vessel).

Note that diabetic ketoacidosis can cause severe abdominal pain that can be mistaken for an acute abdomen (see Chapter 17).

Assessment of a Patient with a Gastrointestinal Complaint

1. First impression. The patient appears to be suffering from an illness rather than an injury. Institute universal precautions (see Appendix F).
2. Ask the patient what is happening. Complete the primary survey in the usual manner, with attention to the airway, adequacy of breathing, presence of respiratory distress, and character of the pulse. Care for any urgent problems discovered.

3. Ask whether the patient has any common gastrointestinal complaints, such as pain, cramps, nausea, vomiting, and diarrhea. Expand on each positive response to find out the time, severity, and frequency at onset; whether there has been a change in the location, severity, or frequency with time; and to obtain a description of vomitus or stools, particularly whether blood or coffee-ground material was seen. Find out what and when the patient ate last, when the last bowel movement was, and in the case of vomiting, how long it has been since the patient has been able to keep food or water down. Ask whether there has been a recent respiratory infection, and if the patient has had chills, fever, painful urination, or a recent abdominal injury.

4. Assess the vital signs and obtain the patient's medical history. Find out whether the patient has had similar complaints before. Inquire about any history of peptic ulcer or gallbladder disease, chronic indigestion, chronic constipation or diarrhea, and whether the patient is on any special diet, has had any abdominal operations, and takes any regular medicines. If the patient is a woman of childbearing age, ask if there have been any missed menstrual periods or other menstrual abnormalities and if there is the possibility of pregnancy.

5. Assess the abdomen (Fig. 16.7) noting any distention, tenderness, rigidity, scars, masses, enlarged organs, or audible bowel sounds. Note the skin temperature, color, and moisture. Tap the costovertebral angles lightly to assess for kidney tenderness.

6. Proceed with the rest of the secondary survey, assessing the remainder of the body, noting in particular whether the throat and tonsils are red or swollen.

Emergency Care of a Patient with a Gastrointestinal Complaint

While reading the following discussion of emergency care of various gastrointestinal complaints, note that there is no effective field treatment for the patient who is vomiting blood, has an abdominal injury, severe rectal bleeding, or who has a severe illness of any type with gastrointestinal symptoms. The patient should be transported to a hospital as soon as possible.

Fig. 16.6 *Organs of the Abdominal Cavity*

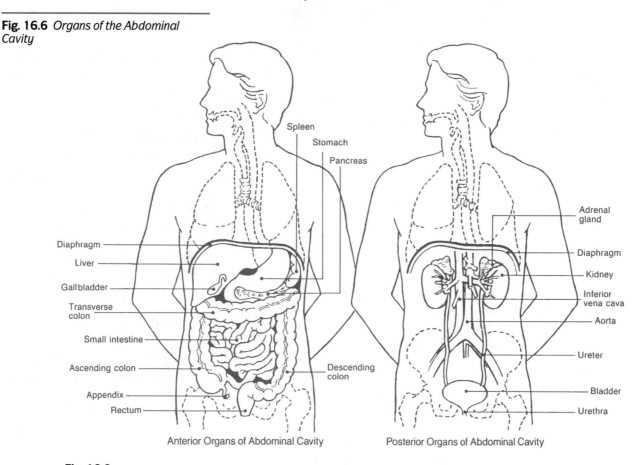

Spleen
Stomach
Pancreas

Adrenal gland
Diaphragm
Kidney
Inferior vena cava
Aorta
Ureter
Bladder
Urethra

Diaphragm
Liver
Gallbladder
Transverse colon
Small intestine
Ascending colon
Appendix
Rectum
Descending colon

Anterior Organs of Abdominal Cavity

Posterior Organs of Abdominal Cavity

Fig. 16.6

Acute Abdomen

1. Keep the patient lying down in the most comfortable position. Most patients will prefer to lie on one side or flat with the knees bent.
2. Do not give the patient anything by mouth. Watch for vomiting, and if it occurs, monitor and clear the upper airway as necessary.
3. Monitor vital signs and record any new developments or changes in signs or symptoms.
4. If shock occurs, elevate the patient's legs 12 inches and give oxygen, if available, at high concentration and flow rate.
5. Since there is no effective field emergency care for an acute abdomen, evacuate the patient to a hospital without delay.

Indigestion

Have the patient try antacids such as Rolaids or Maalox. Avoid over-eating and eating highly spiced or rich foods.

Dehydration

For dehydration caused by diarrhea or vomiting, give the patient liquids by mouth. Electrolyte-containing liquids such as broth, bouillon, or half-strength Gatorade are best.

Later, the patient can try bland foods such as tea, toast, broth, bland soup (chicken noodle or chicken rice), pudding, 7-Up, and Jello.

If the patient cannot keep liquids down, he or she will likely require evacuation to a hospital for intravenous fluid therapy.

Diarrhea

If mild, diarrhea may be controlled by diet alone (see Dehydration above). If diarrhea is moderate, have the patient try nonprescription preparations such as Pepto-Bismol, Kaopectate, or Imodium. If severe, especially with chills, fever, and pus or blood in the stools, evacuate the patient to medical care.

Constipation

Constipation can be alleviated by eating quantities of cooked fruits and vegetables and increasing water intake (especially hot water). If this does not work, try mild, nonprescription bulk laxatives or stool softeners as needed. Do *not* give laxatives to patients with symptoms suggestive of an acute abdomen.

Fig. 16.7 *Assessment of a Patient with a Suspected Acute Abdomen*

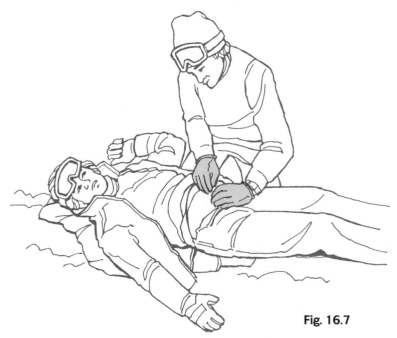

Fig. 16.7

Colic

For the patient with colic, apply heat to the abdomen. If symptoms are severe or prolonged, evacuate the patient to medical care.

Vomiting

If vomiting is mild, wait a few hours and try water, sweet tea, or a carbonated beverage such as 7-Up. If vomiting is severe, evacuate the patient to medical care.

Genitourinary Complaints

Painful Urination

Painful urination (dysuria), usually accompanied by the passage of small amounts of urine at frequent intervals, is a symptom of infection or irritation of the bladder, urethra, or, in the male, the prostate. Patients with serious urinary tract infections also may develop chills, fever, weakness, and pain in the back over a kidney. Occasionally, blood may be seen in the urine.

The emergency care for painful urination is to encourage the patient to drink adequate fluids and consult a physician.

Blood in the Urine

Blood in the urine (hematuria) can be caused by a urinary infection or a tumor or stone in the urinary tract. If there is no pain, a tumor is more likely the cause. If accompanied by dysuria, blood in the urine indicates a urinary infection; if accompanied by colic, a stone. All patients with hematuria should consult a physician.

Incontinence

Incontinence is the uncontrolled passage of urine or feces. This can occur during urinary tract infections if the need to urinate is urgent, in moderate to severe diarrhea, during unconsciousness, epileptic seizures, senility, overuse of drugs or alcohol, following a spinal cord injury, or at times in any severe illness or injury. Incontinence always is of concern and usually causes the patient considerable embarrassment.

The cause may be obvious and require no specific treatment; however, patients with persistent incontinence or newly developed incontinence should see a physician.

Inability to Urinate

Inability to urinate, or "void," can occur in anyone in severe pain, particularly in patients with injuries who cannot sit or stand to void, or who are immobilized in a litter or on a spine board. Painful bladder distention can make it even more difficult to void. Rescue groups should carry lightweight urinals or wide-mouth, screw-top plastic bottles to aid such patients in emptying their bladders. Some normal people are unable to void unless privacy is provided. In elderly men, inability to void is frequently related to urethral obstruction from an enlarged prostate.

Allow the patient as much privacy as possible and the position of choice (sitting or standing) unless prevented by the illness or injury. At times, placing the patient's hand in a pot of warm water or creating the sound of running water by turning on a faucet or pouring water on the ground from a canteen will help. Otherwise, the patient will have to be transported to medical care where he or she can be catheterized.

Abnormal Menstrual Flow

Although average menstrual periods occur at intervals of about 28 days and last five to seven days, there can be considerable variation in interval, quantity, and duration of menstrual flow in normal women. Any vaginal

bleeding aside from the regular menstrual flow is considered abnormal and should be investigated by a physician, although spotting between periods and periods with excessive flow and length are fairly common and usually benign.

The most serious types of abnormal bleeding are associated with pregnancy and can be divided into abnormalities of early and of late pregnancy. If a woman who has missed several periods and possibly has noticed some morning nausea or breast tenderness also has vaginal bleeding, she may be having a **miscarriage**. If she also develops abdominal pain and tenderness, she may be bleeding internally from an **ectopic pregnancy** (a pregnancy in which the fetus grows *outside* of the uterus). A woman who bleeds during the last few months of pregnancy may be entering premature labor or developing another complication of late pregnancy (see Chapter 26).

All of these conditions are potentially serious because of the danger of losing the baby and of severe bleeding and shock. Any pregnant woman with vaginal bleeding should call her obstetrician immediately or be taken to a hospital without delay.

Urethral and Vaginal Discharge

Urethral discharge in females and in males always is abnormal and usually is caused by infection. The patient may be concerned because of the discomfort and the possibility of having contracted a sexually transmitted infection. There is no emergency care other than to recommend consultation with a physician.

A certain amount of vaginal discharge is normal for most women, especially before and after the menstrual period. A physician should be consulted about a vaginal discharge that is abnormally profuse, irritating, discolored, bloody, or foul-smelling.

Miscellaneous Complaints

Vertigo

Vertigo, or "dizziness," means unsteadiness, loss of equilibrium, and a feeling that the "room is whirling." It may be chronic or may occur in acute attacks. The patient may feel normal between the attacks. If vertigo is severe, often it is accompanied by nausea and vomiting. In many cases the patient feels relatively normal when lying flat and still, but any attempt to sit up, move the head, or turn over causes vertigo.

Vertigo usually is caused by a disturbance in the organs that control balance: the inner ear and adjacent parts of the brain. A patient who complains of dizziness should be questioned to distinguish true vertigo from mere "lightheadedness" without the feeling that the room is whirling.

Vertigo is quite common in the elderly, in whom it usually is related to impaired circulation in the inner ear or brain. It also is common in patients with acute or chronic ear diseases such as inner ear infections, chronic deafness, or chronic tinnitus ("ringing in the ears"). Acute attacks of vertigo also can be due to viral infections and allergy; chronic mild vertigo may accompany many serious illnesses and injuries.

Vertigo can be so severe that the patient is unable to turn over in bed or sit up without vomiting. Hospitalization with intravenous feedings may be required. Vertigo also can be seen in head injury (see Chapter 12) and high altitude cerebral edema (see Chapter 18). Persistent vertigo may be an early symptom of a brain tumor. Severe or persistent vertigo should always be investigated by a physician.

Lightheadedness is a feeling of "floating," slight unsteadiness, or faintness, and is most commonly caused by chronic anxiety. It may be accompanied by hyperventilation. In some cases, patients who take medicine for high blood pressure or who have nervous system disturbances that interfere with blood pressure control will feel lightheaded for a few seconds after arising from bed or from a chair.

Headache

Five to 10 percent of Americans suffer from recurrent **headache**, mostly of the vascular (migraine) or sustained muscle contraction (muscle tension) variety. The vast majority of headaches are harmless although uncomfortable.

Common causes of benign headaches are chronic emotional stress, excessive glare, lack of sleep, eyestrain, a respiratory infection, or a hangover. Headaches in outdoor enthusiasts also can be caused by a hard fall while skiing, traction on the neck muscles caused by the weight of a heavy pack, and the effects of altitude.

Migraine headaches usually are recurrent, throbbing, one-sided, accompanied by nausea, and preceded by some type of abnormal visual phenomenon such as blurred vision or bright, moving lights. Muscle tension headaches usually are bilateral, involve the forehead and/or the occiput, and may radiate into the neck and shoulders. Tenderness of the scalp, back of the neck, and the trapezius muscles may be present.

Occasionally, headache may be a symptom of a brain tumor, meningitis, severe high blood pressure, or other serious condition. Patients with newly developed headaches or very severe headaches should see a physician. Patients with headaches associated with a stiff neck, drowsiness, altered mental status, personality changes,

visual changes, a recent head injury, a seizure, or weakness and/or loss of sensation of one side of the body should be taken to a hospital without delay.

People with mild, recurrent headaches should be encouraged to take remedies known to have been effective in the past, which they usually have with them. Common nonprescription drugs such as aspirin, acetaminophen, and ibuprofen usually will control mild headaches.

Pain in the Low Back

Pain in the low back is a common affliction of humankind and a frequent cause of acute and chronic disability. Predisposing factors include the upright stance, poor physical conditioning, poor posture, obesity, pregnancy, and loss of bone calcium in the elderly (osteoporosis).

Although there are many possible causes of low back pain in outdoor enthusiasts, most cases are due to acute compression, bending

and rotational trauma from slips and falls, chronic trauma from carrying heavy packs, and poor lifting techniques. These cause contusions and muscle strains, ligament sprains, and occasionally herniation of the nucleus of the intravertebral disc ("slipped disc").

In most cases, the pain is located across the hips in the area of the sacroiliac joints and the joint between the fifth lumbar vertebra and the sacrum. Frequently, the pain will radiate into one or both buttocks and, if the sciatic nerve is irritated, down the back of the thigh to the knee or ankle. The pain usually is increased by bending, stooping, lifting, twisting, and by actions that increase the pressure of the spinal fluid, such as coughing, sneezing, or straining.

Fig. 16.8 *Assessment of a Patient with a Suspected Sciatic Nerve Irritation*

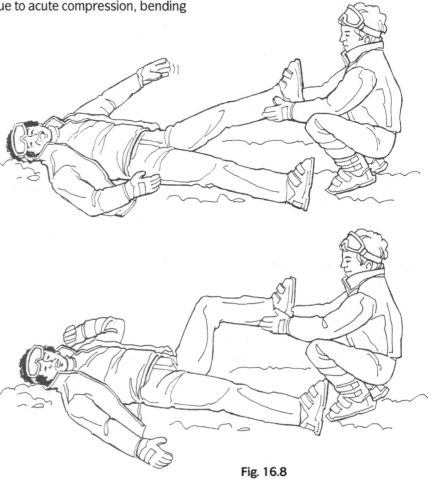

Fig. 16.8

Assessment may show tenderness and tightening of the muscles on either side of the spine in the lumbosacral region. The patient may be unable to straighten up and/or bend forward or to the side. If the sciatic nerve is irritated, lifting the foot with the patient supine and the knee *straight* will cause severe pain in the back by the time the hip is flexed to 30 to 45 degrees; if the knee is *bent,* the hip usually can be flexed to 90 degrees with little or no pain (Fig. 16.8). The most common cause of sciatic nerve irritation is pressure on the nerve roots from a herniated disc.

Acute low back pain may be so disabling that the patient must rest for several days before recovering even enough to self-evacuate without carrying a pack. Comfort can be increased by lying with the knees bent (pillow or rolled parka under the knees) and taking nonprescription analgesics such as aspirin, acetaminophen, or ibuprofen. It also is useful to apply local heat to the back with a heating pad, hot water bottle, canteens of hot water (wrapped to avoid causing burns), or cloths soaked in hot water and placed in a plastic bag. Gentle exercises that straighten the lumbosacral spine, such as touching the knees alternately to the chest while supine, are helpful. In some cases, the patient must be carried out.

Signs of nerve injury such as numbness, tingling, or weakness of the extremity or difficulty with bladder or bowel function indicate a medical emergency, and the patient must be taken to a hospital without delay.

Many back injuries can be prevented by using proper lifting and carrying techniques. Always obtain help when objects are large, bulky, or very heavy. When lifting, use the hips and knees instead of the back. Keep the back straight, face the object squarely with your feet together, and keep the object as close to your body as possible. Never lift when your body is turned to one side or when bending forward with your knees straight (as when removing a suitcase from the trunk of a car). It is easier to carry a heavy load in a pack on your back than in suitcases or duffle bags held by hand.

Scenario #15 (Fig. 16.9)

The following scenario illustrates the emergency management of a patient with a respiratory complaint.

You are enjoying a beautiful day of spring patrolling at High Range Ski Area when a transmission from the base announces a skier in trouble about halfway down the run. No details are given. You stop for a moment to reply that you can respond to the call, then continue down.

After a minute, you see several skiers standing around a man in his 30s who is sitting in the snow. As you approach, you see that he is obviously uncomfortable and breathing heavily. His skis are off. There are no obvious extremity deformities and no blood in the snow. You quickly remove your skis and approach him.

You: "Hi, I'm Ben Schussen of the High Range Ski Patrol. Can I help you?"

Fig. 16.9 *Scenario #15*

Skier: (panting) "Thanks, I'm having a hard time breathing. I don't know why."

You: "Did you fall and hurt yourself?" (reaching for his nearest hand, you remove his glove and assess his pulse. It is regular, strong, and about 100 beats per minute. His breathing is deep and at a rate of about 30 respirations per minute. There are no obvious audible wheezes or other abnormal breathing sounds.)

Skier: "No. I was skiing along and felt a sudden pain in my chest, and now I can't breathe. I had to stop skiing."

You: "Where is the pain?"

Skier: "It was right here" (pointing to his right, upper, anterior chest). "It's better now."

You: "How long did it last?"

Skier: "Just a few seconds."

You: "Does it hurt to breathe at all now?"

Skier: "Not really, but the right side of my chest doesn't feel right."

You: "Were you feeling okay before this happened?"

Skier: "Fine."

You: "Excuse me, I'll call for a toboggan and we'll give you a ride down. Schussen to Summit. I need a toboggan and the oxygen pack on Big Elk, halfway down on the left side of the run." (Summit confirms. You take the patient's skis and make an X in the snow about 20 feet above him.)

You: "What's your name?"

Skier: "Howard Breathing."

You: "Howard, have you ever had anything like this before?"

Skier: "No."

You: "Do you have any history of any heart or lung disease or other serious medical problems?"

Skier: "No."

You: "Have you had a recent cold, cough, or flu?"

Skier: "No."

You: "Are you taking any medicines or drugs for any condition?"

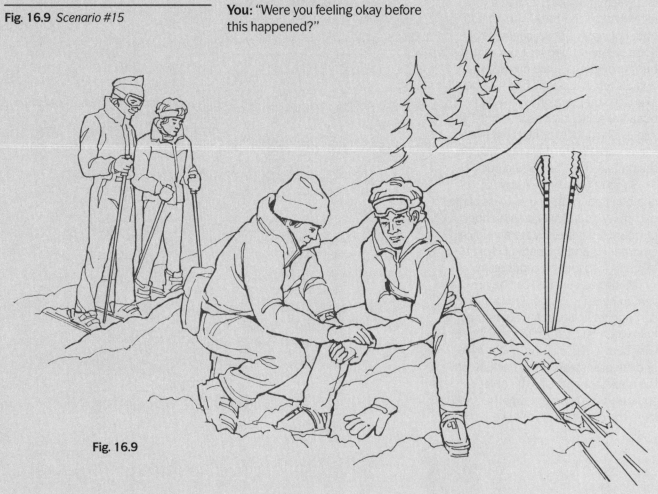

Fig. 16.9

Skier: "No."

You: "Is there anything else medically important that we should know about you?"

Skier: "Not that I can think of."

You: "Howard, while we're waiting for the toboggan, I'm going to check you over and see if we can figure out what is going on." (The skier nods.)

You assess his neck. There are no abnormal lumps or distended veins. Moving downward, you assess the position of the trachea with your forefinger just above the sternal notch. It is in the midline. You open the skier's jacket and place one hand on each side of his chest. Both sides are moving equally as he breathes. You palpate each rib and interspace in turn on each side of the chest. There are no swellings or tender areas.

You: "I don't have a stethoscope, so I am going to listen to your breath sounds with my ear against your chest."

You lift up his turtleneck and put your ear directly on the fabric of his long-john top. You compare the two sides of the chest in several symmetrical areas. The breath sounds are definitely louder on the left side. For some reason, his right lung is not working well. You wonder why. He didn't hurt his chest. Whatever happened, it happened suddenly. He was evidently perfectly healthy just beforehand.

A stir in the crowd announces the arrival of another patroller, Pete, with the toboggan and the oxygen pack. You unzip the pack, take out the non-rebreather mask, and attach the tubing to the output nipple of the oxygen regulator. You open the main tank valve and note that the tank is three-fourths full as registered on the pressure gauge. Turning the regulator valve to 12 liters per minute, you fill the reservoir bag, then turn to the patient.

You: "Howard, I'm going to put this mask over your mouth and nose and give you some oxygen. It should make you much less short of breath."

You attach the mask to his head with the elastic strap. The patient's breathing seems to slow somewhat and becomes less deep after a minute.

You: "Howard, we're going to help you into the toboggan. I want you to sit up rather than lie down, and keep breathing the oxygen."

The patient is taken slowly and carefully to the bottom of the hill and by ambulance to the hospital. A chest X-ray shows a pneumothorax on the left side, very likely a spontaneous pneumothorax of the type that can occur in young people.

Scenario #16 (Fig. 16.10)

The following scenario illustrates the emergency care of a patient with a gastrointestinal complaint.

You and Sandy have decided to try a new outdoor experience this summer. Sandy's mother has agreed to keep the baby for a week while you two float the middle fork of the Tuna River. Since this is your first rafting experience, you have signed up with a rafting company managed by a friend of yours from a ski patrol in a neighboring state. You know that his guides are experienced and well qualified.

The trip will take five days, part of which will be through the deep and narrow Tuna Canyon, where you will have no access to civilization for two days. You have all the personal supplies recommended by the rafting company plus your backpacking first aid kit.

Twenty eager would-be rafters climb into the rafts early the first morning and put in about a day's run from the entrance to the canyon. The first night is spent on a large sandbar. The roar of the river keeps everyone but the guides from sleeping soundly.

The next morning a ranch-style breakfast is prepared by the guides. You notice that Sandy leaves half of her breakfast untouched. When you ask why, she says that dinner the night before bothered her stomach and she is not feeling very hungry, although she feels okay otherwise. She spent a long time at the latrine and mentions to you that she is constipated and her abdomen hurts when she tries to have a bowel movement. After breakfast, camp is packed, the rafts loaded, and the rafters shove off into the swift river.

By late afternoon, Sandy clearly is not feeling well. She has curled up in the bottom of the raft, lying on her side with her hips flexed and her knees drawn up. She looks pale and, when questioned, says that she has a dull ache in her abdomen. You ask her where it hurts; she points to the area around her umbilicus. She finished her menstrual period about two weeks before and thinks she may be having some ovulation pain.

When you reach the next camping place, Sandy crawls into her sleeping bag as soon as the tent is erected. She looks ill to you. You question her more carefully and obtain the information that she started to have mid-abdominal discomfort during the previous night. She has no appetite and feels nauseated. She ate a small amount of breakfast but no lunch, although she has been able to drink water. She does not want any dinner. During the day, the pain spread to involve her right lower quadrant as well. She denies any symptoms of head cold, sore throat, earache, or cough. Her bowel movements were normal until that morning. She has had no pain on urination and has no pain anywhere else in her body.

You take a thermometer out of your first aid kit and take an oral temperature. It is 100.4°F. You warm your hands against your body, then palpate her bare abdomen, starting in the left lower quadrant. There is no tenderness until you move around to the right lower quadrant, where she winces when you apply slight pressure. You lay your ear on her bare abdomen. The bowel sounds seem normal; at least you do not hear the rushes that you have heard in patients with gastroenteritis in the past.

You ask her a few more questions, most of which you think you know the answers to already. She reaffirms that she has never had any serious illnesses, is taking no drugs except for an occasional Tylenol for headache, and was feeling fine before the trip started. She has had no surgery except a tonsillectomy.

Taking a flashlight and tongue blade out of the first aid kit, you look at her throat. It is a normal red color without any white spots. You feel under the sides of her jaw; there are no swellings or tenderness.

Starting to feel uneasy, you seek out Bob, the trip leader, who you know has had wilderness EMT training, and take him aside.

You: "Bob, I'm afraid Sandy has a significant problem. She has had abdominal pain since last night. It started off in the mid-abdomen and then moved into her right lower quadrant. She has no appetite, is nauseated, and has a temperature of 100.4°F. She was constipated this morning and her stomach hurt when she moved her bowels. She's very tender in the right lower quadrant. Her bowel sounds are normal and she has no symptoms of a respiratory or urinary infection. I'm not sure what is going on, but I don't think it's just stomach flu, and I'm afraid it might be serious. Do you have a radio?"

Fig. 16.10 *Scenario #16*

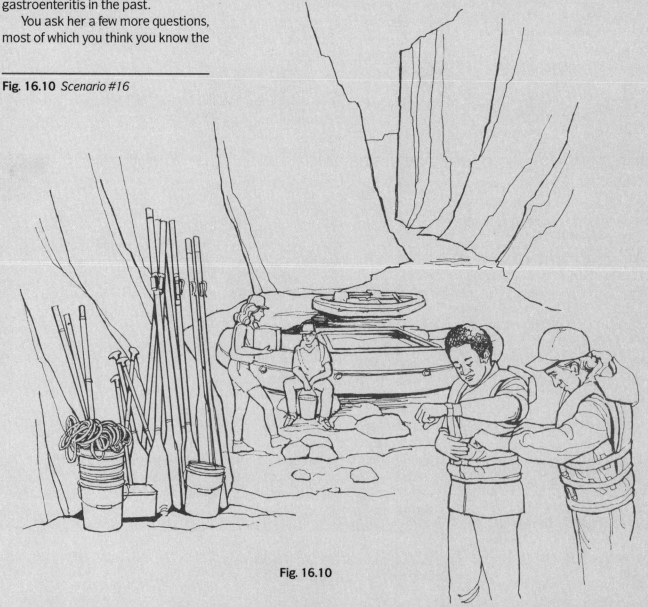

Fig. 16.10

Bob: "No, we don't. The nearest place to get help is when we leave the canyon about 10 miles downstream. We can't get there before noon tomorrow. It will be dark in an hour—we can't continue tonight."

You: "Sounds like we'll have to do the best we can tonight, then get moving at first light. As I recall from my Winter Emergency Care training, we shouldn't give her anything to eat or drink and should get her to a doctor as soon as possible. I don't believe they had a situation like this in mind, though."

Bob: "I'll have a look at her, too." (He goes into the tent and spends a few minutes assessing Sandy. His findings are the same as yours.)

"She has an acute abdomen. In the wilderness EMT course I took, if you couldn't get a patient with an acute abdomen to a hospital right away, they recommended giving small sips of water and antibiotics. We have some Cephalexin in the medical kit and some oral demerol for pain."

You: "That sounds reasonable to me."

You go into the tent and explain to Sandy what is going to happen, trying to keep the worry out of your voice. She swallows an antibiotic capsule and a Demerol pill and manages to keep them down. You can hear Bob talking to the other rafters, explaining the situation while the guides are fixing supper. You stay awake most of the night, listening to her moan occasionally as she sleeps fitfully. She takes an occasional sip of water and on one occasion vomits a cupful into a pan. You inspect the vomitus with a flashlight; it is clear, yellow stomach contents without any blood. Toward morning, she seems more comfortable and falls into a deep sleep for an hour.

You awake with a start. It is still dark, but you can hear Bob moving around outside, clanking pots and pumping the stove. In a few minutes the others are starting to stir. Leaving Sandy, you help with breakfast, breaking camp, and loading the rafts, then get her out of the tent, into a drysuit, and into a raft. She tells you that the pain is better; you reassess her abdomen and find that it is generally tender and slightly distended. She swallows a few sips of water, then vomits it back up. It is getting light as the rafts shove off into the river.

The rest of the trip through the canyon seems to take forever. Sandy is able to keep two more antibiotic capsules down. Finally, you make shore on a sandy beach where a dirt road reaches the river. One of the guides runs off up the road to the nearest house about 2 miles away. Half an hour later, a large four-wheel-drive pickup arrives in a cloud of dust with a friendly rancher at the wheel.

When you arrive at the hospital 20 miles away, Sandy is taken immediately to surgery, where she is found to have an inflamed appendix with a walled-off abscess around an area of perforation. Ten days later, thanks to intravenous antibiotics, she can be flown home.

Chapter 17

Medical Emergencies

A man is as old as his arteries.

—*Pierre J.G. Cabanis*

Because different pathologic conditions can produce similar changes in anatomy and physiology, different illnesses can produce similar signs and symptoms. Emergency care can be directed either at signs and symptoms or at specific illnesses. This chapter examines in detail selected important **medical illnesses** that may present as emergencies in the outdoors. The causes and emergency care of the most common *symptoms* of medical illness are presented in Chapter 16.

Heart Disease

Heart disease continues to be the most common cause of death in the middle-aged and the elderly. It can affect younger individuals as well. The heart's function, its sensitivity to lack of oxygen, and the importance of its blood supply already have been emphasized.

The most common heart disease is **coronary artery disease**, caused by reduction of blood flow to the heart muscle (myocardium) due to **arteriosclerosis**. Arteriosclerosis, also called "hardening of the arteries," leads to the deposit of cholesterol and other materials in the arterial walls, causing them to thicken and scar, and leading to stiffening and narrowing of the arteries (Fig. 17.1). Other less common types of heart disease are caused by heart valve damage, congenital heart abnormalities, infection, and toxins.

Risk factors for the development of coronary artery disease include male gender, a sedentary lifestyle, cigarette smoking, elevated blood cholesterol, hypertension, diabetes, a family history of the disease, and aging itself. While gender, heredity, and aging cannot be altered, risk can be lessened by proper diet, regular exercise, and avoidance of smoking. Diabetes and hypertension can be controlled.

During the early stages of coronary artery disease, the heart may function normally unless stressed by high altitude, unaccustomed physical activity, or strong emotion. Unfortunately, these stresses are not rare in sedentary individuals undertaking a hunting, hiking, or skiing vacation. Ski patrollers, outdoor group leaders, and wilderness rescuers may expect to encounter patients with coronary artery disease.

As coronary artery disease progresses, symptoms occur when the patient is at rest; eventually, symptoms may be present constantly and the patient may enter a state of chronic heart failure or have recurrent chest pain that markedly restricts activity.

The most common forms of coronary artery disease likely to be seen by the rescuer are angina pectoris and acute myocardial infarction.

Angina Pectoris

Angina pectoris (usually called angina) is a characteristic type of pain that occurs when the heart muscle is temporarily starved for oxygen. It usually appears during physical exertion or emotional stress, when the heart requires a larger blood supply than the narrowed coronary arteries can deliver. As the condition progresses, angina may occur at rest or even during sleep.

The pain of angina was described in Chapter 16 under **Chest Pain**. It may be mistaken for indigestion, pleurisy, and other types of chest and upper-abdominal pain. Occasionally, the patient's first attack of angina occurs under the stress of an outdoor recreational experience. However, most patients have been diagnosed previously as having angina and carry medication to use in case of an attack.

Angina can be relieved by measures that reduce the heart's need for oxygen, such as rest, or that increase the heart's blood supply, such as medication. Most drugs used to treat angina either enlarge (dilate) the coronary arteries or slow the heart rate and strength of its contractions, either of which tends to improve the mismatch between the heart's need for more blood and the ability of the coronary arteries to supply it.

The most common medication used to treat an attack of angina is **nitroglycerin**. Nitroglycerin is dispensed as small white tablets that are placed under the tongue as soon as the pain begins. It is absorbed into

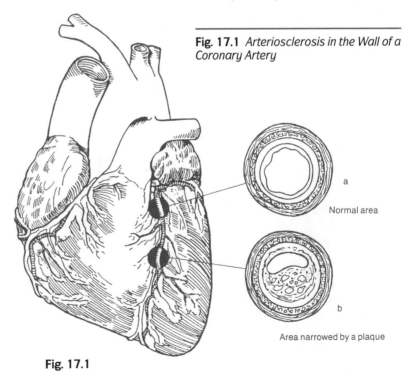

Fig. 17.1 *Arteriosclerosis in the Wall of a Coronary Artery*

a

Normal area

b

Area narrowed by a plaque

Fig. 17.1

the bloodstream through the mucous membrane that lines the mouth. Nitroglycerin should relieve anginal pain within three to five minutes. Other drugs for angina are beta blockers, which prevent pain by slowing the heart and reducing its need for oxygen; long-acting derivatives of nitroglycerin, which cause chronic dilation of the coronary arteries; and calcium channel blockers, which reduce oxygen consumption by the myocardium, increase its oxygen supply, and reduce coronary artery spasm.

The assessment of a patient with angina is described in Chapter 16. The most common locations of anginal pain are illustrated in Figure 16.5 in Chapter 16.

The emergency care of a patient with angina is to encourage the patient to sit down, rest, keep warm, and take any medicine carried for the pain. The rescuer should question the patient to determine whether the patient's immediate plans are realistic, particularly if they include significant physical exertion. Patients with angina should be discouraged from attempting strenuous activities in remote locations because of their limited capacity for exercise. In addition, they are candidates for more serious heart problems such as abnormal rhythms and heart attacks. A mild heart attack may be difficult to distinguish from a severe attack of angina pectoris; if there is any question, the patient should be transported promptly to a hospital.

Many patients with coronary artery disease undergo angioplasty to dilate or surgery to bypass the narrowed portions of the coronary arteries. After these procedures, patients often are able to return successfully to moderately strenuous outdoor activities. Nevertheless, such patients should consult their cardiologists about the advisability of undertaking physical activity where medical assistance is not easily available.

Heart Attack

Because increasing numbers of middle-aged and elderly persons are participating in skiing and other outdoor activities, the incidence of heart attacks at ski areas and other outdoor locations will continue to increase.

Although the term "heart attack" is commonly used for any sudden episode caused by malfunction of the heart, it is usually reserved for a **myocardial infarction**, which means death (infarction) of part of the myocardium. This usually occurs when a blood clot or some other process blocks or narrows a diseased coronary artery in a patient with coronary artery disease (Fig. 17.2). If a blood clot is responsible, in many cases it can be dissolved with special intravenous drugs if the patient can be taken to a hospital within a few hours of onset. The left side of the heart is most commonly involved.

Other types of heart attacks are caused by the sudden onset of a rapid or irregular heartbeat or by sudden failure of the heart muscle in patients with diseased heart valves.

Signs and Symptoms of a Heart Attack

The signs and symptoms of heart attack are caused by the heart's sudden lack of oxygen. This usually causes pain, which triggers anxiety and an autonomic nervous system response. Depending on the size and location of the involved area, interference with the normal regularity and rate of the heartbeat and/or the strength of the heart's contractions may occur. Involvement of a large area of myocardium may lead to cardiogenic shock. **Sudden death** may be the first sign of a heart attack.

1. Pain is similar to that of angina pectoris (see Chapter 16), but usually is more severe and longer lasting. It is described as squeezing, crushing, vise-like, or burning; almost never as sharp or sticking. It often is substernal in location, but may occur in the epigastrium (pit of the stomach), throat, or in the back between the shoulder blades. It frequently radiates

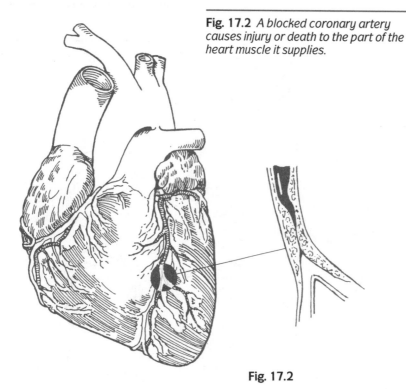

Fig. 17.2 *A blocked coronary artery causes injury or death to the part of the heart muscle it supplies.*

Fig. 17.2

from the chest to the neck, jaw, left shoulder, left arm, and occasionally to the right shoulder and arm or both shoulders and arms. It usually is unrelated to exertion and is *not* relieved by rest or nitroglycerin.

The patient may have had a previous heart attack or previous episodes of angina. Occasionally, a heart attack will occur without pain ("silent" myocardial infarction).

2. The pulse and blood pressure may be normal or abnormal.
3. Changes due to pain, anxiety, and autonomic nervous system response include the following. (Some of these signs and symptoms also are seen in cardiogenic shock).
   a. Fear of death.
   b. Cold, clammy, pale skin caused by constriction of blood vessels in the skin and increased sweating.
   c. Respiratory distress.
   d. Fast or very slow heart rate.
   e. High blood pressure.
4. Changes due to heart muscle damage include the following:
   a. Low blood pressure.
   b. Weak pulse.
   c. Irregular pulse.
   d. Generalized weakness.
   e. Cyanosis.
   f. Signs and symptoms of cardiogenic shock or pulmonary edema (see below).

A patient having a heart attack usually wants to sit up, but occasionally will want to lie down or even walk around.

Complications of Heart Attack

1. **Cardiac arrest**. Cardiac arrest occurs when the heart ceases to pump blood because of either a sudden, rapid, irregular, worm-like twitching of the ventricular myocardium (**ventricular fibrillation**), a heartbeat that is too fast and weak to pump enough blood (**ventricular tachycardia**), or complete cessation of heart contractions (**asystole**).
2. **Cardiogenic shock**. Damage to the myocardium may reduce the heart's output of blood to the point where the blood pressure can no longer be maintained. The signs and symptoms of cardiogenic shock are those of shock (Chapter 6) in addition to those of a heart attack.
3. **Pulmonary edema**. This occurs when the undamaged right side of the heart continues to pump blood *into* the lungs, but the damaged left side is too weak to handle even a normal volume of blood coming *from* the lungs. Blood accumulates in the lungs, increasing the hydrostatic pressure in their capillaries. This forces the fluid part of the blood out into the alveoli. The signs and symptoms of pulmonary edema are discussed in Chapter 16.

The assessment of a patient with a heart attack is described in Chapter 16 under the section on **Chest Pain**.

Table 17.1

Summary of Signs and Symptoms of Heart Attack

1. Pain, usually typical in type and location. Similar to but worse than that of angina pectoris. In some cases, pain may be absent. Pain may not be relieved by rest or nitroglycerin.
2. Anxiety and fear of death.
3. Respiratory distress.
4. Pale, cold and, occasionally, cyanotic skin.
5. Profuse sweating.
6. Pulse that is normal, slow, fast, irregular, strong, or weak.
7. Blood pressure that is normal or abnormal.
8. Patient usually prefers to sit up.
9. Complications:
   a. Cardiac arrest.
   b. Cardiogenic shock.
   c. Pulmonary edema.

Emergency Care of a Heart-Attack Patient

1. Many people have died of cardiac arrest during a heart attack when, with proper treatment, they could have lived normal lives for many years. Therefore, the *most important emergency care* for a heart-attack patient is rapid access to an advanced cardiac life support (ACLS) team that is equipped with a heart monitor, defibrillator, intravenous fluids, intubation equipment, and appropriate medications, and that is in contact by radio with a hospital emergency department. In addition, should cardiac arrest occur, the patient's best chance of survival is to be given basic life support with ACLS available within 15 minutes. In particular, if ventricular fibrillation is present, the best results are obtained if the patient can be defibrillated promptly.

Ski patrols should identify in advance the location of the nearest ACLS team with directions for contacting it when needed. If there is no ACLS team nearby, there may be a team of EMTs trained to use defibrillators (EMT-Ds).

The ACLS team will rapidly transport the patient by ambulance or helicopter to a hospital with an intensive care unit. Therefore, as soon as assessment indicates the possibility of a heart attack, unless urgent care is required, the first step is to *notify the ACLS team.*

These resources may not be readily available in every outdoor situation and may be totally unavailable in the backcountry or wilderness.

2. The patient should remain still in the most comfortable position, which usually will be sitting up, especially if short of breath. Maintain body temperature in the normal range.
3. Give oxygen in high concentration and flow rate, preferably by mask.
4. Keep the patient in a quiet area and shielded from bystanders. Reassure and calm the patient. Watch for the development of complications.

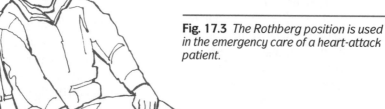

5. If shock develops, it may have to be treated with the patient's head and chest raised (the Rothberg position, Fig. 17.3) because of shortness of breath.
6. If the patient's breathing becomes ineffective, support it with a mouth-to-pocket mask or a bag-valve-mask (see Chapter 19).
7. If cardiac arrest occurs, administer CPR.
8. Treat pulmonary edema by propping the patient up in a seated position and administering oxygen at high concentration and flow rate.

The greatest risk of death is in the first few hours or days after a heart attack, when the risk of cardiac arrest is highest.

In some cases, a patient who suffers a heart attack at an alpine ski area can be transported to a hospital directly by helicopter. If the patient is to be transported from the hill to the first aid room, use of an oversnow vehicle with a large bed should be considered so that CPR is easier to give if needed. The patient should be accompanied by at least two patrollers. Some patrols have devised techniques for administering CPR to a patient transported by toboggan; however, more experience with these techniques is needed to judge their effectiveness. Radio ahead so that the ACLS team can be summoned promptly.

Fig. 17.3 *The Rothberg position is used in the emergency care of a heart-attack patient.*

Vehicles other than ambulances or helicopters should be used to transport heart-attack patients to a hospital only as a last resort. If such a vehicle must be used, it should be a station wagon or van. At a minimum, oxygen, airways, a bag-valve-mask, and suction equipment should be taken along, and two or more patrollers should accompany the patient and driver to assist ventilation or provide CPR, if needed.

Some ski areas have paramedics or physicians on roster and are equipped with intravenous fluids, drugs, and cardiac monitor-defibrillators. While this equipment can buy time, its availability should not be used as an excuse to delay summoning the ACLS team.

The Automatic External Defibrillator (AED) is a recent development that shows promise in decreasing the death rate from cardiac arrest. This battery-operated device is equipped to identify ventricular fibrillation and ventricular tachycardia immediately using two electrodes attached to the patient's chest. It delivers electric shocks automatically, programmed according to local protocols. The first shock can be delivered as soon as eight to 15 seconds from the time the electrodes are attached.

Less than eight hours of training are required to operate this device; the ability to identify electrocardiogram (EKG) patterns is not necessary because the device does it for you. This device would appear to be very useful where large numbers of people are congregated in remote areas such as ski resorts and national parks. Special training, certification, and licensing are required to be able to use the AED.

Conditions that may be hard to distinguish from a heart attack include pulmonary embolus, spontaneous pneumothorax, inflammation of the sac around the heart (pericarditis), a perforated peptic ulcer, disease of

Fig. 17.3

Table 17.2

Summary of Emergency Care of a Heart-Attack Patient

1. Perform the primary survey and deal with urgent problems. Provide airway management, ventilation, or CPR if needed.
2. Contact the EMS system without delay.
3. Keep the patient in the most comfortable position.
4. Give oxygen in high concentration and flow rate.
5. Calm and reassure the patient.
6. Shield the patient from bystanders.
7. Watch for complications. Care for pulmonary edema and cardiogenic shock if they occur.
8. Monitor and record vital signs.

the pancreas or gallbladder, hyperventilation, certain types of indigestion, and inflammation of the muscles or joints of the chest wall (see Chapter 16). Differentiating these conditions from a heart attack may require the expertise of a physician and the facilities of a hospital.

Because a patient with a massive heart attack may die even in the best-quipped hospital intensive care unit, rescuers should be realistic about their ability to resuscitate such patients. Under nonurban conditions, the fatality rate may be as high as 50 percent; the rate may climb to 100 percent for patients who develop cardiac arrest.

Stroke

A stroke, frequently called a **cerebrovascular accident (CVA)**, is caused by interference with the blood supply to a part of the brain, usually because an artery either clots or it ruptures with hemorrhage into the brain substance (Fig. 17.4). Strokes occasionally are caused by a blood clot (embolus) that travels to the brain from another part of the body such as the heart. The underlying cause of most strokes is arteriosclerosis of the arteries that supply the brain, principally the carotid arteries and their branches. Strokes are most common in the elderly and in people with hypertension and diabetes.

The onset of a stroke may be sudden or progress slowly over hours or days, and it may be accompanied or preceded by headache or dizziness. Strokes usually are spontaneous, although they may follow a head injury. The location of the damage in the brain frequently can be suspected from the signs and symptoms, particularly the type and location of impaired sensation and motion.

Minor transient strokes, called **transient ischemic attacks (TIA's),** occur when blood flow through a narrowed brain artery is temporarily inadequate to support the function of the brain area supplied. When the blood flow improves, the signs and symptoms disappear with no lasting neurologic defect.

Signs and Symptoms of Stroke

1. The patient usually has some impairment of responsiveness, ranging from slight confusion to deep coma.
2. One side of the body may be weak or paralyzed. In an unresponsive patient, one side is more limp than the other. The face may show loss of expression and drooping of the involved side.
3. The patient may drool, have difficulty swallowing, or develop slurred speech.
4. Breathing may be noisy because the tongue and throat muscles have weakened. As a consequence, respiratory distress may occur due to partial obstruction of the upper airway.
5. The patient's head and eyes may be turned to one side.
6. The blood pressure usually is normal or elevated.
7. Convulsions (see **Seizure Disorders** below) dizziness, and headache occasionally occur.
8. Patients who have suffered stroke may develop a characteristic speech impairment marked by ability to understand what is said to them but inability to choose the right words to reply (**expressive**

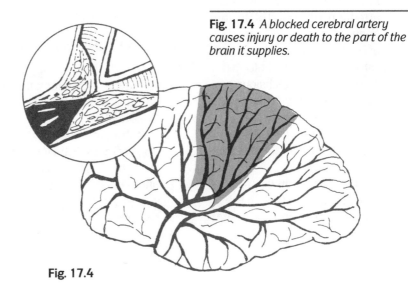

Fig. 17.4 *A blocked cerebral artery causes injury or death to the part of the brain it supplies.*

Fig. 17.4

aphasia). With severe aphasia, the patient repeats one or two words, such as "No!" no matter what is said. With milder aphasia, the patient chooses the wrong word or has a memory lapse when searching for certain words.

Table 17.3

Summary of Signs and Symptoms of Stroke

1. Impairment of responsiveness.
2. Weakness or paralysis, usually of one side of the body.
3. Drooling, difficulty in swallowing, or slurred speech.
4. Difficulty with the airway.
5. The head and eyes turned to one side.
6. Normal or high blood pressure.
7. Occasionally convulsions, headache, dizziness, or aphasia.

Assessment of a Stroke Patient

1. First impression. Is the patient responsive or unresponsive? Is the patient more likely to be suffering from an illness or an injury? Institute universal precautions (see Appendix F).
2. Introduce yourself. Ask, "What's the trouble?" Conduct the primary survey. Pay particular attention to the level of responsiveness, airway, and adequacy of breathing. Open the airway with either the head-tilt/chin lift or jaw-thrust technique as needed. If labored breathing and/or a fast, weak pulse is noted, assess the neck and chest. Care for any urgent conditions found.
3. Perform the secondary survey. Assess the vital signs. In the responsive patient, ask, "What

happened to you?" Obtain the patient's description of the development of the current problem in chronological order. Ask about headache, dizziness, weakness or numbness of extremities, and ability to move. During questioning, note the patient's ability to talk. In the unresponsive patient, question relatives or bystanders.

In the responsive patient, obtain the medical history, including history of illnesses or injuries, and ask about medicines and allergies. Inquire particularly about diabetes, high blood pressure, and any previous episodes like the present one. Ask, "Is there anything else we should know?" In the unresponsive patient, obtain this information from relatives.

Proceed to a general body assessment from head to toe. Pay special attention to the state of the pupils, the symmetry of the face, whether the tongue protrudes in the midline, the patient's ability to move the four extremities, the symmetry of hand-grip strength, and the response to touch and pain. In the unresponsive patient, note whether the sides of the body move spontaneously and whether the patient moves the extremities in response to pain.

Emergency Care of a Stroke Patient

1. Give general care for unresponsiveness as needed (see Chapter 12).
2. Pay strict attention to the upper airway. Even if responsive, stroke patients may be unable to rid their airways of secretions. Suctioning may be required.
3. Give oxygen by mask in high concentration and flow rate.

4. Periodically monitor and record the vital signs and other important signs, particularly the level of responsiveness, state of the pupils, ability to move, and response to touch and pain.
5. Keep the patient lying in the semiprone or NATO position (Fig. 12.3, Chapter 12), preferably with the upper trunk and head slightly elevated.
6. Maintain the patient's body temperature.
7. A patient with stroke who is aphasic or unable to speak may still be able to hear and understand almost normally. Be careful about casual conversation near the patient.
8. Give the patient nothing by mouth initially. If evacuation will be delayed, the patient may be offered small amounts of clear liquids. This should be done slowly and cautiously to prevent choking and should be discontinued if the patient is obviously unable to swallow.
9. Transport the patient to a hospital as soon as possible.

Table 17.4

Summary of Emergency Care of a Stroke Patient

1. Provide care for unresponsiveness if needed.
2. Maintain the upper airway.
3. Use suction as needed.
4. Give oxygen in high concentration.
5. Monitor and record the vital signs.
6. Keep the patient lying down in the NATO position, with the head and upper body slightly elevated.
7. Maintain the patient's body temperature.
8. Give the patient nothing by mouth.
9. Transport the patient to a hospital without delay.

Diabetes

Diabetes is a disease characterized by an absolute or relative deficiency of **insulin**, a hormone produced by the islet cells of the pancreas (Fig. 17.5). Insulin controls the use of glucose by the cells. Because all body cells require glucose to function properly, lack of insulin causes serious disruption of cellular metabolism.

When the body is unable to use glucose for fuel because of lack of insulin, it is forced to use fat. During this type of abnormal fat metabolism, acidic compounds are formed that accumulate faster than they can be used up, causing the blood to become more acidic. In addition, the unused glucose accumulates in the blood and is excreted through the kidneys along with large amounts of water and electrolytes. This accounts for the dehydration, loss of weight, increased urination, and increased hunger and thirst seen in patients with uncontrolled diabetes.

Severe, uncontrolled diabetes may progress to **diabetic ketoacidosis**, a serious condition accompanied by weakness, confusion, stupor, nausea, vomiting, and abdominal pain. Severe acidosis causes the respirations to be rapid and deep. If untreated, diabetic ketoacidosis will progress to **diabetic coma** and death.

There are two types of diabetes: **juvenile** diabetes, also known as labile, type I, or insulin-dependent diabetes mellitus (IDDM); and **adult onset** diabetes, also known as stable, type II, or non-insulin-dependent diabetes mellitus (NIDDM).

Patients with juvenile diabetes produce little or no insulin and require daily injections of insulin and strict avoidance of sugar to control their disease. Juvenile diabetes is more difficult to control and more prone to the development of ketoacidosis than adult-onset diabetes. In an outdoor environment, a juvenile diabetic will go into ketoacidosis quickly if injured or deprived of insulin.

Patients with adult-onset diabetes are able to make some insulin but not enough for their needs. Usually they are overweight, and although their diabetes frequently can be controlled by diet and weight loss, they may require insulin as well. In mild cases, oral medication that stimulates insulin production can be used instead of insulin. Patients with adult-onset diabetes are less likely to get into trouble in the outdoors than patients with juvenile diabetes.

All diabetics are subject to premature development of such complications as arteriosclerosis, impaired vision, high blood pressure, and kidney disease. Because these complications occur sooner in poorly regulated diabetics, most diabetics routinely monitor their blood glucose levels to aid in maintaining strict control of their disease. This is done by measuring the concentration of glucose in a drop of blood with a chemically treated paper strip or an electronic analyzer.

Patients with well-regulated diabetes are able to lead almost normal lives and can participate in skiing, hiking, climbing, and other outdoor sports. Diabetics who require emergency care for their disease usually are suffering from either **hypoglycemia** (insulin shock) or **diabetic ketoacidosis**. Of the two, hypoglycemia is much more common.

Hypoglycemia

When blood glucose falls to abnormally low levels, the signs and symptoms of hypoglycemia, or low blood sugar (sometimes called "insulin shock"), develop. Common causes are when a patient who has taken a normal dose of insulin or an oral antidiabetic agent exercises more than usual or eats too little.

Because the brain is very sensitive to lack of glucose, the first sign of hypoglycemia usually is an alteration of the patient's normal mental status. This may resemble acute alcoholic intoxication.

Signs and Symptoms of Hypoglycemia

1. Personality changes, confusion, stupor, or coma.
2. Signs of sympathetic nervous system hyperactivity such as pale, moist skin and a rapid pulse.
3. Headache, hunger, dizziness, and nervousness.
4. Weakness.
5. Convulsions occasionally occur.
6. The patient usually is wearing a medical-alert tag or bracelet or has a wallet card indicating that he or she is a diabetic.

Diabetic Coma

Diabetic coma occurs in people with previously undiagnosed diabetes and in known diabetics who have taken insufficient insulin or whose insulin requirement is increased because of another illness.

Signs and Symptoms of Diabetic Coma

1. Confusion, stupor, or coma.
2. Rapid, deep respirations.
3. The skin usually is flushed, dry, and warm. The patient may have poor tissue turgor (dry, shrunken, less elastic skin) caused by dehydration.

Fig. 17.5 *Islet Cells of the Pancreas*

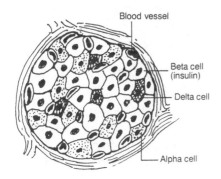

Fig. 17.5

Table 17.5

Summary of Comparison Between Diabetic Coma and Hypoglycemia

Category	Diabetic Coma	Hypoglycemia
Onset	Gradual	Rapid
Sensorium	Confusion, stupor, coma	Same
Respirations	Rapid, deep	Usually normal
Pulse	Rapid, weak	Rapid
Blood pressure	Low	Normal
Skin	Flushed, dry, warm	Pale, moist
Breath	Fruity odor	Normal
Weakness, fatigue	Both	Weakness
Headache	Occasional	Frequent
Hunger	No (except by history)	Yes
Thirst	Severe	No
Convulsions	Rare	Not rare
Shock	May occur	Rare
Abdominal pain	May occur	Rare
Blood glucose (by test strip or glucose meter)	High (>300)	Low (<50)
Treatment:		
General care for unconsciousness	As needed	As needed
Sugar	If in doubt about diagnosis	Yes—urgent
Response to treatment	Slow (in hospital)	Rapid, to sugar

4. A fruity odor to the breath.
5. Weakness and fatigue.
6. In some cases, signs of shock may develop.
7. The patient frequently but not always is wearing a medical-alert tag or bracelet or has a wallet card indicating that he or she is a diabetic.
8. If the ketoacidosis was precipitated by another illness, the signs and symptoms of the second illness usually will be present. This is most frequently an acute, febrile illness such as viral gastroenteritis, influenza, pneumonia, etc. Abdominal pain is common in ketoacidosis itself, however.

Assessment of an Ill Diabetic

1. First impression. Is the patient responsive or unresponsive? Does it look like the patient has an illness or has suffered an injury? Always think of the possibility of hypoglycemia when you see a young, healthy appearing patient with an altered level of responsiveness. Remember that a hypoglycemic patient is more prone to injury. Institute universal precautions (see Appendix F).
2. Primary survey. Assess the airway, breathing, circulation, and bleeding, interrupting assessment as needed to care for urgent problems. In a patient with altered responsiveness, assess the head, pupils, neck, ability to move, and response to pain and touch. Look for a medical-alert tag. Move to the secondary survey as soon as possible.
3. Secondary survey. Assess the remaining vital signs. Question the patient, if possible. Otherwise, question companions as to what happened and whether the patient has any history of medical illness, is taking any medicines, and has any allergies. When assessing the radial pulse, look for a medical-alert bracelet. It is important to find out when a diabetic ate last and whether he or she took insulin or another diabetic medication that day.
4. In a patient with altered responsiveness, *as soon as it is discovered that the patient is a diabetic,* measure the patient's blood glucose if you have the proper equipment and know how to use it. This can be done with a paper blood glucose test strip (Chemstrip bG) or a glucose meter (such as the One Touch II), which may be available in a ski patrol aid room or in a backcountry search and rescue emergency care kit. If you are not able to measure the blood glucose, or if it is low, give the patient sugar while he or she can still swallow. Sugar provides quick relief of hypoglycemia; if the problem is diabetic coma, extra sugar does no harm.

Emergency Care of an Ill Diabetic

1. As emphasized above, if you do not have the equipment to measure blood glucose, give sugar to all diabetics with

altered responsiveness. At times, it may be difficult for even a physician to be sure at first whether a diabetic is suffering from diabetic coma or hypoglycemia; when there is any doubt, *always* give sugar. The source can be a sugary liquid such as orange juice or a soft drink, candy, or a spoonful of table sugar. Tubes or squeeze bottles of concentrated glucose solution are available commercially and are preferred to other sources of sugar. They can be carried in a rescuer's first aid kit or a ski patroller's first aid belt for immediate use. A patient in insulin shock should improve within a few minutes after being given sugar. As soon as the patient is sufficiently alert, give him or her additional food, such as a sandwich or candy bar.

2. If necessary, give general care for unresponsiveness (Chapter 12).

3. A diabetic who recovers from hypoglycemia after being given sugar and food should be encouraged to rest a few hours before resuming normal activity.

4. Some diabetics carry supplies of glucagon, a hormone that raises the blood sugar. If a rescuer is available who is trained and licensed to give injections, one milliliter of glucagon can be injected intramuscularly. This is particularly useful in a partly or completely unresponsive diabetic who is probably hypoglycemic.

5. An unresponsive or poorly responsive diabetic with hypoglycemia can suffer permanent brain damage from prolonged low blood glucose levels. Therefore, a patient who does not recover rapidly after the ad-

ministration of sugar by mouth will need to be given intravenous glucose and should be taken to a hospital without delay. Many EMS ambulance units carry ampuls of 50-percent glucose solution in water for intravenous use.

6. Diabetic coma is a medical emergency. There is no satisfactory field emergency care for a patient in diabetic coma, even if insulin is available. The patient must be taken to a hospital without delay.

Consider the possibility of diabetes in every unresponsive or partly responsive person. If the cause of unresponsiveness is not obvious, look for medical-alert tags and wallet cards *early* in the assessment. (Always have a witness present before searching through a wallet.) A common source of error is a diabetic who has had a few drinks, develops an altered mental status because of hypoglycemia, and is thought to merely be drunk because of the odor of alcohol on the breath.

Seizure Disorders

The term seizure is used for any sudden, transient alteration of normal brain function. Seizures usually appear as abnormal movements or sensations, psychic experiences, or disturbances of autonomic nerve function. They often are recurrent and usually include at least a minimal alteration in responsiveness. They are thought to result from sudden abnormal electrical discharges in the cerebrum.

Seizures accompanied by excessive, abnormal muscular activity are called **convulsions. Epilepsy,** a medical condition characterized by recurrent episodes of seizures, affects about one person in every 200. Although seizures can be caused by head injury, stroke, hypoglycemia, hypoxia, meningitis, brain tumor, and withdrawal from alcohol or sedative drugs, in most cases the cause is unknown.

High fever alone may cause seizures in children.

Most seizures can be controlled by medication so that the patient can live a normal life. However, patients with seizures should be discouraged from engaging in activities where loss of responsiveness or coordination could prove injurious or fatal to themselves or their companions, unless they have a history of reliability, have been seizure-free for at least two years, and have permission from a neurologist. Such activities include climbing, aerial-lift-based skiing, and scuba diving.

Seizures can be of many types, depending on the area of the brain involved. They can be classified into two groups: generalized seizures and partial seizures.

Generalized seizures are seizures that start on both sides of the brain and frequently involve the entire body. Severe generalized seizures involving abnormal muscle movements are called **grand mal seizures,** which are what most people think of when epilepsy is mentioned. Other types of generalized seizures involve only brief losses of responsiveness without muscle movements (absences), muscle jerks without loss of responsiveness (myoclonic seizures), or sudden loss of muscle tone (drop attacks).

Grand mal seizures typically are preceded by an **aura,** a peculiar sensation that can be a sound, sight, or odor. The aura, which always is the same sensation, signals the patient that a seizure is about to occur. Next, the body muscles suddenly contract, frequently causing the patient to cry out hoarsely and fall to the ground with bowed back and rigid arms and legs. This stage, called the tonic phase, is followed within a few seconds by violent, rhythmic contractions of the neck, back, and extremities (the clonic phase). During the attack, which usually lasts only a few minutes, the patient may bite the tongue, be incontinent of urine or feces, or be injured by striking some object. After a seizure, the patient remains unresponsive or sleepy for several minutes to an hour or longer.

Partial seizures start in a localized part of one cerebral cortex, although they may spread to involve larger areas of the brain. There are many types of partial seizures. They may produce localized body movements, abnormal sensations, symptoms of autonomic nervous system activity, automatic behavior, or psychic symptoms, and may or may not involve disturbances in responsiveness.

Assessment and Emergency Care of a Patient with a Severe, Generalized Seizure

If the seizure is witnessed, there is little doubt about what is occurring. Difficulties arise if the patient is discovered in the post-seizure period and the actual seizure was not witnessed. Institute universal precautions (see Appendix F).

1. Because there is no way an impending seizure can be stopped or prevented, and no way a patient having a seizure can be assessed other than by observation, the rescuer should concentrate on protecting the patient from injury. If the patient feels a seizure is about to occur, help him or her lie down in an open area away from obstacles. If possible, a patient in an exposed or dangerous position, such as in water or on a cliff, should be immediately removed or secured in some way.

2. During a seizure, do not attempt to restrain the patient. In the past, it was popular to force an object between the patient's teeth to prevent the tongue from being bitten. Such

attempts are no longer advocated because they generally are useless or even dangerous to both patient and rescuer.

3. Since the patient may be incontinent and, at the least, embarrassed, arrange for as much privacy as possible by screening the patient and discouraging curious onlookers.

4. Breathing may stop temporarily during a seizure but almost always resumes without assistance.

5. After the seizure, the patient may have an altered level of responsiveness, be confused, or be very sleepy. The assessment is the same as that of any unresponsive or partly responsive patient. During the primary survey, open and maintain the airway as necessary. Pay particular attention to assessing for lacerations of the tongue and other injuries caused by the seizure or the fall that accompanied it. Allow the patient to rest until fully responsive and functional.

6. The patient's history is especially important but may not be immediately obtainable. Companions and relatives should be questioned about the possibility of diabetic

hypoglycemia, a recent head injury, history of seizures, any seizure medicine being taken, and whether it is being taken regularly. The patient's companions may know that the patient is taking medicine regularly, but may not realize what it is for. Medicines commonly used for seizures include Dilantin, phenobarbital, Tegretol, Mysoline, Depakene, Zarontin, and Tridione.

7. Patients with grand mal seizures may develop post-seizure paralysis and other abnormalities, which can last for hours or days. At regular intervals, assess and monitor the patient's level of responsiveness, state of the pupils, and ability to move and perceive pain and touch.

8. If the patient has no history of seizures, advise him or her to consult a physician as soon as possible. Even if the patient is a known epileptic, it may be appropriate to suggest that his or her physician be consulted promptly, especially if the seizures seem poorly controlled.

Other types of seizures usually require no emergency care unless the patient is confused and is engaged in

Table 17.6

Summary of Assessment and Emergency Care of a Patient with Severe, Generalized Seizure

1. Protect the patient from injury.
2. Do not restrain the patient or place an object between the patient's teeth.
3. After the seizure is over, perform the primary survey and give general care for unresponsiveness as needed.
4. Obtain the patient's medical history, find out whether the patient has a history of seizures, and whether seizure medicine is taken.
5. Assess the patient for injuries.
6. Allow the patient to rest until fully responsive and functional.
7. Advise the patient to see a physician if there is no history of seizures.

some type of clearly dangerous automatic behavior. The patient should not be physically restrained unless absolutely necessary. Handle such patients as recommended in the section on **Psychology of Dealing With the Ill and Injured** in Chapter 4.

Carbon Monoxide Poisoning

Carbon monoxide is a colorless, odorless gas that is produced by incomplete combustion of carbon-containing substances. Dangerously high levels of carbon monoxide can form whenever fuel is burned in a poorly ventilated space.

When inhaled, carbon monoxide combines with the hemoglobin in red blood cells and renders the cells incapable of carrying oxygen. Symptoms of tissue hypoxia occur when 20 percent of the blood's hemoglobin is combined with carbon monoxide; coma occurs by the time the hemoglobin is 60 percent saturated. (The hemoglobin of heavy cigarette smokers often is as much as 10 percent saturated).

Carbon monoxide poisoning is fairly common. In the United States, it causes several thousand deaths each year, many of them suicides. Carbon monoxide poisoning can be a significant hazard in the outdoor environment, particularly in forest wildfires and when stoves are used in poorly ventilated shelters such as snow caves and igloos. Cooking inside tents can be hazardous during blizzards if drifting snow interferes with ventilation. Many famous polar explorers, including Admiral Richard E. Byrd, S. A. Andree, and Vilhjalmur Stefannson, were killed or narrowly escaped death from carbon monoxide poisoning caused by operating stoves in tightly closed areas. People stranded in vehicles during blizzards also are at risk if the engine is kept running to warm the occupants.

The signs and symptoms depend on the amount of carbon monoxide the patient has inhaled. In mild cases, the patient may be merely dizzy, confused, and have a headache; in severe cases, partial or complete unresponsiveness may result. Sudden respiratory arrest may occur. The classic sign of carbon monoxide poisoning is cherry-red skin, but this is most commonly seen after death. In the living patient the skin may be pale, blue, or pink.

Carbon monoxide poisoning should be suspected whenever a person develops an altered mental status while exposed to fumes from burning carbon-containing substances, especially in a poorly ventilated area. Such persons include firefighters, persons extricated from burning buildings and vehicles, and persons found in dwellings with malfunctioning heating units. Many experts feel that some effects attributed to acute mountain sickness (see Chapter 18) may, in fact, be caused by carbon monoxide from cooking in tents and other shelters. Recognizing this insidious condition may be difficult when all members of the party are affected. Rescuers should suspect carbon monoxide poisoning when all the occupants of a vehicle, dwelling, or other enclosed space have some degree of altered responsiveness without other obvious cause.

The most important emergency care of a patient with carbon monoxide poisoning is to immediately remove him or her from the contaminated area. Fortunately, carbon monoxide is excreted by the lungs within a few hours. Patients with mild carbon monoxide poisoning who have not lost consciousness need bed rest for a minimum of four hours and oxygen at high concentration and flow rate, if available. More severely affected patients may also require support of ventilation, care for unresponsiveness, and transportation to a hospital.

To prevent carbon monoxide poisoning during outdoor activities, avoid cooking in snow caves, igloos, and tightly sealed tents whenever possible. If not possible, provide adequate ventilation by leaving entrances open and, in the case of a snow shelter, making a ventilation hole in the roof the diameter of a ski pole basket (3 to 4 inches). Occupants stranded in vehicles should keep the exhaust pipe cleared of snow and should leave a downwind window partly open whenever the engine is running.

Substance Abuse

Substance abuse refers to the use of mind-altering chemicals without a legitimate medical purpose. These chemicals are self-prescribed and self-administered, usually because they alter perception of the environment and cause artificial exhilaration, tranquility, or disorientation. The substance can be a prescription drug used in excessive amounts or in an illegal manner, an illegal drug, or a nonprescription substance such as ethyl alcohol.

These substances may cause either dependence or addiction; the substance abuser's life may revolve around obtaining and using the drug to the point that career, social functioning, and even simple hygiene are neglected.

Because intravenous drug users often are indifferent to sterile precautions, they are subject to diseases transmitted by dirty needles, including hepatitis and AIDS. Medical personnel find the treatment of drug dependents and substance abusers to be frustrating and frequently unsuccessful. Much crime in this country is committed to obtain money for the purchase of illegal drugs. However, in terms of misery and cost, the most significant form of substance abuse is **alcoholism**.

Before discussing individual substances, it is necessary to define the following commonly used terms:

Drug—Any substance that alters mental or physical function when introduced into the body.

Tolerance—A state in which the body adjusts to the presence of a drug so that increasing amounts are required to produce the desired effect.

Physical dependence—A state in which the drug changes body physiology so that suddenly stopping its use causes well-defined symptoms and signs of withdrawal that tend to be opposite to the effects of the drug itself. Thus, the abuser eventually may take the drug *not* for its mind-altering effects, but to feel *normal*.

Drug dependence (psychological dependence)—A behavioral state in which the abuser becomes obsessed with taking the drug and continues to take it despite obvious physical, mental, or social harm. Most of the abuser's waking hours may be devoted to obtaining and using the drug. Drug dependence may or may not include tolerance and physical dependence.

Addiction—A behavioral state of compulsive drug use where the abuser spends more and more time obtaining and using the drug, usually in increasingly larger doses, with a high tendency to start using the drug again after going through withdrawal. Tolerance usually develops but not necessarily physical dependence. Addiction can be viewed as an extreme form of drug dependence.

Poly-drug abuse—Abuse involving more than one drug. It may occur as an isolated instance, such as when an abuser tries a substitute for an unavailable substance, or on a regular basis. It may be deliberate or accidental, as when an abused substance is adulterated or "cut" with other substances. Poly-drug abuse has become so prevalent that, when presented with a drug-abuse patient, many emergency physicians will presume poly-

drug abuse until proven otherwise. A practical problem for the rescuer is that signs and symptoms may be confusing, misleading, and not typical of any drug or class of drugs.

Designer drug—A substance intended for recreational use that has been modified from an existing, legitimate drug just enough to avoid current legal restrictions. At the present time, such substances are generally modifications of meperidine, fentanyl, mescaline, and methamphetamine (discussed in the appropriate sections below).

Specific Drugs

Alcohol

Alcohol is the most commonly abused drug in industrial nations. In the United States, more than 10 million people are alcoholics, over 200,000 deaths per year are related to alcohol, and the economic costs of alcoholism total billions of dollars annually. Over half of our nation's traffic fatalities and drownings involve alcohol. There is no way to measure the social costs of alcohol in breaking up families and wrecking careers.

Alcohol is a legal drug. Its sale has few restrictions, and moderate alcohol consumption has the tacit approval of society. Unfortunately, many individuals are unable to use alcohol in moderation because it can cause strong psychological and physical dependence.

Alcohol is a powerful central nervous system depressant that interferes with normal judgment, dulls awareness, and increases reaction time. Its so-called stimulatory effects, which usually occur early during the process of intoxication, are caused by interference with the function of the higher brain centers. Acute use of alcohol lowers blood sugar, which can hasten the development of hypothermia. Another physiological effect is dilation of the small blood vessels in the skin, which can cause acceler-

ated heat loss in a cold environment and accounts for the ruddy complexion of the chronic drinker.

Chronic use damages the brain, heart, liver, and other important organs. Alcoholics may develop chronic malnutrition and vitamin deficiencies because of poor appetite and improper diet. Alcohol use during pregnancy may cause fetal alcohol syndrome, characterized by growth retardation, mental deficiency, small head circumference, and other structural abnormalities.

The signs and symptoms of alcohol intoxication are well-known and fall into two patterns: early intoxication, which is characterized by excitement, talkativeness, aggressiveness, and dilated pupils; and late intoxication, characterized by disorientation, slurred speech, and inability to concentrate. This state may progress to stumbling and falling, drowsiness, stupor, and coma.

Chronic alcoholism is found at all levels of society, affecting business and professional people, homemakers, and other "pillars of the community" as well as the destitute. Early in the disease, the patient may appear normal and may deny having any problem with alcohol. A high index of suspicion and careful questioning of the patient and close family members may be necessary to uncover warning signs and symptoms such as solitary drinking, morning shakes, morning drinking, binge drinking, and blackouts (periods of amnesia).

Later in the disease, the chronic alcoholic may be disheveled and unwashed; he or she may experience memory loss, apathy, tremors, jaundice from alcoholic liver disease, chronic indigestion, and chronic diarrhea from the irritant effect of alcohol on the bowel. Alcohol withdrawal in chronic users produces anxiety, tremors, insomnia, nausea, vomiting, seizures, agitation, and hallucinations.

Alcoholics with chronic liver disease (cirrhosis) develop large, dilated veins in the upper stomach and lower esophagus (esophageal varices) because the blood is forced to bypass the injured liver. Severe gastrointestinal hemorrhage can occur if these veins rupture.

Narcotics

Narcotics can be made synthetically or produced from the seeds of the opium poppy. They have been used since antiquity to relieve pain. Legitimate narcotics commonly used in medicine include morphine (Morphine, Roxanol), meperidine (Demerol), fentanyl, methadone (Dolophine), codeine (contained in many combination products such as Tylenol with codeine), oxycodone (Percodan, Tylox), and hydromorphone (Dilaudid). The principal illegal narcotic is heroin. Commonly used "designer" street drugs are the meperidine derivatives MPPP and MPTP, and alpha-methyl-fentanyl ("China white").

Narcotics are central nervous system depressants and powerful respiratory depressants. Tolerance develops rapidly so that increasingly large doses are required to produce the same effects. Narcotics are taken orally or by injection; some—such as opium gum—can be smoked.

The signs and symptoms of narcotic use include lethargy, stupor, slowed pulse and respirations, low blood pressure, and mild hypothermia. Many narcotics cause pinpoint constriction of the pupils (meperidine is an exception). Chronic use causes nasal stuffiness and constipation. Acute overdose may cause coma and death from respiratory failure. MPTP can cause Parkinson's disease.

Withdrawal symptoms may include rapid pulse, anxiety, "gooseflesh," nausea, vomiting, diarrhea, abdominal cramps, frequent sniffling, severe runny nose, and shakiness.

Non-Narcotic Central Nervous System Depressants and Analgesics

These are used legitimately in medicine to produce sleep, for their tranquilizing effects, and occasionally as anticonvulsants. They alter the state of consciousness and relieve anxiety to some extent but do not relieve pain. Some of them can cause euphoria due to suppression of the higher brain centers, similar to the effects of alcohol.

These drugs can be divided into two categories: barbiturates and nonbarbiturates.

Common examples of **barbiturates** include secobarbital (Seconal), amobarbital (Amytal), pentobarbital (Nembutal), and phenobarbital (Luminal). Common **nonbarbiturates** include chloral hydrate (Noctec), glutethimide (Doriden), methaqualone (Quaalude), ethchlorvynol (Placidyl), flurazepam (Dalmane), triazolam (Halcion), alprazolam (Xanax), diazepam (Valium), lorazepam (Ativan), and chlordiazepoxide (Librium). New sedatives and hypnotics are being developed regularly.

The signs and symptoms of overdose include impairment of responsiveness ranging from drowsiness to coma, slow pulse, low blood pressure, slowed respirations, mild hypothermia and, occasionally, seizures.

Acute withdrawal from depressant drugs may cause insomnia, agitation, disorientation, and hallucinations. Occasionally, life-threatening conditions such as shock or seizures may occur.

Central Nervous System Stimulants

These drugs are abused to elevate mood and produce a high. They also may cause seizures, anxiety, hyperactivity, insomnia, agitation, irritability, paranoia, and disorganized behavior. When the drug effects wear off, the user typically becomes depressed, moody, and sleepy. Examples of legitimate, commonly used mild stimulants are caffeine, nicotine, some decongestants, and asthma drugs such as theophylline and its derivatives. Illegal stimulants include cocaine and amphetamines.

Cocaine, the first local anesthetic to be discovered, has since been replaced by better drugs and now has few legitimate medical uses. It is produced from the coca plant, grown in South America. Cocaine is highly addictive, and because of the marked euphoria it produces is one of the most widely abused illegal drugs in industrial nations today. A particularly dangerous form is rock cocaine, or "crack," which is cheap, widely available, and taken by smoking. Other forms are snuffed or injected.

Other effects of cocaine include symptoms of disturbed mental status such as anxiety, panic, paranoia, confusion, and hallucinations; altered motor activity such as tremors and hyperactivity; seizures; dilated pupils; rapid pulse and respirations; and hyperthermia.

Serious complications such as cardiac arrhythmias, heart attack, stroke, psychotic reactions, shock, and gangrene of the intestine occasionally occur. Chronic use can lead cocaine abusers to neglect jobs, families, proper nutrition, and personal hygiene. Withdrawal produces symptoms of exhaustion, depression, and anxiety.

Amphetamines were initially introduced into medicine as mood elevators and appetite suppressants. Examples include amphetamine, methamphetamine (Desoxyn), and dextroamphetamine (Dexedrine). "Ice," a recently introduced smokeable street form of methamphetamine, is highly addictive, similar to "crack" cocaine. Commonly available "designer drugs" also chemically related to the hallucinogen mescaline (see below) include MDA, or methylene-dioxyamphetamine ("Love drug"), MDMA, or methylene-dioxy-methamphetamine ("Ecstasy," "Adam"), and MDEA, or methylene-dioxyeth-amphetamine ("Eve").

Examples of nonamphetamine drugs used as cerebral stimulants or appetite suppressants include methylphenidate (Ritalin), phenmetrazine (Preludin), and diethylpropion hydrochloride (Tenuate).

All of these drugs have significant addictive potential and have few legitimate medical uses at present. Because they promote wakefulness, they are sometimes used inappropriately by truck drivers on long hauls and by students cramming for final exams.

Abusers take these drugs by mouth, injection, or inhalation. They may cause inability to concentrate, rapid heart rate and respirations, increased blood pressure, and such alterations of mental status as irritability, insomnia, anxiety, hyperexcitement, agitation, confusion, hallucinations, and paranoia. Altered motor activity such as hyperactivity and tremors may occur. Serious reactions such as cardiac arrhythmias, seizures, hyperthermia, and coma are seen occasionally. Withdrawal symptoms are similar to those of cocaine.

Cannabis Compounds

Cannabis compounds, probably the most frequently used illegal substances in the United States today, include marijuana, hashish, tetra-hydrocannabinol (THC), and oil of hashish. They are made from the Indian hemp plant, *Cannabis sativa,* and usually are introduced into the body by smoking the dried plant components.

These drugs cause mild euphoria, relaxation, and drowsiness. Side effects include confusion and dream/fantasy states; increased pulse rate; increased appetite ("the munchies"); and impairment of coordination, short-term memory, capacity to do complex work, and time perception. Occasionally, depression, confusion, acute anxiety, and hallucinations can occur. A common sign of marijuana use is reddening of the whites of the eyes. Heavy marijuana smokers can develop chronic carbon monoxide poisoning. Withdrawal may cause anxiety, loss of appetite, irritability, and nausea.

Hallucinogens

These drugs alter the user's perceptions of the environment, sometimes producing hallucinations or delusions. Hallucinogens are a large and growing group of abused chemicals.

Commonly used drugs include lysergic acid diethylamide (LSD), psilocybin (derived from *Psilocybe mexicana* or "magic mushrooms"), mescaline and peyote (from the flowering heads of the *Lophophora williamsii* or mescal cactus), morning glory seeds, STP, and phencyclidine (PCP). The latter, which is widely abused, is characterized by high potency, unpredictable effects, and frequent accidental ingestion since it may be used to "cut" other drugs. Common designer hallucinogens related to mescaline and the amphetamines are MDMA, MDA, and MDEA.

The acute effects of hallucinogen use are unpredictable, but can include euphoria, paranoia, mutism, distorted thought and perception, hyperactivity, gait disturbances, muscular rigidity, decreased pain sensation, and alterations in body temperature. More serious reactions, often called "bad trips," include panic reactions, suicide attempts, violent behavior, psychosis, and other serious psychiatric conditions. Serious accidents can occur when abusers develop misconceptions of their physical abilities and attempt to fly or perform other dangerous activities.

There are no clearly defined withdrawal reactions associated with hallucinogens, although brief recurrences of previous symptoms ("flashbacks") occur occasionally.

Nicotine and Tobacco

Nicotine, an alkaloid found in the plant *Nicotiana tabacum,* is taken by smoking or chewing the plant's dried leaves. Its use has been considered a form of drug dependence since the U.S. Surgeon General's report of 1988. However, the adverse effects of chronic tobacco use are due mainly to substances other than nicotine, such as carbon monoxide; cancer-producing substances such as nitrosamines, aromatic amines, and benzopyrene; and irritating substances such as hydrocyanic acid, nitric oxide, and cresols.

Nicotine causes mild central nervous system stimulation, improves memory, reduces aggression, and causes weight loss by suppressing the appetite for sweets and increasing energy expenditure. Chronic smokers have an increased mortality rate (twice the normal rate in two-pack-a-day smokers). The incidence of serious diseases such as sudden cardiac death, coronary artery disease, stroke, peripheral vascular disease, chronic obstructive lung disease (emphysema), and cancer of the lung, larynx, mouth, esophagus, bladder, and pancreas is increased in smokers. Less serious conditions such as osteoporosis, peptic ulcer, and facial wrinkles also are more common in smokers.

Tolerance and physical dependence develop to some of the effects of nicotine. Chronic smokers who attempt to stop smoking usually experience irritability, anxiety, restlessness, and difficulty in concentrating, which may persist for weeks to months. Nicotine-containing gum and skin patches are available and may be of some use in helping smokers quit.

Assessment of a Patient with Suspected Substance Abuse

Substance abuse is a widespread problem that is not confined to urban ghettos. Outdoor enthusiasts may use marijuana and cocaine while professing to abhor pollution of the environment—their own presumably excepted.

1. First impression. What is most probably going on? Does the patient have an illness or an injury? Institute universal precautions (see Appendix F).
2. Primary survey. Is the patient responsive or unresponsive? What is the level of responsiveness? Open and maintain the airway, assess for breathing, circulation, and obvious bleeding. If the patient is unresponsive, assess the head and neck; if responsive and there are abnormalities of the pulse and/or breathing, assess the chest, abdomen, and pelvis.
3. Proceed to the secondary survey, which is where you will probably be able to find out whether substance abuse is causing the problem. Ask the patient, if responsive, or companions what has happened. Assess the vital signs, particularly the temperature, and obtain information regarding any previous medical problems, drugs or medicines being taken, and allergies.

Substance abuse should be suspected in anyone *whose behavior is inappropriate* or *whose normal state of responsiveness* is altered in the absence of another obvious cause. If the patient does not admit substance abuse, ask pointed questions of any friends or family members who may be present. It is usually wisest to do this out of the patient's hearing.

One danger lies in not thinking of the possibility of substance abuse or in attributing its effects to those of more obvious illnesses or injuries. Another worse danger, however, is to attribute everything you see to substance abuse and miss hypothermia,

diabetic coma, insulin shock, epilepsy, psychosis, a head injury, or other serious condition.

Be aware of and assess for the following common signs and symptoms of substance abuse:

1. **Central nervous system depression**, including mental dullness, lethargy, inability to concentrate, slurred speech, mental depression, apathy, lack of coordination, stumbling, falling, sleepiness, stupor, or coma.
2. **Central nervous system stimulation**, including excitement, talkativeness, aggressiveness, insomnia, tremors, agitation, aimless activity, disorientation, hallucinations, paranoia, and convulsions.
3. Changes in the **appearance of the eyes**. Opiates produce pinpoint pupils; alcohol, barbiturates, and marijuana produce dilated pupils. Unequal pupils suggest a possible associated **head injury**. Alcoholics and marijuana abusers frequently have red eyes caused by engorgement of the blood vessels in the conjunctivae.
4. Changes in the **nose**. Abusers of opiates, cocaine, and other drugs that are taken by snuffing usually have chronic, stuffy noses. Opiate abusers develop runny noses and frequent sniffling during the early withdrawal period. Cocaine abusers may develop perforations of the anterior part of the nasal septum.
5. Changes in the **skin**. Intravenous drug abusers may have multiple, linear, pigmented scars ("tracks") over accessible veins, usually of the forearm and at the bend of the elbow. Alcoholics frequently have ruddy skin and dilated veins over the nose and cheeks.

6. **Psychiatric changes**. Substance abuse may produce extreme agitation, belligerence, paranoia, hallucinations, delusions, panic reactions, amnesia, and psychosis.

Because abusers may lack normal judgment and lose their usual protective instincts and reflexes, they may have to be protected from injuring themselves or others. They may fall, be involved in automobile or machinery accidents, or promote fights and other incidents.

7. **Hyperthermia**. This can occur with the use of amphetamine derivatives (particularly MDMA), hallucinogens, and herbal teas containing certain atropine-like alkaloids.

Emergency Care of a Substance Abuse Patient

The emergency care of a substance abuse patient consists predominately of caring for the effects of central nervous system depression or stimulation as follows:

1. Open and maintain the upper airway. Treat unresponsiveness as necessary (see Chapter 12), using an oral airway and placing the patient in the semiprone (NATO) position.
2. Anticipate vomiting and be ready to suction the airway.
3. The development of respiratory depression is a definite danger; it can occur both with central nervous system depressants and as a late effect with central nervous system stimulants. Monitor the patient closely and use frequent stimulation such as gentle pinching to keep the patient awake. Support ventilation with a bag-valve-mask or pocket mask if necessary.

4. Even though substance abusers rarely go into shock, the patient should be observed for symptoms of shock and treated appropriately if shock occurs.

5. Monitor and maintain the body temperature. Hypothermia or hyperthermia may occur and should be managed as described in Chapter 18.

6. A patient with central nervous system stimulation must be handled calmly. Remain calm, reassuring, and nonjudgmental, and avoid startling the patient. Refrain from arguing. Do not restrain the patient except in an emergency. Remain with the patient until he or she is turned over to the EMS system or another competent authority. Violent patients should be approached very carefully, with several other rescuers (preferably large, strong ones) close at hand in case assistance is needed.

7. If the patient convulses, follow the management outlined for seizure disorders earlier in this chapter.

8. It may be possible to "talk down" a patient who is having a "bad trip." The process, which requires considerable time and patience, is outlined in step 6. Avoid or remove aggravating stimuli such as loud voices, loud music, and bright lights.

9. Arrange for transport to a hospital. Any vomitus and evidence of drug use such as bottles, tablets, and drug paraphernalia should be collected and sent to the hospital with the patient.

Table 17.7

Summary of Emergency Care of a Substance Abuse Patient

1. Open and maintain the airway. Use semiprone position.
2. Provide general care for unresponsiveness, as indicated.
3. Monitor and record the patient's vital signs.
4. Anticipate vomiting and use suction as necessary.
5. If the patient's breathing is depressed, stimulate the patient and support ventilation as necessary.
6. Treat shock, if it develops.
7. Treat hypothermia and hyperthermia, if present.
8. Calm an agitated patient.
9. Treat convulsions if present.
10. Do not leave the patient alone until he or she is turned over to the EMS system.
11. Preserve vomitus, bottles, pills, etc., and send the material to the hospital with patient.

Scenario #17 (Fig. 17.6)

The following scenario illustrates the management of the type of serious medical emergency that may be seen in the nonurban setting.

You are having a late lunch in the Midway Chalet when there is a commotion a few tables away. A middle-aged man has knocked a soft drink cup off his tray and is slumped in his chair. A woman about the same age—probably his wife—rises from her chair and quickly moves around the table to him. The man is holding his hand over his chest, and his face is gray.

You get up and walk over to the pair. As you approach, you can see beads of sweat on his forehead and an anguished look on his face.

You: "Hi, I'm Ben Schussen of the High Range Ski Patrol. Can I help you?"

Patient: "Please!"

Wife: "Something's wrong with my husband. He's never been like this before. Honey, what's wrong?"

Patient: "I have a terrible pain in my chest. I can't breathe."

You: "Where is the pain?"

Patient: "Right here" (indicating the midsternum).

You: "What's your name?" (grasping his wrist and assessing his pulse. It is regular, weak, and rapid; about 100 beats per minute. You estimate his breathing rate at about 20 respirations per minute.)

Patient: "Max Doud."

You: "Have you ever had anything like this before?"

Patient: "No."

You: "How long ago did it start?"

Patient: "Just a few minutes."

You: "What does the pain feel like?"

Patient: "Like someone is squeezing my chest."

You: "Does the pain go anywhere from your chest?"

Patient: "To my left elbow."

You: "Have you ever had any heart trouble or high blood pressure?"

Patient: "Not that I know of."

You: "Excuse me a minute. I'm going to make a quick call on the radio."

You call the Midway patrol shack, not far away, telling the patroller that you have a probable heart emergency, and requesting a toboggan, oxygen, bag-valve-mask, and suction. You ask the patroller on duty to call Dr. Bill Osler, a friend of yours who is signed on for the Doctors' Patrol, and to call the summit and have a patroller bring down the automatic external defibrillator as soon as possible. You also request an ambulance from town.

You: "How are you feeling now?"

Patient: "Pretty bad. The pain's no better."

You: "Would you feel better lying down?"

Patient: "No. This is okay."

If anything, he is looking worse. His breathing is faster and his pulse

---

Fig. 17.6 Scenario #17

faster and weaker. At this point, the Midway patroller arrives with the portable oxygen, bag-valve-mask, and a V-Vac suction unit. You crack the tank and pressurize the gauges.

You: "I'm going to put this oxygen mask on your face and give you some oxygen. This should make you feel better and less short of breath."

Patient: "Thanks, I need it."

You put a non-rebreather mask on the patient's face and turn the flow rate up to 12 liters per minute. The patient looks more relaxed. Suddenly his eyes roll back in his head, he sags back further into the chair, and starts gasping. You have your hand on his radial pulse at the time; suddenly, you cannot feel it.

You: (shaking his shoulder) "Sir, are you okay?"

There is no answer. His wife starts to weep. Quickly, you lift him from the chair, place him supine on the floor, take your pocket mask from your first aid belt, take the mask off his face, and plug the oxygen tubing into the nipple on the pocket mask. He continues to gasp occasionally. You per-

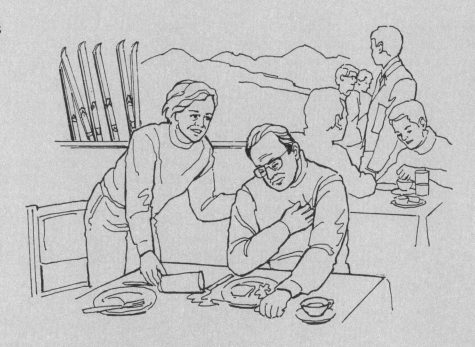

Fig. 17.6

form the head-tilt/chin-lift technique, place the pocket mask over his face, and deliver two rescue breaths. You quickly feel for the carotid pulse. It is absent.

You: "Joe, we have a full arrest" (addressing the Midway patroller, while locating your hand position on the patient's chest). "Call the base and have them send up a Thiokol (a large-bed oversnow vehicle) stat, and make sure that ambulance is on its way from town."

You give 15 chest compressions at a rate of one per second, counting "one-and-two-and...." You give two more rescue breaths, then 15 more chest compressions. By this time, the Midway patroller is back at the patient's side and takes over chest compressions after you give the next rescue breaths. You two intersperse each set of five compressions with a rescue breath using the pocket mask. The patient's color, which had become a ghastly pale blue, is starting to pink up a little.

Dr. Osler comes in the door, followed by the summit patroller carrying the AED. You continue CPR. The physician turns on the defibrillator.

Dr. Osler: "This is a semiautomatic machine with a recording that tells you what to do."

Machine: "Attach electrodes." (Dr. Osler attaches the two electrodes to the patient's chest.) "Assessing. Hands off." (You stop CPR and move away from the patient.) "Shock required." (Dr. Osler pushes the shock button.) "Stand back." (The machine starts to beep. Everyone moves away from the patient. The beeping is replaced by a constant tone. The patient jumps as a 200 joule shock is delivered.) "Check breathing and pulse." (A green light goes on.)

Dr. Osler: "You have a minute to give CPR if there is no pulse." (You assess the carotid pulse; it is absent. You restart CPR.)

Machine: "Assessing. Hands off." (You move away from the patient. The sequence is repeated and the machine repeats the 200 joule shock.)

This time, you can feel a carotid pulse that is soon steady at about 60 beats per minute, and the patient starts breathing again on his own. You attach the oxygen to the bag-valve-mask and two of you start supporting the patient's breaths.

The sound of a diesel motor outside the chalet signals the arrival of the big Thiokol. It is time to load the patient on its flat bed and take him down the hill to meet the paramedics at the base. Dr. Osler, you, and the Midway patroller will ride down the hill in back with the patient and all of your emergency equipment, in case more problems occur. The patient is fortunate that you were right there with him when he arrested and that the defibrillator was available. You have treated three cardiac arrests in your patrol career so far; this is the only one who looks like he may survive.

Chapter 18

Environmental Emergencies

The commanding officer should take the utmost care never to suffer a soldier to sleep, or even to sit down in his tent with wet clothes, nor to bed down in a wet blanket or upon damp straw. The utmost vigilance will be necessary to guard against this fruitful source of diseases among soldiers.

—*Benjamin Rush, M.D.*
  "Directions for Preserving the Health of Soldiers," 1777

There are many hazards in the outdoor environment. Heat, cold, wind, solar radiation, altitude, bodies of water, fire, avalanches, blizzards, and lightning are important causes of injury. Before reading this chapter, please review the elements of adapting to the outdoor environment described in Chapter 1.

Frostbite

Frostbite, the actual freezing of a body part, occurs when the heat produced by the part, the heat carried to it by the blood, and the amount of insulation covering it are insufficient to prevent its temperature from falling below 32°F (0°C). The danger of frostbite is increased by the body's tendency to guard the temperature of vital, internal organs by restricting blood flow to the skin, muscles, and extremities.

Certain body tissues have a higher risk of frostbite than others. The hands, feet, ears, cheeks, and nose all are located far from the heart at the periphery of the body and subject to rapid heat loss because of their large surface-area-to-volume ratio and exposed positions. Other factors that contribute to the development of frostbite include inadequate insulation, wet clothing, fatigue, poor nutrition, alcohol and drug use, smoking, restricted peripheral circulation (because of arteriosclerosis or tight clothing), and contact with metal or hydrocarbon liquids such as gasoline.

Localized cold injury to tissues occurs in two ways: when intra- and extra-cellular ice crystals form, causing direct cell injury, and when blood circulation is interrupted because of blood clots within small blood vessels and red cell sludging due to plasma loss from cold-damaged vessels.

Types of Frostbite

Before a frostbitten area has thawed, frostbite can be classified only as superficial or deep. A patient with **superficial frostbite** (Fig. 18.1) feels a mild tingling or pain followed by numbness. Inspection reveals a gray or yellowish patch of skin, usually on the nose, ear, cheek, finger, or toe. The tissues beneath the area remain soft and pliable. This type of frostbite is common in poorly dressed schoolchildren, cold-weather joggers, and in skiers riding chair lifts on very cold, windy days.

Deep frostbite is a full- or partial-thickness freezing of a body part and most commonly involves the hands or feet. It should be suspected if a painfully cold part suddenly stops hurting when it obviously is not getting warmer. The affected part is cold, solid, wooden, and numb, with pale, waxy skin; it resembles a piece of chicken just removed from the freezer.

After a frostbitten part has thawed, it can be classified into one of four categories depending on the severity of tissue damage (Fig. 18.2), similar to the classification of burns. The first category is superficial frostbite; the other three are degrees of deep frostbite. More than one type of frostbite can occur on a body or body part at risk.

Fig. 18.1 *Superficial Frostbite*

Fig. 18.2 *Categories of Thawed Frostbite*

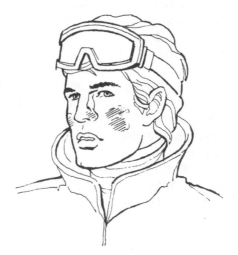

Fig. 18.1

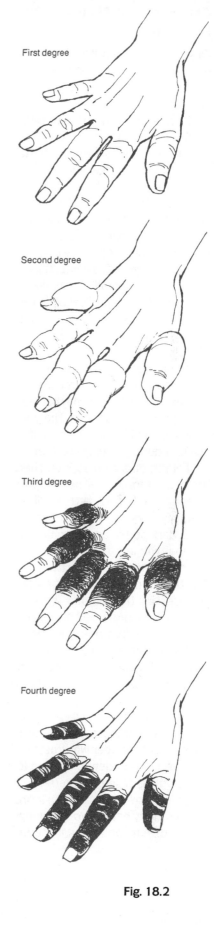

First degree

Second degree

Third degree

Fourth degree

Fig. 18.2

Categories of Thawed Frostbite

First-degree frostbite. The affected part is warm, swollen, and tender. Blisters are either absent or are few and small.

Second-degree frostbite. Blisters form within minutes to hours after thawing and enlarge over several days. They tend to be large, impressive, typically extend to the tips of the digits, and are filled with pink or reddish fluid. Despite its dramatic appearance, second-degree frostbite may heal with little or no tissue loss.

Third-degree frostbite. Blisters are small and contain darker fluid (reddish-blue or purplish) because more severe damage to vessels allows cells as well as plasma to leak out. The blisters are situated more proximally on the digits than in second-degree frostbite. The surrounding skin may be red or blue and may not blanch when pressure is applied. The part is cool and numb; its joints are stiff. Tissue loss during healing is common.

Fourth-degree frostbite. There are no blisters or swelling. The part remains numb, cold, and bloodless. It is gray or white initially but soon turns dark purple and becomes gangrenous within a few days.

Identification of **superficial frostbite** is not difficult. It is made by assessing the patient's signs and symptoms as described above in a setting where frostbite might be expected. The emergency care is to apply direct body heat, e.g., placing a warm hand on a frozen cheek or holding a frozen finger in an armpit (Fig. 18.3). The heat applied need be no warmer than body temperature. Then, the rescuer should consider why frostbite occurred. The patient may need to add clothing or seek shelter.

Deep frostbite is a much more serious injury because of the danger of tissue death and permanent damage to surviving tissue. Experiments have shown that the amount of tissue damage depends on both how *low* the temperature is and how *long* the body part has been frozen. If other factors are equal, frozen parts rewarmed rapidly have less damage than those rewarmed slowly.

Identification of deep frostbite is made by inspecting and palpating the affected body part and by evaluating the patient's symptoms in a setting where frostbite might be expected. The rescuer should keep in mind the possibility of hypothermia also. If the patient is shivering or has an altered mental status, assess as you would for suspected hypothermia (described below).

The preferred emergency care is *rapid rewarming* in a water bath with the water temperature carefully controlled between 102° and 108°F (39° to 42°C). Cooler water rewarms too slowly; warmer water may burn the tissues.

Rewarming should be done *only in a sheltered area* where the patient's entire body can be kept warm. The rescuer will need a suitable thermometer to test water temperature (a standard clinical thermometer may not read high enough) and a vessel that is large enough so that the extremity can be immersed without touching the sides of the vessel. A 20-quart canning kettle is a suitable size for rewarming a foot. Constricting objects such as rings and bracelets should be removed beforehand.

As a rule, rewarming continues for 20 to 30 minutes or until the frozen areas turn deep red or bluish and the color change has progressed distally as far as it will go. Monitor the temperature of the bath and, as the water cools, *remove the extremity,* add hot water, stir, and retest the water temperature *before* re-immersing the extremity.

While the frozen part is being rewarmed, maintain the patient's morale with hot drinks and apply heat to non-frozen body parts to open up circulation to the frozen area. Rewarming usually causes severe pain. Patients with frostbite or who are in danger of frostbite should refrain from smoking or chewing tobacco because nicotine interferes with circulation and retards healing.

One of the worst things that can happen to a frostbitten part is for it to refreeze after thawing. *This always leads to gangrene.* Therefore, protect it against refreezing at all costs. In a patient who can be transported to medical care, apply thick layers of sterile dressings held in place by a loosely applied, self-adhering roller bandage. Leave blisters unopened, separate digits with soft cotton or wool pads, and elevate the part to reduce swelling.

Frostbite frequently occurs in circumstances where the party members are few and subject to severe environmental stress, facilities for proper emergency care are nonexistent—particularly a suitable thermometer and a container large enough for rapid rewarming—and the party's main concern is to escape alive. In this case, either the patient will have to self-evacuate or the party will have to make

Fig. 18.3 *Immediate Care of Superficial Frostbite*

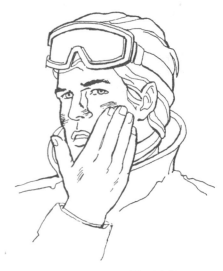

Fig. 18.3

camp and send for help, realizing that a frozen foot or hand will likely rewarm spontaneously and trying to protect it as well as possible from refreezing. At other times, a patient frequently is unaware of a frozen part until it starts to hurt after thawing. By this time it is too late for rapid rewarming. It may be difficult to get a boot back on a blistered and swollen thawed foot if the patient must self-evacuate.

Exercise judgment in deciding whether to rapidly rewarm a frozen extremity in the field. Do not attempt rewarming if the extremity has already rewarmed spontaneously, if you do not have the proper equipment or proper shelter, or if you can obtain medical care soon. Conversely, rapid field rewarming may be advisable if equipment and shelter are available, if the patient can be carried out or evacuated by vehicle or toboggan, and if there is a good chance the part can be protected from refreezing during evacuation.

In the past, it has been recommended that a patient with a frozen foot try to keep it frozen while walking or skiing out to where it can be rapidly rewarmed under proper conditions. Many experienced authorities disagree with this, based on the difficulty of keeping a foot frozen without putting the entire body in serious danger from hypothermia. In any case, the difference in damage between slow and rapid rewarming is not great, *provided that refreezing can be prevented.*

The prevention of frostbite is discussed in Chapter 1.

Hypothermia

Hypothermia, or "exposure," refers to cooling of the body to a core temperature below 95°F (35°C) as determined by a low-reading core thermometer (usually rectal). Hypothermia can occur at temperatures well above freezing; at temperatures below freezing, the patient may suffer frostbite

as well. The combination of cold, wind, and water is especially dangerous, as in being stranded in a blizzard at temperatures near 32°F (0°C) or falling into a mountain stream.

Hypothermia has had a significant impact on human history, especially military history. During World War II, 30,000 British sailors died of hypothermia. Napoleon is estimated to have lost 500,000 troops from cold injury during his Russian campaign. Hypothermia has complicated many natural disasters, such as earthquakes occurring during the cold months of the year. It is a factor in about one-third of the 8,000 drowning deaths that occur yearly in the United States.

When the human body temperature falls progressively, all body functions tend to diminish or slow. The initial drop of one to two degrees triggers shivering, followed by clumsiness, stumbling, falling, slow reactions, confusion, and difficulty in speaking (Table 18.1). The patient frequently is unaware of what is happening. **Impairment of use of the hands** is very serious because it hampers attempts to put on more clothing, set up shelter, or light a fire. At body temperatures below 90°F (32°C), shivering gradually ceases and the muscles become progressively more rigid. The breathing rate and pulse rate slow, and the patient becomes irrational and gradually lapses into a coma. Death may occur at body temperatures below 80°F (27°C).

It is important to think of the possibility of hypothermia when dangerous environmental conditions exist, since hypothermia is an insidious condition that is difficult to recognize in its early stages, and death can occur within two hours of the onset of symptoms. Other members of a party may not realize that a companion is hypothermic because they are becoming hypothermic themselves. When the body is too cold to be capable of shivering, it cannot warm itself without outside help.

Methods for preventing hypothermia are discussed in Chapter 1.

Hypothermia is potentially *lethal*. The mortality rate is greater than 50 percent in severe cases, especially those complicated by injuries or previous illnesses. The most common cause of death probably is **ventricular fibrillation**, which can be spontaneous or precipitated by a sudden jolt to a cold, acidotic heart. However, with proper emergency care, the mortality rate should be low in otherwise healthy patients with core (rectal) temperatures at or above 90°F (32°C).

A patient with severe hypothermia may appear to be dead—the pupils are fixed and dilated, the pulse and breathing imperceptible, and body rigidity may resemble rigor mortis. However, the patient still may be saved with proper emergency care. The dictum "No one is dead until warm and dead" emphasizes that *all* patients with hypothermia deserve an attempt at rewarming.

Ski patrollers should watch for the development of hypothermia in skiers stranded on stalled chair lifts and persons who lie or stand in the snow for long periods, such as accident victims and gatekeepers at ski races. An injury impairs the body's heat conservation mechanisms, making an injured patient more susceptible to cold injury as well. Cold temperatures and high altitude increase the risk of shock, which predisposes the patient to further chilling, making frostbite and hypothermia more likely. Put insulation beneath and over accident victims and protect them from the wind.

Types of Hypothermia

Hypothermia can be divided according to **duration of exposure** into three categories: **acute** (less than one hour), **subacute** (one to 24 hours), and **chronic** (a day or more). These distinctions are somewhat arbitrary but significant because, although at first there is a large difference between the core and shell temperatures, as time passes the core temperature becomes closer to the shell temperature. Also, in acute hypothermia the blood sugar is normal or slightly elevated, and the blood electrolytes and acid base balance (pH) are still normal or only slightly disturbed. In subacute and chronic hypothermia, the blood glucose level is low and the patient becomes acidotic due to shivering and starvation.

Severity of Hypothermia

The severity of hypothermia can be divided according to the patient's core temperature into **mild** (90°F [32°C] and above) and **profound** [below 90°F (32°C)]. This division is useful because emergency care differs according to severity, as described below.

Hypothermia commonly develops in certain well-recognized settings described below.

1. **Immersion hypothermia** is caused by immersion in cold water. It usually is acute or subacute when seen. This type of hypothermia develops rapidly because of the ability of cold water to conduct heat away from the body about 25 times more rapidly than cold air. A similar setting is the combination of cold rain and high wind.
2. **Field hypothermia** occurs outdoors in previously healthy individuals such as off-area skiers, climbers, hikers, and lost hunters. It usually is subacute or chronic because of the time required for search operations, and may accompany injuries occurring outdoors in cold weather.
3. **Urban hypothermia** may occur indoors or outdoors in cities and towns. It usually develops in people with a physical predisposition, disability, or illness. Urban hypothermia usually is subacute or chronic when discovered and has a high mortality rate. Predisposing conditions include those that:
   a. *Increase heat loss* (large surface-area-to-volume ratios in premature infants and newborns; patients with burns or wide-spread skin disorders).
   b. *Interfere with heat production or distribution* (malnutrition, anemia, old age, endocrine abnormalities such as hypothyroidism, shock, heart disease, diabetes, arteriosclerosis).
   c. *Interfere with temperature regulation* (central nervous system disease and injury, and certain drugs).
   d. *Interfere with normal judgment* (senility, psychosis, and drug and alcohol abuse).
   Homeless people are especially at risk of urban hypothermia during cold spells. Many drugs, including sedatives, tranquilizers, Lithium, and beta blockers, can accelerate the development of hypothermia.
4. **Submersion hypothermia** (near-drowning in cold water) is acute hypothermia combined with hypoxia. Cooling due to submersion in water of 70°F (21°C) or below appears to protect the central nervous system from the effects of hypoxia for a limited time; the colder the water, the more the protection.
   The "diving reflex," which was discovered in marine mammals such as the porpoise, also may play a protective role. Immediately after the body or face is immersed in cold water, this reflex slows the pulse, shifts blood flow from the shell to the core, and causes breath-holding. It is present to some extent in man, being more pronounced in children than adults. The activity of the diving reflex, combined with the more rapid cooling rates of smaller individuals, may ex-

Table 18.1

Signs and Symptoms of Hypothermia
(modified from Lathrop)

°F	°C	
99-96	37-35.6	Intense shivering. Impaired ability to perform complex tasks.
95-91	35-32.8	Violent shivering. Difficulty in speaking, sluggish thinking, amnesia.
90-86	32.2-30	Shivering is replaced by muscular rigidity. Exposed skin is blue or puffy. Movements are jerky. Dulled sensorium, but patient still is able to maintain posture and the appearance of contact with surroundings.
85-81	29.4-27.2	Coma, lack of reflexes, atrial fibrillation.
Below 78	Below 25.6	Failure of cardiac and respiratory centers, pulmonary edema, ventricular fibrillation. Death.

plain why survival after submersion hypothermia is higher in children and infants than adults. Rare individuals have survived without neurologic damage after being submerged for periods of 20 to 66 minutes, usually in very cold water.

Assessment of a Patient with Suspected Hypothermia

In the field, it is better to anticipate and watch for hypothermia in patients exposed to dangerous meteorologic conditions so its development can be halted while the patient is still in its milder stages.

Although hypothermia can be suspected from its signs and symptoms, accurate diagnosis depends on documenting a body core temperature below 95°F (35°C), using a low-reading rectal thermometer. However, for obvious reasons, rescuers are reluctant to take rectal temperatures in the field. An oral temperature may be substituted if the patient is responsive; the thermometer should be left under the tongue for a minimum of three minutes. Remember that the temperatures given in this section are *rectal* temperatures; oral temperatures read one degree lower.

Suspect developing hypothermia when a companion shivers, appears clumsy, stumbles, drops things, has slurred speech, and lags behind. Any person who is found ill, injured, or unresponsive outdoors in cold weather or who is removed from cold water should be considered hypothermic until proven otherwise.

1. First impression. Do conditions predispose to hypothermia? Has the patient obviously been injured? What has probably happened? Does the patient have an altered mental status? Institute universal precautions (see Appendix F).
2. Primary survey. Assess the patient's level of responsiveness, airway, breathing, and circulation, and look for obvious bleeding. Remember that in hypothermia the pulse may be weak and very slow and the patient may be breathing only a few times a minute. Take more time than you normally would to assess breathing and pulse. Do *not* start CPR prematurely (see below). Take the patient's temperature.
3. Secondary survey. Before proceeding, take measures to stabilize the patient's body temperature and protect it from dropping further.

Emergency Care of a Hypothermic Patient

The principles of emergency care are to:
1. Prevent further heat loss.
2. Rewarm the patient as safely as possible.
3. Rewarm the body core in advance of the shell, if possible.
4. Treat the patient gently to avoid precipitating ventricular fibrillation.

The application of these principles depends on the patient's core temperature, the equipment available, and the presence or absence of complicating factors such as other illnesses or injuries.

The first priority is to stabilize the body temperature and prevent further heat loss by getting the patient out of the wind or water and into a tent or other shelter. If the patient's clothing is wet, gently exchange it for dry clothing if available. Place the patient in a sleeping bag or place a blanket or spare clothing under and over the patient, and cover the patient's head.

If clothing is wet and no dry clothing is available, wrap something windproof, such as a poncho, around the patient to reduce evaporative cooling. Avoid unnecessary handling, and do not allow the patient to sit, stand, or walk until he or she has been rewarmed. It may be better to cut off wet clothing than to undress a profoundly hypothermic patient. Meanwhile, build a fire or light a stove.

Further emergency care depends on the patient's measured or estimated core temperature. If you do not have a thermometer, consider the patient to have a core temperature of 90°F (32°C) or above if he or she is still shivering and capable of appropriate actions such as zipping an open parka and picking up a dropped mitten. The core temperature is very likely below 90°F if the patient is no longer shivering and, especially, if he or she is partly or completely unresponsive.

Rewarming Methods

Since the numbing effects of cold on skin nerves makes hypothermics less aware of temperature, they are more subject to burns than normal people. During rewarming, always monitor the effects of rewarming devices by testing them on yourself periodically.

Rewarming methods, which can be quite limited in the field, are divided into **fast** and **slow** methods. Fast methods provide large amounts of heat rapidly and frequently are water-based systems because of the high specific heat of water. The 540 calories of heat made available when the temperature of each gram of water drops one degree Centigrade allows a large amount of heat to be transferred from a heat source to the body. Fast rewarming methods suitable for field use include the following:

1. The "hydraulic sarong," a homemade device in which a backpacking stove is used to heat a pot of water, and a bilge pump then circulates the hot water through plastic tubes sewn into a blanket wrapped around the patient's trunk (Fig. 18.4).
2. Hot tubs (available in mountain cabins, etc.).

3. Electric blankets. (Electricity may be available in campgrounds, mountain cabins, etc.)

Fast rewarming methods used in a hospital include hot tubs, electric blankets, machines that circulate warmed fluid through a rubber blanket that is wrapped around the patient, peritoneal dialysis (pumping warmed fluid in and out of the peritoneal cavity), and direct warming of the blood using a heart-lung machine.

Slow methods are more likely to be non-water based. They provide less heat and therefore rewarm the patient more slowly; in many cases their main value may be to prevent further cooling. Methods that can be used in the field include the following:

1. Allowing a mildly hypothermic patient to shiver inside a sleeping bag.
2. Body-to-body contact (one or two rescuers get into a sleeping bag with the patient, all stripped to the waist).
3. Canteens full of hot water.
4. Hot rocks.
5. Chemical heating pads.
6. Devices for delivering heated, humidified air or oxygen to the lungs (Fig. 18.5), such as the UVIC.
7. The Heatpac, a small, lightweight stove that can deliver 250 watts of heat for several hours using a charcoal cartridge for fuel (Fig. 18.6).

Although delivering heated air or oxygen to the lungs would seem to be an ideal way to rewarm the core, studies have shown that the amount of heat actually delivered is small and the main value of the method probably is to prevent heat loss from the airway. If electricity is available, an electric blanket on low can rewarm slowly also.

Slow methods suitable for hospital use include covering the patient with blankets in a warm room and delivering heated, humidified oxygen to the lungs with an anesthesia machine. In a hospital, slow and fast methods usually are combined, i.e., warmed fluid circulating through a rubber blanket plus warmed, inhaled oxygen.

About the only methods available to the *recreational* party are slow, improvised methods: shivering, canteens filled with hot water, hot rocks, and body-to-body contact in a sleeping bag. *Rescue groups* can carry a hydraulic sarong, a Heatpac, chemical heating pads, and devices for airway rewarming.

Mild Hypothermia

A hypothermic whose rectal temperature is 90°F (32°C) or above can be rewarmed by any of the means listed above that are available or can be improvised. Small devices that concentrate heat, such as canteens of

hot water, chemical heating pads, and hot rocks, should be wrapped to prevent burns and placed against areas of high heat loss such as the chest and sides of the neck (Fig. 18.7). If body-to-body warming is used, a healthy "heat donor" should be replaced if he or she becomes cold.

A well-nourished patient in good physical condition who is shivering well can rewarm himself or herself in a sleeping bag out of the wind. Rescue groups usually carry some of the more sophisticated devices listed above.

Under more civilized conditions, rewarming can be achieved with more active rewarming devices such as a hot tub (at 105° to 110°F [41° to 43°C]) or an electric blanket. When the patient is able to swallow, he or she can drink hot, sweet liquids— mainly to boost morale since hot drinks produce negligible increases in body temperature. Alcohol and caffeine should be avoided.

After rewarming, it is best to make camp and allow the patient (and the rest of the party) to rest overnight before proceeding.

Profound Hypothermia

The mortality rate outside a hospital is high for patients who have a rectal temperature much below 90°F (32°C), mainly because of the frequency of ventricular fibrillation and the development of serious metabolic and electrolyte problems that cannot be detected or treated in the field. In-hospital survival is better because personnel can discover, monitor, and treat those problems rapidly and can rewarm the patient under controlled conditions in the intensive care unit (ICU).

Fig. 18.4 *Hydraulic Sarong*

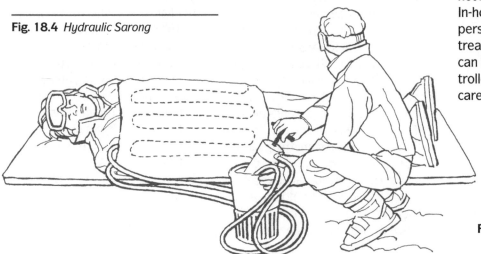

Fig. 18.4

Because of the possibility that these serious complications will develop during rewarming, the best field results are obtained by *preventing further heat loss* and *transporting the patient rapidly to medical care rather than attempting field rewarming*. A patient with a body temperature this low will be relatively stable for a time if treated gently and not allowed to cool further. Prevent further heat loss by one of the slow rewarming methods listed above. Do *not* use fast rewarming methods such as a hot tub or electric blanket on medium or high.

Subacute and chronic hypothermics are dehydrated, partly because cooling increases urinary output. If equipment and properly trained rescuers are available, give the patient warmed intravenous fluids such as 5-percent glucose in half-normal saline.

A patient with profound hypothermia will have slow respirations and a low blood pressure. Because these signs are "normal" under the circumstances, rescue breathing and aggressive treatment for shock are rarely indicated. A pneumatic antishock garment (PASG) is contraindicated except in the patient who also is in hypovolemic shock caused by trauma.

Patients with profound hypothermia may appear to be in cardiac arrest or dead because their pulse and respirations are so difficult to detect. Spend several minutes or longer at-

tempting to detect these vital signs before concluding that they are absent. CPR may actually *precipitate* ventricular fibrillation in a patient with a pulse that is weak or slow enough to be undetectable. Therefore, it should not be given unless *careful* examination reveals *no* signs of life, or ventricular fibrillation is strongly suspected because of a sudden event such as collapse of the patient or loss of a previously detected heartbeat. In very cold patients, CPR may be impossible because the chest is incompressible. An exception to the above is the patient with **submersion hypothermia**. CPR should be started as soon as possible according to standard protocols.

Once begun, CPR should be continued at the normal rate until the patient is hospitalized. Patients with cardiac arrest due to hypothermia have survived after several hours of CPR. This suggests that they may have a more favorable outlook than patients with cardiac arrest due to other causes.

Before transport, make sure the patient is stable, splint fractures, and

Fig. 18.5 *Devices for Delivering Heat to the Body*

Fig. 18.6 *Heatpac*

Fig. 18.7 *Areas of High Heat Loss*

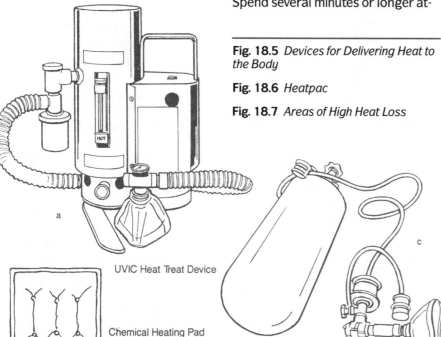

UVIC Heat Treat Device

Chemical Heating Pad

APPLINC Device

Fig. 18.5

b

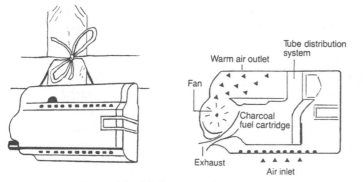

Warm air outlet

Tube distribution system

Fan

Charcoal fuel cartridge

Exhaust

Air inlet

Fig. 18.6

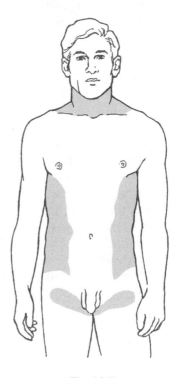

Fig. 18.7

Table 18.2

Summary of Emergency Care of a Hypothermic Patient

A. General measures
   1. Stop further heat loss.
      a. Get the patient out of the wind and into a tent or other shelter.
      b. Build a fire or start a stove.
      c. Add insulation beneath and around the patient. Cover the patient's head.
      d. Replace wet clothing with dry clothing.
   2. Treat the patient gently. Do not allow the patient to sit or stand until rewarmed.
   3. Give hot, sweet liquids after the patient is alert, awake, and able to swallow.
   4. Treat any injuries.
B. Mild hypothermia (core temperature 90°F [32°C] or above)
   1. Raise core temperature by whatever means are available.
      a. Place hot rocks or canteens against high heat loss areas.
      b. Provide body-to-body contact in a sleeping bag.
      c. Use rescue team equipment, i.e., hydraulic sarong, heating pads, Heatpak, airway rewarming devices.
      d. In civilization, use a hot tub or electric blanket.
C. Profound hypothermia (core temperature below 90°F [32°C])
   1. Stabilize the patient.
   2. Keep the patient from cooling further by using one of the slow rewarming methods. Avoid fast rewarming in the field. Use portable devices during evacuation, i.e., Heatpak, airway rewarming devices, heating pads.
   3. Treat dehydration with warmed intravenous fluids if equipment and expertise are available.
   4. Avoid jostling and jolting the patient during transportation.
   5. Avoid CPR unless ventricular fibrillation is highly likely. The exception is near drowning (submersion hypothermia)—follow standard CPR protocols.
   6. If the patient cannot be evacuated, use slow rewarming methods (e.g., body-to-body heat in shelter) and send for help.

treat other injuries using standard methods. Carry the patient slowly and carefully, avoiding sudden jolts. Prevent further cooling during transportation by the use of portable, self-contained, slow rewarming devices that do not require constant monitoring, such as the Heatpak; an airway rewarming device, such as the propane or battery-operated UVIC; or chemical heating pads. A rapid transportation method such as helicopter evacuation is preferable to a long, bumpy toboggan or snow vehicle ride. If possible, take the patient to a hospital with facilities for open-heart surgery.

If a patient with profound hypothermia cannot be evacuated because of the small size of the party, send for help and provide slow rewarming in a tent or snow shelter. The best method probably is body-to-body contact in a sleeping bag. Every situation is different, however, and the course of action depends on the weather, size and physical condition of the party, its equipment, and the terrain and distance involved.

Heat Illness

Localized heat injuries (burns) are described in Chapter 7. Before reading this section, which discusses **generalized heat illness**, please review the section on adapting to the hot environment in Chapter 1.

Generalized heat illness results when the body's heat loss mechanisms are unable to cope with the combination of heat gain from the environment plus internal heat production. This dangerous situation can cause problems in three ways:

1. The body core temperature may rise to dangerous levels *despite normal or increased activity of the heat dissipation mechanisms.* The rise can be caused by excessive environmental heat and humidity or excessive internal heat production (usually due to muscle activity).
2. The body core temperature may rise to dangerous levels *because of faulty heat dissipation.*
3. The body core temperature may be normal or slightly elevated, but the stressed heat dissipation mechanisms may cause illness because of *overactivity, dysfunction, or inadequate replacement of water and electrolytes lost in perspiration.*

Conditions that increase the risk of heat illness include those that:

a. *Increase heat gain* from the environment (large surface-area-to-volume ratios in premature infants and newborns).
b. *Interfere with sweating and the regulation of shell circulation* (extensive burns and widespread skin disorders).
c. *Increase heat production or retention* (overactive thyroid states, excess clothing, muscular overactivity in hot weather).

d. *Interfere with heat transport* from core to shell (old age, heart failure, diabetes, shock, arteriosclerosis, chronic debilitating states, and other causes of poor circulation).

e. *Interfere with normal judgment* (senility, psychosis, drug and alcohol abuse).

Many drugs predispose the user to heat illness by increasing the metabolic rate or interfering with normal sweating, hydration, skin circulation, or body temperature regulation. These drugs include amphetamines, cocaine, hallucinogens, salicylates (aspirin and related compounds), antihistamines, tranquilizers, sedatives, anticholinergics, phenothiazines, antidepressants, and diuretics.

Heat and humidity are a dangerous combination because evaporation of perspiration—a major mechanism of heat loss—is slowed or prevented by high humidity.

There are two types of major heat illness: **heat stroke** and **heat exhaustion**; and two types of minor heat illness: **heat cramps** and **heat syncope**. The division of major heat illness into heat stroke and heat exhaustion is a somewhat arbitrary selection of two points on a continuum; the particular signs and symptoms presented by a given patient ultimately depend on the predominant mechanisms of illness.

Assessment of a Patient with Heat Illness

1. First impression. Suspect heat illness in anyone who becomes ill in a hot environment, particularly if mental status is altered. Institute universal precautions (see Appendix F).
2. Primary survey. Assess level of responsiveness, airway, breathing, and circulation. Care for any urgent problems. Move rapidly to the secondary survey.

3. Assess the pulse, respiratory rate, blood pressure, state of the pupils, and the skin color, temperature, and moisture. If the patient has altered responsiveness, also assess the ability to move and the response to pain and touch. Question the patient or companions about predisposing factors to heat illness, especially concurrent illnesses and drugs being taken.

Heat Stroke

Heat stroke can be divided into two types: **classic** and **exertional**.

Classic heat stroke, seen in the elderly and infirm, is caused by the combination of a hot environment and ineffective mechanisms of heat dissipation. The adverse side effects of the multiple drugs taken by many elderly persons also may be a factor.

Exertional heat stroke is caused by excessive internal heat production from physical activity in warm weather. Wearing too much clothing and lack of acclimatization are frequent contributing factors that hinder heat dissipation. Exertional heat stroke has been common in military recruits and football players and now is being seen in long-distance runners.

Signs and Symptoms of Heat Stroke

1. The skin usually is hot and flushed. Occasionally it is pale or blue, but it always feels hot to the touch.
2. The patient may or may not be perspiring.
3. The pulse is rapid and initially strong; it may become thready later on.
4. The blood pressure may be high, low, or normal.
5. The patient may be confused and complain of weakness, dizziness, headache, and of being very hot.
6. The patient's oral temperature usually is above 105°F (41°C).

7. As the illness progresses, the patient may exhibit:
   a. Signs of injury to the *nervous system*, such as agitation, delirium, stupor, coma, or seizures.
   b. Signs of injury to the *gastrointestinal system*, such as nausea, vomiting, diarrhea, or blood in the stool.
   c. Signs and symptoms of *shock*.
   d. Signs of *bleeding*, because of damaged blood-clotting mechanisms.

Heat stroke is a *true emergency*. The excess heat causes potentially permanent damage to every organ system. The amount of damage is proportional to how high the patient's temperature is and how long it remains elevated.

Emergency Care of a Patient with Heat Stroke

1. Remove the patient from the heat or from direct exposure to the sun.
2. Immediately cool the patient by whatever means are available. Remove heavy clothing; light cotton clothing can be left in place. The fastest method of cooling is to apply ice to the skin. In the hospital emergency department, the patient is loosely covered with a sheet, and cubes of ice from an ice machine are poured over and around the patient (especially between the legs and between the arms and the body). Because ice rarely is available outdoors during environmental conditions that predispose to heat stroke, the most effective cooling method usually is to pour the coldest available water over the patient or to cover the patient (including

the head and neck) with clothing saturated with cold water, and fan him or her to promote evaporative cooling.

Immediate cooling is extremely important and should be started on the spot. *Do not delay*, even if a hospital is nearby. Continue cooling the patient during evacuation and transport. Transport should be in an air-conditioned vehicle if possible. The patient's temperature usually can be brought back to normal within 45 to 60 minutes. To avoid hypothermia, discontinue cooling when the temperature is about one degree above normal.

2. Provide care for unresponsiveness, with particular attention to the airway (see Chapter 12).
3. Frequently assess and record the vital signs, especially body temperature. Watch the patient for a secondary rise in body temperature after cooling has been discontinued.
4. If shock occurs, elevate the patient's lower extremities 12 inches (see Chapter 6).
5. Convulsions and agitation may occur. (These make it difficult to cool the patient).
6. If available, give oxygen in high concentration and flow rate.
7. Transport the patient to a hospital without delay.

Heat Exhaustion

Heat exhaustion is a form of hypovolemic shock caused by varying combinations of excessive sweating, dilation of skin blood vessels, and inadequate replacement of water and electrolytes lost in perspiration.

People who take medications that increase the amount of water and electrolytes lost in the urine (diuretics) may be predisposed to heat exhaustion during periods of hot weather. Other predisposing factors include lack of acclimatization, diseases of the heart and circulatory system, and wearing clothing that is too heavy. Suspect heat exhaustion whenever a person collapses or becomes weak and dizzy in hot weather.

Signs and Symptoms of Heat Exhaustion

1. Thirst, weakness, confusion, cold and clammy skin, a fast or thready pulse, low blood pressure, profuse sweating, restlessness, anxiety, and the other findings typical of hypovolemic shock (see Chapter 6).
2. Blood pressure that may be normal when the patient is lying down but drops when the patient sits up.
3. Normal or slightly elevated body temperature.

Emergency Care of a Patient with Heat Exhaustion

1. Move the patient to a cool environment, and keep the patient lying down until improvement occurs.
2. Remove heavy clothing.
3. If the patient is alert and able to swallow, slowly give up to a quart of an electrolyte-containing commercial sport drink such as Gatorade or Exceed. A solution of a half-teaspoon of table salt dissolved in a quart of tap water can be substituted.
4. If prompt improvement does not occur, transport the patient to a hospital.

Heat Cramps

People who exercise in hot weather can develop heat cramps in active muscles during or after exercise, especially if they replace water without replacing salt lost through perspiration. As much as ⅔ ounce (20 grams) of salt per day can be lost by heavy sweating. The muscles of the abdomen, back, and lower extremities are most frequently involved.

Table 18.3

Summary of Emergency Care of a Patient with Heat Stroke

1. Remove the patient to a cool environment.
2. Immediately cool the patient by any available means.
3. Care for unresponsiveness as needed.
4. Monitor and record the patient's vital signs.
5. Care for shock as needed.
6. Care for convulsions as needed.
7. Give the patient oxygen in high concentration and flow rate.
8. Transport the patient to a hospital; continue cooling en route.

Table 18.4

Summary of Emergency Care of a Patient with Heat Exhaustion

1. Move the patient to cool place.
2. Keep the patient lying down.
3. If the patient is able to swallow, give electrolyte fluids.
4. If improvement is not rapid, transport the patient to a hospital.

Heat cramps can be prevented by drinking electrolyte-containing beverages at regular intervals during strenuous exercise in hot weather. The immediate emergency care for a heat cramp is to massage the muscle and stretch it forcefully in the direction opposite to its contraction. Give the patient a sport drink such as Gatorade or Exceed, or water to which one teaspoon of table salt has been added per quart.

Heat Syncope

Heat Syncope is a mild form of hypovolemic shock that resembles simple fainting (see Chapter 6). It can affect people who sit or stand for long periods in the direct sun or in hot weather. Heat causes an increase in the vascular volume because of increased skin circulation. In addition, the normal return of blood to the heart is partly dependent on muscle action; immobility causes blood to pool in the lower extremities. These mechanisms lead to less blood returning to the heart, a fall in the cardiac output, a drop in blood pressure, insufficient blood to the brain, and, subsequently, fainting.

The signs and symptoms of heat syncope are those of mild, hypovolemic shock (see Chapter 6). Emergency care consists of allowing the patient to lie down and rest in a cool place.

Effects of Altitude and Solar Radiation

With ascent from sea level, solar radiation increases, and environmental temperature, oxygen partial pressure (PO_2), and atmospheric pressure fall. For every 1,000 feet (305 meters) of altitude, the temperature drops about 4°F (2.2°C), the barometric pressure drops 20 mm Hg, and the amount of ultraviolet radiation increases by

about 5 percent. The percentage of oxygen in the air remains constant at 21 percent, but the PO_2 drops so that at 10,000 feet (3,048 meters) only two-thirds of the sea level value remains, and at 18,000 feet (5,486 meters), only half remains.

Acute Mountain Sickness

Before reading this section, please review the section **Oxygen** in Chapter 1.

Ascent to altitude, especially if too rapid to allow acclimatization, has several well-recognized effects on the human body. These are both acute and chronic; the acute ones produce the signs and symptoms of **acute mountain sickness (AMS)**. The effects are due mainly to lack of oxygen, which injures body cells both *directly,* through interference with oxygen-requiring chemical reactions, and *indirectly,* through changes in the circulatory, respiratory, and nervous systems. Cold, fatigue, dehydration, and low barometric pressure also may play a role.

The signs and symptoms of AMS appear to occur in two peaks (Fig. 18.8):

1. An early peak, due to acute hypoxia, that appears soon after altitudes of 7,000 to 8,000 feet (2,134 to 2,438 meters) or higher are reached.

Its severity is related to the rapidity of ascent and the altitude reached. This is called **early AMS**.

2. A later, more serious peak, **advanced AMS**, that appears after a *lag period* of six to 96 hours. This is due to the effect of continued hypoxia in causing certain important changes in the lungs and brain. These changes include the following.
   a. An increase in pulmonary artery pressure due to narrowing of the lung arteries.
   b. Damage to lung capillary walls.
   c. The opening of high pressure shunts in some parts of the lungs.
   d. Brain cell swelling due to cell wall damage.

In the lungs, these changes cause some of the alveoli to fill with fluid, eventually leading to one of the two major, lethal types of AMS: **high altitude pulmonary edema (HAPE)**. In the brain, generalized brain swelling (edema) and increased intracranial pressure eventually lead to the second major, lethal type of AMS: **high altitude cerebral edema (HACE)**.

The signs and symptoms of **early AMS** include fatigue, weakness, headache, loss of appetite, nausea, vomiting, and shortness of breath on exertion. The patient may appear pale

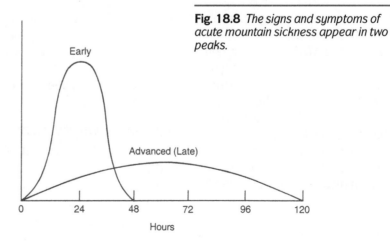

Fig. 18.8 *The signs and symptoms of acute mountain sickness appear in two peaks.*

Fig. 18.8

and ill, and sleep may be difficult for the first night or two. **Periodic breathing** (Cheyne-Stokes respirations) may develop—a condition characterized by regular periods of increasingly deep breathing followed by periods of no breathing during which the patient may stir or awaken with a sense of suffocation. The patient also may hyperventilate (see Chapter 16), which causes symptoms of lightheadedness, dizziness, and tingling of the hands, feet, and mouth.

These distressing symptoms occur in skiers who fly from sea level to the mountains, in mountain hikers, in people traveling in vehicles over high mountain passes, and in passengers in small aircraft without oxygen. The symptoms come on rapidly, and usually disappear quickly upon descent or slowly during one or two days at the same altitude as the affected individual acclimatizes. Rest and a light diet are helpful. Oxygen is useful but generally unnecessary. Occasionally, the symptoms are so severe that the patient must be returned to a lower altitude, usually because of inability to eat or drink due to nausea and vomiting or because of intractable headache.

Recent studies have shown that disturbed sleep at high altitude can be improved by taking one 250-milligram tablet of acetazolamide (Diamox) at bedtime. People who have significant difficulty sleeping at high altitude may wish to consult their physician about obtaining a prescription for this medication.

Advanced AMS is less common than early AMS. The signs and symptoms are similar at first to those of early AMS, but worse. The danger is that one or both of the two major, lethal forms will develop.

HAPE occurs about 10 times more frequently than HACE. Although HAPE has been recognized in the Andes for years, it was largely ignored in North America until 1960, when Dr. Charles Houston reported a case in a cross-country skier and suggested that some patients diagnosed as having pneumonia might have had pulmonary edema instead. Subsequently, extensive studies were carried out by Indian Army physicians in the Himalayas, by Dr. Houston and others on Mount Logan in Canada, and by Dr. Peter Hackett, Dr. Robert Schoene, and others on Mount McKinley.

Advanced AMS has been reported at altitudes as low as 7,500 feet (2,286 meters); however, in the Western Hemisphere, HAPE is uncommon below 12,000 feet (3,658 meters), and HACE is uncommon below 14,000 feet (4,267 meters).

Due to the difficulty in tabulating the total number of people at risk, the incidence of advanced AMS in people who go to altitude is unknown. Dr. Houston has estimated, however, that up to 5 percent of the number of people who go to 12,000 feet or above will develop a dangerous advanced form. This figure is similar to that found in Himalayan trekkers.

Predisposing factors include too rapid ascent, overexertion, and exposure to cold. Children and adolescents seem to be more susceptible than older individuals, but good physical conditioning does not seem to confer immunity to HAPE or HACE. Individuals who automatically hyperventilate at altitude appear to be less susceptible to HAPE and HACE; some high altitude symptoms, such as throbbing headache, can be improved by voluntary hyperventilation. The prevention of AMS has been discussed in Chapter 1.

Signs and Symptoms of the Lethal Types of Advanced AMS

A. High altitude pulmonary edema (HAPE)
  1. Early signs and symptoms:
    a. Dry cough, frequently occurring at night.
    b. Respiratory distress that is made worse by exertion.
    c. Mild chest pain, usually perceived as an ache beneath the sternum.
    d. Weakness.
  2. Later signs and symptoms:
    a. Cyanosis.
    b. Cough that produces large amounts of frothy, pink sputum.
    c. Rapid pulse and respirations.
    d. Audible, gurgling sounds during breathing. When a stethoscope or the ear is placed on the naked chest, wet crackling sounds can be heard when the patient breathes.
    e. Severe respiratory distress.
B. High altitude cerebral edema (HACE)
  1. Early signs and symptoms:
    a. Headache, which is usually throbbing and may be severe.
    b. Nausea and vomiting.
    c. Insomnia.
    d. Cheynes-Stokes respirations.
  2. Later signs and symptoms:
    a. Ataxia (loss of muscle coordination leading to difficulty maintaining balance).
    b. Confusion, which may progress to stupor, coma, and death.
    c. Paralysis of one or more extremities, which may resemble the paralysis seen in stroke.
    d. Blindness.
    e. Convulsions.

HAPE and HACE may occur together, the hypoxia caused by the pulmonary edema tending to make the cerebral edema worse. Many patients with advanced AMS develop retinal hemorrhages, which can be seen with an ophthalmoscope by suitably trained individuals. The patient usually is not aware of the hemorrhages unless they are present in the part of the retina responsible for sharpest vision (macula).

The most important impediment to early recognition of HAPE and HACE is their *insidious onset.* Early signs and symptoms frequently go unrecognized or are ignored by patients and their companions, who also may be suffering from some degree of AMS. By the time a serious problem is suspected, nightfall or bad weather may make evacuation to a lower altitude difficult.

Table 18.5

Summary of the Signs and Symptoms of HAPE and HACE

HAPE
  Cough, respiratory distress, mild chest pain.
  Weakness.
  Later:
  Cyanosis, severe cough with abundant sputum.
  Rapid pulse, severe respiratory distress.
  Audible gurgling sounds in the chest.
HACE
  Headache, nausea, vomiting.
  Insomnia.
  Cheynes-Stokes respirations.
  Later:
  Altered responsiveness
  Paralysis, blindness, convulsions.

Assessment of a Patient With AMS

1. Consider AMS in anyone who is not feeling well at altitudes of 7,000 to 8,000 feet (2,134 to 2,438 meters) or above.
2. Assess the vital signs, especially the pulse and respiratory rate. Compare these with those of other members of the party.
3. Early recognition depends on careful questioning of the patient. Ask about headache, nausea, vomiting, and shortness of breath. Assess the level of responsiveness, and if it is decreased, assess ability to move and perception of pain and touch.
4. Listen to the chest with your ear against the patient's bare skin, or use a stethoscope if one is available. Listen for abnormal sounds such as rattles, wheezes, and bubbly sounds.
5. Assess for ataxia by seeing if the patient can pass the "drunk driver" test: have the patient walk a straight line with one foot in front of the other, the toe touching the heel, or have the patient get up on the knees from a recumbent position without swaying.

Emergency Care of a Patient with Severe or Advanced AMS

1. Descent. The most common practical problem seems to be distinguishing patients with moderately severe, early AMS or mild advanced AMS (that may improve with rest alone) from those with a potentially severe advanced form who require immediate evacuation to a lower altitude.

Symptoms appearing early on the first day of attaining altitude are more likely to be caused by acute hypoxia. A day or two of rest at the *same* altitude (do *not* go any higher) may be appropriate for mildly affected patients *if* their symptoms are not progressive, *if* help is available to carry them down, and *if* they can be carefully observed the entire time, including during the night.

Signs and symptoms that mandate *immediate descent* include the following:
  a. Ataxia.
  b. Audible, bubbly sounds in the chest.
  c. Cyanosis.
  d. Inability to eat or drink due to nausea and vomiting that lasts for more than a few hours.
  e. A rapid pulse or respiratory rate compared to other members of the party, especially if the sign persists after rest.
  f. A sharp decline in general fitness, which is most likely to be seen on the afternoon of the second or third day at altitude.

Descent should be at least 2,000 feet (610 meters) below the initial altitude and preferably to below 10,000 feet (3,048 meters). Descend early, when you first start thinking about it and while the patient can still walk. If the patient can no longer walk, carry him or her in a sitting position.

These guidelines are not absolute. If there is any question about whether to evacuate, always evacuate.

The risk of severe, advanced AMS is quite low after the fifth day at altitude, but symptoms still can be precipitated by stresses such as swimming in a cold stream, a hard fall, hypothermia, or a respiratory infection.
2. Oxygen in high concentration causes temporary improvement but is rarely available outside of first aid facilities or large expeditions. However, because oxygen supplies are always limited, oxygen use should not delay preparations for descent.

Table 18.6

Summary of Emergency Care of a Patient with Advanced AMS

1. Recognize the problem and stop further ascent.
2. Descend rapidly.
3. Give the patient oxygen in high concentration, if available.
4. Keep the patient in the most comfortable position.
5. Treat headache with mild analgesics.
6. Give care for unresponsiveness, if necessary.

3. Allow the patient to stay in the most comfortable position, usually sitting up or lying with the head elevated.
4. Treat headache with a non-prescription medication. Aspirin is preferable to acetaminophen.
5. If the patient becomes unresponsive, provide care for unresponsiveness as described in Chapter 12.
6. A small, portable, hyperbaric chamber, the Gamow bag (Fig. 18.9), has recently been developed and used successfully on many Himalayan expeditions. It weighs about 15 pounds (6.8 kilograms), is big enough to hold a large patient, and is designed for use at ski resorts or expedition advance base camps. The Gamow bag consists of a cylinder-shaped bag of air-tight nylon that opens with a zipper and inflates with a foot or hand pump. It allows the patient to be pressurized 2 to 4 pounds per square inch (PSI) above atmospheric pressure within about six minutes. This is equivalent to a drop in altitude of up to 10,000 feet.
7. A number of drugs are available that have some value in the prevention and treatment of AMS but do not replace descent. They are discussed in Appendix C.

Sunburn, Windburn, and Snowblindness

Humans are more vulnerable to the harmful effects of solar radiation when at high altitudes, on snow, or on bodies of water. This is because exposure is increased by reflection of sunlight from snow or water, while the thin clear atmosphere at higher altitudes filters out fewer of the harmful, ultraviolet rays.

Injury to the skin and eyes is more likely to occur on cloudy days when people often forget to protect themselves, and during the longer days of spring and summer.

Sunburn is a first- or second-degree skin burn caused by ultraviolet light in the medium-wave range (UVB), with a wavelength of 290 to 320 nanometers. Repeated sun exposure over many years may lead to chronic degenerative skin changes such as wrinkling, darkening, thickening, and cancer. These changes, which resemble accelerated changes of aging, can be delayed by avoiding excessive sun exposure and using proper skin protection.

Fig. 18.9 *Gamow Bag*

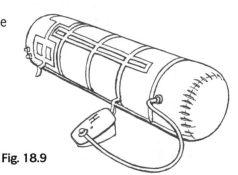

Fig. 18.9

The skin can be protected by clothing or topical sunscreens. Sunscreen preparations come in two basic types: **physical** and **chemical**. Physical sunscreens block sunlight mechanically. They consist of opaque greases containing zinc oxide, talc, or titanium dioxide, and are particularly suitable for limited areas such as the nose and lips. Chemical sunscreens rely on chemical agents to selectively filter out harmful rays. The most effective products now available contain para-amino-benzoic acid (PABA) and its derivatives, benzophenones, cinnamates, salicylates, and oxybenzone. Some preparations contain both physical and chemical sunscreens.

Skin types can be classified into four to six groups according to degree of sun sensitivity. People with type I skin (blue eyes, fair skin, freckles) burn easily and never tan, while those with type IV skin (Hispanics, Asians) tan easily and rarely burn. Types II and III (blonde and brunette Caucasians) fall in between.

Most manufacturers of sunscreen creams, lotions, and lip salves now specify the sun protection factor (SPF) on the label. This number, usually from 2 to 50, refers to how much longer skin protected with the product can be exposed to the sun before becoming red as compared to unprotected skin. People with type I skin should use products with SPF numbers higher than 15; those with type II to III, SPF 8 to 15; those with type IV, SPF 6 to 8. Those with type V skin (Asian and American Indians) and type VI skin (Blacks) rarely need any protection. For practical purposes, maximal protection is given by topicals with SPF 18 to 20; little or no additional benefit is conferred by those with higher numbers.

Because sunscreens with a cream or grease base are better at preventing frostbite and windburn than alcohol-based preparations, they are preferable for use by skiers, high-altitude climbers, and others exposed to cold and wind as well as sunlight. Apply a sunscreen one to two hours before sun exposure and re-apply several times during the day, particularly if sweating is heavy.

Care for sunburn by removing the patient from exposure and applying cool compresses. Later, soothing ointments are useful to control discomfort. A physician should be consulted if the sunburn is extensive or if the skin is blistered.

Windburn is an irritation of the skin that resembles a first-degree sunburn. It is partly due to the drying effect of the low humidity at high altitudes. It can be prevented to some extent by wearing a face mask or by applying a greasy sunscreen. Treat windburn by applying soothing, greasy ointments or lotions. (Greasy sunscreens are useful for both prevention and treatment.)

Snowblindness, which is sunburn of the conjunctiva of the eye, can be prevented by wearing suitable dark glasses or goggles. Because radiation can reach the eye by reflection from the snow, these should have extensions on each side and below (ski goggles, "glacier" glasses or goggles). Dark gray lenses are best; they should transmit only 10 to 15 percent of light. Goggles should be adequately ventilated and have easily replaceable lenses. A separate set of yellow or red lenses is desirable to increase contrast in flat light.

Symptoms of snowblindness develop six to 12 hours after exposure. The eyes feel irritated ("sand in the eye") and are sensitive to light, the conjunctivae are reddened, and there is excessive tearing, swelling around the eye, and pain on eye motion. Emergency care includes covering the eyes or putting the patient in a dark room, applying cool compresses, and using nonprescription pain relievers. In severe cases, the patient should see a physician; medication may be prescribed to relieve the pain and speed healing.

Lightning and Electrical Injury

High-voltage electrical current represents a significant hazard in modern society because of the large number of electrical appliances and their ubiquitous power sources. Each year there are approximately 1,000 deaths from electrocution (including 100 deaths from lightning) in the United States and many more cases of severe electrical burns.

In the outdoors, people are susceptible to injury from lightning during electrical storms and from high voltage power lines, which can be found even in remote areas. Ski areas use large amounts of electric power, and chair lifts are susceptible to lightning strikes, particularly in late spring.

Rescuers need to know how to protect themselves from the dangers of electricity, especially lightning, and how to care for patients injured by electricity.

Ways in which Electricity Causes Injury

1. Injury to the respiratory control center in the brain may stop breathing.
2. Cardiac arrest (ventricular fibrillation or cessation of heart activity [asystole]) can occur from a direct effect on the heart. Alternating current tends to cause ventricular fibrillation while direct current (including lightning) causes asystole.
3. Direct effects on the nervous and musculoskeletal systems can cause pain, paralysis, blindness, numbness, weakness, loss of hearing or speech, and unresponsiveness.
4. Direct effects on the skin, muscles, and internal organs can cause severe, deep burns. Since an electric current tends to travel easily along blood vessels, significant internal damage may be overlooked at first if surface burns are unimpressive.
5. The current can cause strong muscular contractions that throw the patient off balance and can cause injury due to falls.
6. Secondary kidney injury may occur because the kidneys are overloaded with the breakdown products of blood and injured muscle.

Lightning is caused by violent vertical air currents associated with the development of cumulonimbus clouds ("thunderheads"). These are huge, billowing vertical clouds with anvil-shaped tops that may tower to 60,000 feet or more (Fig. 18.10). The air currents produce differences of electrical potential between clouds or between a cloud and the earth. Cumulonimbus clouds usually produce large raindrops, huge snowflakes, or hail; they

---

Fig. 18.10 *Cumulonimbus Cloud*

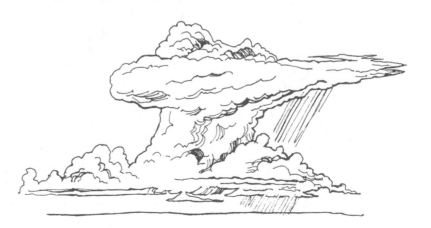

Fig. 18.10

tend to develop during the afternoon or evening in hot, sultry weather. They also can be part of an advancing cold front.

Lightning causes injury in the same way as any other direct electric current, except that the duration of the bolt is so short (.0001 to .001 second) that burns are less severe. The fatality rate in lightning strikes is about 30 percent. A person struck by lightning may suffer a characteristic superficial skin burn that has a pattern resembling a fern leaf (Fig. 18.11). In addition to direct strikes, people may be injured by ground currents and side flashes from nearby strikes. Strikes often cause a person's clothing to explode off the body by instantly converting perspiration or other moisture to steam.

A patient injured by electricity who has not been thrown clear by the jolt must be removed from the source of the current before emergency care can be given. The only safe way to do this is to shut off the power source. The danger to the rescuer is so great that only those with special training and equipment should attempt to remove a hot wire directly from a patient.

Because rubber tires provide good insulation, people trapped in a vehicle near a fallen power line are safe as long as they remain inside the vehicle. If the occupants must be evacuated before the power can be shut off, they should be instructed to jump out, taking care to avoid touching the vehicle and the ground at the same time.

Assessment and Emergency Care of a Patient with an Electrical Injury

1. Because of the danger to the rescuer and the high frequency of pulmonary or cardiopulmonary arrest in the patient who has suffered electrical burns, the first impression, primary survey, and basic life support (see Chapter 4 and Appendix B) are of special importance. Institute universal precautions (see Appendix F). Open the airway with care because of the chance that the patient could have a neck injury from a fall. Because damage to the circulatory and respiratory systems usually is temporary and the patient may be capable of full recovery, continue CPR as long as possible. Give oxygen at high concentration and flow rate if available.

   CPR and rescue breathing are more successful in victims of electric shock, particularly lightning strike, than in patients with other types of cardiac and respiratory arrest. Therefore, in contrast to the usual triage process (Chapter 22), in a multiple-victim accident, patients who are apparently dead should be cared for *first*. Breathing, in particular, may be restored after prolonged respiratory arrest, so do not give up prematurely.

2. The secondary survey is that of the unresponsive patient (see Chapters 4 and 12), with special attention to the vital signs, ability to move, perception of pain, and assessing for burns, wounds, fractures, and other evidence of trauma.

3. Give care for altered responsiveness (see Chapter 12).

4. Dress burns and other wounds, and splint fractures.

5. Take the patient to a hospital as soon as possible.

Prevention of Electrical Injury

Most substances can be divided into **conductors** and **insulators**. Conductors transmit electric currents; insulators resist their flow. Most metals and objects that are wet or contain water (including the human body) are good conductors. Because electric currents tend to follow paths of least resistance, a person can be injured

Fig. 18.11 *Fern Leaf Pattern of a Lightning Burn*

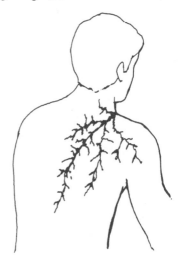

Fig. 18.11

Table 18.7

Summary of Assessment and Emergency Care of a Patient with an Electrical Injury

1. Be aware of possible dangers.
2. Perform a rapid and thorough first impression and primary survey.
3. Give basic life support.
4. Consider the possibility of neck injury and other injuries from falling.
5. Give oxygen at high concentration and flow rate.
6. Give care for altered responsiveness as needed.
7. Perform the secondary survey and care for additional injuries, if present.
8. Monitor and record vital signs at regular intervals.
9. Do not give up too soon on CPR or rescue breathing.
10. Take the patient to a hospital.

when a body part is accidentally positioned in line with such a path so that a circuit is completed. Most urban electrical injuries result from faulty electrical equipment, careless use of appliances, or accidental contact with a power line. Handling an electrical appliance while sitting in a bathtub is particularly dangerous.

Lightning is the main electrical hazard in remote areas. If caught in an electrical storm, avoid bodies of water and take shelter away from high points, exposed ridges, solitary trees, and trees taller than surrounding trees, since all of these attract lightning strikes. If swimming or in a small boat (especially a sailboat), return to shore at the first threat of a storm. Avoid telephones and other electrical appliances during storms. Stay out of small caves where body parts are close to the walls or ceiling, since ground currents may flow through the body instead of taking a longer course along the cave wall. Large buildings and enclosed vehicles usually are safe.

If caught in the open, retreat as far down on the side of a ridge or other exposed area as possible, and move away from ice axes, ski poles, and other metal objects. If golfing, remove cleated shoes. Squat on your heels until the danger is over. This position shortens the body and minimizes ground contact, decreasing the tendency for the body to act as a lightning rod and making it less likely that ground currents will pass through it.

During electrical storms at alpine ski areas, ski lifts and exposed summit structures should be cleared of skiers. Avoid metal structures such as lift towers.

Fig. 18.12 *Rescue Breathing Performed on an Avalanche Victim*

Avalanche Injuries

Even if uncovered within the first half hour after burial, an avalanche victim has less than a 50 percent chance of being alive. If found alive, the patient will be suffering from suffocation and frequently from hypothermia, frostbite, shock, and trauma as well.

As soon as the patient's head is uncovered, open the airway and start rescue breathing unless the patient is breathing spontaneously (Fig. 18.12). Water, snow, blood, and/or vomitus usually must be removed before the airway can be cleared. A portable suction unit is useful under these circumstances and is included in most avalanche rescue caches. A patient in cardiac arrest must be fully uncovered or removed from the burial site before CPR can be given.

Meanwhile, add insulating materials over and around the patient to prevent further heat loss. Although the patient almost always is hypothermic, rewarming usually is impossible during CPR. Give oxygen in high concentration and flow rate, if available.

After breathing and circulation have been restored, perform the secondary survey, manage hypothermia as described previously in this chapter, and treat any fractures or other injuries using the usual techniques.

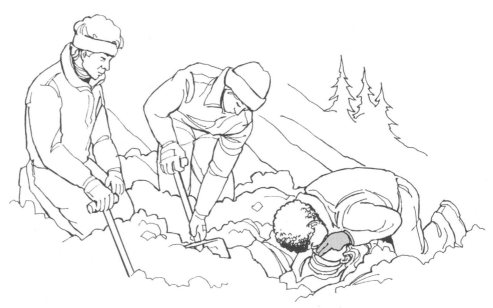

Fig. 18.12

Scenario #18 (Fig. 18.13)

The following scenario illustrates the assessment and emergency care of a patient with a typical environmental emergency.

You have had a busy weekend day as hill chief. It is 5 p.m. and you are waiting for the Midway sweep chief to come off his station so the hill can be closed. There is a commotion outside and the area manager enters accompanied by a worried teenager. "Ben," he says, "This is Sophie Moore. Her boyfriend skied out of bounds off the side of upper Big Elk run around 3 p.m. and hasn't come back. She was supposed to meet him at the cafeteria an hour ago. I'm afraid we need an off-area rescue. The sheriff has asked the patrol to run it."

Nodding your head in agreement, you proceed to question the girl. You find that her boyfriend, Hart Dogge, aged 17, is an expert skier who prefers powder to skipack. He is in good health and good physical condition. They had lunch together and he ate a large meal. He has done some summer backpacking but has had no special training in winter camping or cold weather survival. He was wearing blue jeans, a turtleneck shirt, a pair of ski gloves, and a quilted ski parka, but no hat. She does not think he was carrying any matches or other emergency gear. She was with him when he left the side of the run and followed him about 100 yards before deciding that she had better traverse back to the run. She can show you where they left the run. She wanted him to come back with her, but he insisted on continuing and said he would meet her later at the lodge.

Quickly, you round up two senior patrollers who have taken the advanced ski mountaineering course and brief them on the problem. You place the assistant hill chief in charge of selecting the backup party and someone to cover the radio at the base. You send a patroller after some candy bars from the base lodge and start getting the off-area backpacks and the Heatpak unit out of the off-area cache. You forgot your mountaineering skis, but it sounds like alpine gear will work all right since the topography is all downhill from upper Big Elk to the road. There is a fiberglass Akja toboggan at the summit, and if you can locate the boy it can probably be brought down to transport him if needed.

It is dusk as nine patrollers and the girlfriend get on the lower chair, headed for the top. It is 18°F and the forecast is clear and cold. The plan is for three patrollers to stay at the summit with a radio and the Akja, two to ski all the way down Big Elk looking for tracks coming back into the ski area,

Fig. 18.13 *Scenario #18*

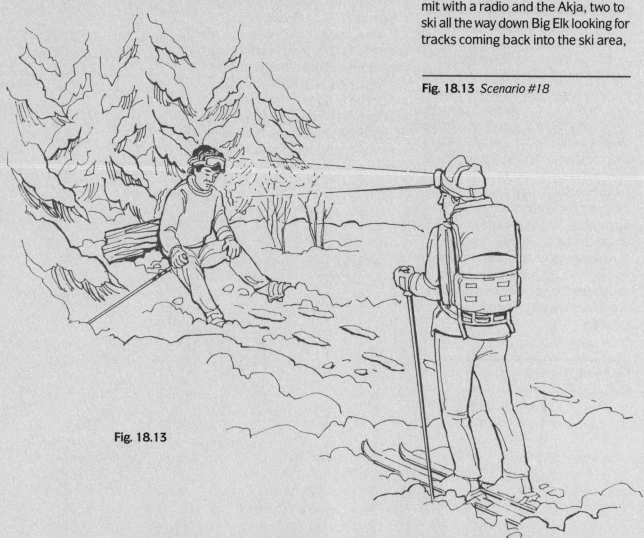

Fig. 18.13

and one to go back down with the girl after she shows you where the boy went. The other three patrollers will follow the boy's tracks. The sheriff's deputies will patrol the road to find the boy if he eventually skis out by himself.

The girl points out where she and her boyfriend skied under the boundary rope on the right-hand side of the run, and there are only their two tracks to follow. You and the other two patrollers turn on your headlamps and ski one after the other down through the dense timber, following the tracks. It is 6 p.m. In a few minutes one set of tracks turns back and starts traversing back toward the run—obviously the girl's tracks.

After about a half hour it is pitch dark. You are down in a deep valley between two ridges and it is getting more level. The tracks continue ahead of you. This boy was definitely a good powder skier; no sign that he has fallen down. After another 15 minutes you are reduced to walking through the deep snow. You report your position at intervals to the summit by radio. The timber is thicker; in some places you can barely get between the small lodgepole pine trees. The tracks start turning to the left, going back uphill. You see some places where the snow is disturbed—the boy probably fell down. He was tiring, and decided to try to climb back up to the run.

Following the tracks uphill is getting harder and harder, and you are getting hungry. You three stop, take your climbing skins from the off-area packs, put them on your skis, and each have a candy bar before continuing.

Suddenly, you find two skis in the snow. He has taken off his skis and started to walk directly uphill in the deep snow. Thank goodness he did not leave his poles, too. You suspect you will find him soon. You report this finding to the summit by radio. In a few minutes, you find you have to take your own skis off in order to follow his trail

because it is so steep. You strap the skis to your packs and steady yourselves with your poles. It is 7 p.m.

The three of you, even though in excellent shape, are breathing heavily as you fight your way uphill through the deep snow. Finally, you reach the top of the ridge and find yourselves in a flat clearing. You put on your skis again and follow the foot-trail in the snow. It is starting to wander from side to side. He is getting tired. You know where you are—in the clearing that drops off from the middle dogleg on Big Elk run, about a quarter mile below the dogleg. He must have been very disappointed not to find the run when he reached the top of the ridge. He would have to climb the next ridge to reach it from here and probably does not have enough strength left. You report the situation to the summit by radio.

Up ahead, you see a dark object in the snow between two trees. The tracks lead to it. Excitedly, you race up to the object. Your headlight beam catches a white face with tousled dark hair. The boy is sitting in the snow, leaning against a log, shivering occasionally. You glance at your watch: it is 8 p.m.

You: "Hello, Hart, are you okay? I'm Ben Schussen from the High Range Ski Patrol."

Patient: (weakly) "Hi, I'm pretty cold."

You: "Well, we're going to get you warmed up and give you a ride down to the road" (assessing the patient's pulse. It is somewhat weak, regular, and 40 beats per minute. His respirations are eight per minute).

You: "Let's take your temperature. Do you think you can keep this in your mouth for a few minutes?"

Patient: "Okay."

You: (taking the hypothermia thermometer out of its case, you shake the mercury down, and place the tip under the patient's tongue.) "Keep your lips tight around this, please."

(You pause and press the radio transmission key) "Schussen to Summit, copy?" (Summit replies.) "We have a 10-23. Need the toboggan. Bring it down to the middle dogleg on Big Elk run, but instead of going to the left, go straight down off area, headed for the road. You'll pick up our tracks in about 400 yards." (Summit confirms.)

You open the off-area pack and take out a waterproof, fleece-lined casualty bag, a long Therm-a-Rest pad, and the Heatpak. One of the other patrollers is digging a small trench to get the patient out of the wind, and the other is gathering wood for a fire. You inflate the pad and place it in the snow, laying the casualty bag on it. Then you look at the thermometer. It reads 91°F. This means a core (rectal) temperature of 92°F. That is cold but not too cold.

You and one of the other patrollers gently help the patient into the casualty bag. His inner clothes are wet with sweat, but the bag is water- and windproof. You assemble the Heatpak, placing a cartridge into the chamber and turning the reversed D cell around so it will power the fan. You light the fuse; a cloud of smoke pours out for a minute and then the device settles down with a hum. You attach the Y-shaped split tubing and push it up under the patient's T-shirt, placing the combustion chamber in its insulated container on his upper thighs. You lace up the casualty bag.

By this time the fire is blazing at one end of the trench. You carefully slide the patient on the pad into the other end of the trench and place a folded space blanket between the fire and the snow so that it reflects the fire's heat toward the patient. His breathing has speeded up and he is more alert.

You: "Do you feel any better now?"

Patient: "I'm starting to feel warmer."

You: "The toboggan will be here shortly."

In about 30 minutes two patrollers can be heard thrashing the heavy toboggan through the dense timber. After they arrive, it takes only a few minutes to load the patient into the toboggan, put out the fire, and start off downhill. As you approach the road, you see the lights of several cars ahead, one of them a sheriff's vehicle with its light-bar flashing red and blue.

The patient and Akja are loaded into a carryall and taken up to the patrol room, about 2 miles away. His parents and Sophie are waiting for him. By the time you arrive, the patient is awake, alert, talking well, and feeling a lot better. His oral temperature is 96°F. It is 9 p.m.

It takes you half an hour to debrief. The patient is sent home with his parents, somewhat subdued when he realizes he will lose his season pass for this episode. The parents are instructed to check in with the emergency department of a nearby hospital when they arrive home. You have a 90-minute drive before you get home yourself and have to be at work at 8 a.m. the next day.

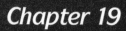

Chapter 19

Advanced
Assessment

Life is short, the art long,
opportunity fleeting, experience treacherous, judgment
difficult.

—Hippocrates Aphorisms I.i

The preceding chapters of this textbook present basic assessment as a relatively rigid protocol to be memorized, practiced, and performed with little leeway for variation. Thus, a reliable framework for examination is presented into which changes due to injury and illness can be incorporated. However, the result is that the reader learns techniques of assessment before learning the changes he or she is supposed to be looking for. This is partly resolved as each new chapter introduces new injuries and illnesses. Now that the reader has a better idea of what to look for, it is time to reexamine the process of assessment, not with the intention of learning many new techniques or changing old ones, but emphasizing what may be found and what it means.

Before reading further, please review Chapter 4.

In the basic assessment algorithm, a major branching point is whether the patient is **responsive** or **unresponsive** (Table 19.1). In the primary survey, assessment and early emergency care of the unresponsive patient (Table 19.2) is similar regardless of whether the unresponsiveness is caused by trauma or by a medical illness. This is because of the overwhelming need for the rescuer to work rapidly, do things in the right order, and give the necessary emergency care for life-threatening disturbances in the respiratory, circulatory, and nervous systems that are common to severe illnesses and injuries.

In the assessment of the responsive patient (Table 19.3), whether the patient is **injured** or has a **medical illness** becomes a major branching point for both assessment and care.

When first notified of someone who needs help, the rescuer may be told what is wrong, i.e., "There is a skier with a hurt knee down on Big Elk Run." Or, you may be told only that "there is a skier down over in the trees on right side of Little Elk Run." In any case, from this point on you start to formulate your first impression, (also called the "scene survey"), which continues to expand from the time you first catch sight of the scene until you are at the patient's side.

You may be able to select which limbs of the algorithm branches to follow as soon as you register the first impression; early into the primary survey you certainly will know which responsiveness branch to follow, but you may have to wait well into the secondary survey before choosing the injury or the illness branch.

The patient's initial location and physical position usually can provide some indication of what happened, whether the patient and/or potential rescuers are in any danger, whether the patient has obviously suffered an injury rather than an illness, and what type of injury to suspect. For example, an unconscious patient wrapped around a tree at the side of a ski run (Fig. 19.1a) or someone who is lying crumpled on a narrow cliff ledge (Fig. 19.1b) is more likely to have been injured than one who has collapsed in a cafeteria (Fig. 19.1c). In the case of a man smelling strongly of alcohol and lying unconscious in an alley behind a bar, the picture is less clear—he may be both ill and injured (Fig. 19.1d).

Do not succumb to the temptation to attribute everything you see to the most obvious cause. Remember that mistakes in emergency care are due more frequently to *lack of thoroughness* than to *lack of knowledge*.

Table 19.1

First Part of Primary Survey

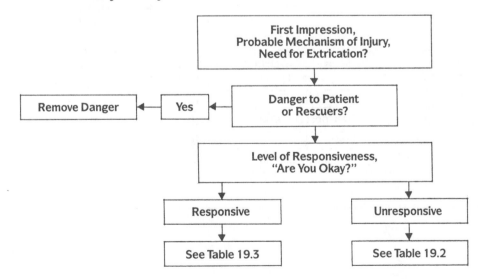

Table 19.2

Primary Survey of Unresponsive Patient

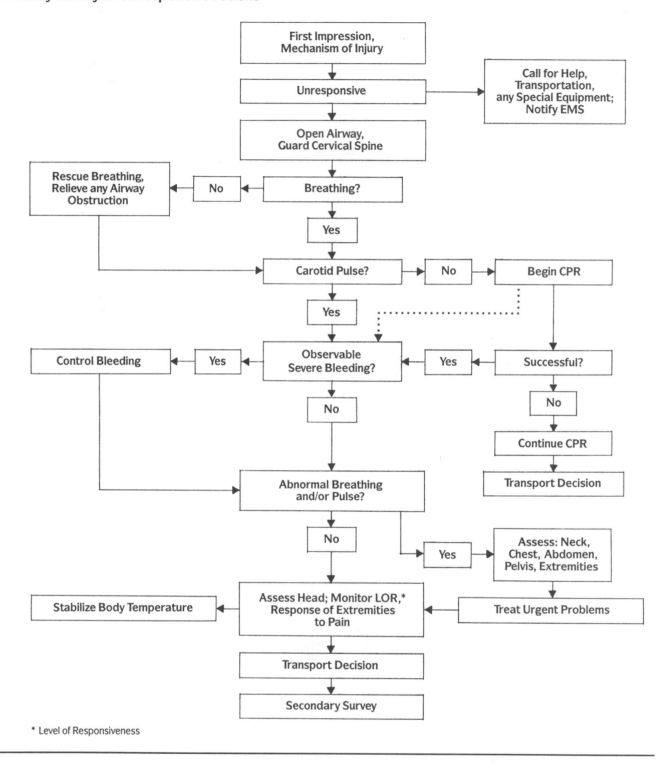

* Level of Responsiveness

Table 19.3

Primary Survey of Responsive Patient

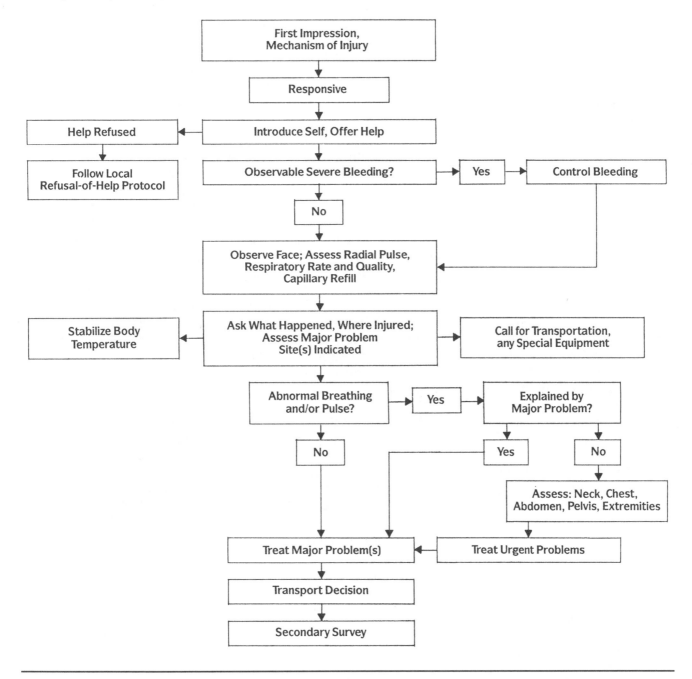

Although clearly injured, the first patient mentioned above may also be a diabetic who skipped lunch, then lost his coordination and skied off the side of the run because of a drop in his blood sugar. The second patient may be an epileptic who fell because he had a seizure while scrambling up a small face. The third patient may have fractured his neck when a sudden disturbance in his heart rhythm caused him to collapse in the cafeteria. The fourth patient may have had a few drinks, been mugged after leaving the bar, and now has an enlarging subdural hematoma of the brain because of a blow on the head.

Hazards to the patient and rescuer are fairly uncommon, but should be considered whenever providing emergency care. They include the following:

1. Environmental hazards such as stormy weather or excessive heat or cold.

2. The danger of falling from an insecure location.
3. Traffic from snow vehicles, land vehicles, and skiers.
4. Structural collapses in natural or man-made disasters.
5. Rockfall or snow avalanche.
6. Rising water.

In the above example, the skier at the side of the ski run is likely in little danger from other skiers or snowmachines, but may be developing hypothermia. The patient on the ledge may be in danger of falling off the ledge or being struck by rockfall (as may the rescuer). The patient in the cafeteria probably is in little danger, aside from his medical condition. The danger to the patient in the alley may be mainly from rescuers who assume he is merely drunk and overlook his head injury.

Despite these preexisting or complicating conditions, the initial emergency care of each patient follows the protocol described in Chapter 4 in the sections **First Impression** and **Primary Survey**. This initial care has a good chance of success because disturbances in airway, breathing, circulation, blood vessel integrity (leading to hemorrhage), central nervous system function, and body temperature are common to many serious illnesses and injuries, and *are cared for in the same way, regardless of cause.*

In the secondary survey, the rescuer should detect any preexisting conditions in a properly conducted interview of the patient or relatives and discover or at least suspect *all* current injuries and illnesses during the whole-body assessment. Remember, what you see at the moment often is the result of inheritance, environment, and lifestyle over many years of life, modified by the effects of the latest episode.

During the first impression, it is important to note your own location relative to the patient's location. This will help you predict any difficulty in reaching the patient, particularly if you are pulling a toboggan or carrying a litter. As you get closer, you can usually tell whether the patient is either **obviously responsive** or **possibly unresponsive**, and you should be able to spot any **blood** on the snow or ground.

You probably will not be able to tell if the patient is **partly responsive**, **definitely unresponsive**, or whether an unresponsive patient is **breathing** until the primary survey begins. Be sure to institute universal precautions (see Appendix F), especially in the case of trauma or obvious bleeding. This means putting on a pair of rubber gloves, at a minimum, and having your pocket mask or mouth shield handy before starting the primary survey.

This chapter examines assessment step by step, noting possible abnormalities that may be found and discussing what they may mean. The assessment of the patient with an illness will be discussed in detail. The primary survey of the unresponsive patient has been covered thoroughly in Chapter 4 and will not be repeated here. Also, to avoid repetition, the secondary surveys of both **responsive** and **unresponsive** patients will be discussed together; it will be assumed that the reader knows a patient with altered mental status may not respond to questions or commands and may not indicate that a body area is injured except by moaning or flinching when the part is touched or moved.

Always remember that an injured or ill patient may vomit. In an unresponsive patient, vomiting is a serious complication since vomitus that is not expelled completely may block the airway or be aspirated into the lungs. A hand-operated or portable battery-operated suction device is invaluable, but you usually will not have one with

Fig. 19.1 *The patient's location and physical position help the rescuer form the first impression.*

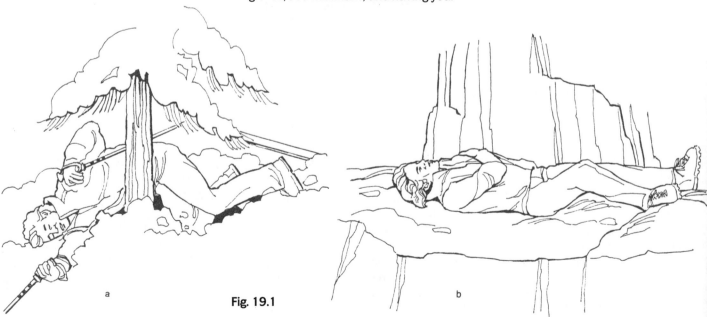

a

Fig. 19.1

b

you when you first arrive at the scene. However, if retching occurs, roll the patient immediately to the side, using the one-rescuer logroll (see Fig. 12.4, Chapter 12).

A primary goal of assessment is to determine whether the patient has any illness or injury that represents a "threat to life or limb." Such illnesses and injuries include the following (not listed in order of importance):

A. Immediate or potential **"threat to life"**:
   1. Head injury, especially with altered responsiveness of five minutes or more, or an open skull fracture.
   2. Unresponsiveness due to any cause.
   3. Shock due to any cause.
   4. Fracture of the femur, pelvis, or of two or more long bones.
   5. Flail chest, sucking chest wound, tension pneumothorax, or any other chest injury with respiratory distress.
   6. Any illness with respiratory distress.
   7. Cervical spine injury, especially with paralysis, loss of sensation, shock, or labored breathing.
   8. Open wound of the abdomen.
   9. Traumatic amputation of the arm, forearm, thigh, or leg.
   10. Crush injury of the abdomen or pelvis.
   11. Heart attack, especially with cardiac arrest.
   12. Stroke.
   13. Anaphylactic shock.
   14. Internal bleeding.
B. Less serious illnesses and injuries representing the danger of **serious disability**, or **"threat to limb"**:
   1. Major eye injuries.
   2. Injury to the blood or nerve supply to an extremity.
   3. Crushing injury to an extremity.
   4. Hip, knee, or ankle dislocation.
   5. Fractures or fracture-dislocations near the elbow or knee.
   6. Open fractures.
   7. Back injury, especially with weakness, paralysis, or loss of sensation.

After identifying an injury or illness that represents a threat to life or a danger of serious disability, transport the patient as soon as initial emergency care and splinting have been performed and the patient is stable, and arrange for an ambulance or helicopter to provide rapid transport to a hospital.

Primary Survey of the Responsive Patient

In the primary survey, as described in Chapter 4, approach the patient, make eye contact, introduce yourself by giving your name and the name of your organization, and ask if you can be of help.

If the patient accepts help, the first priority is to institute universal precautions if there appears to be any chance of contact with the patient's blood or other secretions (see Appendix F). Next, control any obvious hemorrhage. Then, ask the patient, "What's wrong?" or "What happened?" The patient usually will respond by telling you the chief complaint. Conduct the following actions while listening:

1. Grasp the patient's wrist, assessing the rate, rhythm, and strength of the radial pulse.
2. Note the temperature, color, and moisture of the skin of the wrist.
3. Assess the capillary refill time.
4. Note the respiratory rate and any cough or labored breathing.
5. Listen for any abnormal sounds connected with breathing.
6. Inspect the patient's face for facial expression, skin color, and moisture.

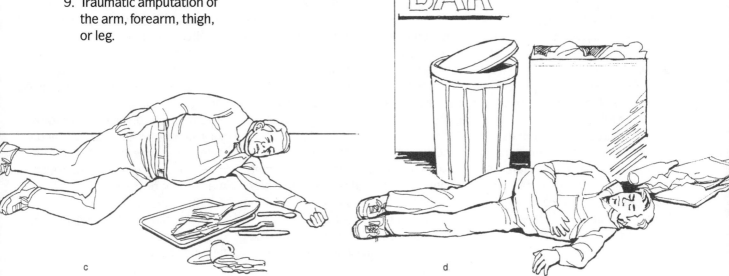

7. Note the patient's vocal inflections and emotional state.

A patient in pain will have an expression of anxiety or discomfort. A patient with severe pain or a significant illness usually will be pale and sweaty as well. A normal pulse and breathing rate will help distinguish the patient with a lesser injury or illness from one with a severe, painful, or life-threatening one. By this time you also will have established whether the patient probably does or does not have an adequate airway, breathing, circulation, and level of responsiveness, and whether there is any visible bleeding.

If the chief complaint leads you to suspect a possible neck or back injury, caution the patient not to move, and stabilize the head and neck as well as possible considering the amount of help available and other, more urgent considerations.

In the **injured** patient, first assess the site of injury. Then, if the patient has labored breathing or a fast, irregular, and/or weak pulse that not are explained by the initial injury, immediately assess the head, neck, and chest. If changes in breathing and pulse still are not explained, assess the abdomen, pelvis, and extremities in a search for additional serious injuries or evidence of external or internal bleeding. If you suspect a **head injury**, assess the patient's head and neck, the state of the pupils, and the ability to move the extremities and feel touch and pain (see **Secondary Survey of the Unresponsive Patient** below). Monitor the level of responsiveness, the state of the pupils, ability to move, and response to touch and pain at regular intervals.

In the patient with an **illness**, it is more important to explore in detail the patient's chief complaint(s) and medical history before moving further into the survey. Ask the patient how long it has been since he or she felt entirely well, and try to reconstruct in chronological order the events leading up to the illness. The most important signs and symptoms of illness are **pain** in some area (including headache), **fever**, and **variation from normal body functions**, usually of the circulatory, respiratory, gastrointestinal, and/or genitourinary systems.

Significant symptoms that arise from these variations include weakness or severe fatigue, unexplained weight loss, fever or chills (usually described as the sensation of being hot or cold), sore throat, runny nose, earache, cough, chest pain, shortness of breath, pus in the sputum or in the nasal discharge, palpitations, pain or difficulty on swallowing, loss of appetite, heartburn, sour stomach, nausea, vomiting, diarrhea, change in bowel habits, abdominal pain or cramps, painful urination, and blood in the bowel movements or urine.

Further explore each positive response to determine major characteristics of the symptom, such as the time of day, manner, and circumstances of onset; how long it has been present; whether there has been a change in type or location; whether it is improving or worsening; whether it is constant or intermittent; whether it is associated with body position or activity (such as walking, breathing, lying down, turning over in bed, coughing, eating, moving the bowels, or passing flatus); whether anything makes it better or worse; and whether the patient has had similar symptoms in the past.

If the patient complains of **pain**, ask him or her where it hurts, and then to elaborate, including time of onset, location at onset, change in location or severity with time, radiation, character (dull, aching, crushing, sharp, burning, stabbing, crampy, constant, intermittent), and severity. Also note whether the pain changes in response to breathing, coughing, motion, or change in position, and whether the patient has had similar pain in the past.

By the time you have elicited this type of detailed description of the pain, you should have a good idea of what is causing it. Refer to Chapter 16 for a discussion of **Common Medical Problems**, including chest pain, abdominal pain, and headache.

Headache is a common human affliction. It can be a nonspecific part of most serious diseases and injuries or can occur with stress, lack of sleep, or a hangover. It also can be an integral part of a serious condition such as high altitude cerebral edema, severe high blood pressure, meningitis, or a head injury.

If the patient complains of headache, ask about the location and duration of the pain, whether it is recurrent, what time of day it develops, whether it changes with a change in body position or activity, and whether it is steady or throbbing. Determine whether the headache is accompanied by nausea or abnormal visual symptoms such as blurring or moving lights (suggestive of migraine or vascular headaches), whether the neck is stiff, whether the patient is subject to headaches, and what the patient thinks may have caused the current headache, e.g., missing a meal. Inquire about any recent blow to the head, and be sure to take the patient's blood pressure.

If the patient has a **fever** and/or an acute **infection** is suspected, it is important to find out what part of the body is involved. **General** symptoms of infection include chills, fever, headache, backache, weakness, and aching all over. If a patient with a fever has any **wounds**, they should be inspected for signs of wound infection.

Symptoms of an **upper respiratory infection** include a stuffy and/or runny nose, sore or scratchy throat, hoarseness, and cough. The cough may be dry, or material may be coughed up. Ask what the sputum or nasal discharge looks like. If it is yellow or green, a significant bacterial infection may be present.

Symptoms of a **lower respiratory infection**, such as pneumonia or severe bronchitis, include a higher fever more likely to be associated with shaking chills, more weakness and general discomfort, more cough, and possibly pain on one side of the chest made worse by cough or deep breathing. Blood as well as pus may be seen in the sputum. It is important to tell whether the material the patient produces is coughed up from the lungs or is material from the nose and sinuses that is spit out.

Another common febrile illness is **gastroenteritis**. This is characterized by fever, aching all over, and various combinations of nausea, vomiting, and diarrhea. You may be able to hear loud abdominal gurgles with the naked ear, and the patient may complain of abdominal pain or cramps.

A **urinary tract infection (UTI)** is another important cause of fever and is due to an infection in the bladder, prostate (in men), or a kidney. Most patients with a UTI will complain of pain on voiding and of passing small amounts of urine at frequent intervals. Shaking chills are common. Pain across the small of the back also is common; if it is worse on one side, the kidney on that side may be involved.

If the patient complains of a **stiff** or **sore neck**, ask whether there has been a recent neck injury or history of arthritis of the neck. Ask the patient to touch the chin to the chest. Inability to do this in a patient with fever may indicate meningitis.

If the patient has **difficulty breathing**, ask about recent chest injury, cough, sputum production, coughing up blood, fever, chills, wheezing, ankle swelling, palpitations, chest pain, and a history of heart disease, emphysema, or asthma. Recent onset of shortness of breath in a previously healthy patient should make you suspect acute, de novo conditions such

as pneumonia, high altitude pulmonary edema, or a spontaneous pneumothorax. More slowly developing shortness of breath in a patient with known heart or lung disease may indicate heart failure, especially if there is edema of the ankles. In a patient with emphysema, suspect further deterioration in lung function. A history of asthma may indicate an asthma attack, usually obvious because of audible wheezing.

If the patient has **abdominal pain**, ask about the time of onset, location of the pain at onset, the type of pain (dull, crampy, sharp, etc.), whether it has moved or changed in type or intensity, and the relationship of the pain to eating (especially eating spicy foods), passing flatus, or moving the bowels. Inquire whether the pain is new or is a recurrence of similar pain felt in the past. Ask about the presence of nausea, vomiting, constipation, or diarrhea, how long since the bowels moved last, and any activity that makes the pain better or worse. Ask about a history of ulcer, gallbladder disease, or colitis, and whether the appendix has been removed. Ask when the patient last ate and, in the case of vomiting, when the patient was last able to keep food or liquids down.

Common abdominal pain syndromes include the following:

1. The acute onset of upper abdominal pain, fever, nausea and perhaps vomiting, and diarrhea as part of a viral infection.
2. Upper abdominal pain, sour stomach, and heartburn following a large or spicy meal.
3. Right lower quadrant pain caused by appendicitis.
4. Severe epigastric pain improved by antacids or milk due to an ulcer or inflammation of the stomach.
5. Right upper quadrant pain due to gallbladder disease.
6. Chronic left lower quadrant ache due to chronic constipation or colitis.

If the patient has **nausea** or **vomiting**, ask about duration, frequency, characteristics of the vomitus, and the presence of blood or "coffee grounds" material (digested blood) in the vomitus. Also ask whether abdominal pain is present and what the relationship of the nausea and vomiting is to the pain, particularly whether the pain gets better or worse before or after vomiting. Ask about how long it has been since the patient has been able to keep anything down, which will give you some idea of the patient's state of hydration and nutrition.

Most nausea and vomiting is caused by viral gastritis, but it also can accompany an ulcer, acute mountain sickness, a severe headache, or overindulgence in food and alcohol. Remember that nausea and vomiting can be associated with *any* severe illness or injury.

If the patient has **diarrhea**, ask about the duration, whether the patient has had chills and fever, the number and type of bowel movements, whether the bowel movements contain pus or blood, and the relationship of abdominal pain to moving the bowels.

Most diarrhea that lasts longer than a few hours is caused by a specific bowel infection—usually a virus but occasionally *Giardia lamblia* or a dysentery organism.

If the patient has **chest pain**, ask the patient to describe the pain, specifically the type (sharp, squeezing, dull, pressure); location (beneath the sternum, over the lower ribs, over the heart); characteristics of onset; duration; whether the pain worsens with coughing or deep breathing or is brought on by exertion; and whether it radiates to the neck, jaw, back, shoulder, or arm, particularly the left shoulder and left arm. Ask whether the patient has had similar chest pain before and whether there is a history of lung disease, angina, or heart disease, particularly coronary artery disease. The general topic of chest pain is discussed in Chapter 16.

If the complaint is about **weakness**, ask the patient to explain what is meant by weakness. Ask if the patient is actually tired rather than weak, whether the weakness is chronic or of recent onset, and whether it is general or confined to an arm, a leg, or one side of the body. It is important to know whether the patient is capable of normal activities or if the weakness prevents sitting, standing, or walking.

Ask if sleeping habits have been normal or have changed, and whether the onset of the weakness coincided with the onset of a febrile illness such as a head cold or influenza, an injury, an operation, missing one or several meals, or a disease of the circulatory, respiratory, gastrointestinal, or urinary system. Weakness of sudden onset that involves one or more extremities usually is caused by injury or illness affecting the nerves supplying the weak parts and, in the case of weakness of one side of the body, may mean a stroke. General body weakness can accompany many injuries and illnesses, can be due to overwork and lack of sleep, or, if chronic, psychoneurosis. However, general weakness also can be caused by a subtle medical condition such as anemia, newly developing diabetes, chronic kidney disease, hidden malignant disease, or a low thyroid state.

If the patient complains about **difficulty voiding**, ask the patient what is meant by that. Elderly men with enlargement of the prostate gland have difficulty starting and stopping the urinary stream and have to get up at night frequently to void. Women who have borne several children may have trouble with urine leaking involuntarily on coughing or laughing. Pain on urination and frequent voiding of small amounts usually indicates the presence of an infection.

Secondary Survey

The secondary survey of a **responsive patient with a medical illness** begins with reassessing and recording the following:

1. Pulse.
2. Capillary refill.
3. Breathing rate.
4. Temperature.
5. Blood pressure.
6. Skin color, temperature, moisture, and turgor of the skin. To assess turgor, or skin hydration, pinch a fold of skin on the forearm or abdomen into a ridge with the finger and thumb and see how long it takes to return to its original state. If the patient is well hydrated, the skin is elastic and returns quickly; if the patient is dehydrated, the ridge subsides slowly. Poor turgor also is seen in chronic illness, malnutrition, old age, and other causes of atrophic skin.

Then, the patient is interviewed (as outlined in Chapter 4 and expanded below) about the following:

1. The patient's medical history.
2. Allergies.
3. Medicines or drugs taken.
4. "Anything else we should know about you?"

A total body assessment is conducted (see Chapter 4). In the head-to-toe assessment of the patient with a **medical illness**, the rescuer should:

1. Examine the throat with a flashlight and tongue blade (or spoon handle), looking for redness, pus on the back of the throat, enlargement of the tonsils, and white spots on the tonsils.
2. Feel under the back of the jaw for enlarged, tender lymph nodes.
3. Listen to the breathing for rattles, wheezes, and other noises.
4. Observe for respiratory distress.

5. Palpate the abdomen for tender areas, and listen for audible bowel sounds.
6. Palpate the costovertebral angles for tenderness.
7. Look at the feet and ankles for evidence of swelling.

The first part of the secondary survey of the **unresponsive patient** consists of assessing and recording the vital and other important signs.

As emphasized above, there is one situation in which the pupils and response to pain should be assessed as part of the primary survey, immediately after the airway, breathing, bleeding, and circulation have been assessed. That is when the patient with a head injury is unresponsive or has an altered mental status. Assess the pupils for equality and response to light using a flashlight. Assess the extremities for response to pain on both sides by pinching the patient's thumbnail and ankle skin or big toenail hard between your index finger and thumb. The patient's response to pain, usually by withdrawing the extremity or pushing your hand away with the other hand, should be equal on both sides.

If one pupil is larger than the other and/or the arm and leg on one side (usually the side opposite to that of the enlarged pupil) are weaker than on the other side, the signs are said to be "lateralized." Lateralization indicates that there is great likelihood of serious bleeding inside the head. Since this type of bleeding can frequently be treated successfully by immediate surgery, a *neurosurgical emergency* exists and the patient must be transported without delay to a hospital with a neurosurgeon.

In the head-injured patient, the level of responsiveness, pupils, and pain response should be reassessed at 15-minute intervals to detect any deterioration in the patient's condition, especially the onset of lateralization.

All of the vital and other important signs are interrelated; changes in one are frequently accompanied by changes in some or all of the others. These signs are *dynamic, not static.* A single determination means little in an injured or ill patient. The signs must be reassessed at regular intervals to monitor possible progression of an illness or injury, and to detect deterioration in the patient's level of responsiveness.

Pulse

The carotid artery pulse is the easiest to feel during the primary survey, but the radial pulse usually is more convenient for monitoring in the patient *who does not require CPR.* The pulse should be correlated with the skin temperature, color, and moisture, the blood pressure, and the capillary refill time. If the radial pulse is palpable, the blood pressure is at least 80 mm Hg systolic.

A strong pulse at a normal rate is good evidence that unresponsiveness may be caused by uncomplicated head trauma or a medical condition such as a stroke, drug overdose, or seizure. With a strong, normal pulse, unresponsiveness is unlikely to be caused by shock or a severe injury.

A weak, fast pulse should be correlated promptly with the capillary refill, skin examination, and blood pressure (if you are carrying an apparatus to measure it). The patient probably is in shock if the blood pressure is normal or low; the skin perfusion abnormal as shown by delayed capillary refill; the breathing rate increased; and/or the skin cold, pale or blue, and moist.

If you have no blood pressure apparatus, consider a rising pulse rate in an injured patient as the most reliable early sign of shock. If you detect vital sign changes suggesting shock, immediately reassess the airway and do a body assessment for external bleeding and bleeding into the chest, abdomen, pelvis, or thigh (from a femur fracture). Remember that a trauma patient may have multiple injuries. The more injuries, the greater chance of shock.

A slow pulse should be correlated with the body temperature and skin color, since it is seen in hypothermia, but it also can be seen in serious head injuries, high spinal cord injuries, and some types of heart disease. In cold weather, the skin temperature may be low, even in normal people.

A rapid pulse in a patient with normal skin color, moisture, and temperature may indicate a primary heart problem with an abnormally fast heart rate. A rapid pulse in a patient with red, hot skin and an elevated temperature is characteristic of significant infection, or in a hot environment, of heat stroke.

The level of responsiveness usually is altered in heat stroke but also may be altered in infection. Infections that can cause altered responsiveness include pneumonia, septicemia (blood stream infection), and meningitis.

Capillary Refill and Blood Pressure

The capillary refill time is a measure of **skin perfusion**, (i.e., the rate of blood flow through the small skin vessels). It can be altered by conditions that alter general body circulation, such as shock, but also by local factors that alter flow, such as skin cooling and local injury.

Capillary refill should therefore be correlated with other signs, such as the pulse rate, blood pressure, skin characteristics, and the location of any injuries. Capillary refill is reassuring when normal but less helpful when prolonged, since delayed capillary refill can be caused by insignificant factors such as exposure to cold weather as easily as to serious illness or injury. It is related to the blood pressure; however, determination of capillary refill time is not a substitute for taking the blood pressure. Delayed capillary refill may indicate **early shock**, since it is prolonged by compensatory mechanisms that support the blood pressure and body core circulation such as constriction of skin vessels, and may be abnormal while the pulse and blood pressure are still normal.

The blood pressure also should be correlated with other vital signs. High blood pressure can be seen in chronic hypertension, in stress (caused by painful injuries), occasionally in strenuous exercise, and in head injury. Normal blood pressure does not rule out the early stages of shock and many other serious conditions. Low blood pressure accompanied by a normal pulse and breathing rate can be seen in many healthy persons, especially endurance athletes. Low blood pressure accompanied by a fast and/or weak pulse and rapid respirations indicates the likely presence of a serious disease of the heart and/or circulatory system, such as a heart attack or shock.

Respirations

An **increased** respiratory rate should alert the rescuer to the likelihood of low blood oxygen, fever, or a disturbance in lung integrity or respiratory dynamics. The amount of effort required to breathe should be noted. Normally, both the rate and depth increase together, but in the case of a chest injury, each breath may be shallow with only the rate increased, especially if it hurts to breathe.

Hypoxia and fever increase the respiratory rate and depth through reflex action on the breathing control center in the brain. Lung disease or injury increase the rate, either through the resulting hypoxia or through nerve impulses coming directly to the breathing center from the abnormal lung tissue.

A **decreased** respiratory rate is seen in hypothermia, severe hypoxia, brain damage due to stroke, increased intracranial pressure, head injury, and in some types of drug overdose (from narcotics, barbiturates and other central nervous system depressants). In these cases, the depth of breathing may or may not be abnormal.

During the primary survey, if the airway is open, investigate abnormal respirations immediately by assessing the level of responsiveness, and the head, neck, and chest.

Ineffective respirations are respirations that do not bring enough air into the lungs to oxygenate the blood. Respirations may be ineffective because they are too slow, too fast, and/or too shallow. Respirations of less than 10 per minute or more than 30 per minute are ineffective because they are too slow to move enough air or too fast to allow the lungs to fill properly between breaths. Respirations of less than 12 per minute or more than 20 per minute may or may not be ineffective, but should be considered ineffective if they are shallow as well. Other signs of ineffective respirations are **cyanosis** and **altered mental status**. If in doubt, assume that respirations are probably ineffective, especially if the patient has a chest injury or a chest infection.

Support ineffective respirations by ventilating the patient with the pocket mask or bag-valve-mask. Add oxygen if available, at high concentration and flow rate. (However, oxygen alone without ventilating the patient is not enough). Oxygen by nasal cannula is insufficient for these patients. In the unresponsive patient, the rhythm of respirations should be the same as the patient's own respirations at first, so that you are assisting rather than competing with the patient.

Use an oropharyngeal airway in the patient without a gag reflex. Grad-

ually increase the volume delivered and the respiratory rate to maintain a volume of about 800 milliliters (1.5 pints) and a rate of 16 to 20 per minute. Be sure that the patient's skin color is good and that the chest rises and falls well with each breath.

In the responsive patient, explain what you are going to do and tell the patient that it will make him or her feel better. Start by matching the patient's breathing volume and rate, and gradually increase the volume after every few breaths until you are providing a volume of about 800 milliliters at a rate of 16 to 20 breaths per minute. Monitor the patient's alertness and skin color.

Agonal respirations are another type of ineffective respiration. These are seen in dying patients, including those with cardiac arrest. There are two types of agonal respirations. In one, the patient takes very shallow breaths, opening the mouth with each breath, but the chest does not lift. In the other, the patient takes an occasional deep breath, frequently opening the mouth wide or lifting the head or chin with each breath.

If the patient has had a cardiac arrest, do *not* mistake agonal respirations for adequate respirations. Provide rescue breathing or assisted ventilations with a pocket mask or bag-valve-mask to these patients according to standard CPR protocols.

Temperature

The patient's temperature should be taken by thermometer. This rarely is done in the field, but is usually left until the patient has been moved to the ski patrol first aid room or other shelter (as is the measurement of blood pressure with a sphygmomanometer).

In the unresponsive patient, a rectal temperature is preferred. The only situation in which taking the temperature in the field might make a difference is in hypothermia or heat stroke. Since the range of an ordinary

clinical thermometer usually is between 94° and 108°F, a special low-reading thermometer is required to diagnose hypothermia.

The technique of estimating a hypothermic patient's temperature without a thermometer is discussed in Chapter 18.

Level of Responsiveness

During the first impression or early in the primary survey, the rescuer will have designated the patient as responsive or unresponsive, based on the patient's response to the question, "Are you okay?" (**V** on the AVPU Scale, Chapter 3). During the secondary survey, if not sooner, the patient unresponsive to a verbal stimulus should be graded on the AVPU Scale based on the response to pain as either **P** or **U**. This is done by noting whether the patient *reacts* (by moaning, opening the eyes, moving the head, withdrawing the extremity, or pushing away the examiner's hand) or *does not react* to pressure on a fingernail or a painful pinch. The sensitive skin of the inner arm or inner thigh is a reliable and usually accessible area to pinch.

In any patient with altered responsiveness, after you have assessed the airway, breathing, and circulation, and looked for obvious bleeding, the next step is to assess the head, including the equality of the pupils, and all four extremities for response to pain.

The level of responsiveness, as well as other vital and important signs, should be reassessed at 15-minute intervals, recorded, and the record given to the appropriate personnel when the patient arrives at a hospital or is turned over to the EMS system.

Interview of Witnesses and/or Family Members
(Fig. 19.2)

In the unresponsive patient, the rescuer may have time to ask bystanders what happened while conducting the primary survey and taking the vital signs.

In the case of an **accident**, the rescuer will hear the following types of descriptions:

1. "'A' was skiing fast and close to the side of the run. He looked like he caught an edge, crashed, and hit a tree."
2. "'B' was skiing down the middle of the run when this 'hot dog' ran into him."
3. "'C' was looking over the edge of the cliff when he slipped and could not stop himself."

Next, extract the essentials of the accident to reconstruct the story in an orderly, usually chronological, fashion. Ask the witnesses the types of questions listed below. Build on each answer to formulate the next question, so that the story unfolds in a logical manner.

1. "How long ago did it happen?"
2. "Did you actually see it happen?"
3. "Did you see how 'A' ('B' or 'C') landed?"
4. "Did you see him hit his head?"
5. "What happened after that?"
6. "Was he unconscious right away or later?
7. "Did he vomit?"
8. "Did he move after the accident?
9. "Did he seem to be moving all four extremities?"

10. "Was he feeling okay before the accident?" "If he was not okay, what specifically did he complain of?" "Has he been sick lately?" (with the flu, etc.). "Did he complain of anything else?"
11. "Did he eat or skip breakfast (or lunch)?"
12. "Did he have any trouble sleeping last night?"
13. "Was he partying last night?"

In the case of an **illness**, the rescuer will hear the following types of descriptions:

1. "'A' didn't seem to be feeling very well this morning, and we had to wait for him a lot. We were waiting for him at the bottom of Big Elk when we saw him sitting down in the snow. We hollered to him but he didn't answer. We hiked back up the hill and by the time we reached him he was lying down and wouldn't say anything."
2. "We gatekeepers were all feeling pretty cold during the first run of the race. The wind was blowing and it was really snowing hard. 'B' seemed to be all right, but then we noticed that he was just sitting there and not checking off the racers. By

the time we got to him he was lying down and we couldn't get him to talk."
3. "We've been camping for two days. 'C' must have had something for supper last night that made him sick. He was up and down all night vomiting and couldn't hold anything down this morning. He was so weak we were worried, so we packed up and started to move out. He had to stop several times due to diarrhea. Finally, he just laid down and we couldn't get him moving, so we made camp again and sent someone out for help."

In caring for a person with an illness, as with an accident, try to reconstruct the events leading up to the present situation. In the case of unresponsiveness due to a medical illness, the possibilities are much more diverse than with an injury. In addition to obtaining general information from the patient's companions, question them about the important medical signs and symptoms the patient may have manifested, as outlined above in the **Primary Survey of the Responsive Patient** with a medical illness.

Next, obtain information about the patient's **medical history, allergies**, and any **regular medicines** taken. This information usually is not

---

Fig. 19.2 *Interviewing Witnesses*

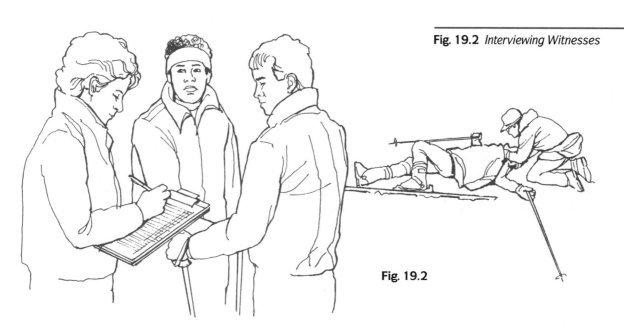

Fig. 19.2

obtainable from casual acquaintances —friends or family members are much more helpful—but you should try anyway.

Examples of important elements of the medical history related to unresponsiveness include the following:

1. Diabetes. Could the patient be hypoglycemic or in diabetic ketoacidosis? Whenever a history of diabetes is obtained in a patient with an altered level of responsiveness, the patient should be given sugar immediately if able to swallow.
2. Epilepsy. Could the patient have had a seizure and now be in a post-seizure state of temporary unresponsiveness, or could the patient have fallen during the seizure and suffered a head injury?
3. High blood pressure or transient ischemic attacks (TIA's) of part of the brain. Could the patient have had a stroke?
4. Coronary artery disease. Could the patient have had a heart attack with unresponsiveness due to temporary interruption of circulation to the brain?
5. Excessive drinking, the inappropriate use of medicines, or the use of recreational drugs. Has the patient overindulged in alcohol or taken an overdose of another drug?
6. Depression. Has the patient tried to commit suicide by overdosing with some drug?
7. Peptic ulcer. Could the ulcer have bled or perforated, causing shock with altered mental status?
8. Chronic obstructive lung disease. Could the patient have developed lung failure?
9. Fever, headache, or stiff neck over the previous few days. Could the patient have meningitis or another serious infection?

Even though the patient may clearly have had an accident with a head injury as the immediate cause of the unresponsiveness, a preexisting illness may have contributed to the accident.

The importance of identifying any allergies lies in the possible relationship of unresponsiveness to an anaphylactic reaction. Usually this is caused by taking a medicine, eating a food, or being stung by an insect to which the patient is allergic.

Asking about any medicines or illegal drugs taken regularly reinforces information from the patient's medical history as discussed above. *Always ask for what condition(s) the patient is taking the medicine.* Medicine for heart disease, blood pressure, or cholesterol alerts you to the possibility of heart attack or stroke. The importance of antiseizure medicines, insulin, or pills for diabetes is obvious. Tranquilizers and sleeping pills may interfere with judgment and coordination and, if taken in excess, can cause unresponsiveness. Patients taking antidepressants may be subject to suicide attempts. Many different types of medicines, including tranquilizers, antidepressants, blood pressure medicines, and antihistamines, can interfere with body temperature regulation and predispose patients to heat stroke or hypothermia. Medicines that block the action of adrenalin (beta-blockers) are widely used to treat heart disease and high blood pressure. Patients taking beta blockers have slow heart rates even when seriously injured or in shock.

Finally, ask the friend or family member, "Is there anything else you can think of that we should know in order to help?"

Next, proceed to a thorough, systematic whole body survey, as described in Chapter 4, stopping at any point where immediate care is required for bleeding or any other serious condition.

The whole body survey is performed by exposing each area in turn, and using the senses—sight, touch, hearing, and smell—to detect any abnormalities.

Things to **look** for include the following:

1. Facial expression.
2. Skin color and moisture.
3. Open wounds, bleeding, impaled objects, exposed internal organs.
4. Scars.
5. Abnormal discharges.
6. Bruises.
7. Swellings, including edema of the feet and ankles.
8. Deformity, asymmetry, abnormal position, abnormal shortening (compare the two sides of the body).
9. Missing or displaced body parts.
10. Abnormality of superficial veins.
11. Capillary refill time.
12. Symmetrical chest expansion.
13. Amount of effort required to breathe.
14. Abdominal distension.
15. Movement of extremities.
16. Medical-alert tags and bracelets.
17. Jewelry on injured extremities.

Things to **feel** for include the following:

1. Skin temperature and moisture.
2. Tenderness.
3. Enlarged lymph nodes.
4. Swellings.
5. Indentations.
6. Deformities. (Compare the two sides of the body.)
7. Crepitus.
8. Subcutaneous emphysema.
9. Abdominal masses.
10. Deviated trachea.
11. Peripheral pulses.

Things to **listen** for include the following:

1. Abnormal sounds during breathing or talking, such as wheezes, stridor, rhonchi, frequent coughing, hoarseness, and a weak voice.

2. Audible bowel sounds.

Things to **smell** for include the following:

1. Alcohol.
2. Fruity odor of diabetic ketoacidosis.
3. Urinous odor of kidney failure.
4. Odor of urine or feces (incontinence).

Body Survey

The Head

To assess the head, look at the skin of the face first. Pale or grayish skin that is cool or cold indicates that blood flow through the skin is reduced. This occurs when the blood is conserved for more important parts of the body (as in shock), to conserve heat (as in hypothermia), and as a reflex in fainting or stressful situations (as in fear, anxiety, and pain).

The skin will be moist if there is moisture from rain or melted snow on it, if the body is trying to cool itself by perspiring (as in exercise, fever, or a hot environment), or if there is reflex sweating caused by pain, fear, anxiety, or shock.

Red skin means that the blood flow through the skin is increased, and the skin usually will feel warm or hot. However, the skin can be both red and cool in exposure to wind and cold air (due to their local irritant effect on exposed skin), after alcohol consumption in cold weather, or if the body has cooled itself by losing heat through increased skin circulation.

The skin will be blue (cyanotic) if there is an increased amount of unoxygenated hemoglobin in the blood. This occurs when diseases or injuries affecting the circulatory or respiratory systems *prevent normal oxygenation* of the blood (as in decreased cardiac output due to heart attack, abnormal heart rhythm, or heart injury; flail chest, pneumothorax, lung contusion, and pneumonia; and shock). Blue skin

also may occur if the circulation is so slow because of local conditions that there is time for the cells to remove more than a normal amount of oxygen from each unit of blood, such as in cold exposure.

Look at the face as a whole. It may be puffy in a chest injury that obstructs veins that drain the head; in heart failure; and in patients who take cortisone derivatives. The face will appear thin in patients with malnutrition and other types of chronic illness.

Look at the patient's expression. Seriously ill people have an anxious, drawn appearance. Determine whether the patient looks depressed, tearful, excited, sad, frightened, or relaxed and happy.

Is the face symmetrical? Asymmetry in a trauma patient may mean a contusion with swelling or a fracture of the nose, facial bones, or jaw. Inspect the face for open wounds, impaled objects, bleeding, swelling, bruises, scars, and areas of tenderness. Inspect and palpate the scalp as well (Fig. 19.3). Swellings usually are caused by an accumulation of blood, plasma, or tissue fluid. Soft spots usually are caused by tissue destruction from blunt trauma, without much bleeding. Indentations may indicate a depressed skull fracture. Look for white scalp in the depths of a deep scalp wound, and for visible brain tissue (glistening pink or gray material), which means an open skull fracture.

Next, inspect the skin around the eyes for swelling or bruising. These tissues are delicate; blood from injured vessels spreads easily into the upper and lower lids (black eye). Bleeding into the orbits from a skull fracture resembles a black eye but usually involves both eyes and has a sharp margin where the spreading of the blood through the skin is limited by the attachment of the eye fascia to the bone around the rim of the orbit ("raccoon eyes"). A patient with bruising around the eye should be assessed carefully for injury to the eyeball itself.

Determine whether the patient is wearing contact lenses. Look for bleeding into the conjunctiva (white of the eye). Are the pupils normal in size, round and regular, and equal to each other? Shine a flashlight into each eye to see if both pupils constrict. Remember that an occasional patient will have a glass eye, which a hasty examination can cause you to overlook at first. Look for anything unusual behind the pupil (such as blood).

Trauma to one eye can cause an unequal, irregular, or unresponsive pupil on that side. A recessed eyeball may mean a fractured orbit; a protruding eyeball, an orbital hemorrhage or a trauma-caused enucleation. A dilated, enlarged pupil may indicate a brain injury, usually on the same side; this type of pupil may or may not respond to light. If both pupils are abnormally dilated or constricted, think of the effects of such drugs as barbiturates, opiates, or marijuana. In the responsive patient, test gross vision by holding up several fingers and asking the patient how many fingers are seen.

Next, look at the nose. Is it swollen, bruised, flattened, or pushed to

Fig. 19.3 *Assessment of a Head Laceration*

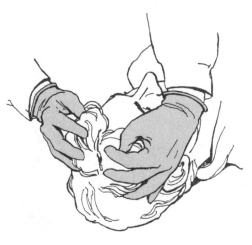

Fig. 19.3

one side? Is there bleeding from one or both nostrils? The most common cause of a nosebleed in an unresponsive patient is direct injury to the nose; less commonly, a skull fracture. Bleeding from the nose should raise the possibility that the patient may vomit swallowed blood. Airway obstruction caused by bleeding or swollen tissues may also occur. Clear fluid draining from the nose may be mucus, or it may be spinal fluid. Do not attempt to stop it.

Inspect both ears, looking for blood or other discharge. Although blood from a scalp wound may run down into the ear, definite bleeding or a clear or pinkish discharge from the ear should make you suspect a skull fracture with leakage of blood or spinal fluid. Again, do not attempt to stop spinal fluid drainage. If in doubt, allow a few drops to fall on a piece of white cloth to see if a bull's-eye pattern with a red center and a pink rim develops. Look for bruising behind the ears, also a sign of a skull fracture ("Battle's sign").

Use both hands to carefully palpate the face and the sides and back of the head for swellings, deformities and, in the responsive patient, tender areas. Compare one side with the other. Deformities may indicate fractures of facial bones with impending danger of airway blockage from swelling and bleeding.

Inspect the mouth with a flashlight and tongue blade or spoon handle, opening it with the crossed-finger technique, if necessary. Look for loose dentures, foreign objects, bleeding, and open wounds. Look at the upper and lower jaws for broken, loose, avulsed, or missing teeth, and for deviations in the even rows of teeth. Compare one side of the mouth with the other. Note whether the lower jaw is properly aligned under the upper jaw when the mouth is closed. If not, there probably is a fracture of the lower or upper jaw.

In a responsive patient, listen to the patient's voice. Hoarseness or a weak voice may mean injury or infection (laryngitis) of the larynx or damage to the nerves in the neck and chest that supply the larynx.

Smell the patient's breath. Important odors are alcohol, the fruity odor of acetone in diabetic ketoacidosis, and the urinous odor of kidney failure (uremia).

The Neck

As with the head, inspect the skin for color, moisture, bruises, swellings, scars, open wounds, impaled objects, and bleeding; and look for asymmetry, deformities, and the amount of engorgement of the superficial veins. These veins usually stand out

in recumbent patients but may be flat in patients with hypovolemic shock. They usually are markedly distended in those with heart failure or mechanical interference with heart muscle function, such as pericardial tamponade.

Use both hands to palpate both sides of the neck simultaneously. Start by feeling under the posterior jaw on both sides for enlarged lymph nodes, which are round, almond-sized and almond-shaped swellings that may be tender. Feel for deformities, lumps, and swellings as you move your hands downward. Air in the soft tissues of the neck from a ruptured larynx or trachea gives a characteristic crackling feeling (subcutaneous emphysema). Look for a medical-alert tag. Check the sternal notch to see whether the trachea is in the midline (Fig. 19.4).

The Chest

For adequate assessment of the chest, bulky outer clothing must be opened or removed. This may not be advisable in cold, windy weather or if it is snowing or raining, but should be done as soon as shelter is reached. T-shirts, undershirts and turtlenecks can be pulled up; bras should be left in place.

First, look at both sides of the chest for symmetry, obvious deformities, bruises, swellings, scars, open wounds, impaled objects, bleeding,

Fig. 19.4 *Assess the position of the trachea by pushing an index finger in on one side of the sternal notch.*

Fig. 19.5 *To adequately assess the chest, compare one side with the other.*

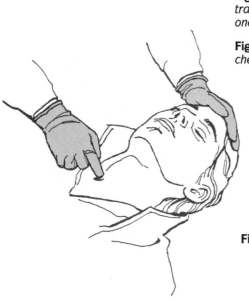

Fig. 19.4

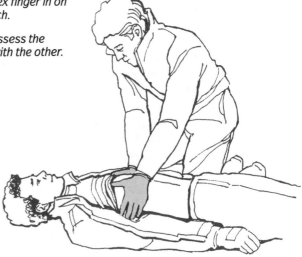

Fig. 19.5

and equal movement during breathing. Place one hand on each side of the lower chest and note whether your hands move symmetrically as the patient breathes (Fig. 19.5). Note the breathing rate, depth, and amount of effort required to breathe. If you discover a section of chest wall on one side that does not move well with respiration or that moves in instead of out on inspiration (flail chest), stop the assessment at this point and stabilize it. If air is heard whistling in and out of an open wound during breathing (sucking chest wound), stop the assessment at this point and seal it. In serious chest injuries, *be alert for the development of inadequate ventilations* and *support* them with the bag-valve-mask or mouth-to-pocket mask.

Ask the responsive patient to point out any painful areas. Next, start at the clavicles and proceed downward. Palpate the sternum and all the ribs and the spaces between them in turn to detect deformities, swellings, tenderness (especially over the ribs), and the crackling feeling of subcutaneous emphysema. A patient with a rib fracture usually will complain of pain on deep breathing and coughing and will be able to point to the area of fracture. Generally you will be able to locate the fracture site by finding

point tenderness with your finger over the injured rib. It is best to examine both sides of the chest simultaneously so that they can be compared, but this may be difficult in the field.

Listen for audible wheezes (asthma or bronchitis), rattles (bronchitis or pulmonary edema), frequent coughing (bronchitis or pneumonia), or a crowing sound on inspiration (laryngitis, foreign body).

The Abdomen and Pelvis

To adequately assess the abdomen and pelvis, the rescuer must open or pull up the patient's upper body garments or pull down the lower body garments (Fig. 19.6). Again, this may not be advisable in inclement weather, but should be done as soon as shelter is reached.

Ask the responsive patient to show you the location of abdominal pain, if any. Starting at the costal arches and moving downward, look for scars, open wounds, exposed internal organs, impaled objects, bleeding, bruises, swellings, scars, abdominal distention (swelling or enlargement), and exposed bone in pelvic injuries.

Abdominal distention may be seen in abdominal injuries, peritonitis, intestinal obstruction, and, occasionally, in severe constipation. If the patient has any scars and is responsive,

ask what type of operation(s) caused the scar(s). If the patient has abdominal pain and the appendix has been removed, the pain is not likely to be caused by appendicitis. If an open wound is discovered, especially if part of an internal organ is protruding, stop the assessment and care for it.

Use the pads of your fingertips to examine the four quadrants of the abdomen in a clockwise manner, starting with the right upper quadrant.

Palpate the abdominal wall to find tenderness, rigidity of the muscles, localized swellings, masses, enlarged organs, and tightening of the abdominal muscles over a tender area ("guarding"). Palpate the area above the pubis to discover a distended bladder in a patient unable to pass urine. (Ask the responsive patient when he or she last urinated.) With trauma, an area may be tender or painful because of injury to underlying abdominal organs, to the abdominal wall itself, or to both.

In both illness and injury, the location of abdominal pain and tenderness provides a clue to the possible organs involved. In compression ("blunt") trauma, discomfort in the right upper quadrant indicates the possibility of liver injury, discomfort in the left upper quadrant indicates the possibility of spleen injury, and discomfort above the pubic bone suggests injury to a distended bladder (or uterus in the case of a pregnant woman). Bowel injury or injury to blood vessels can cause discomfort in any area. Generalized pain and tenderness may indicate peritonitis from a ruptured hollow organ or intra-abdominal bleeding, either of which can produce localized discomfort at first, spreading to generalized discomfort later.

In the uninjured patient, discomfort in the right upper quadrant may indicate gallbladder or liver disease; discomfort in the right lower quadrant suggests appendicitis. Left lower

Fig. 19.6 *Remove or open clothing to adequately assess the abdomen and pelvis.*

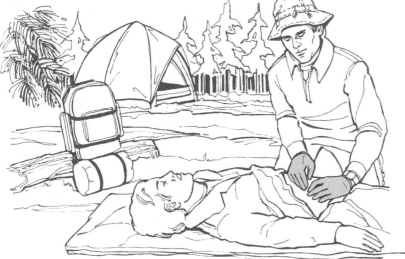

Fig. 19.6

quadrant discomfort can be seen in gastroenteritis, diverticulitis, chronic constipation, and colitis. The most frequent cause of discomfort in the left upper quadrant is an accumulation of gas in the colon or stomach.

In the injured patient, gently press the sides of the pelvis toward each other with a rotary motion, and then backward to see if this causes pain—a sign of a fractured pelvis.

Listen for audible bowel sounds, usually heard as gurgling sounds coming in intermittent rushes. These mean excessive bowel activity, which may be caused by hunger, gastroenteritis, or the bowel attempting to work its contents past an area of obstruction. If you suspect a lower abdominal or pelvic injury, inspect the perineal area for evidence of bleeding from the urethra or vagina. (Have a witness of the same sex as the patient present while you do this.)

Smell for abnormal odors, such as the odor of urine or feces in incontinence or the fecal odor of vomitus in some patients with intestinal obstruction.

The Lower Extremity

Exposing the lower extremities for assessment in the outdoor environment is difficult, and it may be preferable to wait until shelter is reached. If necessary, trousers and slacks can be pulled down below the hips; skirts can be pulled up. It may be difficult to pull up the legs of tight-fitting garments such as stretch pants and tights.

Open fractures and other open wounds should be exposed completely in the field, even if this means cutting open expensive clothing or opening seams with a seam ripper (Fig. 19.7). In most cases, footgear and socks should be removed after shelter is reached to expose injuries to the ankles and feet and to assess pulses and nerve function in the lower extremities. However, properly applied splints should be removed only if absolutely necessary.

For a detailed discussion of the practical problems associated with the field assessment of circulation and nerve supply in lower extremity injuries, refer to **Assessment of Musculoskeletal Injuries** in Chapter 8.

Starting at the groin area and moving downward, look at the exposed skin of the thighs, knees, legs, ankles, and feet for scars, open wounds, impaled objects, bleeding, bruises, swellings, deformities, and unusual positions. If in doubt, compare the two extremities.

If you find blood, always search for the source. It usually will be coming from a nearby open wound, but occasionally it will come from a wound in another part of the body. Care for any open wounds found during the secondary survey immediately, first by controlling any bleeding with direct pressure and then by covering the wound with a sterile compress. If the wound is part of an open fracture, splint the fracture before continuing with the survey.

Starting at the groin area and moving downward, feel the skin, muscles, and bones for tender areas, swellings, depressions, and crepitus. Locate and palpate the femoral, dorsalis pedis, and posterior tibial pulses. Assess extremity perfusion by the capillary refill test in a toenail.

Tenderness, swelling, and/or bruising over the hip, knee, ankle joint, or foot may mean a contusion or sprain; if deformity is present, a dislocation. Ankle deformity frequently means a fracture-dislocation. Tenderness, swelling and/or bruising over the shaft of the femur, tibia, or fibula may mean a contusion or fracture. A fracture is almost certain if deformity, marked swelling, shortening, or crepitus is present. If the knee is involved, gently palpate the patella, especially the tendons at its upper and lower borders; the lateral and medial ligaments of the knee; and the lateral and medial hamstring tendons. Tenderness of one or more of these structures will indicate which part of the knee joint is injured. Deformity above the knee joint may mean a supracondylar femur fracture.

If the ankle is involved, gently and carefully palpate the Achilles tendon, the lateral and medial malleoli, and the ligaments that connect the malleoli with the foot. Tenderness of these structures means a sprain or fracture; deformity, marked swelling, or crepi-

Fig. 19.7 *Open fractures and other open wounds should be exposed during assessment of the lower extremity.*

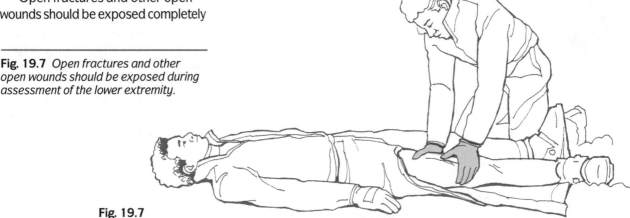

Fig. 19.7

tus means a fracture or fracture-dislocation is likely.

Assess nerve function in the lower extremity by asking the responsive patient if he or she can feel the legs and feet, and if they feel normal, numb, or tingly. Test for sensory function by scraping the skin of the thighs, legs, and feet with a fingernail. Ask the patient to flex and extend the hip, knee, and ankle, and wiggle the toes. However, do *not* ask the patient to move the joint above or below the site of a possible fracture, or the limb above or below the site of a possible dislocation or severe sprain. In all the above maneuvers, compare the two sides of the body.

Test the major nerves of the lower extremity specifically by asking the patient to do the following:

1. Tighten the quadriceps muscle (femoral nerve).
2. Dorsiflex (pull proximally) the big toe (peroneal branch of the sciatic nerve).
3. Indicate whether he or she can feel a fingernail scraped across the sole of the foot (tibial branch of the sciatic nerve).

In the unresponsive patient, observe for spontaneous movement of both lower extremities. Test for ability to move in response to pain by pinching the skin of the inner thigh, rubbing the skin over the tibia hard with your knuckle, or pinching the nail of the great toe firmly.

The Upper Extremity

To assess the upper extremity, remove bulky outer clothing, if possible, or at least open it and slide it off the shoulders. Roll up sleeves to expose as much of the extremity as possible. Again, if you suspect an open fracture or other open wound, remove the clothing completely, by cutting or opening along a seam, if necessary. After reaching shelter, expose and assess closed fractures and other injuries. Remove properly applied splints only if it is absolutely necessary.

Starting at the shoulders and moving distally, look at the skin of the shoulder, arm, elbow, forearm, wrist, and hand for scars, open wounds, impaled objects, bleeding, bruising, swelling, deformities, abnormal shortening, and unusual positions. If in doubt about whether abnormalities are present, compare with the opposite, normal extremity. Look for a medical-alert bracelet.

As with the lower extremity, the rescuer must find the origin of any blood, control bleeding, dress open wounds, and splint open fractures before continuing the secondary survey. Be sure to remove watches, bracelets, and rings from an injured extremity before swelling occurs. Give them to the responsive patient, a family member, or other responsible companion. (It is best to have a witness present when this is done.)

Starting at the shoulder and moving distally, palpate the shoulder, arm, elbow, forearm, wrist, and hand, looking for abnormal swellings, tender areas, depressions, and crepitus (Fig. 19.8). Tenderness, swelling, and/or bruising at a joint suggests a sprain; severe pain or deformity as well means a dislocation is likely. Tenderness, swelling, and/or bruising along the shaft of the clavicle, humerus, radius, ulna, or bones of the hands or fingers suggests a contusion or fracture; if deformity and/or crepitus is present as well, a fracture is almost certain.

The clavicle is easy to assess since its entire length can be felt under the skin. Compare the two shoulders—the point of each shoulder should be equally rounded. A step-off deformity at the place where the rounding of the shoulder begins means that the patient has an acromioclavicular separation; a squared-off shoulder may mean a dislocation of the shoulder joint. (Feel for the head of the humerus in the armpit.) Deformity above the elbow may mean a supracondylar fracture of the humerus.

Feel the radial pulses at the wrists, and check perfusion in both extremities with the capillary refill test. Ask the patient to flex and extend the shoulder, elbow, wrist, and fingers, and to squeeze both of your hands simultaneously so you can compare the two grips and test strength. However, as with lower-extremity injuries, do *not* ask the patient to move the joint above or below a possible fracture, or the limb above or below a dislocation or severe sprain. Test sensation by gently pinching or scraping the skin of the arm, forearm, and dorsum of the hand with a fingernail. In all the above maneuvers, compare the two sides of the body.

To conduct a rapid test for the function of the major nerves of the upper extremity, ask the patient to do the following:

1. Raise the arm to the side (axillary nerve). If this is not advis-

Fig. 19.8 *Assessment of an Upper Extremity*

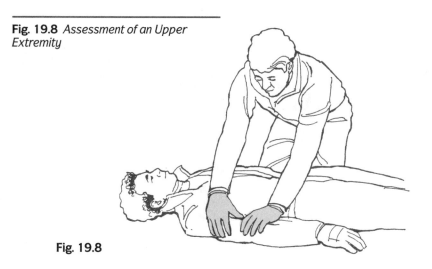

Fig. 19.8

able because of a shoulder dislocation or other injury, place your hand on the deltoid muscle and ask the patient to tighten it as though the arm were being abducted. Even though the patient will not move the shoulder because of pain, if the axillary nerve is intact you should be able to feel the deltoid muscle contract.

2. Tighten the biceps (musculocutaneous nerve).
3. Make a tight fist with the wrist cocked up, then open the fist with the fingers widely spread (radial, ulnar, and median nerves).

Another way to confirm the function of the median and ulnar nerves is to test sensation at the tip of the index finger (median nerve) and little finger (ulnar nerve).

In the unresponsive patient, observe for spontaneous movement of both upper extremities. Test for ability to move in response to pain by pinching the skin of the inner arm or pinching a fingernail hard with your thumb and forefinger. Compare the reactions of the two sides of the body.

The Back

For adequate assessment of the back, the patient must be lying prone or on the side, and the back must be exposed with the clothing pulled either up or down. If the patient is already prone or on the side, assess the back before turning the patient unless urgent problems detected during the first impression or the primary survey require immediate turning into the supine position for basic life support.

If the mechanism of injury or abnormalities found during the back assessment make you suspect a neck or back injury, the non-urgent patient should not be moved until enough help arrives to do it by safe methods.

If you suspect a back or neck injury in the supine patient, conduct detailed assessment of the back at the time the patient is logrolled for placement on a long spine board in order to avoid unnecessary logrolling. While waiting for help to arrive, you can start the back assessment by sliding your hand under the neck and back and palpating each spinous process in turn from above downward for step-off deformity, abnormal prominence, swelling, and tenderness (Fig. 19.9). At times, bleeding will be detected in this way as well, so it is best to wear rubber gloves.

Beginning at the back of the neck and moving footward, inspect the skin of the neck, back, and buttocks for scars, open and closed wounds, impaled objects, lumps, swelling, bleeding, deformities, and unusual positions. Feel the neck, back, and buttocks for swellings, tenderness, deformities, or unusual positions.

Pay special attention to the spinous processes of the vertebrae. Tenderness, swelling, and/or ecchy-mosis anywhere on the back suggests a contusion; if over a spinous process and especially if there is a deformity, the patient is considered to have a spine injury. Tenderness in one or both costovertebral angles suggests a possible kidney injury or infection.

Management of Stress

After completing your training and becoming an emergency care provider, you will be exposed to scenes and involved in activities unlike any you have experienced before. You will see patients who are in great pain, who are anxious, and who may be uncooperative, critical, or hysterical. Occasionally, you may see horribly disfiguring and gruesome injuries. Rarely, someone will die.

You will find these experiences hard to deal with at first, but remember that your reactions of concern, grief, and sorrow are normal. Even physicians, nurses, and emergency medical technicians who deal with serious events on a daily basis have trouble controlling their feelings occasionally. As you become more experienced, you will develop a professional approach to emergency care that will help you deliver competent care and show concern without becoming emotionally involved to the point where you are inefficient or ineffective.

Common reactions that follow association with a death or serious injury may include the following:

1. Psychological reactions such as sadness, guilt, lack of enthusiasm, insomnia, inability to concentrate, irritability, lack of motivation, a desire to quit emergency care activities, and a lack of interest in family and friends.
2. Physical sensations such as headache, backache, fatigue, indigestion, decreased appetite, and loss of weight.
3. Persistent thoughts about death, suffering, or pain.

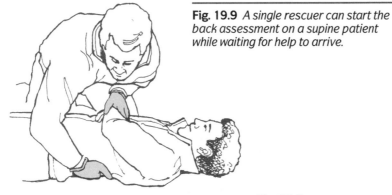

Fig. 19.9 *A single rescuer can start the back assessment on a supine patient while waiting for help to arrive.*

Fig. 19.9

4. Unintentional recalls ("flashbacks") of the stressful experience.
5. Feelings such as "If only I had done something differently."

Do not keep these feelings to yourself. Discuss them with your co-workers, many of whom will have had similar experiences. If these feelings are persistent or severe, you may be developing a state called "burn-out" due to the cumulative effects of stress from your emergency care activities plus other types of stress from your job or personal life. In this case, it is wise to seek psychological counseling as soon as possible since the longer the symptoms last, the harder they are to treat.

Although the rewards of being able to help suffering patients are great, you must realize that patients tend to regress to a more dependent and infantile state where they are not always cooperative or grateful for your efforts. Occasionally, you may be unjustly criticized by a patient or his or her friends or relatives.

Over the past few years medical workers have realized that certain types of events produce severe stress reactions. These include mass-casualty incidents, multiple deaths, and particularly gruesome or tragic deaths. The Critical Incident Stress Debriefing (CISD) program has been developed to aid caregivers in dealing with these incidents so that the process of normal grieving is facilitated and significant psychological problems prevented. A CISD program should be started as soon as possible after the event. Most localities with well-developed EMS services have a CISD team, which can be contacted through your local hospital emergency department.

During the incident debriefing, all involved persons should be present. The event will be reviewed, including the mechanisms and resulting injuries or illnesses, critical decisions and why they were made, and suggestions for handling of similar incidents in the future. All team members should share their feelings, anxieties, anger, and guilt, if any; free discussion is encouraged. Remember that "only people who avoid love can avoid grief. The point is to learn from it and remain vulnerable to love." (Richard W. Swanson, M.D.)

Determination of the Probable Occurrence of Death

Although a legal pronouncement of death can be made only by a physician or other legally constituted authority, a rescuer can tell from a properly performed patient assessment whether death has likely occurred or is obvious. Factors to consider include the following:

1. The mechanism of injury was such that a lethal injury would be anticipated. Or, the death was preceded by a period of obvious severe illness with the symptoms of pneumonia, heart attack, pulmonary or cerebral edema, or serious infection. Death may have been anticipated because of a previous diagnosis of terminal cancer, far advanced heart or kidney disease, a severe stroke, or other illness incompatible with prolonged life.
2. The patient exhibits signs of death, which can be divided into early and late. (Remember that the hypothermic or near-drowning victim may look dead and still be salvageable.)
   a. Early signs:
      (1) Evidence of lethal injury such as decapitation; severe head injury; massive open wounds of the head, chest, or abdomen; consumption of the body by fire; or a severing injury of the trunk.
      (2) Careful assessment that shows no respirations, pulse, or detectable heartbeat over a period of several minutes.
      (3) No response to painful stimuli.
      (4) Widely dilated pupils that do not respond to light.
      (5) Pale, cool skin; blue lips and nails.
      (6) Rapidly glazing eyes.
      (7) Relaxed body sphincters, evacuation of body wastes.
   b. Late signs:
      (1) Rigid limbs and trunk (rigor mortis). The rescuer is not able to straighten bent body parts (also may occur in severe hypothermia).
      (2) Mottled, bluish, or purple skin, especially the parts closest to the surface on which the body is lying (livor mortis or lividity).
      (3) Odor of decay (may be difficult to distinguish from odors caused by bowel incontinence in someone who is still alive).

Do not start CPR and other emergency care in the case of lethal injury, rigor mortis, livor mortis, or body decomposition. If there is a question, however, give emergency care including full resuscitation. If emergency care has already been started, even though you believe the patient is dead, you generally must continue the care until the patient is pronounced dead. To stop it is to risk being charged with abandonment (see Appendix A) unless other factors such as rescuer exhaustion or danger to rescuers supersede.

Scenario #19 (Fig. 19.10)

The following scenario illustrates the assessment of a patient with a serious medical problem.

As part of a family reunion, you have agreed to take six cousins from the East on a four-day backpacking trip into the high country northeast of Grandstone National Park. They have all hiked parts of the Appalachian Trail but before now have never been above 6,000 feet for very long.

You sent them a list of gear to bring, and they have done quite well with the aid of L.L. Bean and Eastern Mountain Sports: everyone has a pair of serviceable boots, a poncho or rain parka, and a pile jacket. By borrowing from your friends and ransacking your basement equipment room, you have two big tents and enough Therma-Rests and sleeping bags for everybody. The cousins all look like they will make up in enthusiasm for anything they may lack in experience.

You are able to get everyone and all the gear into your king-cab pickup and your four-door sedan. You leave the vehicles at the Lady-of-the-Lake trailhead. You take the lead and ask Joe, who used to be a ski patroller at Mount Scree in Vermont, to herd the stragglers from the rear. You set a steady, rhythmic pace and stop at regular intervals to admire the view and the many small meadows with their colorful patches of elephant-head, rosecrown, yellow monkey-flower, and some type of purplish composite that you have never been able to identify. Everyone is somewhat short of breath from the altitude, but no one lags behind.

Camp that night is at the lower end of Lower Aerie Lake, at an altitude of 9,500 feet. Several of the group have their spinning gear out as soon as they spot the huge brown trout in the deep water at the bottom of a small cliff nearby, but it is shrimp-hatch time and they do not have any luck.

You prepare a masterpiece for supper: fresh pasta from Bernadelli's in town, with their famous homemade sauce, freeze-dried vegetables, garlic bread, and pistachio instant pudding. Everyone is in their sleeping bag by 8:30 p.m., with plans for fishing the next morning for grayling in an inlet creek and scrambling up Wolverine Peak for a view of the entire mountain range.

You usually do not sleep well your first night at altitude, and this night is no exception. You hear some stirring from the other tent several times, and once a flashlight beam plays briefly on the side of your own tent. It sounds like someone is walking up the path to where you have established a latrine. You are in a deep sleep when you are suddenly awakened by a disturbance at the tent entrance.

Fig. 19.10 *Scenario #19*

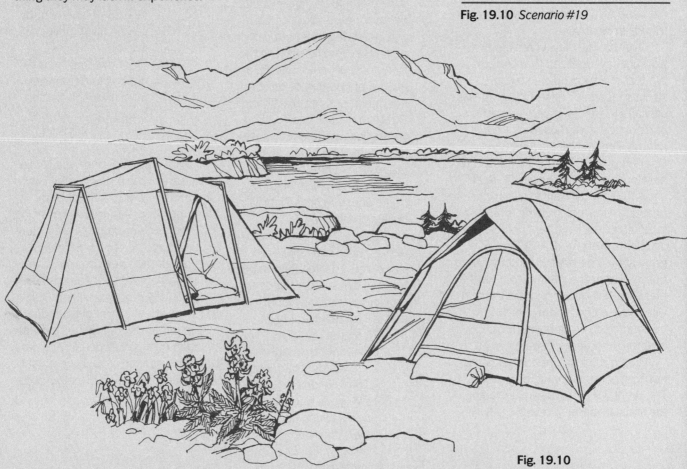

Fig. 19.10

"Ben, come out here, please. Something is wrong with Bill." It is Joe, with a worried look. You pick up your pile jacket, strap on your camp sandals, and squirm out through the entrance. The sun is just up over the ridge to the east. You glance at your watch: it is 6 a.m.

Joe tells you that Bill got up several times during the night to go out and is now lying in his sleeping bag. He is complaining of being short of breath and weak.

You crawl into the tent, a four-person, center pole relic from past expeditions. Cousin Bill, a 36-year-old computer programmer from Massachusetts, is lying on his side. There is enough light for you to see his face, which is pale with beads of sweat on the forehead. He looks anxious.

You unzip the bag, reach in, and grasp his wrist. "Joe, get me your flashlight, please." Bill's pulse is regular, strong, and 110 beats per minute. He is breathing at a rate of 24 respirations per minute. You test the capillary refill in a fingernail; it is normal.

You: "Bill, what's wrong?"

Bill: "I'm not sure. I'm very weak and can't get my breath."

You: "When did it start?"

Bill: "I was okay when I went to bed… maybe a little tired from the walk in. I woke up about midnight and had to move my bowels in a hurry. On the way back from the latrine I was more short of breath and my legs felt pretty weak. For a few minutes I wasn't sure I would make it back to the tent. I felt better after I got back into my bag and went back to sleep. I guess it was two hours later, I had to get up and have another bowel movement. On the way back I was weak and short of breath again. I got back to sleep, but I'm not feeling any better. I'm still weak and short of breath, and starting to feel sick on my stomach."

You: "Do you have any headache or dizziness?"

Bill: "No headache, but I feel dizzy."

You: "Do you mean you're light-headed, or do you actually have trouble with your balance? Is the tent going around in circles?"

Bill: "Light-headed, I guess."

You: "What was the bowel movement like? Did you look at it? Was it diarrhea? Did you have any cramps?"

Bill: "It was soft but not diarrhea. I couldn't see much, it was too dark and my flashlight battery is weak. No cramps."

You: "Have you had a cold, sore throat, chills, fever, nausea, vomiting, or diarrhea during the last week or so?"

Bill: "No."

You: "Have you had any other changes in your bowel habits?"

Bill: "The bowel movements have been pretty dark the last few days."

You: "Have you had any indigestion, like heartburn or sour stomach?"

Bill: "Some sour stomach. I've used a lot of Rolaids the last two weeks."

At this point, you are puzzled. His airway, breathing, and circulation seem to be basically all right, but stressed, with a fast heart rate and breathing rate. You know that you should think of acute mountain sickness in anyone who is not feeling well above 7,500 feet. Also, there is a lot of stomach flu going around, but it does not sound like a typical case of that. You need to assess his neck and chest.

Pulling down the neck of his T-shirt, you look at the neck. The veins are not distended. You do not feel any tender nodes under the jaw. There are no swellings or tender areas. The trachea is in the midline.

Pulling the T-shirt up around his neck, you look at the chest. Both sides are moving symmetrically as he breathes. You put your ear to both sides of the chest. You do not hear any rattles, wheezes, or other noise. The breathing sounds are loud and equal on both sides. Where do you go from here? Better assess the abdomen.

With the tips of your fingers, you palpate the abdomen, starting in the right upper quadrant, asking each time you push in with your fingers, "Does this hurt?" When you reach the epigastric area, he winces. You can hear some loud gurgles. There are no other tender areas.

You have a feeling that you are forgetting something. **A**irway, **B**reathing, **C**irculation: That's it! **C** stands for bleeding as well as circulation. "Joe, do me a favor. Run up to the latrine and tell me what Bill's bowel movement looks like. Seriously." Joe is back in a few minutes.

Joe: "There is a lot of reddish-black bowel movement in the latrine."

The picture is falling together. Bill probably has an ulcer and is bleeding from it. You remember reading about bleeding ulcers in *Outdoor Emergency Care.*

You: "Bill, have you ever had an ulcer?"

Bill: "I had one three years ago, but it cleared up with Tagamet."

You: "Does this feel anything like that ulcer?"

Bill: "Maybe so."

You: (wracking your memory) "This sour stomach you mentioned, what happens when you eat?"

Bill: "It gets better, but then comes back in an hour or so."

You: "Are you taking any regular medicine besides the Rolaids?"

Bill: "No."

You: "Have you had any other medical problems in the past? Any allergies?"

Bill: "No."

You: "Anything else we need to know about you?"

Bill: "I've always been healthy, but more tired lately. Probably because we've been awfully busy at work. I had a hard time getting off to come on this trip."

After this, you start feeding Bill some reconstituted powdered milk and instant Cream of Wheat, and give him some Mylanta you have in your first aid kit. You send Mike, who runs marathons, out to the roadhead on the double to call for a helicopter, not forgetting to give him the car keys.

As it turns out, Bill has only one more bowel movement, his pulse slows and his color returns to some extent before he is helicoptered out to a hospital early that afternoon. A duodenal ulcer is found on esophagogastroscopy. It was not bleeding actively by then, so your emergency care may have helped. You resolve to leave Bernadelli's famous pasta sauce off future menus.

Scenario #20 (Fig. 19.11)

The following scenario illustrates the assessment of a patient with multiple injuries.

It is a beautiful June day in the Granite range. High Range Ski Area has been closed for six weeks, but you are still not ready to quit skiing. You, your wife Sandy, and two other couples have just driven up the switchbacks of the Whitetail Highway to 10,000 feet where there is not only plenty of snow but plenty of steep chutes to ski.

You have several vehicles so that you can leave one about six switchbacks below at 8,000 feet on the highway to ferry you back after you have skied the Granite Creek Headwall. You hoped to have it to yourselves, but there are five other cars at the turn-off by the top of the headwall. It is only 7 a.m., so the snow is still in good condition. There will be time to make a dozen runs before it turns to mush in the hot, June sun.

Several other skiers are getting into their bindings as you brake to a stop. It takes a few minutes to limber up and get into your own bindings.

Fig. 19.11 *Scenario #20*

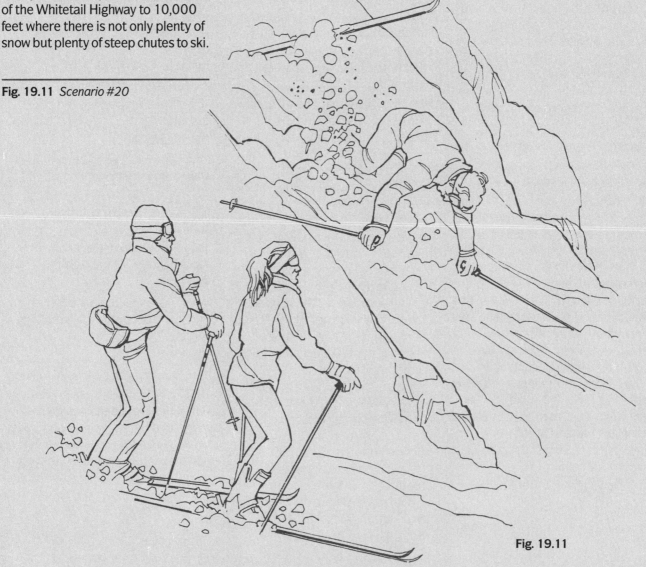

Fig. 19.11

The right-hand chute is narrow but in excellent condition as you jump-turn down the 50-degree section at the top and break out into the wider, easier terrain below.

You are puffing some when you reach the bottom. Your wife is right behind you, demonstrating the smooth, effortless technique that you have always been a little envious of. The other four arrive a few minutes apart. It is obvious that they have not forgotten how to ski.

At the end of the third run, you are feeling it a little in your quads. You skid to a stop and look up the chute. Sandy is half-way down, lookin' good. She joins you, breathing easily in the thin air. As you both look uphill, the next skier is coming down. You do not recognize him—he must be from one of the cars with the number 6 licence plates, from the University.

As you watch, he suddenly loses his balance during a turn, falls forward, and starts to cartwheel. Both skis fly off. His poles must still be with him, but there is such a cloud of snow you are not sure. You hear Sandy gasp as he hits a small rock outcrop and launches into the air, picking up speed as he hits the snow headfirst. From there he tumbles over and over, bounces off one side of the gulley, and finally slides to a halt about 30 yards above you. You and Sandy both kick off your skis and run toward him. As you run, you reach behind you to make sure your first aid belt is still there.

The skier is a young man, probably in his early 20s. He is not moving. As you reach his side, you take in the scene rapidly. There is some blood on the snow near his head. His cap is gone, and his eyes are closed. You are not sure he is breathing. His right thigh is twisted at an unusual angle.

You steady his head with your hand, shake his shoulder, and call loudly: "Buddy, are you okay?" There is no answer. His face is pale with beads of sweat on his forehead. With a quick motion, you release your first aid belt. "Sandy, please get out two pairs of rubber gloves from that black film can on the left."

You move around behind him and stabilize his head and neck while you thrust his jaw forward. You bend your ear to his mouth and nose and are relieved to hear the air moving in and out. You feel for his carotid pulse under the neck of his pullover; it is strong and around 100 beats per minute. You can see his chest lifting; his breathing rate is about 20 respirations per minute. Looking at his dark hair, you see blood trickling through the hair on the right temporoparietal area of the scalp and running down his cheek. Sandy has a pair of gloves on; she takes over the airway and neck stabilization while you put on the other pair.

Reaching into the first aid belt, you retrieve an oral airway, a flashlight, and a tongue blade. You check the airway for size by placing it against his cheek. You open his mouth with the two-finger technique and use the tongue blade to push the tongue out of the way; he does not gag. There is no blood in his mouth, and his teeth look normal. You slip the oral airway in place.

Quickly, you assess the eyes and pupils; both pupils are round and respond to the light of your flashlight, but the right one is slightly bigger than the left. "Uh-oh! Better do the AVPU," you think. You pinch the skin of his inner arm through his jacket; he stirs and moans. Next, you pinch the nail of his right index finger hard, then the nail of his left index finger; he withdraws the right hand but not the left. You repeat the hard pinch on the skin of both lower legs; he moves the right leg slightly but not the left. The capillary refill time is longer than two seconds. He has a bad head injury and is probably starting to lateralize, but he also seems to be in early shock. You know that head injuries by themselves do not cause shock; there must be something else going on.

Turning back to his head, you assess the scalp and easily find a large laceration oozing blood. Gently feeling the scalp around the laceration, you cannot feel any depression or irregularities.

By this time, one of the other two couples has arrived, and you recruit the wife, Jenny, to hand you a sterile compress from the plastic bandage bag, which you place over the laceration. Mike, her husband and a fellow patroller, has his fanny pack off and a pair of gloves on. He puts direct pressure on the wound while you turn to the rest of the head and face.

There is no blood in either ear. The sides of the jaw are symmetrical. Moving to the neck, you run your fingers down the spinous processes of the seven cervical vertebrae, failing to find any step-off deformities or lumps. Anteriorly, the veins are flat, there are no open wounds, bruises or swellings, and the trachea is in the midline.

You notice that his breathing rate has increased, it is now 28 respirations per minute. You recheck the carotid pulse, which is weaker and 120 beats per minute. Moving quickly to the chest, you open his jacket and place a hand on each side of the chest. Both sides expand equally. Lifting his pullover, you run both hands down the ribs on each side while you inspect the skin. There are no wounds, bruises or swellings of the upper chest, but when you reach the lower chest there is a large bruise over the lower right ribs. Moving down to the abdomen, you notice he moans when you press on his right upper quadrant beneath the costal angle. You press the sides of the pelvis together and backward; they seem solid and he does not moan.

Proceeding downward to the lower extremities, you run your hands over both thighs. The mid-right thigh is swollen beneath his jeans, and he moans again when you press on the swollen area. The lower extremities are otherwise normal.

At this point, you see the other couple approaching, accompanied by two young skiers—probably the patient's friends. You reflect a moment. You have a skier who took a bad fall with lots of kinetic energy, bounced off some rocks, cartwheeled, and tumbled. He is responsive only to pain, has a large scalp laceration and a maybe an early blown pupil on the right. His left side is not moving as well as his right in response to pain. To you, this indicates a bad head injury that is getting worse. In addition, he has a rising pulse and respiratory rate, evidence of injuries to the lower right chest and upper right abdomen, and a probable right femur fracture. He has plenty of reasons to be going into shock; take your pick: possible lung and liver injury, let alone the femur. He probably should be hyperventilated to reduce his rising intracranial pressure, and you remember that you have your pocket mask along.

You: "Pete, get the pocket mask out of my first aid belt and take over for Mike. Hold some pressure on that head wound. Mike, give him mouth-to-mouth with the pocket mask at about 30 deep breaths per minute."

The two friends have arrived. "Hi," you say, "I'm Ben Schussen from the High Range Ski Patrol. Is this man a friend of yours?"

Friend: "Yes. He's Oliver de Place. He's a senior at the 'U.' What happened to him?"

You: "He took a bad fall and tumbled all the way down the chute. He's unconscious, badly hurt, and going into shock. He has injuries to his head, chest, abdomen, a probable femur fracture, and a possible neck injury. Do you have a car parked down there at the turnout?"

Friend: "Yes."

You: "This is an emergency. I need you to get in your car and drive as fast as you can to the restaurant at the entrance to the canyon, just before the switchbacks start up. Call the county sheriff and tell him about your friend, where he is, that he fell about 1,000 feet down the Granite Creek Headwall, what injuries he has, and that he is going into shock. We need the advanced life support ambulance from the town hospital with a doctor or paramedic, and some help from the sheriff's office right away. Tell them we need a spine board, traction splint, oxygen, bag-valve-mask, suction, a litter, and at least six people to carry him out to the road. We need a LifeFlight helicopter from the city to meet us in town. Can you remember all that?"

Friend: "You bet. I'm writing it down. I'm on my way."

As he leaves, you finish the secondary survey by assessing the patient's upper extremities and running your hand behind his back from the base of neck to the tailbone. With Pete's help, you remove both boots and check the pulses in both feet. They are easy to find and strong. Then you take a pair of paramedic shears from your fanny pack and cut his right pant leg open to the hip. There is a large swelling in the middle of the thigh; no blood or open wounds anywhere.

You, Pete, Mike, and Sandy then align the patient into the anatomical position, straightening his right lower extremity with axial traction. While maintaining the extremity traction and head/neck stabilization, the four of you roll him carefully a quarter turn onto his side while Jenny places several parkas on the snow under him.

You talk to the patient's other friends and are able to get some sketchy details about his medical history. He has no illnesses, is on no medicines, has no allergies, and has always been healthy although somewhat impulsive and carefree. He has

been skiing two seasons, has never taken any lessons, and this is the first time he has skied the Headwall. His favorite summer sport is motorcycle racing.

The patient is evacuated without incident to town on a long spine board, with a traction splint on his right lower extremity. He is flown immediately to City Hospital where he spends the next five weeks, two weeks of it in the surgical intensive care unit on a ventilator. For some reason, he did not fracture his neck. He requires brain surgery for removal of a right subdural hematoma followed immediately by a laparotomy to sew up a laceration in his liver. His fractured femur is treated with an intramedullary nail a week later. In three months, he is back on his motorcycle.

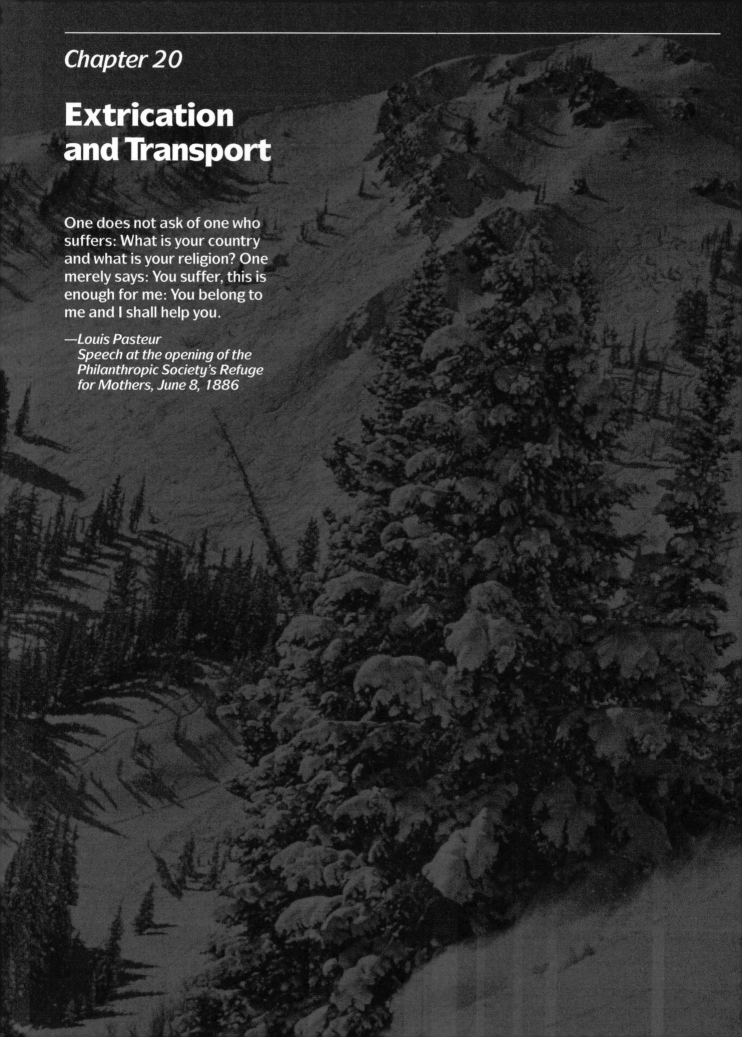

Chapter 20

Extrication and Transport

One does not ask of one who suffers: What is your country and what is your religion? One merely says: You suffer, this is enough for me: You belong to me and I shall help you.

—*Louis Pasteur*
  Speech at the opening of the Philanthropic Society's Refuge for Mothers, June 8, 1886

The preceding chapters of this textbook present the assessment and emergency care of patients, regardless of their physical location. This chapter describes techniques for obtaining access to, extricating, transferring, packaging, and transporting patients who may be found in remote areas, unstable positions, and awkward locations (Fig. 20.1).

This entire process, together with techniques for *locating* the patient, frequently is called **search and rescue (SAR)**. After the patient has been located and accessed, the principles of emergency care are the same as those presented in previous chapters but may have to be modified somewhat to fit unusual situations.

Search and rescue operations begin with a search for the patient, often a complicated and time-consuming process. In the United States, most searches are conducted by a management plan called the Incident Command System. This plan, originally developed for fighting forest fires, is widely used by government agencies. After being located, the patient must be **rescued**, which involves the other techniques listed above. Search techniques are beyond the scope of this book; rescuers interested in studying them should consult standard SAR manuals such as those published by the National Association for Search and Rescue (NASAR).

After being located and given initial emergency care, the patient frequently must be removed from the original location to a more convenient place where further emergency care can be given and the patient can be packaged for transport. This process, called **extrication**, involves delicate techniques designed to move the patient *without causing further injury to either the patient or the rescuers*. Extrication can tax the strength, skills, and ingenuity of the rescuer. The patient may be found tangled in machinery or a thicket, or in an awkward

position and/or tight location such as in a wrecked vehicle, tree well, hole, or cave. Close approach may be difficult, conventional alignment of deformities may be impossible, and there may be no room to bring in splints or spine boards. Or, the patient's location may be dangerous or unstable, such as on a narrow ledge, on an avalanche slope, or in a partially collapsed building.

After extrication, the patient is **transferred** to a spine board if injury is suspected, then to a transportation device such as a litter or toboggan. In the next step, **packaging**, the patient is positioned properly in the transportation device, padded, strapped in securely, and protected from the elements and hazards such as rockfall by various types of insulation and shielding. After being packaged, the patient is **transported** to definitive medical care.

Overview of the Rescue Process

When first sighting the patient, note the location and position compared to your own, and determine the fastest and most efficient way to reach the patient with all necessary equipment.

Also note hazardous aspects of the scene that may endanger the patient and/or rescuers. The patient may be in a precarious position in imminent danger of such hazards as falling, drowning, suffocating, burial, or being crushed in a structure collapse. Rescuers may run the same risks in

Fig. 20.1 *A Patient being Lowered Down a Steep Snow Field*

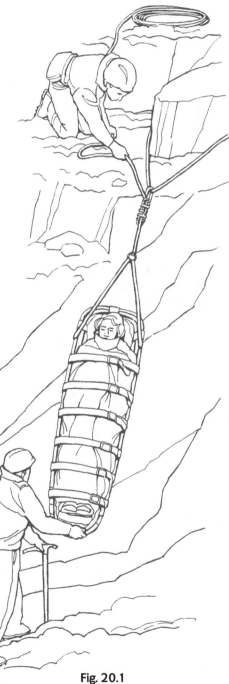

Fig. 20.1

attempting to reach the patient. Rescuers may endanger the patient by accidentally knocking down loose objects such as rock or dislodging the patient from an unstable position. As a general rule, a patient should not be approached from directly above or directly below unless there is no alternative. The safest route of access may be difficult to determine.

Specific hazards can include potential rockfall, steep slopes, heavily traveled ski runs, technical terrain, snow avalanches, slippery rocks in the middle of rivers, whitewater, flash floods, approaching storms, forest fires, weakened structures, moving machinery, and heavy vehicular traffic.

Remember that, despite altruism, your first responsibility should be to yourself, second to your fellow rescuers, and third to the patient. Hazards to the patient frequently are hazards to the rescue team as well. In extreme cases, rescue may be impossible.

If the terrain is unique, steep, or technically challenging, search and rescue should be conducted *only* by rescuers *with training and experience in this environment;* otherwise, special rescue teams should be called in. Such teams available for problem environments include search dog units and mountain, cave, whitewater, mine, and urban disaster rescue teams.

Hard hats should be worn routinely in situations where falls or injuries from falling objects such as rocks or building materials could occur. It may be necessary to work quickly to reach shelter in advance of an approaching storm. Dangerous slopes may have to be crossed to reach a person buried in an avalanche; rescuers may be endangered if unstable slopes feed into the avalanche track above the site (Fig. 20.2). Gaining access to the patient may require cutting away trees and brush, moving rocks and other obstacles, prying or cutting open vehicles, and using special techniques such as rappeling.

After the patient has been reached, urgent care should be given at the scene using the standard techniques of assessment and emergency care discussed in previous chapters.

Fig. 20.2 *Rescuers may be endangered if unstable slopes feed into the avalanche track above the site.*

Impedances may have to be cleared by sawing, cutting, prying, or digging before transportation equipment can be brought in and the patient can be extricated. It is best, when possible, to remove the impedance from the patient, *not* the patient from the impedance.

The scoop stretcher, short spine board, vest-type devices, and special litters such as the SKED stretcher (see Chapter 8) have been designed for difficult extrications (Fig. 20.3). However, it may be faster and cause less movement of injured parts for trained rescuers to use special lifts, slides, and carries to move the patient a short distance to where long spine boards, traction splints, and other conventional devices can be used.

In general, a patient should not be moved until all necessary emergency care, especially basic life support, has been given, all injured parts have been immobilized, enough help is available, and it is clear that the patient will not be injured further if moved. Circumstances, however, may require that the patient be moved sooner. The various techniques for moving a patient are divided into **emergency** and **nonemergency moves**.

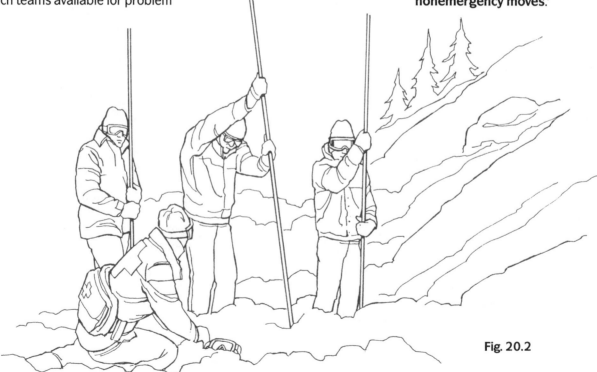

Fig. 20.2

Principles of Extrication

As taught by Dr. Peter Goth and his colleagues of Wilderness Medical Associates, there are six basic anatomical positions in which a patient may be found (Fig. 20.4): three main positions—1, 2, and 3; and three variations—1a, 2a, and 3a.

Position 1: The patient is supine, in the neutral, anatomical position with the back straight, the eyes facing forward, and the extremities straight with the palms against the sides of the thighs. This is the position the patient must be aligned into before being immobilized on a long spine board.

Position 1a: The patient is supine, but the head, neck, back, and extremities may be rotated, bent, or in any position other than the anatomical one.

Position 2: The patient is on the side, but in the neutral, anatomical position with the back straight, the eyes facing forward, and the extremities straight. This is the position the patient must be in when rolled onto the side in the logroll.

Position 2a: The patient is on the side but with the head, neck, back, and extremities in any position except the anatomical position.

Position 3: The patient is prone but in the neutral, anatomical position, except that the head is usually turned to the side.

Position 3a: The patient is prone with the head, neck, back, and extremities in any position except the neutral, anatomical position.

The ultimate goal of extrication is to have an injured patient, especially one with a suspected neck or back injury, *in position 1* on the ground or on a long spine board.

As discussed in Chapter 8, the spine can be thought of as composed of two long bones and three joints. The bones are the cervical and thoracolumbar segments of the spine; the joints are the joint between the skull and the first cervical vertebra, the joint between the seventh cervical and first thoracic vertebrae, and the joint between the fifth lumbar vertebra and the sacrum. Proper immobilization of an injured spine requires that all three of these joints be immobilized.

Think of a flat surface on which a patient lies as a flat **spinal plane**. As the patient lies supine in the anatomical position on the flat surface, the occiput, shoulders, upper back, buttocks, sacrum, calves, and heels are in contact with this plane. The three important reference points to keep in mind are the **head, shoulders**, and **hips**. The goal is to align the patient so that these three points are in line with each other, at right angles to the spine, and related to each other as though the patient were lying on

---

Fig. 20.3 *Extrication Tools and Litters*

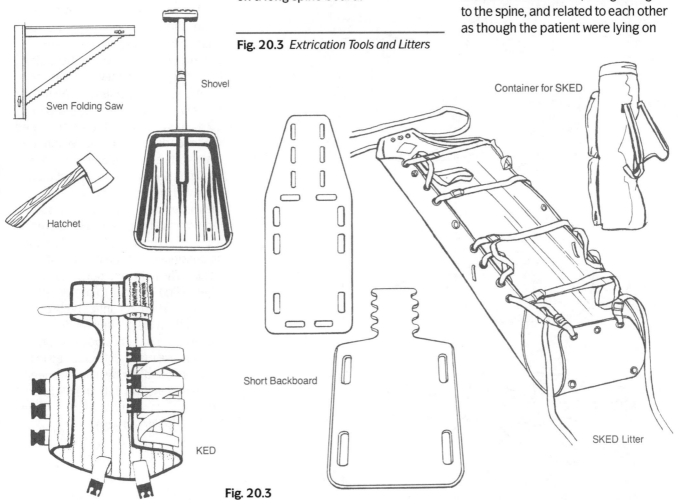

Sven Folding Saw

Shovel

Hatchet

KED

Short Backboard

Container for SKED

SKED Litter

Fig. 20.3

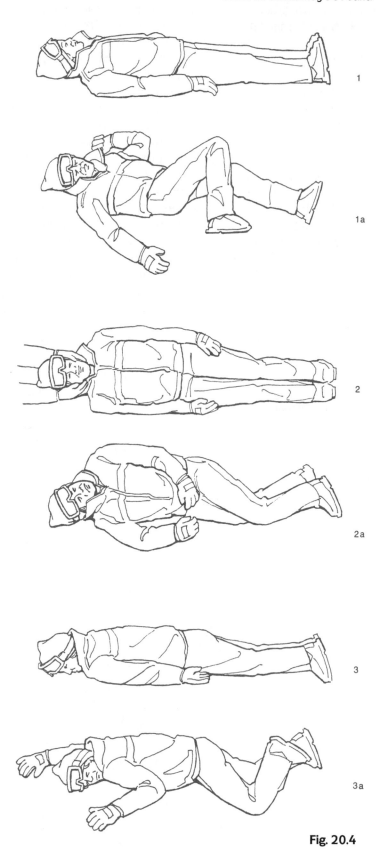

Fig. 20.4 *Basic Anatomical Positions in which a Patient may be Found*

1

1a

2

2a

3

3a

Fig. 20.4

this spinal plane in the neutral, anatomical position; and that they remain so during any movement of the patient.

If this can be accomplished, the three joints of the spine will be stabilized, there will be little or no motion of the areas of the spine between the joints, and the spine itself will remain splinted. Keep the concept of the spinal plane in mind at all times when moving the patient, so that the three reference points can be kept in proper relationship to each other.

At least four (but preferably six) rescuers are required to align the patient: one at the patient's head, one at the shoulders (or at each shoulder), one at the hips (or at each hip), and one at the legs. All rescuers should move smoothly, steadily, and in unison under the command of the *leader*, either the rescuer at the patient's head or the one at the site of the severest injury.

The three reference points—the head, shoulders, and hips—are stabilized manually *at all times*. The patient's body is moved either axially, by sliding, or vertically, by lifting or lowering, but *not* sideways. All movement is in short increments of 6 to 12 inches and is started and stopped at the leader's command. When the limbs or the head and neck must be straightened, only one joint at a time is moved in one plane at a time, while the three reference points are stabilized manually. All body parts are aligned into position 1, 2, or 3 as early as possible unless pain or resistance occurs. The head and neck usually are aligned first in order to protect the airway. Parts that cannot be brought into anatomical position at first because of the patient's position or location are manually stabilized in the position found during all movement of the patient and until the patient reaches a place where there is room for the rescuers to work.

The maneuvers should be performed rapidly but not hastily. Also, the number of positions should be kept to a minimum and generally should progress from 3 to 2 to 1. For example, a patient in position 3a is aligned as closely as possible into position 3, then logrolled into position 2 and then into position 1 as described in Chapter 13. A patient in position 2a is aligned into position 2 and then logrolled into position 1. A patient in position 1a is aligned into position 1. A patient in position 1 is lifted a few inches off the ground or logrolled into position 2 in order to be placed on a long spine board. A rigid collar is applied as soon as possible, i.e., when the head has been moved into a neutral, in-line position in relation to the torso and the collar can be applied with minimum movement of the head and neck.

The most difficult extrication problems are those in which a patient is in a closely confined area not much larger than his or her body, or located so that body parts are held in non-anatomical positions by being jammed against other objects, such as a foot (Fig. 20.5a) or the head (Fig. 20.5b) against a tree. In this case, the entire body must be moved before all the body parts can be aligned. If enough of the body can be accessed and the ground surface is reasonably smooth, this can be done by sliding the body axially. Otherwise, or if the patient is in a hole, usually it is best to raise the body high enough so that a long spine board or similar rigid object can be slid underneath. This is done by a multiple-rescuer direct ground lift, described in Chapter 13 and repeated below. Belts, cravats, or nylon webbing may be useful as lifting straps.

Before lifting or sliding the patient, try to align the patient as closely as possible into position 1, 2, or 3. Parts that cannot be aligned must be stabilized in place. While moving the patient, maintain stabilization of the three reference points and maintain all other body parts in either their aligned or original positions. After the patient is on the board, complete further alignment into the neutral, anatomical position (position 1).

The same principles apply when removing a seated patient from a vehicle.

It is important to pay attention to footing and balance, especially on slippery rocks, icy stairs, and wet or snowy inclines. Movements must be made *smoothly* and in unison with fellow rescuers. During multiple-rescuer lifts and carries, one rescuer should be designated as the *leader*—usually the rescuer stabilizing the head and neck —and all movements should be made on agreed-upon signals from the leader.

The safety of the rescuers is an important consideration in any move. Every rescuer should know how to lift and carry heavy loads in order to avoid

Fig. 20.5 *Non-anatomical Positions in which a Body may be Jammed*

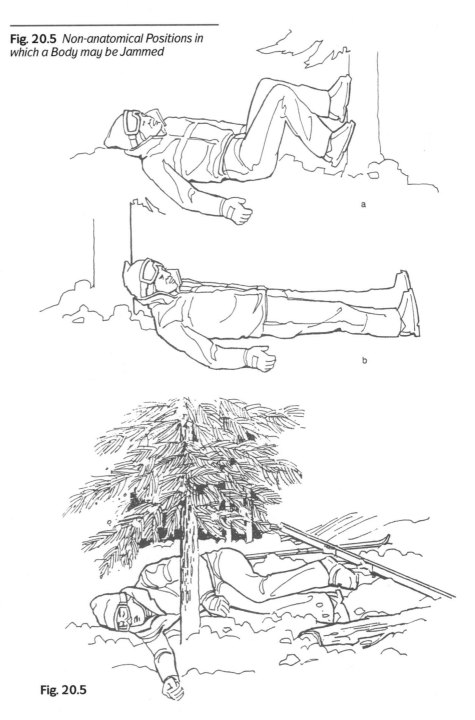

Fig. 20.5

injuring the back or another body part. It is unwise to lift or carry too heavy a load without adequate assistance. The back is vulnerable to injury during common mishaps such as lifting and twisting to the side with the feet mired in mud or snow, or lifting while bending forward (as when moving a cooler from the trunk of a car).

Lift with the *hips* and *legs* rather than the back. Keep the back straight; do not twist or bend forward or to the side (Fig. 20.6). Hold the load as close to the body as possible, and avoid sudden jerky movements.

Fig. 20.6 *Proper Lifting Procedure*

Fig. 20.7 *Fireman's Drag*

Fig. 20.8 *Fireman's Carry*

Fig. 20.7

Fig. 20.8

Emergency Moves

Emergency moves are used when there is an immediate need to move the patient whether or not enough help is available. These moves may be necessary in such circumstances as immediate danger to the patient

Fig. 20.6

or to the rescuers, approaching bad weather, inability to access the patient for care, the need to move the patient to a flat, level surface for CPR, or the need to gain access to other patients with life-threatening injuries. The main danger of an emergency move is *aggravating a spine injury.*

If there is no time to immobilize injuries before moving a patient, the spine and other injured areas should be protected as much as possible by using the multiple-rescuer direct ground lift and transfer (described below), provided enough help is available, or by an axial slide.

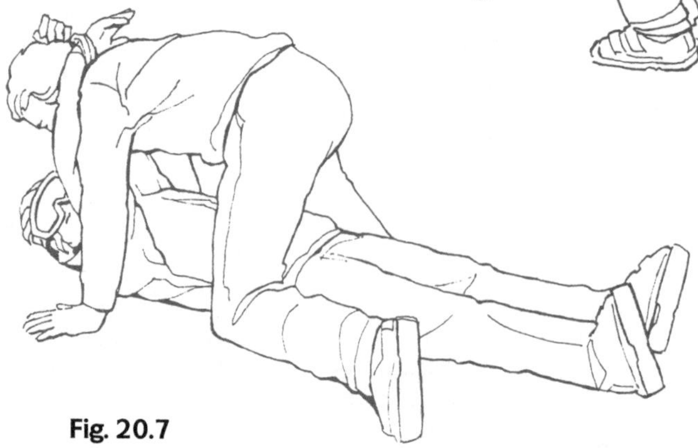

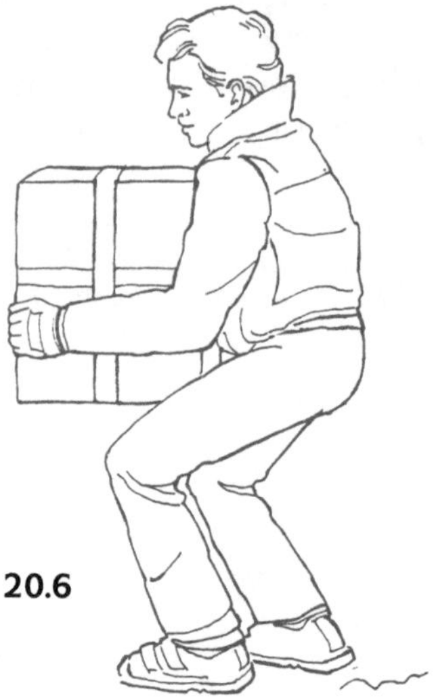

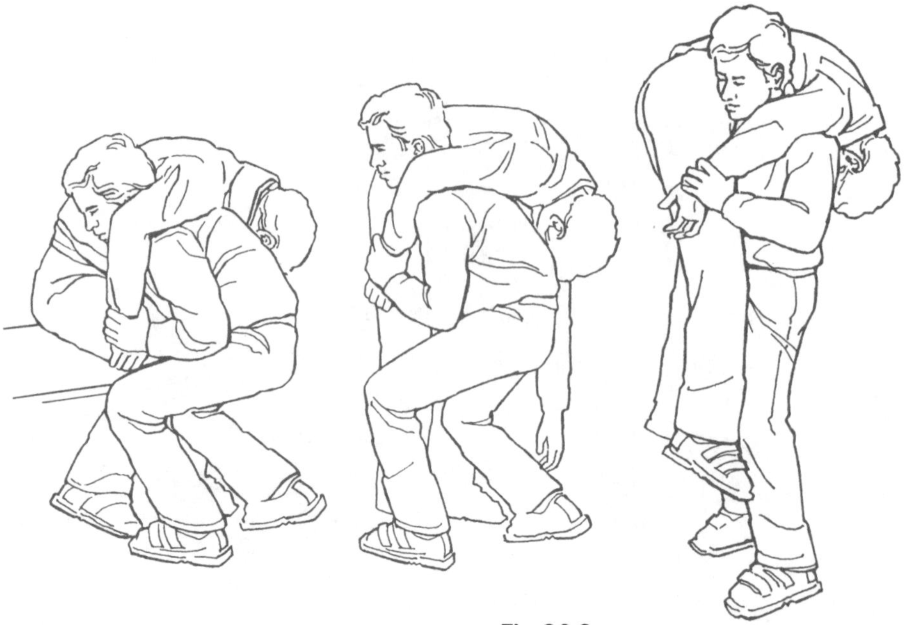

Nonemergency Moves

When the need to move is not urgent, the patient should be stabilized *before* being moved. This means that the primary survey is completed, urgent care given, bleeding controlled, fractures splinted, the neck and back stabilized, and body temperature maintained. Enough help and all needed equipment should be at hand.

Lifts and Carries

Lifts and carries can be divided into the following categories: emergency versus nonemergency, spine injury versus no spine injury, and single rescuer versus multiple rescuers.

Emergency, One-rescuer Techniques—Spine Injury Unlikely

These techniques are used only when there is a bona fide emergency and no time to obtain assistance.

Fireman's Drag

As the name implies, this carry was devised for removing a patient from a burning building.

Roll the patient onto the back and tie the wrists together with a cravat or belt. Face the patient, kneel straddling the patient, raise the patient's arms, and place them around your neck and shoulders so the patient's hands are behind your neck. As you raise your shoulders and begin to crawl, the patient's trunk is lifted clear of the ground and the patient's legs are dragged along the ground between your knees (Fig. 20.7).

Even though this carry is one of the least desirable from the standpoint of patient comfort and safety, it is useful for removing a patient from a low, confined space where there is room for only one rescuer and for removing a patient from a smoke-filled room, since the freshest air is near the floor.

Fireman's Carry

Stand facing the patient, who must be standing or sitting, and grasp both the patient's wrists. Bend your knees into a partial squat and pull the patient toward you so that he or she is slung across your shoulder with the hips and legs anterior and the chest and head posterior (Fig. 20.8). Keep holding on to the patient's wrists, and walk with your legs spread apart for increased stability.

Human Crutch

A person who is conscious and not seriously ill can be assisted in walking to safety. Have the patient put one arm around your shoulders while you put an arm around the patient's waist (Fig. 20.9a). If two rescuers are available, they should flank the patient and each put an arm around the patient's waist; the patient puts his or her arms around the rescuers' shoulders (Fig. 20.9b).

Front Cradle

A strong rescuer can carry a small, light patient in his or her arms. Place one arm around the patient's upper back with the hand under the armpit and the other arm under the patient's knees. The patient's near arm goes around your neck (Fig. 20.10).

Back Carries

In difficult terrain, a one-person carry is easier if the patient can be placed on a strong rescuer's back. The patient must be responsive and without serious injuries. A seat can be fashioned

---

Fig. 20.9 *Human Crutch*

Fig. 20.10 *Front Cradle*

from a long nylon sling about 15 feet long (Fig. 20.11) or from a climbing rope (Fig. 20.12).

To fashion a sling seat, find the midpoint of the sling and put it over the middle of the patient's upper back, running each end under an armpit and around to the patient's chest anteriorly. Cross the ends and run them up and over your shoulders like rucksack straps. Then cross the ends anteriorly over your chest, and run them around your sides and between the patient's legs. Cross them again and run each end around the patient's opposite buttock and up around your waist where they are tied. Use padding under the webbing around the patient's buttocks to increase comfort. The patient's arms come forward over your shoulders and the wrists are tied together. Carry the patient in a piggyback fashion, walking bent slightly forward, holding the patient's wrists with one hand and supporting yourself with an ice ax or pole in the other hand. Two additional rescuers should walk one on each side to help steady you and the patient, if necessary.

To fashion a seat from a climbing rope, double the rope and wind it into

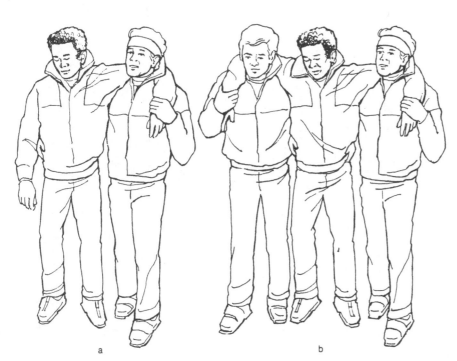

a   b

Fig. 20.9

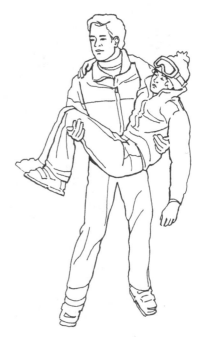

Fig. 20.10

two large coils by passing the doubled rope under your feet and over a hand held at waist level, leaving about 16 feet of rope at the two ends. Secure the coils with a large coil or knot in the middle. Then separate the coils and lay them side by side on the ground. The patient sits down and inserts one foot in each coil; the coils are pulled up so that the patient is sitting on the knot. The rescuer squats, inserts an arm through each coil as if putting on a backpack, and stands up, assisted by helpers. The loose ends are crossed over the patient's back and held by the rescuer to stabilize the patient. The patient is carried piggyback on the rescuer's back. An assistant walks on each side to steady the rescuer.

One-person back carries are tiring for the rescuer and uncomfortable for the patient. They should not be used for long-distance carries: they are best suited for moving patients short distances over very rough terrain or for short vertical stretches when both the patient and the rescuer are belayed.

Emergency One-rescuer Moves—Possible Spine Injury

Long Axis Drag

Roll the patient into the supine position. As mentioned above, this is difficult for the single rescuer because the patient must be rolled without twisting the neck or back (Chapter 4).

The patient can be pulled by the feet or trousers and dragged feet first (Fig. 20.13). To drag a patient head first, extend both arms above the head, cradle the head in the neutral position between your arms, and pull the patient by the wrists. It is preferable to pull the patient on a sheet of material such as a poncho or space blanket, if this is available (Fig. 20.14). Roll the patient (if found non-supine) onto the material or place the material under the patient by first pleating or tightly rolling it lengthwise, leaving one-third flat. Place the rolled side of the material alongside the patient and push it under the patient's body, then pull it from the opposite side so

that it unrolls under the patient. If done properly, it unrolls so that the patient ends up at its center.

Emergency Two-rescuer Moves—No Spine Injury

Seated Carries

A conscious patient without serious injuries who is unable to walk can be carried in a seated position by two rescuers using either a two-handed or four-handed seat (Fig. 20.15). The patient's arms go around the rescuers' shoulders (Fig. 20.16).

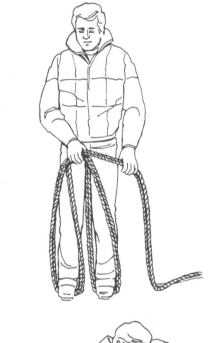

Fig. 20.11 *Nylon Webbing Carry*

Fig. 20.12 *Rope Coil Seat*

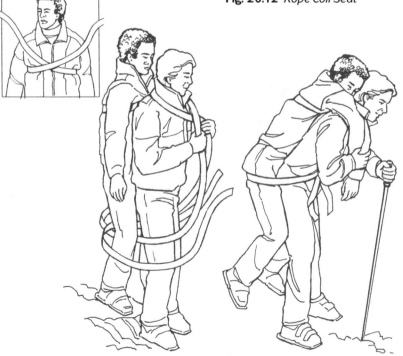

Fig. 20.11

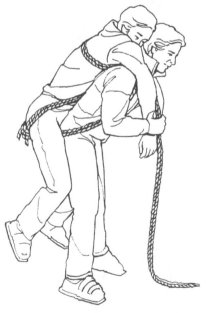

Fig. 20.12

Fore-and-Aft Carry

An unconscious patient with no serious injuries can be moved as shown in Figure 20.17. The first rescuer raises the patient to a sitting position, squats or kneels behind the patient, and wraps his or her arms around the patient's chest under the armpits. The second rescuer faces away from the patient, kneels between the patient's legs, and places a hand under each of the patient's knees. On command, the rescuers both rise.

Nonemergency Moves—One or Two Rescuers

In nonemergency situations, patients with minor injuries may be carried by one or two rescuers as described above for emergency moves. In general, nonemergency moves are best deferred until more help arrives, especially if the patient has injuries that are more than trivial.

Fig. 20.13 *Drag without a Tarp*

Fig. 20.14 *Placement Procedure and Drag on a Tarp*

Fig. 20.15 *Hand Positions for Two-handed and Four-handed Seats*

Fig. 20.16 *Seated Carry*

Nonemergency Moves— Multiple Rescuers

Direct Ground Lift and Carry— No Spine Injury

This method requires at least three rescuers. The rescuers kneel at the patient's least-injured side. One rescuer is positioned at the patient's shoulder, one at the hip, and one at the knee (Fig. 20.18). A fourth rescuer, if available, kneels at the patient's opposite hip (Fig. 20.19). Additional rescuers can kneel at the patient's feet and opposite shoulder. All rescuers kneel on the knee closest to the patient's feet.

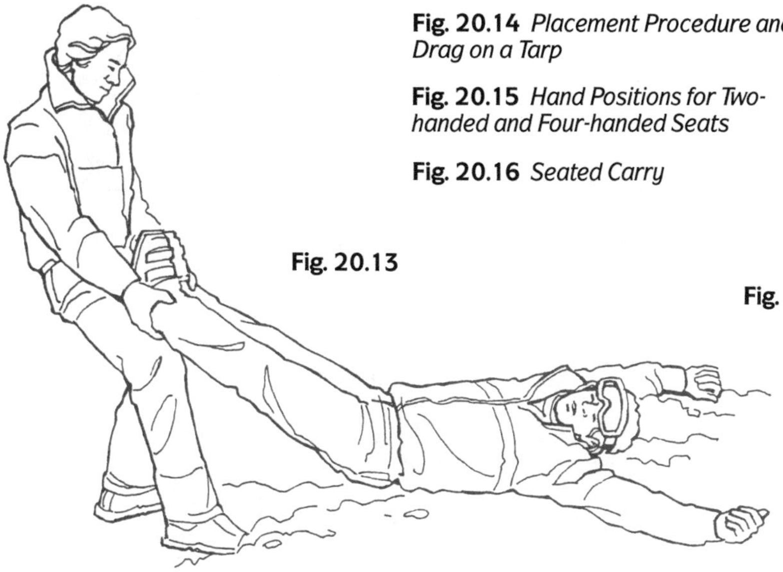

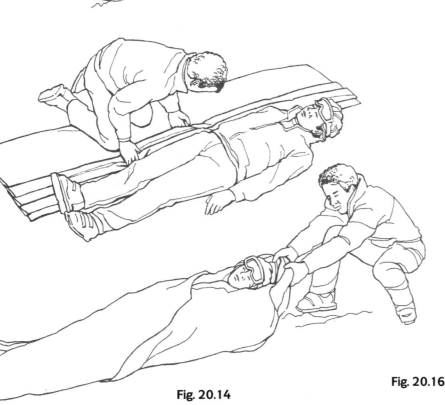

Fig. 20.13

Fig. 20.14

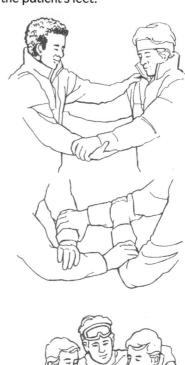

Fig. 20.15

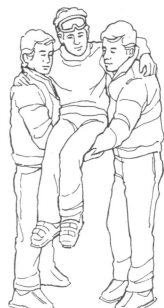

Fig. 20.16

To better coordinate lifting and moving the patient, the rescuers' arms should touch each other as much as possible and should interlace with those of the rescuers on the opposite side.

The first rescuer puts one arm under the patient's head, neck, and shoulders and the other arm under the patient's upper back; the second rescuer puts one arm under the patient's lower back and the other arm under the patient's upper thighs or buttocks; and the third rescuer puts one arm under the patient's lower thighs and the other arm under the patient's legs or ankles. A fourth rescuer, if available, puts one arm under the patient's midback and the other under the patient's midthighs from the patient's opposite side.

On command, the rescuers simultaneously lift the patient to knee level (Fig. 20.20). At this point, one of the rescuers or an assistant can slide a litter or toboggan under the patient and, on command, the patient can be lowered into it (Fig. 20.21). If the rescuers must first carry the patient some distance, they simultaneously stand on command, roll the patient's body toward the chests of the first three rescuers, and walk in unison. The procedure is reversed to lower the patient to the ground or into a litter.

Direct Ground Lift and Carry— Possible Spine Injury

This method is similar to the direct ground lift and carry with no spinal injury, except that at least four (but preferably six) rescuers are required. The rescuer at the patient's head is the leader, who maintains manual stabilization of the head and neck during the procedure and calls out the commands.

Fig. 20.17 *Fore-and-Aft Carry*

Fig. 20.18 *Direct Ground Lift for a Patient with no Spine Injury*

Fig. 20.19 *Direct Ground Lift Using a Fourth Rescuer*

Fig. 20.20 *The first rescuer coordinates a simultaneous lift.*

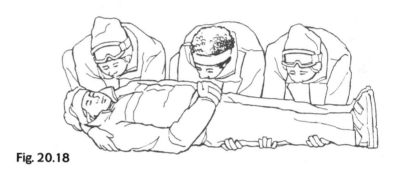

Fig. 20.18

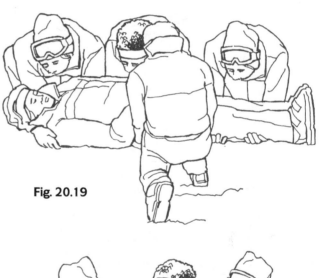

Fig. 20.19

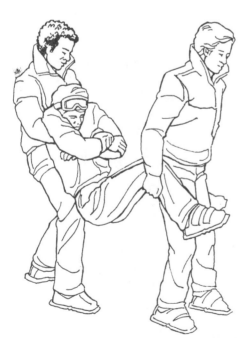

Fig. 20.17

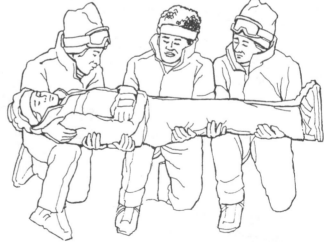

Fig. 20.20

The technique also is used to lift a patient out of a hole so that a spine board can be slid underneath. The patient can be in any one of the six basic positions described above in **Principles of Extrication**, although position 1 is the preferred position. A patient in one of the three "a" variations should be aligned into one of the three main positions as much as possible before being moved. However, if the patient is in a hole where this cannot be done, he or she should be lifted with all body parts maintained in the position found, placed on a long spine board, and then aligned into position 1.

When only four rescuers are available, the first rescuer stabilizes the head and neck; the second rescuer places one hand under the patient's shoulders and the other under the patient's upper back; the third rescuer places one hand under the patient's lower back and the other under the patient's upper thighs or buttocks; and the fourth rescuer places one hand under the patient's lower thighs and the other under the patient's calves (Fig. 20.22a). If six rescuers are available, the first rescuer stabilizes the head and neck; two interlace their hands from each side to support and stabilize the patient's shoulders and upper back; two interlace their hands from each side to support and stabilize the patients hips and lower back; and the sixth rescuer supports the patient's legs (Fig. 20.22b).

All rescuers should have a mental image of the *spinal plane* whenever the patient is moved so that, during movement, the head, shoulders, and hips are maintained in line with each other, at right angles to the spine, and parallel to the plane (or, if previously unaligned, in the position found). On command, the rescuers simultaneously lift the patient a previously specified distance, usually 6 to 12 inches. At this point, a long spine board is slid under the patient and, on command, the patient is lowered onto it.

If the rescuers must carry the patient a short distance, they simultaneously stand on command and walk in unison. The procedure is reversed to lower the patient to the ground or onto a long spine board.

The direct ground lift is safer than the carry. Ideally, this maneuver should be used *only* to lift a patient high enough so that a long spine board can be slid underneath, or to lift and carry a patient a minimal distance to a long spine board.

Fig. 20.21 *Technique of Lowering a Patient into a Litter*

Fig. 20.22 *Direct Ground Lift for a Patient with a Suspected Spine Injury*

Extremity Lift, Fractures Splinted—Two or More Rescuers

Ski patrollers frequently use this lift to move a patient with a splinted lower extremity from the first aid room to a nearby vehicle. It is more suitable for minor lower-extremity sprains and fractures than for major, painful injuries.

Two patrollers help the patient stand and provide support from either side. The patient balances on the uninjured foot and puts one arm around each patroller's neck. The patroller on the side of the injury supports the splinted extremity.

The patient, supported and partially carried by the patrollers, then hops to the waiting vehicle (Fig. 20.23).

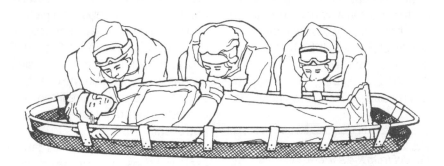

Fig. 20.21

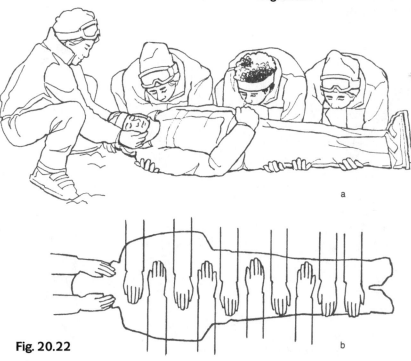

Fig. 20.22

The patient should be oriented so that the splinted leg will be along the back of the seat. To load a patient into the back seat of a four-door vehicle, open both rear doors so a third patroller can enter the far door to help pull the patient onto the seat (Fig. 20.24). If a station wagon or suburban is available, the patient can be loaded into the rear compartment in a similar manner.

Stretcher to Bed Transfer or Vice Versa—No Spine Injury

If the patient is lying on a sheet or blanket, it can be used to lift the patient from a stretcher on the floor to a bed. At least four rescuers are required.

The stretcher is laid next to the bed and two rescuers are positioned on either side (Fig. 20.25a). The sides of the sheet are rolled to provide a better grip. On a signal, the rescuers lean back slightly, lift the patient to bed level (Fig. 20.25b), and transfer the patient to the edge of the bed (Fig. 20.25c). During this transfer, the two rescuers holding the side of the

Fig. 20.23 *Technique of Assisting a Patient from the Patrol Room*

Fig. 20.24 *Technique of Positioning a Patient in a Vehicle*

sheet nearest the bed move toward the patient's head and feet respectively, so that the patient's side rests on the edge of the bed. Then, these rescuers, while maintaining their hold on the sheet, move to the opposite side of the bed and pull the sheet toward them, moving the patient to the center of the bed (Fig. 20.25d).

This procedure is easier if an adjustable-height stretcher such as a gurney is used (Fig. 20.26). A multiple-rescuer direct ground lift also can be used.

Canvas Stretcher or Blanket Lift and Carry—No Spine Injury

Many ski patrols use a heavy canvas stretcher with eight handles to transfer a patient from a toboggan to a first aid room cot (Fig. 20.27). The stretcher is laid flat inside the sleeping bag or blanket roll in the toboggan pack, and the patient is placed directly on it when loaded into the toboggan. On arrival at the first aid room, the sleeping bag is opened and the canvas stretcher and patient are lifted and carried to the cot by four or more patrollers.

A strong sheet or blanket can be used as a substitute for the canvas

stretcher. The sides should be rolled tightly lengthwise to fit the contours of the patient's body. Two or three patrollers are stationed at each side. They should space their hands evenly along the sides of the blanket and grasp it tightly. On command, the patrollers lean back slightly, lift the patient to waist level, and carry the patient to the cot (Fig. 20.28).

To slide a sheet or blanket under a patient from the side, pleat it lengthwise for two-thirds of its width and place the pleated side alongside the patient (Fig. 20.29a). Logroll the patient about 45 degrees away from the blanket, push the pleated side of the blanket as far under the patient as possible (Fig. 20.29b), and roll the patient back onto the pleats and then 45 degrees to the opposite side. Next, pull the blanket under the patient so that it is smooth (Fig. 20.29c). This should position the patient in the center of the blanket.

Litters and Stretchers

Litters and stretchers include toboggans; rigid litters such as the Stokes and its plastic and fiberglass modifications; semirigid litters such as the SKED; short and long spine boards;

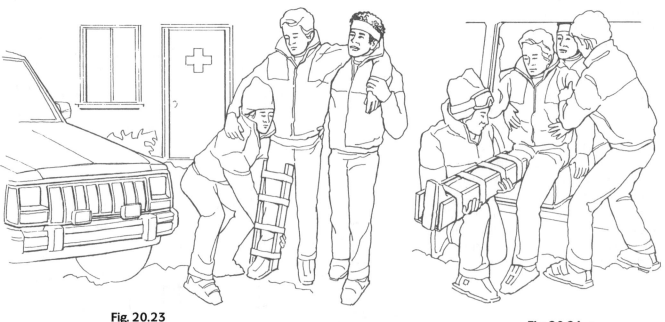

Fig. 20.23

Fig. 20.24

scoop stretchers; adjustable, wheeled cot-stretchers such as the gurney; soft stretchers; and improvised litters. Soft stretchers, except for the canvas type described above, are rarely used in modern emergency care because they do not protect an injured spine. Spine boards and scoop stretchers are discussed in detail in Chapters 8 and 13, and toboggans in Chapter 20.

Fig. 20.25 *Using a Blanket Lift to Transfer a Patient from a Stretcher to a First Aid Cot*

Rigid and semirigid litters (Fig. 20.30) are used by search and rescue groups for lowering, raising, and transporting patients. These include the familiar wire basket Stokes litter and heavy-duty plastic and fiberglass modifications such as the Ferno-Washington, Thompson, Jakes, Cascade, and SKED litters. Some newer versions can be broken down for easier transport to the accident site. Rigid and semirigid litters are adequate for stabilizing patients with neck and back injuries if used with a short backboard or vest-type device such as the Oregon spine splint II or Kendrick extrication device (KED).

Most litters have handholds or nylon loops for lifting and carrying. Carrying a litter over a boulder field or along a rough trail is a tiring exercise that requires many trained rescuers, preferably in two or more teams of six to eight. The teams should be rotated frequently, and the rescuers

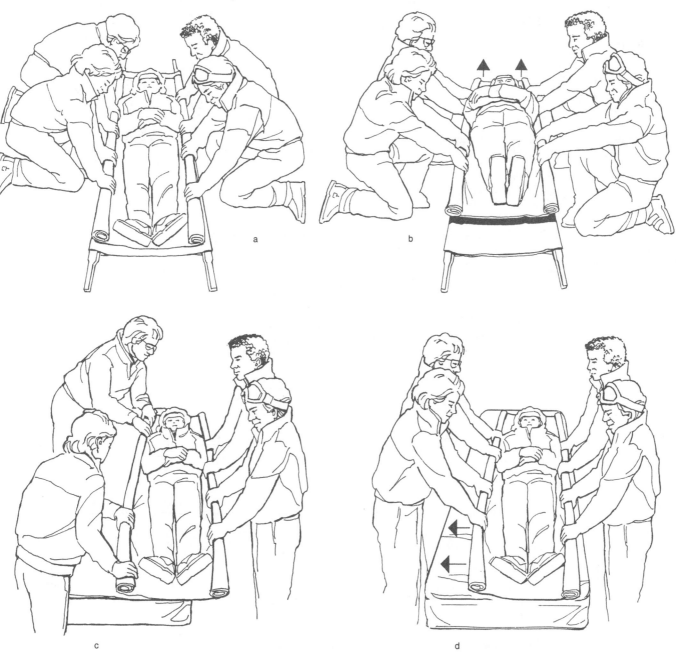

a b

c d

Fig. 20.25

Fig. 20.26 *Adjustable-height Wheeled Stretcher*

Fig. 20.27 *Canvas Stretcher*

Fig. 20.28 *Blanket Litter Carry*

Fig. 20.29 *Technique of Sliding a Pleated Blanket Under a Patient*

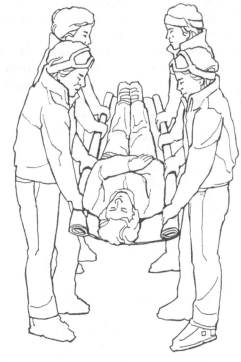

Fig. 20.26

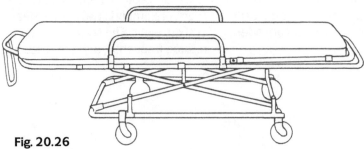

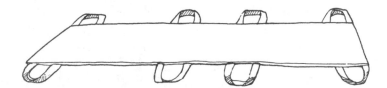

Fig. 20.27

Fig. 20.28

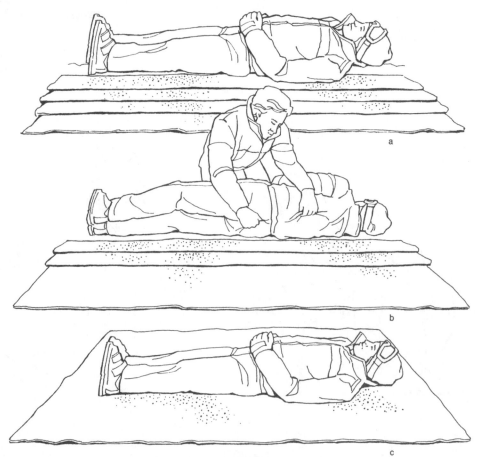

Fig. 20.29

should switch from one side of the litter to the other at regular intervals.

The most comfortable way for rescuers to carry a litter is to shift the strain from the hands and arms to the shoulders using long nylon slings. One technique is to form slings for each rescuer from 15-foot pieces of 1-inch tubular nylon tied into a loop with a double overhand knot (see Appendix G). The rescuer places the loop over the head so it rests on the outside shoulder (the shoulder farthest from the litter) and inserts the inside arm through the loop. The loop is pulled across the rescuer's chest, inserted through a litter handhold, brought in front of and over the inside shoulder, then down across the back to the waist, where it is held by the outside hand (Fig. 20.31). This method distributes the weight of the litter fairly evenly across both shoulders.

Three to four rescuers are needed for each side of the litter; additional rescuers can precede the litter to clear away obstacles, warn the party of hazards, and set up belays, if necessary. The litter should be belayed down steep or very rough slopes. As a convenience, a detachable wheel can be mounted on the litter when traversing easier trails (Fig. 20.32).

Adjustable, wheeled cot-stretchers such as the gurney (Fig. 20.26) were developed for ambulance use. The height of these stretchers can easily be changed to the best position for patient transfer, transport, and ambulance loading—a useful feature for ski patrol first aid rooms. Adjustable stretchers can be elevated to bed level, making it easier to carry out assessment and emergency care. The patient's trunk and legs can be independently raised or lowered as needed.

Improvised Stretchers and Litters

Improvised stretchers and litters tend to be uncomfortable and are insufficiently rigid for patients with spine injuries. They should be limited to short-distance moves.

An emergency soft stretcher can be improvised from two long poles and a **blanket** or several **jackets or parkas**. The blanket is folded as shown in Figure 20.33. If parkas are used, they should all be about the same size. Zip them closed and insert the poles, one on either side, inside the parkas and through their arms (Fig. 20.34). The poles can be carried by one or two rescuers at each end and other rescuers at the sides.

An easier method is to tie the ends of the poles to backpacks, preferably packs with external frames.

Fig. 20.30 *Rigid and Semirigid Litters*

Fig. 20.31 *Technique of Carrying a Litter with a Nylon Sling*

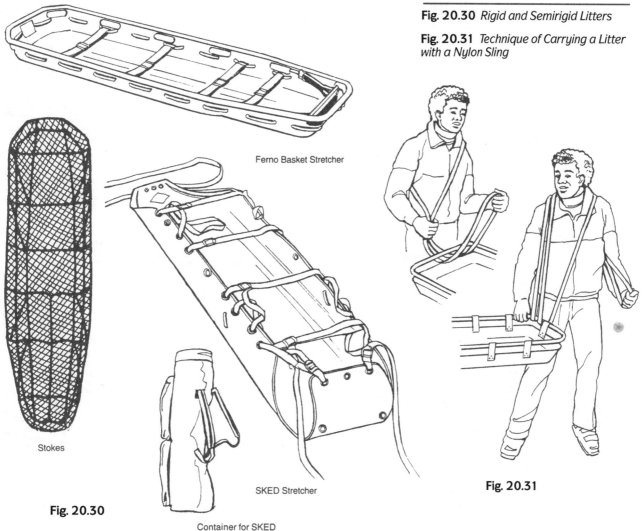

Ferno Basket Stretcher

Stokes

SKED Stretcher

Container for SKED

Fig. 20.30

Fig. 20.31

The packs are then worn by rescuers in the usual manner. The poles should be long enough so that the rear rescuer can see his or her feet while walking.

Stretchers also can be made from **climbing ropes** or **pack frames**. The National Outdoor Leadership School recommends improvising a semirigid litter using two pack frames tied end to end, strengthened with one or two additional frames as illustrated in Figure 20.35. This type of litter can be carried alone or tied to two poles as described above.

A rope stretcher can be improvised from a 150-foot climbing rope. Uncoil the rope and locate the center. Then, lay 16 180-degree bends on the ground, eight on each side of the center of the rope (Fig. 20.36). The total distance between the first and last bend should be slightly longer than the patient's height, and the distance between bends should be slightly longer than the patient's width. Bring the two free rope ends around, one on each side of the stretcher. Tie a clove hitch in these ends at the site of each bend, and insert the end of the bend about 2 inches into the hitch to form a loop.

After all bends have been inserted into a hitch, thread the remaining rope ends through the loops until no rope is left. Snug up the clove hitches, tie off the ends, and lay an Ensolite pad or sleeping bag on the stretcher. A rescuer should try out the stretcher to locate uncomfortable areas; these should be padded before the patient is placed in the stretcher. Four to six rescuers can carry the stretcher, or it can be tied to poles as described above.

Fig. 20.32 *Stokes Litter with Detachable Wheel*

Fig. 20.33 *Technique of Using a Folded Blanket as a Stretcher*

Fig. 20.34 *Stretcher Made from Two Parkas*

Fig. 20.35 *Stretcher Made from Pack Frames*

Fig. 20.36 *Rope Stretcher*

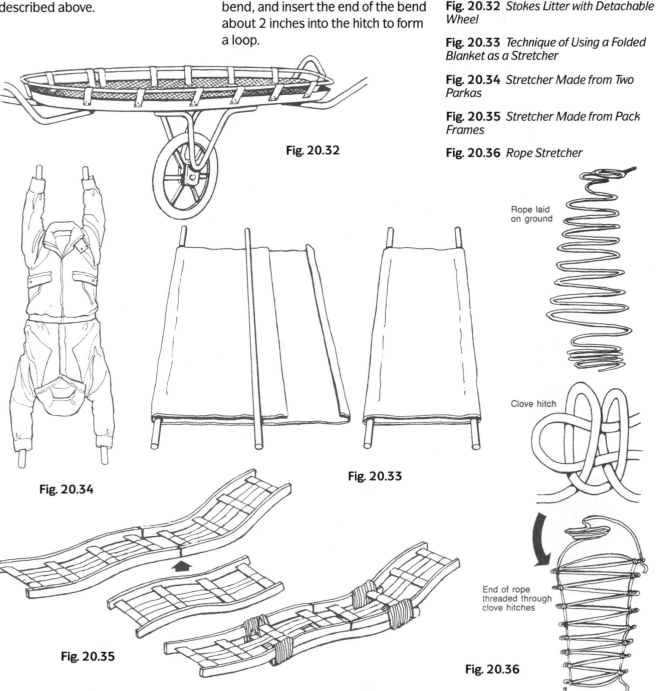

Fig. 20.32

Fig. 20.34

Fig. 20.33

Fig. 20.35

Rope laid on ground

Clove hitch

End of rope threaded through clove hitches

Fig. 20.36

Rescue from a Difficult Position or Remote Location (Figs. 20.37 and 20.38)

After locating the patient, the first rescuer to arrive surveys the scene for possible hazards to the patient and rescuers. Upon reaching the patient, form a first impression and perform the primary survey, identifying and giving care for life-threatening conditions such as respiratory or cardiac arrest, serious bleeding, a flail chest, a sucking chest wound, shock, etc., as described in previous chapters of this textbook. Treat these conditions immediately. Stabilization of the patient's body temperature also is an important priority.

Next, identify less critical injuries and medical conditions and care for any wounds or fractures. If the patient is unconscious because of trauma, or if injuries to the neck or back are suspected, stabilize the patient's head and neck during these initial proce-

dures, apply a rigid collar, and do not move the patient unless there is enough help to use proper techniques.

During assessment and care, protect the patient against wind, cold, rain, snow, strong sun, excessive heat, rockfall, and other dangers. A hard hat, dark glasses, extra clothing, sleeping bag, ponchos, tarps, and/or rescuers' backpacks may be needed.

These emergency procedures are ideally carried out before the patient is moved, unless there is difficulty accessing the patient or there is significant hazard to the patient or rescuers. While waiting to extricate and transport the patient, perform as much of the secondary survey as possible.

Meanwhile, other rescuers should prepare the extrication route. In the case of a skiing accident, the patient may be entangled in trees, dense brush, snowmaking equipment, a snow fence, or a crowd of other skiers; or may have slid into a gully or tree well. In other situations, a patient may be found jammed between boulders, in

a crevice, in a crevasse, on a ledge, in a narrow cave passage, or on a rock in midstream. It may be necessary to cut trees, move rocks, shovel snow, chip away ice, or set up lowering, raising, or traversing rope systems. Axes, saws, shovels, and special technical rescue equipment may be required.

The patient should be moved from the accident site only after he or she has been stabilized and the route has been prepared. This movement must be carried out so that no further injury is caused and existing injuries are not aggravated.

It usually is possible to extricate a patient from a tight or awkward location by using a multiple-person lift, slide, or lift and carry. Be careful to stabilize deformed body parts in place during extrication until the patient is transferred to a long spine board or you reach a place where

Fig. 20.37 *Rescue of a Patient from a Remote Location*

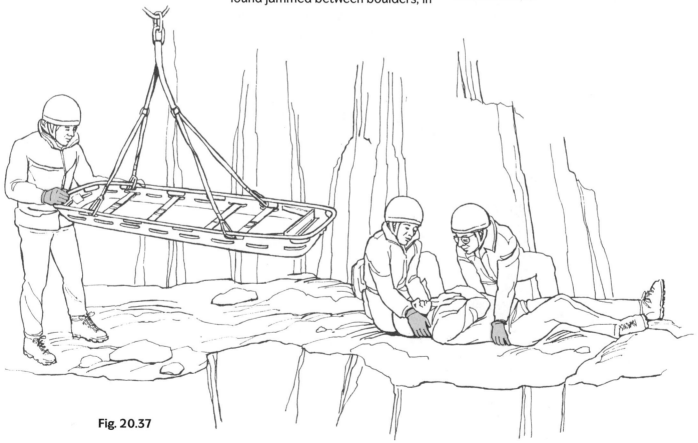

Fig. 20.37

there is room to align and splint them properly. Occasionally, it may be preferable to apply a short backboard, vest-type device, or scoop stretcher before moving the patient. The SKED stretcher, a narrow, semirigid litter, is lightweight and useful for tight places such as cave passages. Small fixation splints such as the SAM splint; compact traction splints such as the Sager and Kendrick traction device; and cravats, slings, and swathes can be used to splint injuries either before or after the patient is extricated.

Occasionally, a litter or long spine board cannot be brought close to the patient. If the patient must be carried a short distance, use at least a three-person direct ground lift and carry. An alternative is to drag the patient in the direction of the long axis of the body as described above.

After reaching stable ground, conduct the secondary survey to detect additional injuries and other problems. Avoid unnecessary exposure of the patient's body to inclement weather.

When a rescue party must make a long approach on foot to the scene of an accident, it is difficult to carry a full-sized long spine board. Many rescue groups use the combination of a vest-type device and a sturdy litter to immobilize a neck or back injury.

After giving all necessary emergency care and reaching stable ground, place the patient into a toboggan, litter, or other transport device, protect the patient from the elements and hazards (e.g., rockfall) with suitable insulation and shielding, and strap the patient in securely. Since emergency care in the field is primitive with even the best equipment, do not delay transporting the patient to definitive medical care. Allow the patient to urinate or defecate, if necessary, before being packaged (See Appendix C for a discussion of extended care of the patient in a wilderness situation.).

Transport requires sufficient manpower and must be done with deliberate speed, yet in a gentle and safe manner so that the patient is not jarred or jostled unnecessarily and injuries are not aggravated. It may be necessary to control onlookers and crowds.

When a prolonged backcountry evacuation is required, maintain radio contact with the authorities or send runners ahead to alert them. If there is insufficient manpower to transport the patient fast and safely, it may be preferable to make camp and send for help. Arrangements should be made as far in advance as possible if a rendezvous with a helicopter or ambulance will be required.

Fig. 20.38 *Rescuers Removing a Patient from a Wrecked Car*

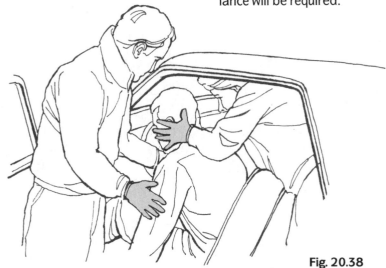

Fig. 20.38

Scenario #21 (Fig. 20.39)

The following scenario illustrates a typical extrication problem.

You and three friends have planned a day of rock climbing. At the last moment, Lucky comes down with vomiting and diarrhea, so you and the other two friends drive to the Rosebud Lake road and park at a turnout just past a bridge over Rosebud Creek. From there it is about ¼ mile to the base of the Central Spire, through a small woods and up a boulder field.

Instead of climbing in two teams of two as originally planned, you will have to climb in one team of three. To save time, you decide to alternate leads and leave a fixed rope to protect the third man. He follows, self-belayed by two jumars while the first man belays the second man up the next pitch.

Spike leads the first pitch, an easy 5.6, belayed by Tom, then gives Tom an upper belay while Tom climbs the first pitch, secures the fixed rope, and continues up the second pitch, belayed by Spike. Meanwhile, you follow the fixed rope and join Spike at the top of the first pitch, retrieve the fixed rope, and keep going to join Tom at the top of the second pitch.

The second pitch is a harder 5.8 to 5.10 to the right of a wall. The middle part involves a 40-foot traverse to the right along a narrow ledge, an area of tricky climbing on some loose rock, and then some small faces alternating with small ledges leading back toward the wall. You clean the Friends and chocks as you go, afterwards noting that the rope you are trailing is now hanging straight down about 30 feet to the left of the bad section. After you join Tom, you have a fleeting feeling that you probably should have left some of the protection in for Spike to take out.

You tie off Spike's fixed rope securely to the anchor, call to Spike that it is ready, then belay Tom up the next pitch. You notice some motion on Spike's rope, then it tightens and you know he has started up. Tom's pitch is easy, and in 10 minutes you hear his "Off belay!"

Suddenly, you hear a cry from below. Looking over, you see Spike hanging free in his harness next to the wall. He yells something; you can hardly hear it over the noise of the creek in the valley, but it sounds like "Help!" You call to Tom: "Spike's hurt! Come back down!" In a few minutes, Tom has rappeled back down to join you.

Fig. 20.39 *Scenario #21*

You: "What's wrong?"
Spike: "My shoulder."

You and Tom rappel down to Spike and pull him over to a small ledge, where he can stand. Tom threads a descending ring onto two slings and ties them around a nearby horn. As soon as the anchor is ready, you clip Spike into it. Spike is holding his left forearm with his right hand.
You: "What happened?"
Spike: "I fell off that loose stuff over there and pendulumed into the wall. I hit my shoulder. It hurts bad and I can't move it."

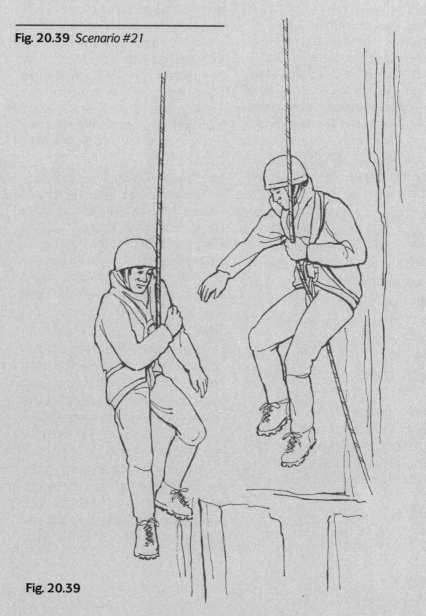

Fig. 20.39

You: "Did you hurt anything else? What about your head and neck? You sure took some fiberglass off your helmet."

Spike: "I bounced my head off the wall, but my head and neck feel okay."

You: "What about your back?"

Spike: "It feels okay."

You: "Let me see you move your fingers." (Spike wiggles the fingers of his left hand.) "Can you squeeze my hand?" (Spike does so.) "Can you feel this?" (scraping your fingernail over the skin of the back of Spike's left hand. Spike says he can.)

You assess the injured shoulder. Running your finger from the sternum to the point of the shoulder along the clavicle, you note that the surface of the clavicle is smooth, regular, and non-tender. When you get to the shoulder, you note that the point of the shoulder is sharp and squared off. You suspect an anterior dislocation. Placing your fingers into the axilla, you feel a rounded knob, which you know must be the head of the humerus.

Spike: (groaning) "This is really sore. I gotta sit down."

You: "Okay, I'll steady you. Be careful you don't slip. Can you feel this?" (You pinch the skin over the left deltoid muscle and then the right.) "Does it feel the same on both sides?"

Spike: "Yes."

You: "Can you move your shoulder at all?"

Spike: "No."

You: "Because it hurts, or because it's weak?"

Spike: "Because it hurts."

You: "I think your shoulder may be dislocated. Let me check a few other things, then we'll get you splinted and out of here."

You quickly assess the head, neck, and back while asking Spike if he hit his chest or pelvis. He denies any pain anywhere else. His pupils are round, regular, equal, and respond to light. The mouth is normal, there is no obvious bleeding from the mouth or nose and no obvious facial injuries. You do not remove the helmet, since he will still need it for evacuation. There is no tenderness or swelling of the neck, particularly over the spinous processes. There is no tenderness or obvious deformities of the back either, especially the spinous processes of the vertebrae, which you examine through his jacket.

You open your small backpack and take out a long length of 1-inch nylon webbing, two triangular bandages, and a spare pile jacket. You fold the jacket into a tight bundle and place it between Spike's arm and his chest. You make a sling out of one bandage and cradle his left arm in it, then fold the second bandage into a wide cravat and secure his arm to his chest with it.

You: "Spike, you can't rappel with your bad shoulder. Since I'm the biggest, what we're going to do is make a harness with this sling so that you can sit on my back. Tom is going to belay the two of us while we rap off to the ground. Good thing we have a spare rope. If we tie two of the ropes together, they'll reach."

Spike: "Okay."

Meanwhile, Tom has retrieved and coiled the two ropes, taken the third rope out of his pack, and uncoiled it.

You: "Spike, stand up where you are. Tom is going to do the harness. I'll back up to you so Tom can strap you on my back."

Tom centers the sling at the middle of Spike's upper back, then runs an end around each side of the chest under the armpit and crosses the ends over Spike's chest. You back up to

Spike and half-squat so he can straddle your back. Tom runs an end over each of your shoulders, then across your chest like an X, through Spike's legs, around his hips, and across your waist where you tie the ends securely. The system feels solid. Tom slips the end of one of the two 150-foot ropes through the descending ring on the anchor, ties the two ropes together, and throws the coiled ends of the ropes out into space. They reach easily to the ground. You tie the belay rope to your harness and Spike's harness. Tom sets up a belay using a Munter hitch. You set up your rappel with a figure-8 belaying device clipped to your harness and slowly back to the edge while Tom keeps you tightly on belay. Leaning backward, you brace your legs widely apart as you walk over the edge.

All goes well—Spike is solidly attached to your back and able to balance himself with his feet as you descend. You lean to the opposite side to keep his injured shoulder away from the rock. Fortunately, it is a sheer wall most of the way to the ground, without any loose rock. You reach the ground without incident, and within a few minutes, Tom rappels down to join you.

It takes about half an hour to negotiate the boulder field; Spike walks slowly and carefully and is supported as necessary by the two of you. A few minutes later, you are in the car and headed for town.

Scenario #22 (Fig. 20.40)

The following scenario illustrates the extrication of an injured skier from a difficult location.

It is the first of March at High Range Ski Area. Several storms in a row have dumped 3 feet of powder snow on the mountain's 8-foot base, and continued cold temperatures have kept it in good condition. Early Saturday morning, the parking lot is full of the 4 x 4 vehicles of the powder hounds. The lines waiting for the lifts to start are as long as you have ever seen them.

You are looking for some good skiing yourself, especially on pre-sweep, and you are not disappointed. You have first duty at Summit, but after that you plan to make at least one run down through the trees in Powder Park, the best ungroomed area on the mountain. First duty is quiet and you are standing outside the hut, ready to get into your bindings when your replacement arrives. He is covered with snow, and you know where he has just been.

About halfway through the Park, you hear a shout and catch sight of a

wildly gesticulating skier. Curious, you leave the untracked area and ski toward her across an area of powder-covered bumps. She is pointing into a clump of trees where a set of tracks leads toward a huge spruce whose lower branches are buried in snow.

Skier: "Sir, my friend is down under that tree and can't get out. Can you help him?"

You nod your head and motion for her to follow you. As you approach the tree, you see that the tracks appear to ski right into the closest lower branches, which are bare of snow. The tracks disappear in a hole in the snow underneath the branches.

You pole up to the hole, part the branches, and look into the gloomy snow well that surrounds the trunk of the tree. A young man is upside down in the well, his skis tangled in the lower branches and his head buried in the snow. One ski pole is still attached to his right wrist by its strap and the other is nowhere in sight.

You quickly get out of your skis, lower yourself into the hole, bend

down, and start digging the snow away from his face. Out of the corner of your eye, you note that his right arm seems to be bent at a peculiar angle.

You: "Sir, are you okay?"

There is no answer. Quickly, pulling off your gloves, you thrust his jaw forward, opening his airway, and place your ear close to his mouth and nose. You hear a faint gasp and a cough; he is breathing slowly. You quickly open your first aid belt and put on a pair of rubber gloves, then open his mouth with the crossed-finger technique and perform the finger sweep. There is no snow in his mouth. You palpate his carotid artery; the pulse is strong, regular and about 100 beats per minute.

You key your lapel mike: "Schussen to Summit, copy?" Summit replies. "There is an accident in Powder Park, just to the left of the opening of the lower chute. I need a toboggan, long spine board, KED, oxygen, suction, two snow shovels, an ax and saw, and at least six patrollers."

You turn to the patient again. "Sir, are you okay?" There is a moan. His eyes remain closed but he is now

Fig. 20.40 *Scenario #22*

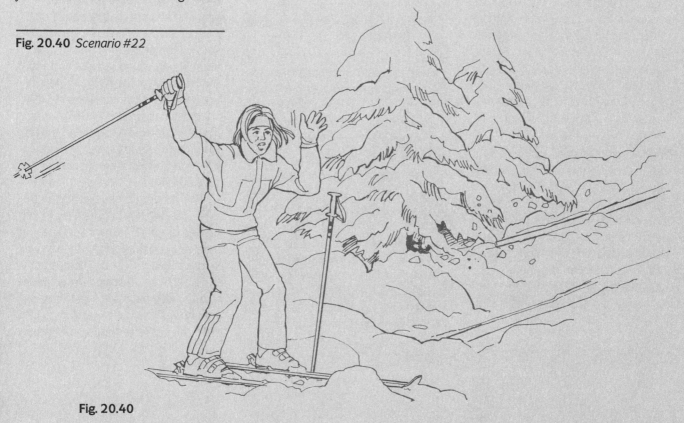

Fig. 20.40

breathing well and his pulse is strong. You call to his friend, asking her to take your skis and make an X in the snow with them to guide the other patrollers. You keep his jaw thrust forward with one hand while you enlarge his breathing space some more with your other hand. Since the patient is moaning, he probably has a gag reflex and will not tolerate an oral airway. You shift yourself around to where you can stabilize his head and neck better. It is quite a trick— this is the first time you have tried it on someone who is hanging upside down like a side of beef in a locker. While waiting, you introduce yourself to the patient's friend and explain what you are doing.

After what seems like hours, the toboggan arrives, followed shortly by a crowd of fellow patrollers. After surveying the scene and receiving a short briefing from you, one of them takes the shovel and starts to enlarge the entrance to the well, being careful not to dislodge any snow that is supporting the patient. The patient's skis are left on for the moment since they are wedged into the branches and are supporting the patient's legs. The oxygen backpack and portable hand-suction unit are brought up, and one of the patrollers crowds into the hole with you, ready to use them. Fortunately, the oxygen tubing is about 6 feet long. The patroller places a non-rebreather mask on the patient's face and adjusts the flow to 10 liters per minute.

You: "I think the best course of action is to dig out this hole until we can get in here to raise the patient enough to slide the spine board under him. We have to assume that he has both a neck injury and a head injury. I haven't had time to look closely, but I think his right arm may be broken. Bill, take a look at the arm and then get ready to stabilize the shoulders

and arms with Pete. Mike and Sue, you get ready to stabilize the hips. Jack, as soon as you have enough snow shoveled out of the way, stabilize the legs and get his skis off. Bill, after you check the arm, better get the ax and saw and clear away those lower branches. Careful that you don't jar him. Before anyone else comes down into the hole, get that spine board in here."

In just a few minutes, the hole is big enough so you can maneuver. You have the patient's head and neck stabilized manually, there are two patrollers stabilizing the shoulders and arms, two the hips, and one the legs. Bill had assessed the right arm and reports that there is a swelling and some crepitation in its mid-portion. The skis are off, having been removed very carefully since they were partly supporting the patient's legs. The spine board is down in the hole and the patient's friend is ready to slide it in place under him.

You: "The idea is to lift and pivot his body like a log until he is horizontal, face up, and the spine board can be slid under him and its ends braced on the sides of the hole. I'll call the signals. We'll move him about 12 inches at a time, pivoting around his hips, so that his legs will rotate down and the rest of his body will rotate up until he is horizontal. As you move him, bring his legs together and his arms to his sides. Keep the shoulders and hips at right angles to the spine, and keep the spine straight. Okay, everybody ready, raise his upper body 12 inches on three. One, two, three!"

The patient's upper body is raised 12 inches toward the horizontal and the legs lowered 12 inches. "Another 12 inches, on three," you say. "One, two, three!" Slowly and smoothly, the patient is pivoted into the face-up, horizontal position, the spine board is slid under him, and he is lowered onto it. Mike takes a regular adult-size Stifneck collar out of the spine board stuffsack and applies it to his neck.

By now the patient is starting to stir and moan and his eyes are open. The six of you carefully carry him a few feet on the board out into the open snow where there is room to work, while you maintain manual stabilization of his head and neck.

Mike quickly does a secondary survey of the patient's body and, finding no injuries except the right arm fracture, takes a SAM splint from his fanny pack, doubles it, shapes it into a trough, and applies it to the side of the patient's right arm, fixing it in place with 2-inch Kling. The patient's extremities are aligned and he is strapped to the board with padding under the back of his head, under the small of his back, and on both sides of his legs. The splinted right upper extremity is secured to his body with two cravats, using a modified sling and swathe arrangement. Since the toboggan has to go down a steep chute to get out of the Park, across-the-shoulder crisscross straps and groin straps are put in place in addition to the standard four straps.

Relieved of your duty at the head and neck, you get a flow sheet form out of your first aid belt and start filling it out. You reassess the vital signs: he has a strong, steady pulse of 90 beats per minute, he is breathing well at 16 respirations per minute, his pupils are round, regular and equal, and he is a V on the AVPU scale, since he opens his eyes and looks at you when you call his name. Before being strapped down, he had been moving all four extremities spontaneously and withdrawing them when you pinched them.

The toboggan has been brought alongside and the tarpaulin and sleeping bag opened. The boarded patient is placed into the toboggan, and the sleeping bag is closed. The patient and board are strapped in securely because you have a rough toboggan run ahead; if he has to vomit you plan to tip the entire toboggan on its side and use the V-Vac. There was some discussion as to whether he should be head uphill or head downhill; the former opinion prevailed because of his altered mental status, the original breathing problem, and the steepness of the route.

In a few minutes, the patient is on his way to the base with Mike skiing beside him while monitoring his airway, breathing, oxygen, and watching for early signs of vomiting. There is one steep, narrow part of the chute where the toboggan will have to be belayed down, but fortunately the patroller who brought the toboggan remembered that in Powder Park you *always* bring along a lift evacuation sack with 150 feet of goldline, a longhorn figure-8 belaying device, some sling, and a locking carabiner.

Scenario #23 (Fig. 20.41)

The following scenario illustrates the extrication of two injured people from a difficult location.

It has been a pleasant spring day with a warming snow pack, rivulets at the base lodge, and mud in the parking lot. You and two other patrollers are among the last to leave. You are putting your skis on the car when you see two skiers come out of the Bierstube and climb into a red sedan. Mud flies as they accelerate out of the parking lot, turn onto the road, and disappear down the mountain at a high speed.

As you enter the final curve before turning onto the main highway, you see a car in the borrow pit ahead, taillights still on and nose against a large tree at the edge of the road. It looks like the red sedan. You pull over to the side of the road and turn on your emergency blinkers. The three of you jump out of the car with patrol first aid belts in hand and approach the accident site. The snow is heavy, damp, and about 2 feet deep.

The front end of the two-door sedan is crumpled against the tree. There is a figure in each bucket seat: the driver, who is bent forward over the steering wheel, and the passenger, who has slid slightly forward on the seat and is lying on his left side with his head and chest on the seat, his left knee bent, his left hip flexed and internally rotated, and his abdomen and left lower extremity under the dashboard. Neither is wearing a seatbelt and neither is moving. There is a star-shaped crack in the driver's side of the windshield. You do not smell any gasoline.

You try to open the driver's door; it is locked. Jan is trying the right door. It is not locked, but it is bent and will not open. You give Joe your keys and ask him to get the lug wrench out of the trunk of your car. The car is stable as it rests against the tree, and it appears safe to try to access the two individuals.

You open your first aid belt and take out a pair of rubber gloves and

Fig. 20.41 Scenario #23

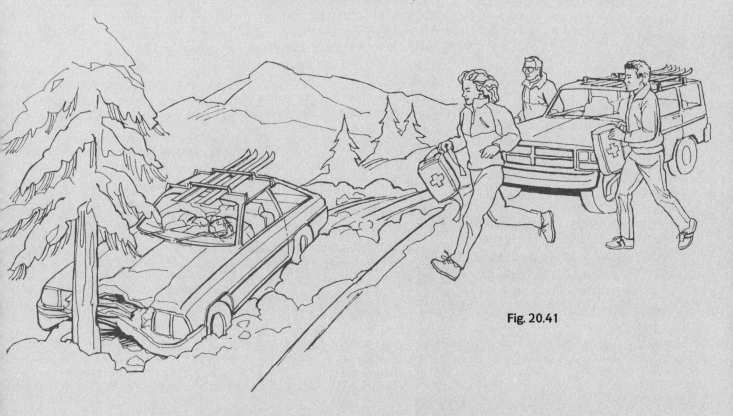

Fig. 20.41

a roll of 2-inch adhesive tape. Quickly, you tear off four long strips and lay them on the left rear window in the form of an eight-pointed star. Using the sharp end of the lug wrench, you give the window a hard blow at its lower rear corner. The tempered glass turns white as it fractures into multiple, small pieces, most of which stay in place. With the blunt end, you knock a large hole in the glass so you can reach in and flip the front door latch open with the end of the lug wrench. The door opens easily.

You reach in across the driver to turn off the ignition and notice that the top of the steering wheel is cracked and bent forward. There is a distinct odor of beer in the car. Neither patient has stirred, but you can see that the driver is breathing. There is a pool of blood on the top of the dashboard in front of the steering wheel. You now quickly pull on the rubber gloves.

Jan squeezes into the rear seat. She moves to the right side behind the passenger, reaches forward, and opens the window of the passenger door. You follow her, then reach forward over the back of the driver's seat to stabilize the driver's head and neck manually. There is a large cut on his forehead from which blood is dripping down his face. The skin of his face is cool and moist. Jan helps you pull the driver back against the seat while you use the jaw-thrust technique to improve his airway.

You: "Sir, are you okay?"

The driver stirs and moans. His eyes remain closed. He is breathing rapidly and shallowly at 24 respirations per minute. You feel for his carotid pulse; it is regular, strong, and 100 beats per minute.

Jan puts on a pair of rubber gloves, leans forward over the back of the seat, and says loudly to the passenger, "Sir, are you okay?" He moans and his eyes open.

Jan: "I believe he said 'No.'"

A pair of headlights approaches from the rear.

You: "Joe, stop that car. Have them call from the nearest phone and get an ambulance. Tell them we have a car accident up here with two victims, both with possible head and neck injuries."

The car slides to a stop and Joe recognizes two lift operators from the ski area, both reliable. Joe delivers the message and they pull away.

Jan: "This patient is breathing well at 16 per minute. He has a good carotid pulse at 90 per minute. He responds to verbal stimuli. His skin is cold and clammy. There is no obvious bleeding that I can see." (She is manually stabilizing the patient's head and neck.)

You: (speaking to Joe) "Jan and I have to keep these folks stabilized and maintain their airways. Please finish the primary survey and do a body survey on them while we're waiting for the ambulance. Start with this one because he has a big cut on his forehead, is bleeding, and has labored breathing. Don't forget your gloves."

Joe leans in the door and assesses the driver's head, announcing his findings as he goes. The driver's breathing, although rapid, appears to be adequate. The carotid pulse is still regular and 100 beats per minute. There is a 2-inch cut on his forehead from which blood is still dripping. Joe finds no other open or closed wounds, aside for some bruising of the right upper and lower eyelids. He takes a sterile compress from his first aid belt, applies it to the wound, and anchors it with a 2-inch self-adhering roller bandage around the patient's head.

Because of the abnormal breathing, Joe then assesses the neck, chest, and abdomen. The neck shows no open or closed wounds and no deformities. Joe opens the patient's jacket and pulls up his turtleneck shirt. There are no obvious open chest wounds, but there is a large ecchymosis in the center of the chest. Fortunately, both

sides of the chest are moving equally as the patient breathes.

Joe unfastens the driver's ski pants and assesses the abdomen. There are no obvious open or closed wounds, no distension, and the patient does not flinch when Joe presses on all four abdominal quadrants. Joe presses the iliac crests together and then backward. There is no crepitus and the patient does not flinch.

Joe does not attempt to expose the driver's lower or upper extremities but palpates them through the clothing. There are no obvious swellings or deformities. Both radial pulses and the capillary refill in a finger of both hands is normal. The driver moves all four extremities in response to a painful stimulus. Joe slips a hand behind the patient's neck and back and runs it down as many of the spinous processes as he can. He notices no deformities or swellings.

Moving around to the right of the car, Joe reaches in the window, and with some difficulty performs the ABC's on the passenger. His breathing is adequate at a rate of 16 respirations per minute, and the carotid pulse is still strong and regular at 90 beats per minute.

There is no obvious bleeding. There are no abnormalities of the neck or chest. Because of the patient's position, the abdomen cannot be assessed yet. There is a large, blue area of swelling on the patient's forehead. The pupils are normal and both respond to light. The mouth and nose appear normal. There are no obvious abnormalities of the upper extremities or back.

Joe: "There is a dent in the dashboard near this man's knee. His hip is flexed and internally rotated. I'll bet he has a dislocation of the left hip."

You hear the sound of a siren in the distance and in a few minutes the headlights and flashing red lights of the ambulance from town appear around the bend ahead, followed by a highway patrol car. The ambulance pulls to a halt on the other side of the road. You recognize the two attendants as Skip and Cliff, an EMT and a paramedic you have worked with before. They are both good people.

You: "Hello, guys. We have two patients here. The driver is partly responsive, responds to verbal stimuli. His pulse is 100, breathing is 24 and labored. He has a large laceration on his forehead and a steering wheel injury to his chest. The passenger is also partly responsive, responding to verbal stimuli. His pulse is 90; his breathing 16. He has a bruise on his forehead and a possible dislocated left hip. Neither one was wearing a seat belt."

After a rapid survey of the scene, Skip and Cliff unload the extrication kit, trauma bag, oxygen apparatus, two long spine boards, two vest-type devices, a portable oxygen tank, and a wheeled cot-stretcher from the ambulance. Cliff puts on a pair of rubber gloves and removes a rigid collar from the trauma bag. While you continue to maintain stabilization of the driver's head and neck, Cliff quickly repeats your primary and secondary surveys, finding no additional abnormalities of the head, anterior neck, chest, abdomen, and extremities.

At first, you can not help feeling some resentment at Cliff's repeating the assessment that you have just done and reported on to him, but then you remind yourself that this is standard procedure whenever a patient is turned over from one part of the EMS system to another.

The compress over the head laceration shows some blood at its center, but there is no active bleeding coming from beneath the compress. Cliff palpates the patient's back and posterior neck through the clothing. There are no deformities or other abnormalities. He then applies the rigid collar and brings over the oxygen tank,

attaching a non-rebreather mask to the patient's face with the oxygen flow turned to 12 liters per minute.

Meanwhile, Skip has sprung the lock of the passenger's door with a pry bar and opens the door, providing good access to the patient. As Jan continues to stabilize the head and neck and Joe the patient's trunk, Skip repeats the primary survey and body assessment, including the abdomen and both upper and lower extremities. He finds nothing that Joe did not find in his initial survey and agrees with Joe's assessment of the probability of a dislocated left hip. A rigid collar is applied, a second oxygen apparatus brought in, and oxygen started by rebreather mask at 12 liters per minute.

Just then, you note an increase in the driver's breathing rate. You call to Cliff, who repeats the primary survey. The driver's breathing rate is now 30 per minute, and his carotid pulse is 120 per minute. He has to be extricated as soon as possible; there is no time to apply a vest-type device. Cliff calls to Skip, who with the aid of Joe brings the wheeled stretcher and a long spine board over to the car. Skip forces the left door as far forward as possible, springing its hinges.

While you continue to stabilize the driver's head and neck, Cliff supports the driver's chest and Skip frees the driver's legs from the pedals. Skip then carefully moves into the back seat and the three of you rotate the driver so that his back is facing the open doorway, his hips and knees are bent, and his feet are between the bucket seats. You carefully maintain his head and neck in line with his trunk during these maneuvers.

Joe moves the stretcher with the board on it so that one end is at the door opening. He raises it to seat level and slides the end of the board under the driver's buttocks. The driver's chest and abdomen are carefully lowered onto the board and slid axially until the body is centered and the

legs can be straightened and lowered onto the board. Oxygen is continued at 12 liters per minute.

The driver is reassessed. He continues to be responsive to verbal stimuli. His pulse has slowed somewhat, probably because he is now supine. His capillary refill time is prolonged. His respirations are unchanged; his blood pressure is taken and is 100 over 90. Despite the likelihood of compression injury to the anterior chest, both sides of the chest continue to moved symmetrically, and his skin color is good. No open or closed abdominal wounds or tender areas are discovered. Responses to pain in his four extremities are normal and symmetrical; he is also noted to move all four spontaneously.

Meanwhile, Jan and the highway patrolman are applying a vest-type device to the passenger. The device is slipped between the seat and the patient's back and the patient's body secured to the device by the body side-flaps, thoracic straps, and right groin strap. The left groin strap of the device is not fastened because of the flexion and internal rotation of his injured left hip. The back of his head is padded to maintain the head and neck in the neutral position and the head secured by the head side-flaps and foam straps across the forehead and the rigid collar.

By this time, the driver has been moved on the board over to the ambulance and placed on the squad bench. The passenger is placed on a long spine board by carrying the wheeled stretcher back over to the righthand door, placing it in the snow, laying the second board on it, raising the stretcher to seat level, and shoving the foot of the spine board carefully under the patient's buttocks. The patient, with the vest-type device in place, is then carefully rotated to the side with his back facing the open door, slid onto the lower end of the spine board, laid flat, and slid headward until he is in the middle of the spine board. The dislocated left hip is carefully stabilized in place during this maneuver.

The passenger is reassessed as well as can be done with the vest-type device in place before being strapped securely to the spine board. Special attention is paid to the lower abdomen and pelvis, which could not be assessed well in the patient's original cramped position.

The passenger's pulse and breathing rate are unchanged and his blood pressure is 140 over 90. Reassessment of his pupils, head, and neck shows no changes. The abdomen shows no open or closed wounds, no distension, and no areas of tenderness. Aside from the obvious left hip injury, no other abnormalities are found in his four extremities. The ambulance's pulse oximeter shows that the blood oxygen saturation of both driver and passenger are normal on 12 liters of oxygen per minute.

Skip is driving and Cliff is in the back of the ambulance. Since he will be very busy with two patients, they have asked you to come along to the hospital and help Cliff. You agree; Jan and Joe will meet you at the hospital. As the ambulance drives off, a tow truck from town arrives to remove the wrecked vehicle.

Chapter 21

Ski Injuries

There was blood upon his
   bindings,
There were brains upon his skis.
Intestines were a-hanging from
   the highest of the trees.
We scraped him up from off
   the snow
And poured him from his boots.
Well, he ain't a-gonna race
   no more.

—*Traditional ski song*

A comparison between recent data and data collected 15 to 20 years ago reveals changes in both the **ski injury rate** and the **relative frequency** of certain types of ski injuries. The overall alpine injury rate has been steadily falling to its current level of about three accidents per 1,000 skier visits in the United States, and even less elsewhere (0.5 to 1.0 per 1,000 in Scandinavia).

While ankle fractures and sprains are now less frequent, lower leg fractures and knee injuries have become relatively more frequent, probably because higher, stiffer ski boots transmit forces to a different and more proximal area of the lower extremity. Leg fractures at the level of the top of the boot (boot-top fractures) continue to be common, but the incidence of spiral fractures of the tibia and fibula has decreased, apparently because of the reduction of friction between modern ski boots and bindings and from advances in lateral toe release technology.

Soft-tissue injuries continue to occur at high rates although the incidence of lacerations has been reduced by the widespread replacement of safety straps by ski brakes. The relative incidence of upper body injuries, which currently make up 50 percent of ski injuries, continues to rise. These include head injuries, shoulder sprains and separations of the acromioclavicular joint, shoulder dislocations, sprains of the hand and fingers, and fractures of the ribs, clavicle, arm, and forearm. Skier's thumb is the most frequent upper body injury and one of the top two most frequent ski injuries, depending on incidence of reporting.

Knee sprains, long the most common serious ski injury, have decreased somewhat in overall frequency. However, the incidence of severe sprains, especially complete tears of the anterior cruciate ligament, has more than doubled. These serious injuries, a permanent threat to an active life-style, can occur without a fall. Wearing high, stiff boots seems to increase their incidence. The mechanisms of many anterior cruciate ligament injuries have recently been identified. They include the following:

1. External rotation of the lower leg on the thigh during a forward fall.
2. Thrusting forward of the tibia by the top of the boot during a backward fall.
3. Internal rotation of the hyperflexed knee caused by catching the inside edge of the tail of the ski while sitting back.

Knee injuries present a constant challenge to equipment manufacturers to design a binding that will provide better knee protection, and to ski instructors to perfect techniques that will help prevent knee injuries.

An ominous development has been the increase in serious injuries to multiple areas of the body, including various combinations of injuries to the head, spine, chest, and abdomen that resemble the injuries seen in motor-vehicle accidents. This worrisome trend, noted both in Europe and North America, is probably a by-product of improvements in equipment, technique, and slope grooming, which have led to higher speeds involving greater kinetic energy and more dangerous types of trauma, especially deceleration trauma; and slope crowding, which has led to more frequent collisions. As a consequence, ski areas now emphasize better hill design and more effective policing of hazardous skiing habits.

The equipment used in skiing and the characteristics of the body movements involved in skiing produce injury patterns not seen in other sports. The ski boot is designed to hug the foot and is fixed tightly to the ski by the binding. This allows the boot to reflect movements of the lower extremity accurately and transmit them to the ski. However, movements of the ski are transmitted back to the boot and lower extremity. Modern alpine skiing technique is possible because the heel is held down rather than being free to lift off the ski. But, if the skier suddenly changes momentum or direction, the lever action of the ski magnifies the resulting forces that act on the extremity. Release bindings are designed both to free the boot from the ski before these forces exceed the body's threshold of injury and to withstand the smaller forces produced during normal skiing without releasing.

An ideal binding would allow both the heel and toe to release to either side and upward, and the foot to release in a roll-out fashion to either side. No currently available binding is capable of releasing under all test conditions without injury to the lower extremity. The difficulty seems to be in designing a binding that will provide release in multiple directions without releasing prematurely. Intermediate and expert skiers tend to choose the convenience of step-in bindings that release laterally at the toe and upward at the heel and that prevent premature releases. Beginners are advised to select a multi-directional release binding.

Despite the most sophisticated advances in ski boot and binding technology, skiing technique, and ski hill design, there probably will always be an irreducible number of skiing accidents. Nonetheless, skiing is relatively safe when compared with other sports. Injury rates of three per 1,000 participants per year in alpine skiing and less than one per 1,000 in nordic skiing can be compared with injury rates of 21.7 per 1,000 participants per year in football, 18.6 per 1,000 in basketball, 9 per 1,000 in soccer, 9 per 1,000 in bicycling, 1.2 per 1,000 in tennis, and 0.9 per 1,000 in swimming (rates calculated from National Safety Council figures). Also, only about one in 500 falls while skiing produces a significant injury.

Types of Ski Accidents

There are two basic types of ski accidents: **falls** and **collisions** (Fig. 21.1). Collisions occur in many different ways and can injure almost any part of the body. Falls can be divided into two general types: **rotational** (twisting) and **nonrotational** (nontwisting). The specific type and extent of any injury produced by a fall depends on the type, magnitude, and direction of the resulting forces and whether these forces are concentrated on one or more body parts in a manner that exceeds their threshold of injury. The type of equipment (i.e., high, low, stiff, or soft boots, ski poles held with straps around the wrists) may be important, as well as the skier's physical condition, flexibility, weight, and bone structure. Another important factor is whether the bindings release normally, prematurely, or not at all.

A **rotational fall** most commonly rotates the foot *outward* and forces the leg outward at the knee, e.g., when a skier catches an inside edge while falling forward or to the side (Fig. 21.2). This fall can sprain or rupture the medial or anterior cruciate ligaments of the knee, sprain or fracture the ankle (usually the lateral malleolus), or fracture one or both bones of the leg. If the leg is fractured, the fracture line usually spirals around the shaft(s) of the bone(s) in contrast to the more horizontal fracture line produced by a nonrotational fall. A less common type of rotational fall rotates the foot *inward,* e.g., when a beginning skier crosses his or her ski tips. This type of fall can cause fractures and sprains of the ankle, particularly the medial structures; fractures (usually spiral) of the leg bones; and knee sprains.

A **nonrotational fall** typically occurs when a skier falls forward over the ski tips, tending to bend the leg over the front edge of the boot (Fig. 21.3). This can sprain the ankle or knee, rupture the Achilles tendon, fracture the ankle, or cause a boot-top lower leg fracture.

Landing on an outstretched hand may sprain the hand, wrist, or shoulder; dislocate the shoulder; or fracture the clavicle, arm, forearm, or hand.

A skier wearing high, stiff boots or who sits back may suffer a boot-top fracture during a *backward* fall as well. The lack of an upward toe release in most modern bindings contributes to the possibility of this injury. The repeated impact of a stiff, poorly padded boot top against the outer leg can cause an isolated fibular fracture.

Lacerations and contusions can be caused by collisions or by blows from a ski or pole during a fall. A sharp pole tip can cause puncture wounds, and blows from the butt of a pole grip can cause serious eye injuries.

The shoulder, forearm, hand, or fingers can be fractured or dislocated if a pole basket is caught in a tree when the pole straps are around the skier's wrists (Fig. 21.4). Skiers who use breakaway pole grips or who do not use wrist straps can avoid this injury, but these precautions will not prevent **skier's thumb** (also called "gamekeeper's thumb"), which occurs when a skier tries to break a fall with an outstretched hand while holding onto a ski pole (Fig. 21.5). The pole grip holds the thumb so that it is easily bent back on impact, spraining or fracturing the medial structures of the first thumb joint (metacarpophalangeal joint). When standard ski poles are used, the only way to prevent this injury entirely seems to be for skiers

---

Fig. 21.1 *Two Basics Types of Ski Accidents*

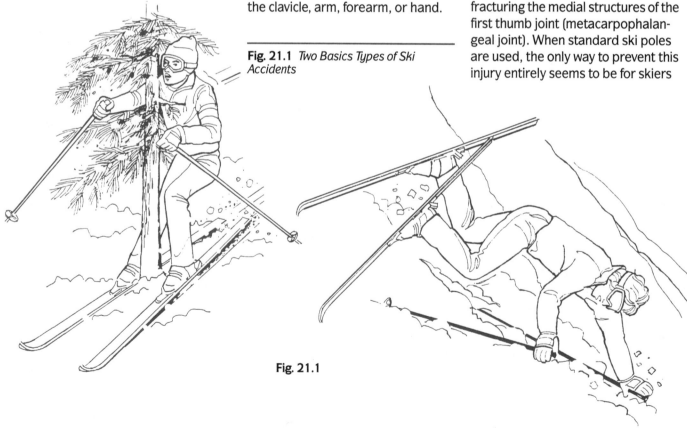

Fig. 21.1

to learn to discard their poles during a fall. The development and widespread use of poles with a saber or handlebar grip probably would reduce the incidence of skier's thumb.

The late ski safety expert Gordon Lipe called attention to a common cause of medial knee ligament injury unrelated to binding malfunction. The skier falls forward between the skis while skiing in the stem or wedge position. The ski and boot press sideways into the hill, preventing binding release, the knee hits the snow, and the skier's body rotates over the knee, tearing the ligament (Fig. 21.6). It may be possible to prevent this injury by teaching beginning skiers to fall to the side rather than falling forward between their skis. Devices that prevent ski tips from crossing also are useful.

The tibia and fibula, like other bones, are viscoelastic structures, behaving like a viscous liquid under some stresses and like an elastic solid under others. A slow, twisting force of 60 to 70 foot-pounds is sufficient to cause a spiral fracture of a man's tibia. However, if the force is applied quickly, it must be considerably greater before the tibia will break. This phenomenon, combined with the lesser likelihood that bindings will release in a slow fall, explains the relatively high rate of fractures occurring to beginning skiers during slow, twisting falls compared to the lower rate of fractures from hard falls suffered by experts who "load" the tibia at a much more rapid rate.

Other studies have shown that the amount of comminution (number of fragments) produced when a bone breaks is related to the magnitude of the forces involved. A high-speed fall generating a large amount of kinetic energy that has to be dissipated by the lower leg will cause more comminution of the fractured bone and more injury to the soft tissues than a fall involving lesser forces.

Likelihood of Injury

Currently, more than 55 million skier visits are recorded in the United States each year. There are approximately 160,000 ski injuries in the United States each year, many of which are trivial. Deaths and serious injuries are rare, deaths occuring at an annual rate of one for each million skier visits.

According to engineering professor Jasper Shealy, Ph.D., these incidents are not randomly distributed through the skiing population, but like fatal automobile and industrial accidents they tend to involve a small subset of males in their late teens to mid-20s with the "young adult male immortality complex" (YAMIC).

For data on ski injuries to be meaningful, their sources must be specified.

Fig. 21.2 *Rotational Fall*

Fig. 21.3 *Nonrotational Fall*

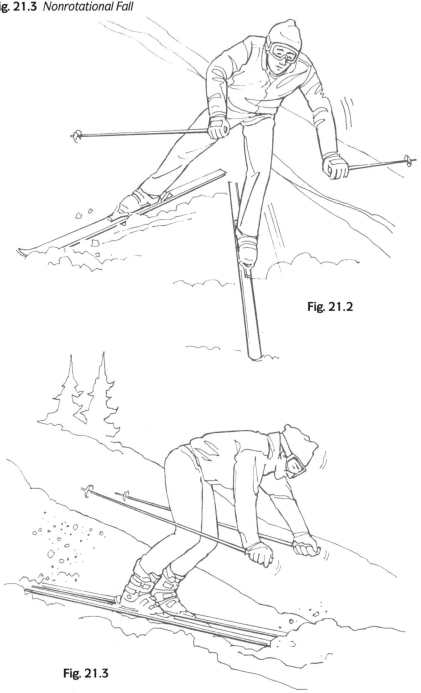

Fig. 21.2

Fig. 21.3

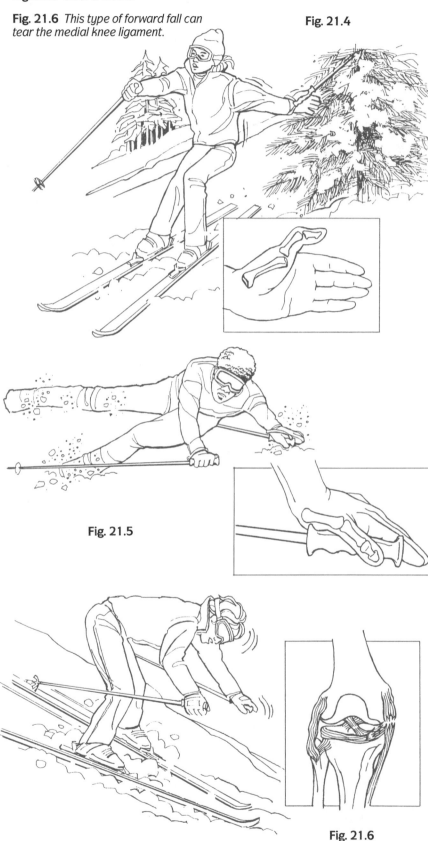

Fig. 21.4 *A skier can be injured if a pole basket catches on a tree.*

Fig. 21.5 *Skier's Thumb*

Fig. 21.6 *This type of forward fall can tear the medial knee ligament.*

Fig. 21.4

Fig. 21.5

Fig. 21.6

It is necessary to know whether the injuries occurred at a single ski area or at several areas, during a single year or over several years, and if snow conditions were typical or unusual. Injury rates at a small, weekend ski area with a single T-bar lift may differ from injury rates at a large, destination ski resort or at a resort that serves a large, metropolitan area.

In addition, because only 25 to 50 percent of injuries are reported to the ski patrol, it is important to state the distance from the ski area to the nearest large town or medical center and indicate whether data came from the ski patrol, a local medical clinic, or both. It also is important to indicate whether the services of the patrol are free, as in the United States, Canada, Japan, New Zealand, and Australia, or whether a fee is charged, as in most of Europe.

Any comparison of injury rates in different classes of skiers must take certain variables into account. For example, fractures and other serious injuries are more likely to be reported than trivial injuries. Also, beginning skiers, children, ski school students, women, and older people are more likely to report their injuries than are younger people, expert skiers, and men.

Nevertheless, certain general statements can be made. *Ability* and *experience* are probably the most important factors in determining a skier's likelihood of injury. The decline in overall injury rate over the last 30 years probably has resulted because of increased numbers of older and more experienced skiers on the hills, better teaching methods, better slope grooming, shorter skis, better bindings, better rental equipment, and the use of ski brakes and antifriction devices.

Beginning skiers, women, and children have proportionally more injuries than experienced skiers, men, and adults. The higher incidence of injuries during the late afternoon is largely because more skiers are on the hill at that time, although fatigue, poor lighting, and deteriorating snow conditions undoubtedly play a role. Skiing in large groups or when the slopes are crowded also seems to increase the injury rate, which is lowest on weekdays. In alpine ski racing, almost half the injuries occur on the last third of the course, a statistic that probably reflects the importance of fatigue as a contributor to ski injuries.

Certain types of snow conditions are associated with higher injury rates. These include heavy, wet snow, which increases knee sprains and other rotational injuries; icy conditions, which are associated with more upper body injuries due to falls; deep powder, and breakable crust.

The various types of nordic skiing continue to be much safer than alpine skiing. Although the informal nature of nordic skiing makes data collection difficult, injury rates are estimated to be about 0.5 per 1,000 skier visits.

In nordic skiing, most injuries result from falls while going downhill. Injury to the upper body occurs more often than to the lower extremity. However, as in alpine skiing, the most common serious injury is the knee sprain. Thumb, forearm, shoulder, and ankle injuries also are common. Fractures of the lower leg and femur and serious head and trunk injuries may occur occasionally. In track skiing, devices that restrain lateral motion of the heel on the ski (e.g., heel wedges and heel locators) increase the lower-extremity injury rate.

In backcountry and telemark skiing, the use of higher boots and more rigid bindings results in a higher proportion of lower-extremity injuries than the use of three-pin bindings and low nordic boots. Skiing in convertible mountaineering bindings with the heels locked down would be expected to produce lower-extremity injuries similar to those of alpine skiing. If a

releasable three-pin binding were developed that could release as reliably as alpine bindings, it would be expected to further reduce the low nordic injury rates. Nordic skiers with previous experience in alpine skiing have a lower injury rate than those without it; the reverse is not true.

Modern alpine bindings are safer than the old cable bindings, but the perfect binding has yet to be invented. Such a binding would have to be inexpensive, simple to install, and easy to adjust and maintain. It would have to release during a fall but not during a hard turn, release equally well during all types of falls, and be unaffected by dirt, snow, ice, or corrosion.

Increasing Skiability and Preventing Accidents

1. Stay in good physical condition, preferably all year long. See Chapter 1 for suggested exercise programs to build endurance, agility, balance, and quadriceps strength. Mountain biking, stair climbing, balance boards, and ski-simulation machines are particularly useful.
2. Purchase good equipment and keep it tuned and repaired. Get the best bindings you can afford. Keep ski edges sharpened and ski bottoms repaired and waxed.
3. Learn the mechanics of your bindings and keep them properly maintained, lubricated, and adjusted. Keep bindings clean and free of snow and ice. Spray them regularly with a silicone lubricant.
4. Test toe and heel releases regularly for proper setting (Fig. 21.7).
   a. Toe release testing method:
      (1) Put on your boots and buckle them tightly.
      (2) Put one ski on a flat surface (snow, a rug, etc.) and place the proper boot into its binding.

(3) Bend your knee, put the ski on its inside edge or against a wooden block, and twist inward at the toe. Release should occur without excessive pressure. Repeat the test with the ski on its outside edge, twisting outward at the toe. Take off the ski.
(4) Put the other ski on the flat surface, place the other boot in its binding, and repeat step (3).
   b. Heel release testing method:
      (1) Perform steps (1) and (2) above.
      (2) Push the knee toward the tip of the ski. Do

Fig. 21.7 *Binding Release Check*

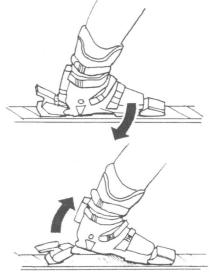

Fig. 21.7

not have anyone stand on the rear of the ski because a hard lunge may injure the Achilles tendon if the heel does not release. It is useful to hold onto a set of railings during this maneuver. The heel piece should release without undue pressure.

(3) Repeat these steps with the other ski.

5. Use antifriction devices.
6. If necessary, obtain cants, which improve skiing ability because the skier will edge better and catch fewer edges. Most modern boots (especially the more expensive ones) have built-in canting adjustments.
7. Cover bindings to protect them from dirt and corrosion, especially when carrying skis on top of a vehicle.
8. Use ski brakes instead of safety straps to decrease the likelihood of being hit by a windmilling ski during a fall. Powder skiers should use powder cords to avoid lost skis, and all skiers who use ski brakes should be careful not to accidentally release a binding while riding on an aerial lift.
9. Take skiing lessons, especially adult racing lessons that will teach you to carve turns. You can always afford to ski better.
10. Do not put ski pole straps on your wrists unless you need to pole uphill. To avoid skier's thumb, train yourself to get rid of your poles in a fall.
11. Do not ski on slopes or in snow conditions that you do not know how to handle.
12. Ski carefully at intersections, slow speed areas, and crowded areas. Do not stop unexpectedly.

13. Do not use alcohol, tranquilizers, sleeping pills, or any drugs that interfere with alertness (such as antihistamines) or co-ordination before or during skiing.
14. Do not skip meals during skiing or other strenuous physical activity. High carbohydrate meals and snacks are the best fuel for replenishing and maintaining muscle glycogen.
15. When you are tired or cold, go to the chalet, rest, and have a snack.
16. Dress for conditions. Carry spare clothing in a backpack or in your vehicle. Carry emergency equipment when nordic skiing or skiing out-of-area (see Chapter 1). At a minimum always carry matches and a sturdy knife.
17. Be familiar with the area where you are skiing. Carry a map of the area.
18. Avoid skiing alone in isolated areas. If you must ski alone (because it is part of your job, etc.), carry a radio.
19. Follow the Skier's Responsibility Code, and urge others to do the same.
    a. Ski under control and in such a manner that you can stop or avoid other skiers or objects.
    b. When skiing downhill or overtaking another skier, avoid the skier below you.
    c. Do not stop where you obstruct a trail or are not visible from above.
    d. When entering a trail or starting downhill, yield to other skiers.
    e. Always use devices to help prevent runaway skis.
    f. Keep off closed trails and posted areas, and observe all posted signs.
20. Other ski equipment: Goggles should be unbreakable, ventilated to avoid fogging, and equipped with light-sensitive or interchangeable yellow and dark lenses. The dark lenses should filter all but 2 to 15 percent of the sun's ultraviolet rays.

Ski pole length should be determined by the height and experience of the skier. To avoid eye injuries, the top of the pole grip should be at least 25 square centimeters in surface area (12 square centimeters for children). If pole straps are used, they should be a break-away design. The pole tip should be hollow and round to provide a good grip on ice.

Wear hard hats during giant slalom and downhill races, and when "timber-bashing."

Snowboarding, a relatively new downhill, oversnow sport, is contributing its share to injuries likely to be seen by the ski patroller. There are estimated to be well over 1 million snowboarders in the United States.

During snowboarding, both feet are fixed to the board so that the lower extremities do not move independently as they do in skiing. Also, since the snowboard is relatively short (4 to 5 feet in length), it turns easily as the snowboarder turns. Consequently, most snowboarding injuries are due to deceleration forces—collisions and falls—in contrast to alpine skiing in which most injuries are due to rotational forces. Soft-tissue injuries such as contusions and lacerations are common. There are relatively more upper-extremity injuries in snowboarding than in skiing. The most frequent lower-extremity injuries are ankle sprains and fractures, as compared with skiing in which the most common ones are knee sprains. Since a snowboard is steered with the back leg while most of the weight is on the forward leg, most lower-extremity injuries occur to the forward leg.

Table 21.1

Summary of Methods of Increasing Skiability and Preventing Accidents

1. Stay in good physical condition year-round.
2. Get good equipment and take care of it.
3. Know your bindings and test them regularly.
4. Use antifriction devices.
5. Use cants if necessary.
6. Cover bindings when carrying skis on top of a vehicle.
7. Use ski brakes instead of safety straps.
8. Take ski lessons to improve your skiing.
9. Keep ski straps off your wrists.
10. Avoid slopes and snow conditions you cannot handle.
11. Ski with care when other skiers are around.
12. Avoid alcohol and drugs while skiing.
13. Stay well nourished while skiing.
14. Rest, warm up, and eat when tired and cold.
15. Dress for conditions. Have spare clothing handy.
16. Be familiar with your ski area.
17. Do not ski alone.
18. Follow the Skier's Responsibility Code and urge others to do the same.

Several snowboarders have died recently when they were unable to extricate themselves after falling in deep powder.

Snowboarders can prevent injuries to some extent by wearing the type of padding worn by skateboarders, and by wearing hard-shell boots instead of soft boots or tennis shoes—at least on the forward foot.

The **mono-skier** uses a wide ski with two conventional ski bindings side by side. Problems can occur if one binding releases and the other does not. A study by Binet in Europe showed that mono-skiers had more lacerations and ankle injuries than traditional skiers and more upper body injuries than snowboarders.

Approach to the Injured Skier

Unless there are specific local instructions to the contrary, the first patroller on the accident scene is considered to be in charge. The patroller places his or her crossed skis upright in the snow several yards above the accident to caution other skiers and to help toboggan handlers find the accident (Fig. 21.8). Assess the patient and give urgent care as described in Chapter 4. Place warm clothing over him or her.

If it will be necessary to call for a toboggan, first determine the need for special equipment such as a spine board or traction splint. If a radio is unavailable, send a responsible skier to the nearest phone or lift shack to notify the patrol. Make sure that the messenger can accurately describe the patient's location. In confusing areas, use map coordinates. If the patient is critically injured, radio ahead so that an ambulance or helicopter can be summoned.

The toboggan generally is brought to the patient from the side and is parked securely in a safe location below the patient. It should be close enough to aid loading yet not so close that it interferes with emergency care. Anchor the unloaded toboggan with skis or a rope belay if it must be left unattended. On very steep hills, it may be easier to load the patient into a toboggan parked *above* rather than *below* the patient. Before loading the toboggan, turn it so that its head end is nearer to the part of the patient's body that will be downhill during transport.

In a patient with a lower-extremity injury, whether the ski boot should or should not be removed on the ski hill

Fig. 21.8 *Approaching an Injured Skier*

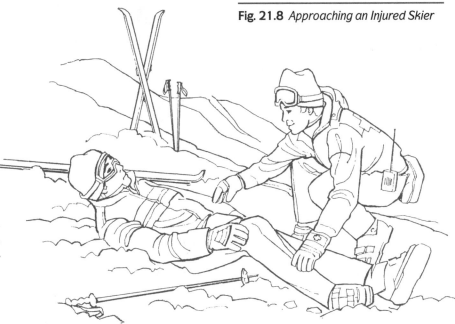

Fig. 21.8

has been the subject of considerable discussion in the past.

The major arguments in favor of removing the boot are that circulation and nerve supply to the foot cannot be assessed directly with the boot in place, and that patrollers are better able, because of their experience, to remove the boot than emergency department personnel. The major arguments against removing the boot are that the boot protects against the cold, provides additional support and, in the case of a femur fracture requiring a traction splint, distributes the pressure from the traction harness over a larger area of the foot, causing less pain and danger of pressure injury. Furthermore, circulation and nerve function on the hill can probably be assessed satisfactorily in almost every case by merely asking the patient whether he or she can feel the toes and wiggle them. Even if the answer is "no," any problem with circulation or nerve function that the patroller can improve on the ski hill will respond to alignment and splinting alone. In any event, transportation becomes a high priority and removing the boot on the hill would only delay this.

Most experts feel that the boot should not be removed on the hill, but should be loosened slightly by being unbuckled and rebuckled in a looser mode, and that a fixation or traction splint should be applied over the boot.

Positioning the Patient in the Toboggan

The general rule is to position the *injury uphill* to keep the patient's weight from jamming the injured extremity against the end of the toboggan during a downhill ride. However, no rule is absolute, and the patient's comfort should be a strong guide in how to position the patient.

Positioning Guidelines

1. *Head downhill* for patients with shock, hypothermia, lower-extremity injuries, and abdominal injuries (unless they are short of breath).
2. *Head uphill* for patients with injuries to the head, face, neck, chest, and upper extremity, as well as for patients who are short of breath, unconscious, or suspected of having a heart attack, and perhaps when the terrain is very steep.
3. *On the injured side* for a unilateral chest injury.
4. *Semiprone* or NATO position (Fig. 5.14) for patients with nausea and vomiting and for patients unresponsive for non-traumatic reasons.

When a patient has suffered multiple, serious injuries, a head or chest injury may indicate a head-uphill position, but the presence of shock may indicate a head-downhill position. The rescuer should be guided by the most life-threatening condition, even though some requirements conflict with others.

After splinting and providing other emergency care, lift the patient into the toboggan (Fig. 21.9), being careful not to aggravate injuries (see Chapter 20). Placing the patient directly on a canvas litter will make removal from the toboggan easier. Wrap the patient

---

Fig. 21.9 *Preparing a Patient for Downhill Transportation from a Ski Slope*

in a blanket or sleeping bag covered with a tarp or other snowproof and windproof cover, and strap the patient in securely. Toboggan straps should not put pressure on the site of injury. A jacket or first aid belt can be used as a pillow, if necessary. If the patient is to be put on a long spine board, consider beforehand how to manage vomiting. Either the spine board or the entire toboggan will have to be tipped to the side. In the former case, the spine board cannot be strapped in place in the toboggan.

Take the toboggan down the hill to the first aid room by the safest, smoothest, and shortest route. Avoid jostling and bumping. Strap the patient's skis and poles to the side of the toboggan opposite the injury with their tips pointing toward the patient's feet, or have a patroller carry them. Never leave a loaded toboggan unattended.

Oversnow Rescue Techniques and Equipment for Nordic Patrollers and Ski Mountaineers

Cross-country skiers and ski mountaineers can become sick or injured in difficult or isolated terrain. Members of nordic patrols and other winter rescue groups should be familiar with the techniques of backcountry oversnow rescue and toboggan handling taught by appropriate units of the National Ski Patrol.

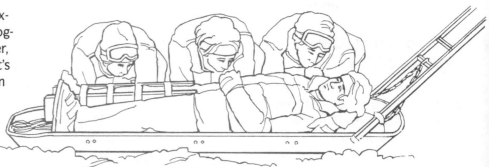

Fig. 21.9

If the site is accessible by snowmobile or helicopter, the best practice often is to stabilize the patient and send for such help. Otherwise, the patient will have to be moved by a toboggan, which can be brought to the site or built from available materials.

A toboggan loaded with a heavy patient can be very difficult to pull uphill or handle in deep snow with insufficient manpower. Toboggans should be belayed on steep terrain and dangerous sidehills.

Commercially-made Backcountry Toboggans

Commercially-made toboggans are available from many different manufacturers and come in various sizes. Backcountry toboggans, which are lighter and smaller than those used by alpine ski patrols, usually have two long front handles and are pulled by a single skier by means of a backpack-type waist belt; some models have detachable rear handles as well.

Some toboggans have detachable shoulder straps and are light enough to be carried on the back of a single skier. Others break into two halves for packing purposes. Otherwise, the toboggan will have to be pulled to the scene.

When transporting a patient, one or more ropes should be attached to the front of the toboggan so that additional skiers can help pull, and other skiers should guide the toboggan from the rear, using the rear handles or a tail rope. This is especially important on sidehills, in difficult snow, when going uphill, or on steep downhill stretches.

A disadvantage of most practical backcountry toboggans is that they are too small to satisfactorily transport a patient with a back or neck injury.

Improvised Backcountry Toboggans

Improvised toboggans are made from one or more pairs of skis held together by a frame that forms a platform to which the patient can be strapped. Several types of frames are commercially available; they also can be improvised from pack frames or stout branches (Fig. 21.10).

Improvised toboggans usually are weaker, more difficult to handle in snow, and more difficult to pull over long distances than commercially available toboggans. However, they do save time, especially over short hauls, if it would otherwise be necessary to send out for a toboggan. The commercial frames for use with skis are much lighter to carry than commercial toboggans.

There are two general types of improvised toboggans. One type is made from a long, narrow, flat piece of aluminum flashing or heavy plastic that is carried rolled into a cylinder in the backpack. To assemble, unroll the piece so that it is flat, and bolt a pair of skis to the top surface, where they act as splints to maintain the shape of the toboggan (Fig. 21.10a). A second type is made of one or two pairs of skis held side-by-side by a commercial frame (Fig. 21.10b) or a frame of poles, branches, and ski poles fastened to the top surface of the skis (Fig. 21.10c).

Improvised toboggans are handled like commercial toboggans. Front and back handles can be improvised from ski poles with the basket end tied to the front and back of the toboggan. Ropes should be available so that extra rescuers can help pull the toboggan uphill or help slow it on downhill stretches.

Fig. 21.10 *Improvised Backcountry Toboggans*

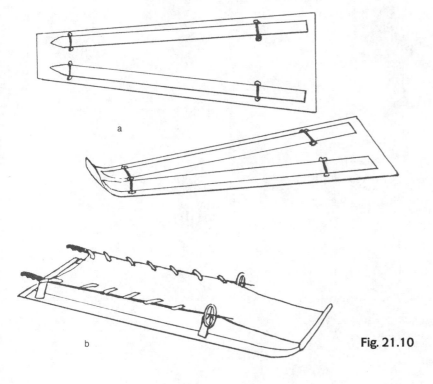

Fig. 21.10

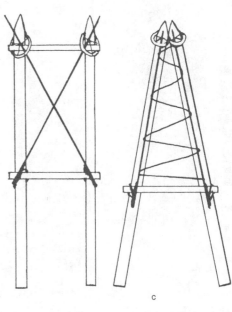

Chapter 22

Triage

Good fortune will elevate even
petty minds, and give them
the appearance of a certain
greatness and stateliness, as
from their high place they look
down upon the world; but the
truly noble and resolved spirit
raises itself, and becomes more
conspicuous in times of
disaster and ill fortune.

—*Plutarch*
Eumenes

The French word **triage** means "to choose" or "to sort out." In emergency care, triage refers to the technique of handling a disaster with so many patients that the capabilities of the rescuers are *initially overwhelmed* and the resources of the community are stretched to the limit or exceeded. This type of disaster is called a **multiple-casualty incident (MCI)**. A basic characteristic of the MCI is that there are more patients than rescuers.

MCI's may range in complexity from single-vehicle accidents involving two or more people; through multiple vehicle, bus, and train accidents involving dozens or scores; to tornados or earthquakes involving hundreds or thousands. When limited resources do not allow everything possible to be done for every patient, rescuers must be guided by the principle of *doing the greatest good for the greatest number*.

Another characteristic of the MCI is that as time goes on, more rescuers and other resources arrive, and more attention can be paid to patients with less chance of survival.

In a single patient with multiple injuries, triage also can refer to the proper order in which to treat each injury.

Triage in the outdoors follows the same principles as triage under urban conditions, except that terrain, weather, equipment, manpower, communication, and distance from definitive medical care often make the rescuer's decisions more difficult and may require modifications of standard triage protocols.

In any MCI, there are three general types of patients:

1. Those who will live no matter what is done.
2. Those who will die no matter what is done.
3. Those for whom what is done will make a difference.

In triage, the rescuer identifies and concentrates time and effort on patients of the third type, remembering always that *life takes precedence over limb*.

The most experienced and best-trained rescuer should be in charge of triage. Priorities for both care and transportation to a hospital must be set for each patient while keeping in mind that, in isolated areas, emergency care can be given, but early transportation may be impossible.

By international convention, four color-coded categories of priority have been established.

Triage Categories

Red

Red is the category for first or immediate priority patients. Usually these patients have injuries to the circulatory and/or respiratory systems.

Red priority patients include the following:

1. Patients in whom hypoxia or shock is either present or imminent.
2. Patients in whom survival is highly probable with immediate care and rapid transportation to a hospital.
3. Patients who can be stabilized without constant attention.

Note that patients with severe head injuries and major crushing injuries of the chest and abdomen *usually do not* meet these criteria.

Red priority patients include those with the following conditions:

1. Obstructed upper airway.
2. Respiratory distress due to shock, flail chest, sucking chest wounds, closed pneumothorax, tension pneumothorax, respiratory tract burns.
3. Major external or internal hemorrhage.
4. Open abdominal wounds.
5. Pericardial tamponade.
6. Burns of 20 to 90 percent of the body surface.

7. Head injuries showing progression.
8. Any injury with shock present or imminent.

Yellow

Yellow is the category for second or delayed priority patients. Yellow priority patients are considered urgent but not as urgent as red priority patients, based on injury type, less rapid progression of the injury, or less chance of survival. They are more likely to have severe injuries to the musculoskeletal and/or nervous systems. Usually, yellow priority patients are able to wait longer than red priority patients before being transported.

Yellow priority patients include the following:

1. Patients who are seriously injured but not yet hypoxic or in shock, and who appear to be able to wait without serious risk for 45 minutes or longer before being transported to a hospital.
2. Patients who have a poorer chance of survival than the red patients, especially if they need constant attention.

Stabilize yellow priority patients, give as much necessary care as possible, and transport them after the red priority patients have been transported.

Examples of yellow priority patients include those with the following conditions:

1. Severe burns covering less than 20 percent or more than 90 percent of the body surface.
2. Back or spinal cord injuries.
3. Multiple fractures.
4. Pelvic or femur fractures without shock.
5. Open fractures.
6. Stable abdominal injuries.
7. Eye injuries.
8. Catastrophic head or chest injuries.

Green

Green is the category for patients whose injuries have third or lowest priority. They may be ambulatory or even uninjured and are regarded as able to wait several hours before being transported to a hospital.

Green priority patients include the following:
1. Patients with minor injuries that do not present a risk to life.
2. Patients that can be stabilized with a minimum of emergency care.
3. Patients who are uninjured but need to be "accounted for" because of their presence at the MCI scene.

Green priority patients include those with the following conditions:
1. Localized soft-tissue injuries.
2. Single, closed fractures.
3. Uncomplicated or minor burns (usually less than 10 percent of the body surface).
4. Most psychological problems.

Black

Black is the category for nonsalvageable patients.

Patients in the black category include the following:
1. Patients who are dead.
2. Patients who die during emergency care.
3. Patients who have lethal injuries and no chance of survival, even in a hospital.

Examples of patients in the black category include those with the following conditions:
1. Cardiac arrest.
2. Absent respirations not responding to opening the airway.
3. Decapitation or severage of the trunk.
4. Massive, especially open, injuries of the head, chest, or abdomen.
5. Incineration.

Triage Technique

In triage, the task is to sort a large number of patients as rapidly and accurately as possible, concentrating first on identifying and caring for patients with critical *yet correctable* conditions, and then on setting priorities for transportation. Priorities may change as the condition of each patient changes and as more help arrives, so that more attention can be given to those with less chance of survival.

Standard techniques of first impression, primary survey, and secondary survey are too time-consuming for triage and must be replaced by techniques that are rapid, effective, easily taught, and easily remembered. An excellent technique is the START (Simple Triage and Rapid Treatment) plan, developed at Hoag Memorial Hospital Presbyterian, Newport Beach, California. This plan, designed to be used by the first rescuer or rescuers responding to a multiple-casualty

Table 22.1

Summary of Triage Categories

Priority	Handling	Color Code	Description	Examples
1	Immediate	Red	1. Hypoxia or shock is present or pending. 2. Survival is likely with rapid care and transport. 3. Care is not time-consuming.	Upper airway obstruction, chest wounds with respiratory distress, major bleeding, open abdominal wounds, pericardial tamponade, shock, progressing head injuries, burns of 20 to 90 percent.
2	Delayed	Yellow	1. Serious injuries are present without hypoxia or shock. 2. Able to wait more than 45 minutes before transport, or chance of survival is less than red priority patients.	Burns less than 20 percent or more than 90 percent, back or spinal cord injuries, multiple or major fractures, stable abdominal injuries, eye injuries, severe head or chest injuries.
3	Hold	Green	1. Injuries are not a risk to life. 2. May be ambulatory. 3. Minimum of emergency care is needed. 4. Able to wait several hours before transport.	Closed fractures, minor burns, non-disruptive psychological problems, localized soft-tissue injuries, uninjured to be accounted for.
4	Dead	Black	1. Vital signs are absent or soon to be absent.	Cardiac arrest, respiratory arrest, obvious lethal injuries, obvious death.

incident (MCI), allows the rescuers to rapidly identify salvageable, high-risk patients and provide basic salvaging maneuvers. It includes five steps:

1. Identify patients with *minor injuries* who are not at risk.
2. Assess each patient's ventilation and provide appropriate salvaging maneuvers.
3. Assess each patient's circulation and provide appropriate salvaging maneuvers.
4. Assess each patient's mental status.
5. Identify those who, for practical purposes, are *dead*.

Immediately upon reaching the MCI site and determining the presence of any hazard to rescuers, the first rescuer indicates a large tree or other easily identifiable object and shouts: "All of you who can walk, move over there!"

This step immediately sorts out most of the green priority patients—the "walking wounded," and allows concentration on the remainder.

Beginning with the *nearest* patient, the rescuer carries out a rapid **survival scan** of each patient, spending only a minute or two with each. Rubber gloves should be put on if possible. After examining the patients and providing any necessary salvaging maneuvers (described below), the rescuer should tag each patient with the appropriate triage category identification tag (Fig. 22.1) or colored tape. If these are unavailable, the initial of the appropriate color (R, Y, G, or B) should be written on a piece of adhesive tape and attached to the patient's forehead.

The survival scan begins with a rapid observation of the patient's **breathing**. The patient is then classified as not breathing, breathing normally, or breathing more than 30 times a minute (about twice the normal rate).

While evaluating breathing, the rescuer should check the airway. If necessary, clear the airway of foreign material and open the airway with the head-tilt/chin-lift or jaw-thrust technique. In these circumstances, the usual cautions about guarding the cervical spine may have to be ignored. Patients who are not breathing despite an open airway are immediately classified as dead or nonsalvageable (black). Patients who are breathing normally are not classified at this step. Patients who are breathing more than 30 times per minute are classified as red priority.

Because there is insufficient time to count respirations, rescuers should learn to detect a respiratory rate of over 30 times per minute by observing others simulate this rate until they can detect this degree of significant tachypnea at a glance. If there is doubt, the patient is still assigned red priority.

Patients with slow respirations also may be at risk, but they usually can be classified more precisely after their mental function is assessed. The rescuer cannot remain with the patient to maintain the airway; time may permit only simple techniques such as positioning the patient or inserting an oral airway (if available) before moving on to the next step or the next patient. If necessary, recruit one of the walking wounded (green priority patients) to maintain the airway. Patients with airway problems are also classified as red priority.

The next step for patients who are breathing normally is to assess their **circulation** by palpating the radial pulse at the wrist. If the pulse is very weak or cannot be felt, the patient should be tagged red priority. If the pulse is palpable, it is considered normal. If the pulse is weak or not palpable, rapidly check the patient for bleeding, and elevate the patient's legs 12 inches. If external bleeding is found, have the patient or one of the walking wounded apply direct pressure (Fig. 22.2).

In patients with normal breathing and a normal radial pulse, the next step is to assess the **mental status**. By this time, the rescuer has had a chance to see whether these patients can follow simple commands. If in doubt,

Fig. 22.1 *Triage Identification Tag (front and back)*

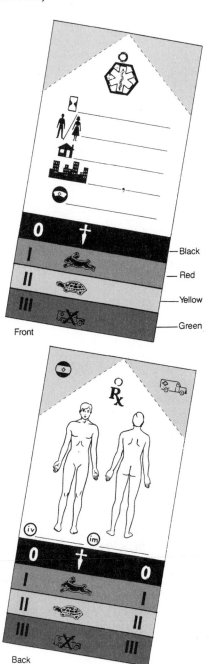

Front

— Black
— Red
— Yellow
— Green

Back

Fig. 22.1

Table 22.2

Algorithm

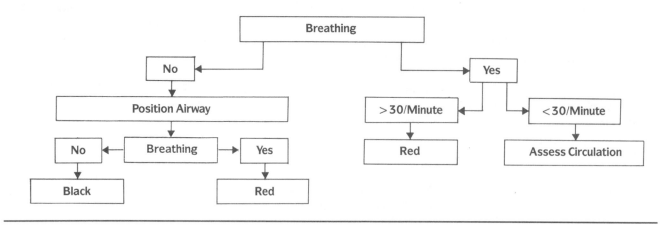

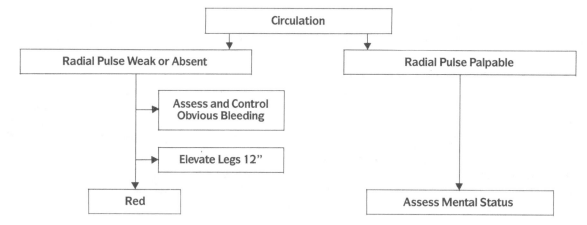

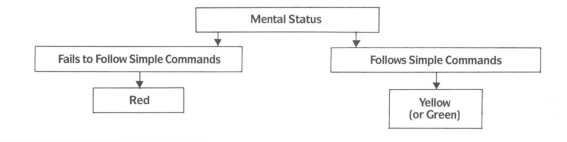

ask the patient to open or close his or her eyes or to squeeze your hand. Patients who are unable to follow the commands are classified as red priority; those who are able are triaged as yellow priority. Unconscious patients are rolled into the semiprone (NATO) position to keep the airway open (Fig. 22.3).

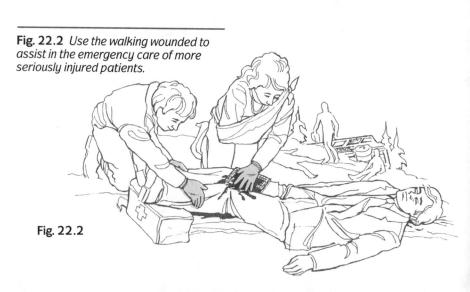

Fig. 22.2 *Use the walking wounded to assist in the emergency care of more seriously injured patients.*

Fig. 22.2

Table 22.3

Comparison Between Standard Assessment and Triage Assessment

Standard Assessment

1. **A**—Open the airway and guard the cervical spine. Ask, "Are you okay?"

2. **B**—Assess breathing. Give rescue breathing if required.

3. **C**—Assess circulation and bleeding. Assess the carotid pulse. Control bleeding if required. Give CPR if necessary. If the patient has a rapid/weak pulse and/or labored breathing, assess the neck, chest, abdomen, and pelvis.

4. **D**—Check for disability. Look for injuries to the musculo-skeletal and nervous systems.

5. **E**—Expose.

Triage Assessment

1. Open the airway and ignore the cervical spine.

2. Assess breathing. Do not give rescue breathing. (Have green priority patient keep the airway open if needed).

3. Assess the radical pulse. If it is weak or absent, check for bleeding, and elevate the patient's legs 12 inches. Do not give CPR. (Have a green priority patient put direct pressure on the bleeding site if necessary).

4. Assess the mental status. Can the patient follow simple commands?

5. Conduct further assessment and provide care when time and additional help permit.

After an initial evaluation of all patients is completed, and as additional rescuers arrive, patients assigned to the red group can be transported. Patients designated yellow and those in the red group who are awaiting transportation can be monitored and given more extensive assessment and care. Patients whose condition has deteriorated are moved to a higher priority category.

Another triage device, the CRAMS Scale (Table 22.4), is useful in assigning patients to one of two clearly divided groups, one with a score of 6 or less and a high mortality rate (62 percent), and the other with a score of 7 or more with a low mortality rate (0.15 percent).

In some cases, factors other than the type of injury may influence the category to which a patient is assigned.

Fig. 22.3 *Technique of Rolling an Unresponsive Patient to the NATO Position*

An injured rescuer or relative of a rescuer is automatically assigned to the red category regardless of the severity of injuries. This is done to minimize distraction and maintain rescuer morale. An injured child, hysterical patient, or patient with a hysterical relative also should be assigned a higher priority than the injury might otherwise warrant.

As more rescuers arrive, the first rescuer on the scene assumes the job of triage officer. He or she assigns the new rescuers to handle direct patient assessment and care and begins to organize the scene and the transportation process. When more experienced people arrive, the job of triage officer can be transferred to one of them.

The ambulance dispatch center or hospital emergency department needs to know brief details of the type of multiple-casualty incident, the number of victims, and their injuries. Requests for ambulances, additional equipment, and help must be relayed to the proper sources. If there are many patients, a second triage and treatment area should be set up away from the disaster site and close to the transport area, protected from the weather, and furnished with lighting

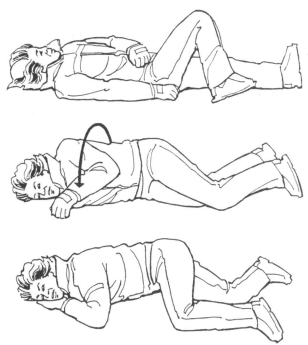

Fig. 22.3

Table 22.4

CRAMS Scale

(**C**irculation, **R**espiratory, **A**bdomen, **M**otor, **S**peech)

Category	Score
Circulation:	
Normal capillary refill, blood pressure above 100 systolic.	2
Delayed capillary refill, blood pressure 85 to 99 systolic.	1
No capillary refill, blood pressure below 85 systolic.	0
Respiration:	
Normal.	2
Abnormal (labored, shallow, or rate above 35 per minute).	1
Absent.	0
Abdomen:	
Abdomen and thorax not tender.	2
Abdomen and thorax tender.	1
Abdomen rigid, thorax flail, or deep, penetrating injury to either the chest or abdomen.	0
Motor:	
Normal (obeys commands).	2
Responds only to pain, no posturing (extension or flexion).	1
Postures or gives no response.	0
Speech:	
Normal (oriented).	2
Confused or inappropriate.	1
No speech or makes unintelligible sounds.	0

Significance of CRAMS Scale: A score of 6 or less indicates a critically ill person (62 percent of overall mortality rate even in a hospital, and an expected mortality rate close to 100 percent if the patient does not reach a hospital within two hours). A score of 0 means the patient is essentially dead or will be dead within a few minutes. A score of 7 or above is favorable, with an overall hospital mortality rate of 0.15 percent.*

*Clemmer, et. al., *Journal of Trauma*, 25:188, 1985.

if necessary. For efficiency, the patients should be grouped together by category. Since more help is available, rescuers can initiate emergency care based on standard principles while waiting for transportation to arrive.

One of a rescuer's more difficult jobs is dealing with the emotions of seriously injured patients and of their friends and relatives, who may not understand why a certain patient is being "neglected" by being placed in a lower category.

Triage of a Single Patient with Multiple Injuries

By now, you have studied basic and advanced assessment, basic life support, and the care of injuries and illnesses of various organ systems. You are ready to draw this information together to provide the proper sequencing of emergency care for a patient with multiple injuries. It goes without saying that all such patients should be taken to a hospital as soon as possible. If transportation is ready and waiting, rescuers *should not spend any more time in the field than necessary to stabilize the patient.*

EMS personnel use the concept of the "golden hour," which refers to the average amount of time that elapses before a patient with serious or multiple injuries starts to deteriorate rapidly. For every 30-minute period following this first hour, the patient's chances of survival are cut in half. To increase the patient's chances of survival, the rescuer must be knowledgeable, experienced, able to work quickly and efficiently, establish priorities, and improvise when necessary. There will be no time to go back and reread the emergency care manuals; important things must be done right the first time.

Be aware of the dramatic appearance of a seriously injured person and of the normal tendency to feel panic and inadequacy when faced with several simultaneous, life-threatening problems in one or several individuals.

Providers of prehospital emergency care should remember also that their job is to buy time for the patient until a hospital is reached or an ambulance or helicopter arrives. Emergency department personnel and advanced life support attendants have extensive training and sophisticated equipment; they deal with serious injuries every day. Arrangements for their involvement should be started as soon as it is apparent that a serious accident has occurred.

Life-threatening injuries usually involve the **circulatory**, **respiratory**, and/or **nervous** systems. Fortunately, the assessment techniques you have already learned are designed to help you discover and care for these injuries immediately. *You do not have to learn anything new;* you basically need to practice your assessment techniques until you automatically will do the right things in the right order *right away.* Frequently, the most difficult task will be to concentrate on doing what you have been taught despite the distracting effects of dramatic but noncritical injuries such as bloody lacerations or extremity fractures. Since most musculoskeletal injuries are *not* life-threatening, their management is *not* part of the ABC's.

The first impression is very useful in determining the mechanism of injury and predicting what you might find. Refer to Chapter 9 for common patterns of injury and Chapter 19 for an in-depth discussion of assessment. Do not forget to institute universal precautions (see Appendix F).

No matter how much blood there is on the ground, the first consideration is always the **airway** and assessment of **breathing** and **circulation**. As soon as the airway is open and adequate breathing and a heartbeat are confirmed, move immediately to investigate where the blood is coming from, and care for active, external **bleeding**. Ignore any large, non-bleeding or slowly bleeding wounds for the moment. By this time, you usually will know the patient's level of responsiveness, which, if decreased below the normal, alert level, suggests either a head injury or lack of perfusion of the brain due to shock. If the patient has a fast, irregular, and/or weak pulse, or labored breathing, and these are not explained by what has already been discovered, move next to assess the neck, chest, abdomen,

and pelvis. Look for evidence of the following:

1. External injuries that interfere with the normal breathing process, such as a sucking chest wound or flail chest.
2. Internal injuries that might be causing interference with heart or lung function, such as pneumothorax, tension pneumothorax, hemothorax, or cardiac tamponade.
3. Internal bleeding with shock—such as in any of the injuries listed above as well as in open abdominal wounds, evidence of blunt trauma to the abdomen, or a fractured pelvis.

If shock still is not explained, assess the thighs for a fractured femur. Finally, assess the extremities and back for evidence of fractures, open and closed wounds, and evidence of spinal cord trauma. Multiple fractures can cause shock as easily as a fractured femur or pelvis.

When assessing and opening the airway, use the jaw-thrust technique since every seriously injured patient is considered to have a cervical spine injury. Use the finger-sweep method or suction to remove any obstructing material such as snow, vomitus, or blood. Meanwhile, stabilize the head and neck as well as possible and, when time permits, apply a rigid collar. Perform the Heimlich maneuver if necessary to removed a foreign body from the airway. If the patient is unresponsive and has no gag reflex, put an oral airway in place.

If the airway cannot be maintained with the above techniques, particularly if there is an injury to the neck or face, it will probably be necessary to use advanced airway maintenance with an endotracheal tube, which is a tube introduced through the mouth or nose into the trachea and used with a bag-valve-mask; or cricothyroidotomy, which is a tube introduced into the trachea through the membrane

between the cricoid and thyroid cartilages. If no one at the scene is trained in these techniques, the patient will probably suffocate unless taken immediately to a doctor or hospital.

A sucking chest wound or flail chest can be treated in the field with simple techniques described in previous chapters. A pneumothorax, tension pneumothorax, and cardiac tamponade require advanced techniques such as the ability to introduce needles and tubes into the chest. Oxygen, if available, is always useful and should be given in high concentration and high flow rate.

If the patient is not breathing, give artificial ventilation, using a pocket mask or a bag-valve-mask with added oxygen. If the patient is breathing ineffectively, support ventilations. An oral airway should be in place in any unresponsive patient without a gag reflex. CPR will be required if the patient has no pulse, although it usually is ineffective in a patient with cardiac arrest due to trauma, even in a well-equipped hospital.

Control bleeding with direct pressure. A pressure bandage is useful when not enough help is available to keep manual pressure on the wound. A physician or paramedic treats shock with intravenous fluids and/or a PASG; a rescuer without these special skills has very little to offer in the field other than controlling external bleeding, giving oxygen, supporting ineffective ventilations, and elevating the patient's legs.

Experience with the prehospital management of trauma in rural areas has shown that the two most useful, advanced skills are the abilities to perform endotracheal intubation and give intravenous fluids.

By following the ABC's, the rescuer will have dealt by now with the conditions that pose an immediate threat to life *that can be cared for in the field.* The next consideration is **disability**, which refers to the rescuer's search for injury to the patient's nervous and musculoskeletal systems. Reassess the patient's level of responsiveness, and assess the state of the pupils, ability to move, and perception of pain and touch. The AVPU Scale or Glasgow Coma Scale (see Chapter 4) is useful in recording and monitoring the level of responsiveness. Remember that an altered level of responsiveness frequently is due to hypoxia. Hypoxic patients may be agitated or belligerent rather than obtunded.

Assess the patient's extremities and back for additional open and closed wounds and fractures. Protect external wounds with sterile dressings. Remember to **expose** the patient, which refers to removing enough clothing from the chest, abdomen, and extremities so that you can discover all injuries to these areas. This part of the ABCDE's—except for exposure needed to locate the site of and care for external bleeding—frequently should be delayed until the patient reaches shelter, especially in inclement weather. At an alpine ski area, full exposure usually takes place only in the first aid room.

Because of the need for rapid transport, it is almost always preferable to immobilize the multiple-trauma patient on a long spine board rather than to treat individual fractures and other extremity injuries separately. This saves time, is the best care for spine and spinal cord injuries, and is effective for most fractures or other injuries that may be present. An exception is a **femur** fracture which, because of the need to control bleeding into the fracture site, usually should be managed separately with a traction splint.

Scenario #24 (Fig. 22.4)

The following scenario provides an example of triage in action.

You are a professional ski patroller at Destination Ski Area, a large area served by a gondola as well as multiple chair lifts. You are patrolling a high bowl above the gondola, when you hear over the radio that there has been a derailment. Eight gondola cars have fallen to the ground.

You arrive at the first gondola car and see nine victims inside. You point to a spot outside, and say, "All of you who can walk, move over here." Three of the nine are able to do so. Your survival scans reveal the following. (The patients are not listed in the order in which you scanned them.)

1. A middle-aged woman who is screaming hysterically. She has a large lump on her forehead and a fractured wrist. Her respirations and pulse are normal. She tells you that she hurt her head and wrist when the gondola fell.
2. A middle-aged man who is lying in the gondola wreckage, unconscious, breathing normally, groaning, and spontaneously moving all four extremities. His pulse is palpable and strong.
3. An elderly man with an obvious crushed chest. He is not breathing and has no detectable pulse.
4. A young woman who is lying quietly. Her skin is pale, cold, and clammy, her respirations are rapid and shallow, and her pulse is fast and weak. She complains weakly of abdominal pain.
5. An obnoxious middle-aged man who is yelling, cursing, and threatening to sue the ski area. He does not appear to be hurt.
6. A young man who is lying quietly on his side, complaining of pain in the back between the shoulder blades. His breathing is normal, and his pulse is palpable and strong. He says he cannot move his legs.
7. An elderly woman who appears basically healthy and vigorous for her age. She is in respiratory distress and is complaining of chest pain. Her pulse is strong and fast, and her breathing rate is above 30 per minute. A brief inspection of the pain site discloses a flail segment of the chest wall.
8. A middle-aged woman who seems calm and does not appear to be injured.
9. A teen-aged girl who is lying quietly. Her respirations are shallow, irregular, and more than 30 per minute, although they improve somewhat with the jaw-thrust technique. Her pulse is rapid and weak, and the skin of her wrist is cold and clammy. She does not respond to your voice.

You assign patients 4 and 7 to red priority because of impending shock and hypoxia, respectively, and because with simple care and rapid transport they should survive. You assign patients 2 and 6 to yellow priority because, although seriously injured, they appear to be stable enough to wait for transport. You classify patient 3 as black priority and patients 1 and 8 as green priority.

Since patient 8, who is calm, appears to be sensible, you ask her to try to quiet patient 1; if this is unsuccessful, you plan to move patient 1 to yellow priority. You plan to move

Fig. 22.4 Scenario #24

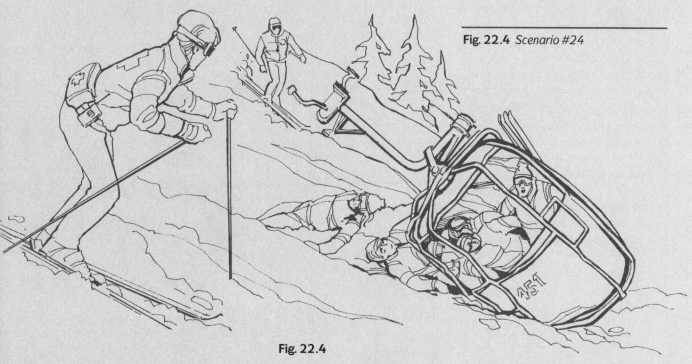

Fig. 22.4

patient 5 up to the red category for immediate transport to get him out of everyone's hair (otherwise you would assign him to green priority because he appears uninjured). Then you decide to try a rapid, tactful request for his help to see if this will calm him down by giving him something to do.

You assign patient 9 to yellow priority because, although her survival scan would indicate that she is red priority, her chance of survival is less than patients 4 and 7, and she will require more care than they do. As soon as more help arrives you can move her up to red priority.

You perform basic salvage maneuvers on patients 4, 7, and 9. These actions include a rapid search for external bleeding and elevating the legs 12 inches for patient 4, and stabilizing the flail chest for patient 7. For patient 9, you open the airway, elevate the legs 12 inches, and conduct a rapid search for external bleeding. You recruit green priority patients to manually stabilize patient 7's flail chest and maintain patient 9's airway. As soon as more help arrives, you plan to spend your time caring for and preparing transportation for patients 4, 7, and 9, and monitoring patients 9, 2 and 6. Later you will arrange transport for patients 1, 8, 3, and 5.

Scenario #25 (Fig. 22.5)

The following scenario illustrates the management of a patient with multiple injuries.

You are patrolling the summit on a calm day two days after a severe storm that covered High Range Ski Area with 2 feet of heavy powder. The Drainage, a steep, heavily forested, ungroomed area to the north, has just been opened after the patrol has skied it without finding any evidence of unstable snow.

You are ready to go off duty when the phone rings. It is the hill chief: "Ben, there has been an avalanche in the Drainage at the narrow, run-out chute. We have a report of a person buried. Mike is on his way up on a snowmobile with a witness. Vikki is coming with her avalanche dog. Get ready to take a hasty party down as soon as you get some patrollers off number 2 chair. Be careful."

You quickly take six transceivers out of the avalanche locker in the summit shack, then leave on a run headed for the shed where the avalanche gear is stored. You know exactly where the Drainage slid; it slid there once before, many years ago. Your radio sputters with an announcement from the hill chief, directing all available patrollers to report to the summit for an avalanche search.

Opening the shed, you pull out four shovels, some flagging, and the large bundle of probe poles, carrying them over to the side of the lift unloading ramp. Returning to the summit shack, you get the oxygen backpack from the closet. You see two patrollers on a chair, ready to unload; you wave them over. The whine of the snowmobile announces the arrival of Mike and the witness, a young man in his late 20's who is pale but calm. Leaving word with the lift operator, you distribute transceivers, probes, and shovels. Then, shouldering the oxygen backpack yourself, you follow the witness into the Drainage.

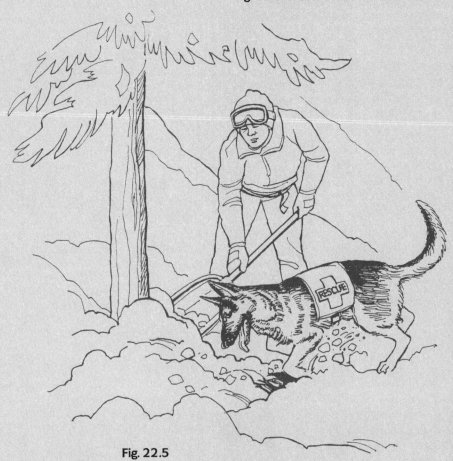

Fig. 22.5 *Scenario #25*

Fig. 22.5

The heavy powder is hard going, but in less than 10 minutes you arrive at the top of the chute. There is a 2-foot fracture line above an icy base with a large pile of debris at the bottom. The witness points out where he last saw the victim, a young man in his early 20's named Harold Slab. You mark the point-last-seen with flagging, then carefully make your way down the icy avalanche bed to the upper margin of the debris pile.

Your assessment has been that the area above the chute is stable since it has been well skied by the patrol. You four patrollers spread out and slowly descend toward the toe of the avalanche, looking for clues, kicking at the snow, and probing at likely areas. After 10 minutes, you reach the toe without finding any sign of the victim.

A shout from the top announces the arrival of Vikki with Loki, a four-year-old German shepherd. Vikki takes off her skis, gives the command "Check it out!" and they start to descend the chute, the dog ranging from side to side, sniffing the snow. They reach the toe of the slide without finding anything, then start up again. The dog stops suddenly above a large tree at the north side of the slide and starts to dig and bark.

Everyone converges on the spot with shovels and probes. You take off the oxygen backpack, then start to dig carefully to the side of the dog and uncover the tail of a ski. The dog is called off and two of you dig rapidly, uncovering part of the patient that appears to be the right thigh and hip. The patient's body is wrapped around the tree trunk. The right thigh is twisted and bent at an abnormal angle. Now that you have oriented the way the patient is lying, it is easy to locate the head.

There is an ice mask around the face; he is not breathing. As soon as enough space is excavated around the patient's head, you start rescue breathing using a pocket mask from your first aid belt. After two rescue breaths, you assess the carotid pulse. It is faint but present at 120 beats per minute. You continue rescue breathing.

Bill radios the base to report the successful find. He is told that there is a toboggan on the way down from the summit. He asks the base to request a LifeFlight helicopter, which should arrive about the time the toboggan reaches the base with the patient.

Bill then retrieves the hand-powered suction unit from the oxygen backpack and lays it at your side, attaches the bag-valve-mask to the tank with a length of tubing, and starts oxygen flowing into the bag-valve-mask at 12 liters per minute. You remove the pocket mask from the patient's face. Bill deftly inserts an oropharyngeal airway into the patient's mouth, then fits the mask over the patient's face and holds it there, stabilizing the head and neck with both hands. You start squeezing the ventilation bag at a rate of one breath every 5 seconds. There appears to be chest rise beneath the patient's parka with each ventilation. Meanwhile, the others have completely uncovered the rest of the body and removed the patient's skis.

Mark begins an assessment. The neck appears normal; no open wounds or tracheal deviation. Assessment of the chest reveals that the right side is flattened compared to the left and there is some crackling on palpation of the skin over this area. You ask Mark whether there is paradoxical motion of the right side of the chest, and he replies that there is good chest rise on each side with the ventilations. You remember that paradoxical motion only occurs when the patient is breathing normally, not when he is being ventilated.

The abdomen appears normal. The right thigh is angulated at its midpoint with the leg and foot rotated externally and a definite bulge in the midthigh area compared with the left.

The radial pulse is palpable but weak, and is still 120 beats per minute. You remark that this means his blood pressure is at least 80 mm Hg.

Mark assesses the patient's back by running his hand up and down it. There are no obvious deformities although the mechanism of injury suggests the strong possibility of neck and/or back injury. A blanket is carefully pushed under and around the patient.

You: "Mark, call Base and have someone bring down a backboard and a traction splint if they're not already on the way."

A shout from the top of the chute announces the arrival of the toboggan and two more patrollers. Mark reaches the toboggan handler by radio, suggesting that the toboggan be belayed down to the accident site. Fortunately, operating procedures require that every toboggan that goes into the Drainage carry a climbing rope, anchor sling, and a large figure-8 carabiner for belay purposes. By the time this is done, three patrollers arrive carrying a long spine board and a Sager splint. One patroller is assigned to act as avalanche lookout while the other two make their way to the accident site with their equipment.

The Sager splint is applied to the patient's left lower extremity and traction is initiated. The extremity straightens and rotates into the normal, anatomical position in the splint. You and Bill continue to ventilate the patient, maintaining manual stabilization of his head and neck, and stopping every few minutes to see if he has started to breathe on his own. The is some discussion about stabilizing his flail chest, but you point out that the positive pressure generated by the bag-valve-mask makes this unnecessary.

After the traction splint is in place, the long spine board is laid next to the patient and six of you raise the patient carefully out of the hole without changing his position. The board is slid under him and he is carefully aligned into the anatomical position on the board. A rigid collar is applied.

By this time the patient is starting to moan and stir. He is strapped down securely to the board with four main straps plus over-the-shoulder straps and groin straps, then lifted into the toboggan. Again, there are different opinions about whether his head should be uphill or downhill. The conclusion is that his head should be uphill, because the respiratory system is probably compromised more by his respiratory arrest and crushed chest than his circulatory system is by his probable hypovolemia and hypothermia.

The board is moved forward in the toboggan so that there is room for the oxygen tank and a patroller at the rear by the patient's head. Since you have the biggest hands, you are elected to man the bag-valve-mask. You have practiced using one hand to stabilize a patient's head and neck and keep the mask in place while squeezing the bag with the other hand in the past, and you know you can do it. Since the first 200 yards of the route to the base is steep, you fashion an "umbilical cord" with a short length of 1-inch webbing and tie yourself to the rear of the toboggan so that you will not fall forward.

The toboggan is slowly belayed down the remaining 50 yards of the avalanche debris and arrives at the base 10 minutes after reaching the gentler slopes 150 yards beyond. By this time the patient is starting to breathe irregularly on his own. You continue to support him with the bag-valve-mask. His blood pressure is taken in the first aid room and is 90 over 40. His pulse is 105 beats per minute. You hear the throbbing of the helicopter rotor becoming louder in the distance.

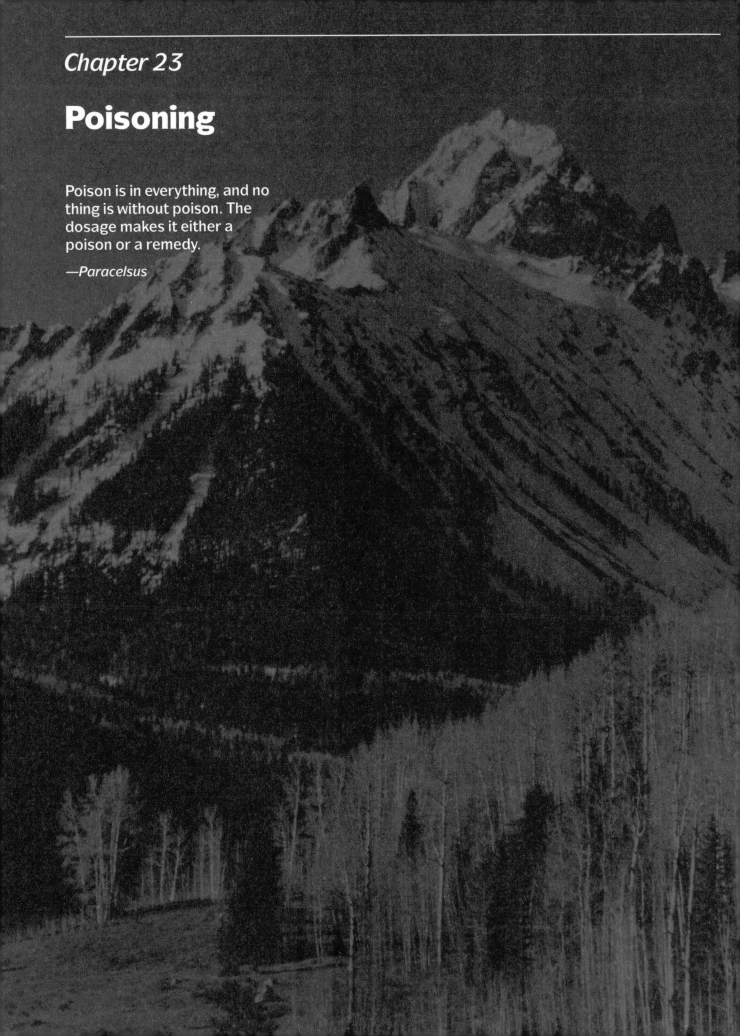

Chapter 23

Poisoning

Poison is in everything, and no thing is without poison. The dosage makes it either a poison or a remedy.

—*Paracelsus*

Poisons (Fig. 23.1) are substances that damage the body directly or through chemical actions that interfere with normal metabolic processes. Poisons may be substances foreign to the body, such as lead and arsenic; normal body constituents present in excessive amounts, such as vitamin D; or familiar medicines taken in overdose, such as aspirin. They also can be compounds that are produced naturally by the body but for some reason are not detoxified or excreted. For example, in patients with chronic kidney failure, the normal byproducts of metabolism accumulate to toxic levels.

Many poisons are present naturally in the environment, such as the elements arsenic and selenium in soil and poisonous chemicals found in certain mushrooms and higher plants. Some types of seafood, such as California mussels, are safe to eat at some times of the year and poisonous at others, usually because they have ingested seasonal toxin-containing microorganisms and concentrated the toxins in their tissues. Other poisonous creatures introduce toxic materials into the body through stings, bites, and appendages such as spines.

Poisonous substances can enter the body through ingestion, inhalation, injection, or absorption through the skin or mucous membranes. Since there are so many possible sources of poisoning, details of recognition and emergency care are hard to remember. Therefore, when every minute counts, call experts in regional poison control centers and hospital emergency departments for up-to-date, specific recommendations.

This chapter discusses poisoning in general, emphasizing the importance of early access to the EMS system and rapid transport to a hospital. It also discusses the assessment of a patient with suspected poisoning and provides suggestions for care when expert advice and rapid transport

Table 23.1

Common Signs and Symptoms of Poisoning

1. Inappropriate behavior, or disturbances of responsiveness ranging from hyperactivity and excitement at one extreme to slight confusion, stupor, and coma at the other.
2. Suspicious materials, such as bottles, vials, pills, spilled liquids, chemicals, syringes, needles, and the remains of food and drink.
3. Unusual odors associated with the patient.
4. Convulsions.
5. Shock.
6. Gastrointestinal symptoms such as abdominal pain, nausea, vomiting, and diarrhea.
7. Excessive salivation or sweating.
8. Abnormal pulse and/or respirations.
9. Dilation or constriction of pupils.
10. Redness, blistering, stains, or burns on the skin, especially around the mouth.
11. The patient or witnesses report that the patient has ingested, inhaled, or injected a substance (even when other signs and/or symptoms are absent).

cannot be obtained. Chapter 24 discusses the specifics of poisoning and other injuries resulting from contact with hazardous animals and plants.

In the United States, more than five million poisonings occur each year, causing about 10,000 deaths. *Few specific antidotes for poisons exist,* and these few are available only at a hospital. Therefore, the cornerstone of emergency care for poisoning is *to transport the patient to a hospital as soon as possible.* In the hospital, poisoning is treated by removing the poison where possible, preventing its further absorption, curtailing its conversion to an active form, enhancing its excretion or conversion to an inactive form, and/or counteracting its clinical effects.

In urban areas, most poisonings occur in the home as a result of the ingestion of drugs or household chemicals, usually accidentally but occasionally with suicidal intent. Toddlers who get into their elders' medications make up a large percentage of accidental, household poisonings. In the outdoors, most poisonings occur as the result of ingestion of or con-

tact with poisonous plants or animals or their products.

It is important to keep *all* medications, household cleansers, weed killers, pesticides, and other chemicals safely out of the reach of children—preferably by locking them away. As in most emergencies, prevention is best. Prescription medicines should

Fig. 23.1 *Poisonous Substances*

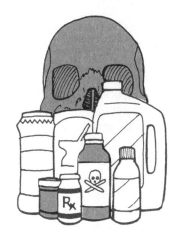

Fig. 23.1

be in kept in their original containers, which should be childproof. Medications kept at the bedside should be only in small amounts for use during the night. Empty soft drink bottles and food containers should not be used to store household cleansers and other chemicals because someone who thinks the original contents are still in the container may accidentally ingest the harmful substance.

Assessment and Emergency Care of Possible Poisoning

If a victim of poisoning is to receive proper emergency care, the rescuer must first provide any urgent care necessary, next suspect poisoning, then identify the poison, and finally provide care for the poisoning itself.

Emergency care for poisoning includes both **general** and **specific** measures. General measures include basic life support, care for unresponsiveness, shock, and convulsions, and rapid transport to a hospital. Specific measures include contacting the regional poison control center or emergency department for specific instructions, removing or diluting the poison, slowing its absorption, or speeding its elimination.

The most important parts of the assessment and general care include the following:

1. Register the first impression. If the patient is in an urban environment, note the obvious presence of spilled pills or liquids, bottles of medications, containers of household chemicals, strange odors, and other clues. If the patient is in an outdoor environment, note such things as leftovers from a recent meal containing the remains of seafood, mushrooms, wild plants, etc. Note whether the patient is obviously responsive.
2. Perform the primary survey and give urgently required care for airway, breathing, and circulation problems.
3. Care for unresponsiveness and convulsions, as required (see Chapters 12 and 17).
4. Question the patient, family member's or witnesses about recent events leading up to the current problem. The patient may admit to inhaling, ingesting, or injecting a toxic substance. Is the patient taking any regular medications? Does the patient have any significant preexisting medical illnesses, including psychiatric disorders such as depression? In the backcountry or marine environment, has the patient consumed any wild food or been bitten, stung, or otherwise injured by any hazardous creature? Look for and ask specifically about any of the common signs and symptoms of poisoning (Table 23.1).

   Once poisoning is suspected or confirmed, it is important to attempt to identify the poison even though there are general measures that are useful for most types of poisons. However, at this point, contact the EMS system, even if the patient does not appear very ill. Since the actions of some poisons are delayed, the patient may appear entirely normal when first seen. Inspect any drug or chemical labels to identify the toxic substance. If possible, find out *what* substance was taken, *how much* was taken, *by what route, when,* and *why.*
5. After contacting the EMS system, and while waiting for the ambulance, contact the nearest poison control center or call the nearest hospital emergency department. The poison control center number can often be found in the telephone directory or can be obtained by calling the operator or dialing 911. Poison control centers are staffed 24 hours a day by experts with up-to-date information who can recommend immediate emergency care measures to carry out while awaiting the ambulance. The staff will need to know the age, size, general health, and weight of the patient, a description of the drug or poison, when and how much was taken, and the time and distance to the nearest hospital.

   Containers of most prescription drugs are labelled with the name, strength, and number of dose units (tablets, ounces of liquid) of their contents. The labels of chemical containers usually list their contents and frequently include recommendations for immediate emergency care in case of poisoning. However, since these recommendations may be inaccurate or outdated, they should be followed only if you are not able to contact a poison control center or emergency department. If you must take the patient to the emergency department by private vehicle, always call ahead to alert emergency department personnel, who can give you instructions for immediate care. Also, always call the poison control center.
6. When you call the poison control center or hospital emergency department, *write down* any instructions given over the phone for immediate care, then follow them.
7. Save suspicious material (see Table 23.1), vomitus, etc. to

Table 23.2

Summary of Assessment and General Care for Poisoning

1. Survey the scene and conduct the primary survey.
2. Provide basic life support and any other necessary immediate care.
3. Obtain the patient's medical history from the patient or witnesses: what was taken, how much, by what route, when, and why.
4. Call EMS for an emergency ambulance.
5. Call the regional poison control center or hospital emergency department.
6. Provide any immediate care recommended by poison control center or hospital personnel.
7. Save containers, poisonous substances, vomitus, etc., and send this material along with the patient to the hospital.
8. Monitor the patient's condition frequently.
9. Provide airway, suction, ventilation, CPR, and treatment for shock and convulsions as needed.
10. See that the patient is taken rapidly to a hospital.

---

send to the hospital with the patient for later analysis. If medication is involved, save the container(s) and document the exact number of pills or amount of fluid remaining.

8. Monitor and record vital signs and changes in the patient's condition frequently (every 10 to 15 minutes).
9. Monitor breathing and be ready to maintain the airway, give suction, provide and assist ventilation, give CPR as needed, and treat for shock and convulsions if necessary.
10. See that the patient is taken rapidly to a hospital.

Emergency Care of Specific Poisons

Ingested Poisons

These poisons include medications, alcoholic beverages, household chemicals, contaminated food, parts of plants, etc. Because of the variety of substances that can be ingested, it is best to follow the directions of the emergency department or poison control center personnel. However, if you

are in an outdoor environment without a telephone or radio, or if transport time to a hospital will be long, there are some general principles that can be followed immediately.

The principles are to **dilute** the poison with milk or water, **remove** it by inducing vomiting, and **absorb** any remainder by giving the patient activated charcoal. Dilution also provides something for the stomach to "act on" during vomiting.

There are some exceptions to these principles. Do not dilute in the case of petroleum products, since swallowing and overdistention of the stomach may cause vomiting, and if aspiration occurs, serious chemical pneumonia may result. Also, do not dilute in the case of patients with an altered level of responsiveness because their ability to swallow is usually impaired.

Do not induce vomiting in patients who are more likely to aspirate because of an altered level of responsiveness, convulsion, or lack of a gag reflex. Do not induce vomiting in the case of strong acids (such as sulfuric acid, hydrochloric acid, phenol) or alkalis (such as lye), since they are corrosive and may cause additional injury when they come back up. For

reasons mentioned above, vomiting is also undesirable if petroleum products have been swallowed. If more than one hour has elapsed since ingestion occurred, vomiting is unlikely to be beneficial and should not be induced.

Do not give activated charcoal in the case of ingestion of strong acids or alkalis or in patients with an altered level of responsiveness who are unable to swallow.

Emergency care of a patient who has ingested poison includes the following:

1. If the patient is awake and alert, the first step is to have him or her drink milk or water to dilute the poison. The amount is one to two glasses, depending on the patient's size. (Larger amounts may increase the risk of speeding the passage of the poison from the stomach into the duodenum.)

   Next, induce vomiting by gagging the patient with a tongue blade or spoon handle (Fig. 23.2). If gagging the

---

Fig. 23.2 *Vomiting can be induced with a spoon handle.*

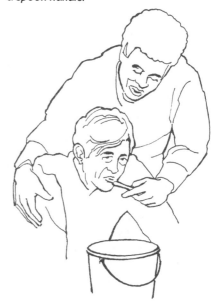

Fig. 23.2

patient does not induce vomiting, give syrup of ipecac, if available. The dose is two tablespoonfuls for an adult or one tablespoonful for a child over one year. Syrup of ipecac will almost always cause vomiting within 15 to 30 minutes. When the patient vomits, guard the upper airway by turning a recumbent patient onto the side and using suction as necessary.

2. Activated charcoal (nonprescription) is a strong inactivator of many poisons. If activated charcoal is available, give it *instead* of inducing vomiting when ingestion has occurred *more* than one hour previously, or *after* inducing vomiting in order to absorb any remaining poison when ingestion has occurred *less* than one hour previously. Stir 50 to 100 grams of activated charcoal into a glass of water for the patient to drink. Premixed activated charcoal containing sorbitol (a mildly laxative sweetener) is also available (follow directions on container).

Some authorities feel that activated charcoal should be given *first* in most patients instead of inducing vomiting. Other authorities caution that giving syrup of ipecac may cause protracted vomiting that will delay giving activated charcoal.

Inhaled Poisons

Inhaled poisons include smoke, industrial gases such as chlorine and hydrogen sulfide, and natural gases such as carbon dioxide and methane, which may accumulate in harmful amounts in wells and caves. One of the most commonly inhaled poisons is carbon monoxide (see Chapter 17).

Inhaled poisons cause damage by directly irritating the lung, by replacing oxygen in the air, or by acting as general body poisons.

The first step in emergency care is to remove the patient from the contaminated atmosphere (Fig. 23.3). Frequently, there is considerable danger to the rescuer, and all necessary precautions must be taken, including the use of lifelines and self-contained breathing apparatuses (SCBA). In many cases, patient extrication should be done only by specially trained and equipped personnel. Do not become a victim yourself.

Give oxygen in high concentration and flow rate, if available.

Injected Poisons

Injected poisons include a variety of drugs that are deliberately injected, as well as stings and bites of flying insects (bees, wasps, and hornets) and arachnids (spiders, scorpions, mites, ticks), snakebites, and puncture wounds from the spines of marine animals.

General principles of emergency care include removing all watches, rings, and bracelets from an involved extremity before swelling starts. Give them to the patient or a family member to keep in a pocket. (This should be witnessed and documented.) Place a cold pack on the injection site to slow absorption, except in the case of snakebite. Do *not* immerse an extremity in ice.

Injected poisons are rapidly absorbed, which makes them difficult to remove by suction. However, at least some of the poison may be removed by treating subcutaneous and intramuscular (*not* intravenous) injections with a recently developed commercial negative pressure device such as the Sawyer Extractor (Fig. 23.4), if this can be started within five minutes after the poison is injected (three minutes for snakebites). Its use should never delay transport of the patient to a hospital.

Contact Poisons

Contact poisons include chemical substances such as acids and alkalis, and natural substances such as the sap of poison ivy, poison oak, and poison sumac.

The first principle of emergency care is to remove the substance from the skin. If the material is dry, first dust it off, then flush the area with copious amounts of water. Rinse off non-dry materials thoroughly with water, and then wash the area with soap and water.

Fig. 23.3 *The fireman's drag can be used to remove a patient from a contaminated area.*

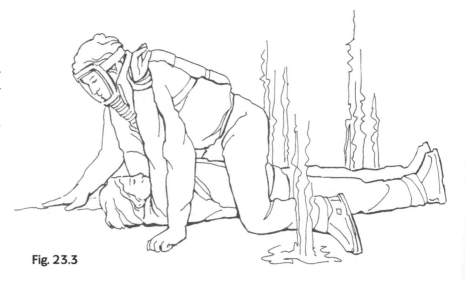

Fig. 23.3

Table 23.3

Summary of Emergency Care of a Poisoning Victim

1. Ingested poisons. Follow the directions of the poison control center or emergency department personnel. If no directions are available:
   a. Dilute the poison with milk or water (unless it is a petroleum product or the patient is unable to swallow).
   b. Induce vomiting (except in the case of strong acids or alkalis, petroleum products, if the patient is unresponsive or convulsing, or ingestion occurred more than one hour previously).
   c. Give the patient activated charcoal (unless the poison is acid or alkali, or the patient is unable to swallow).
2. Inhaled poisons
   a. Remove the patient from the contaminated atmosphere. Protect yourself.
   b. Give oxygen at high concentration and flow rate.
3. Injected poisons
   a. Remove watches, rings, or bracelets.
   b. Place a cold pack on the injection site.
   c. Use a negative pressure device, if available.
   d. Provide specific treatment for snakebite (see Chapter 24).
4. Contact poisons
   a. Remove substance from the skin. Use different techniques for different substances.
   b. Remove contaminated clothing, including footwear.
   c. Provide care for eyes as described in Chapter 12.
   d. Dress open wounds.

In the case of lye, dry lime, elemental sodium, or other materials that react with water, dust off the material thoroughly and then remove the rest by flushing with a strong jet of water from a hose or large faucet.

Elemental phosphorus catches fire when exposed to air. It should be washed off while the affected body part is immersed in water.

Remove contaminated clothing as soon as possible, including shoes and socks. If the eyes are involved, follow the guidelines in Chapter 12.

Cover open wounds with sterile, dry dressings. Do not use salves or creams.

Fig. 23.4 *Sawyer Extractor*

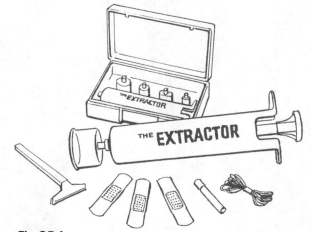

Fig. 23.4

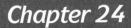

Chapter 24

Hazardous Plants and Animals

Beware the Jabberwock, my
son! The jaws that bite, the
claws that catch! Beware the
Jubjub bird, and shun The
frumious Bandersnatch.

—Lewis Carroll
  (Charles Lutwidge Dodgson)
  "Jabberwocky"

Chapter 23 discusses the general topic of poisoning, the general characteristics of ingested, inhaled, injected, and topical poisons, and their assessment and emergency care. This chapter discusses specific plant and animal hazards, together with any characteristics of their assessment and emergency care that differ from the generic ones listed in the preceding chapter. The emphasis is on emergency care where contact with a poison control center or hospital emergency department may not be possible and transport may be delayed.

Poisoning by Plants

Several thousand cases of plant poisoning occur every year in the United States. Because many domestic and wild plants or their parts are poisonous, only persons with training and experience in plant identification who are *thoroughly familiar* with the poisonous as well as the edible plants native to the area should eat or even taste unfamiliar plant materials. This is especially true of mushrooms. Observing wild animals eating a certain plant is no sign that it is safe for humans.

Teaching anyone to identify specific types of poisonous plants is beyond the scope of this book, since there is considerable local variation. An excellent reference is the *AMA Handbook of Poisonous and Injurious Plants*, by Kenneth F. Lampe and Mary Ann McCann, published by the American Medical Association, Chicago, 1985.

If plant poisoning is suspected, bring the plant or a stem with the leaves attached to the hospital with the patient, protecting yourself as necessary. If berries, nuts, fruit, fruit pits, or bark were eaten, bring samples of these for identification and laboratory analysis if necessary. Be able to tell the emergency department physician what was eaten, how much was eaten, and how long ago it was eaten. Save any vomited material and bring it along with the patient.

Unless the patient has no gag reflex, has diminished responsiveness, or is having convulsions, the initial emergency care for all cases of toxic plant ingestion consists of diluting the poison, inducing vomiting, and giving activated charcoal (if available) as described in the section on ingested poisons in Chapter 23.

Common Reactions and Their Emergency Care

Most poisonous plants can cause more than one class of reaction. Usually nausea, vomiting, and/or abdominal pain occur at first, followed later by central nervous system and/or circulatory disturbances. Since few specific antidotes for plant poisonings exist, emergency care is empiric and consists of treating the signs and symptoms. If the plant or its parts were eaten at a communal meal, more than one person may be ill.

Common reactions and their emergency care include the following:

1. **Circulatory disturbances**. Heart abnormalities and early or developed shock may occur. Provide emergency care as you would for a patient having a heart attack (see Chapter 17) or in shock (see Chapter 6).
2. **Gastrointestinal disturbances**. Little can be done to treat symptoms such as nausea, vomiting, diarrhea, and cramps. If transport will be delayed, prevent dehydration by having the patient drink water and electrolyte-containing fluids after the vomiting stops. If possible, save the initial vomitus and take it to the hospital with the patient.
3. **Central nervous system symptoms**. Emergency care depends on the major manifestations, which range from convulsions, excitement, and hyperactivity at one extreme to depression, mental confusion, stupor, and coma at the other. As needed, give basic life support (see Chapter 4 and Appendix B), provide general care for unresponsiveness (see Chapter 12), and care for convulsions (see Chapter 17).
4. **Skin irritation.** Symptoms can include itching, redness, burning, swelling, blister formation, and rash. As soon as possible, wash the area thoroughly with soap and water to remove the offending substance. Repeat several times, being sure to rinse off all soap. A soothing nonprescription lotion such as Calamine or a topical steroid may be applied later, if desired.

Persons whose occupations require exposure to poison ivy and similar plants, such as U.S. Forest Service employees and rural fire fighters, should monitor the availability of new barrier creams being developed that contain organoclay, activated charcoal, and linoleic acid derivatives. Be

---

Fig. 24.1 *Dieffenbachia*

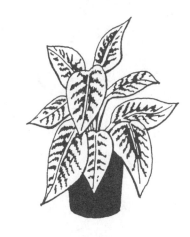

Fig. 24.1

aware of the danger of respiratory system irritation from exposure to smoke from burning poison ivy.

5. **Swollen mucous membranes**. The common houseplants *Dieffenbachia,* or dumb cane (Fig. 24.1), and *Caladium* can cause a unique problem. If the plant is placed in the mouth, it causes the mucous membranes to swell, which makes swallowing and talking difficult and may obstruct the upper airway. Emergency care includes keeping the upper airway open and administering oxygen.

Hazardous Animals
Stings and Bites of Arthropods

The phylum Arthropoda contains many members that are annoying or dangerous to man. Such arthropods include members of the following groups:

1. Class Insecta
   a. Order Hymenoptera (bees, wasps, hornets, yellow jackets, ants).
   b. Order Diptera (mosquitos, biting flies).
   c. Order Lepidoptera (caterpillars).
   d. Order Coleoptera (blister beetles).
   e. Order Hemiptera (true bugs).
2. Class Arachnida (spiders, scorpions, ticks, mites).
3. Class Chilopoda (centipedes).

Dangerous Insects

Insects are the most numerous of the higher orders of creatures. The stinging apparatus of most stinging insects (Fig. 24.2) is a small, hollow spine resembling a hypodermic needle. This projects from the end of the abdomen and is attached internally to a venom sack. Since the honeybee's stinger is barbed and cannot be withdrawn after it is embedded, the honeybee can sting only once because it is disemboweled when it flies away after stinging. All other hymenoptera can sting repeatedly. Some, such as the fire ant, can both sting and bite.

Local symptoms of an insect sting or bite include sudden pain followed by swelling and redness. A white, itchy swelling resembling a hive may develop at the site. The honeybee's stinger frequently remains embedded in the wound and should be removed by gentle scraping with a knife blade so that the venom sac attached to its end does not squeeze more venom into the wound (Fig. 24.3). Additional emergency care is given as listed in the section on injected poisons in Chapter 23. If available, a small amount of moistened baking soda or unseasoned meat tenderizer (Adolph's, etc.) applied to the wound may provide some pain relief.

Some persons are allergic to the venom and may develop severe local reactions or anaphylactic shock (see Chapter 6). Assist these persons in using a "bee sting kit" if they have one along, and transport them quickly to the emergency department. Basic life support may be required.

Fig. 24.2 *Examples of Stinging Insects*

Fig. 24.3 *Technique of Removing a Honeybee Stinger*

Fig. 24.4 *Examples of Biting Insects*

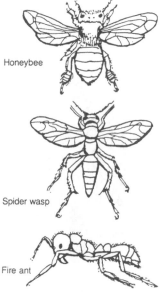

Honeybee

Spider wasp

Fire ant

Fig. 24.2

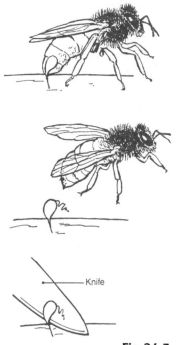

Knife

Fig. 24.3

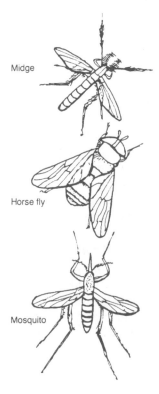

Midge

Horse fly

Mosquito

Fig. 24.4

Contact with stinging insects can be minimized by storing garbage away from living areas, by eating food inside tents and other shelters, and by not wearing brightly colored clothing or perfumed skin preparations (cosmetics, after-shave lotions, etc.) while outdoors in infested areas. Give hives and nests a wide berth. When confronted by aggressive stinging insects, remain calm and avoid loud noises and "shooing" motions. If pursued by swarms, seek refuge in tents or vehicles, or jump into a body of water. If you do plan to swat, swat to kill!

Although mosquitos, black flies, and other biting flies (Fig. 24.4) can carry serious diseases such as encephalitis, malaria, yellow fever, and sleeping sickness, in North America these insects generally are more of a nuisance than a menace. Their bites, unless multiple, usually do not require treatment. Soothing, nonprescription lotions (Calamine, etc.) can be used for local symptomatic relief. Bites can be prevented by using chemical insect repellents containing N,N-diethyl-3-methylbenzamide (DEET) and by wearing tightly woven protective clothing with long sleeves, long trouser legs, and tight cuffs. Avoid over-application of DEET, especially in children. Tents and other sleeping quarters should be protected by suitable netting.

Certain caterpillars, such as the puss, saddleback (Fig. 24.5), and gypsy moth, have irritating hairs that can cause an uncomfortable rash. Emergency care consists of removing the hairs with adhesive tape and applying a soothing lotion.

Blister beetles (Fig. 24.6) contain cantharidin, a substance that is very irritating to human skin. Emergency care consists of washing the area with soap and water and applying a soothing lotion.

Some members of the order Hemiptera (Fig. 24.7) can inflict a painful bite that is treated like a bee sting (see above).

Dangerous Arachnids

There are only two spiders in North America that are dangerous to humans: the black widow and the brown recluse.

The female black widow spider is the only one of the two sexes that is poisonous. This shiny black spider spans about 1 inch with its legs extended and is characterized by a red hourglass marking on the underside of its abdomen (Fig. 24.8a). It spins a nondescript scraggly web and prefers to live in garages, basements, outbuildings, and woodpiles. One or more brown egg cases often are visible in the web. The spider is shy and bites only if disturbed. Black widow spiders occasionally spin webs under the seats of outhouses and may bite the nether parts of unsuspecting users if webs are disturbed by falling excrement.

A black widow bite may be overlooked because it is seldom painful at first. As the effects of the toxin appear, the patient experiences severe muscle spasms, chest tightness, respiratory distress, dizziness, nausea, vomiting, and burning of the soles of the feet. The abdominal muscles may develop boardlike rigidity that can resemble an acute abdomen. Although most patients recover with symptomatic care, the toxin can be dangerous to small children and the elderly. Intermittent application of an ice-pack to the site of the bite

---

Fig. 24.5 *Saddleback Caterpillar*

Fig. 24.6 *Blister Beetle*

Fig. 24.7 *Blood-sucking Bug*

Fig. 24.8 *Poisonous Spiders*

Fig. 24.9 *Scorpion*

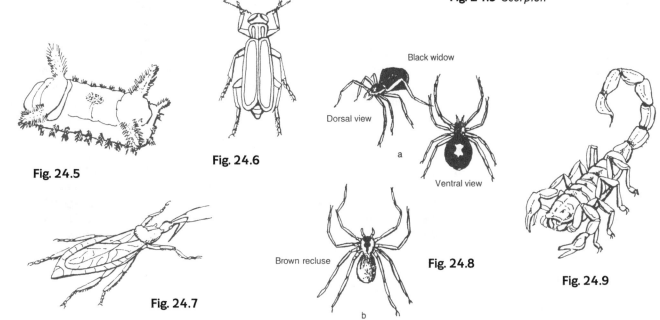

Fig. 24.5

Fig. 24.6

Fig. 24.7

Black widow

Dorsal view

Ventral view

a

Brown recluse

Fig. 24.8

b

Fig. 24.9

seems to be beneficial. Since field emergency care is limited and since antivenin is available, the patient should be taken to the emergency department without delay.

The brown recluse spider is found mainly in the southern United States, although it occasionally is carried to other areas in the personal belongings of travelers. This dull brown spider has a smaller body than the black widow, often with a characteristic violin-shaped marking on its cephalothorax (Fig. 24.8b). It inhabits dark, sheltered areas such as basements, vacant buildings, and woodpiles. The bite is painful and soon ulcerates. The ulcer enlarges over several weeks and heals very slowly. The most effective field emergency treatment is to apply continuous ice packs to the bite, which controls the pain and may limit the spread of the venom. Heat should *not* be applied. The patient should be taken to the emergency department.

Scorpions (Fig. 24.9) are found primarily in the southwestern United States. They have a long, jointed tail-like posterior abdominal projection with a stinger at its tip. The stings of most scorpions are no worse than a

bee or wasp sting, causing only localized pain, redness, and swelling. However, one species, the Arizona scorpion (*Centruroides exilicauda*) has a venom that can cause a severe systemic reaction with muscle spasms, convulsions, shock, and heart irregularities due to autonomic nerve stimulation. It is a slender, yellowish-brown, nocturnal scorpion with a small swelling at the base of the stinger.

The emergency care for a scorpion sting is the same as for any injected poison. If a sting by the Arizona scorpion is suspected, the patient should be taken to a hospital as soon as possible. It may be necessary to provide basic life support and general care for unresponsiveness and convulsions (see Chapters 4, 12, 17, and Appendix B.)

Prevention of spider bites and scorpion stings consists mainly of avoiding contact with these creatures. It is unwise to walk barefoot, especially at night, or to place hands, feet, and other body parts in uninspected places. When camping in the desert or tropics, shake out clothing, footgear, and bedding before use to remove unwanted tenants.

Although ticks (Fig. 24.10a) can carry serious diseases, they usually are more of a nuisance than a hazard. The incubation period of such tick-borne diseases as Colorado tick fever, Rocky Mountain spotted fever, and Lyme disease is long enough so that the outdoor traveler usually is back home before the disease develops. One exception is tick paralysis, an interesting disease characterized by extreme fatigue and weakness of the arms and legs. If a member of a party traveling in tick country complains of these symptoms, conduct a thorough search for an attached tick. Removing the tick usually cures tick paralysis within 24 hours.

If you develop any obscure illness or one with high fever, arthritis, or a rash, always inform your physician of

any recent contact with ticks or travel in tick-infested areas. Lyme disease, in particular, may have an incubation period so long that tick exposure has been forgotten.

Embedded ticks should be removed with forceps rather than with the fingers. To avoid leaving the mouthparts of the tick in the wound, remove a small area of surrounding skin along with the front end of the tick, using a sturdy pair of splinter forceps (Fig. 24.10b). The forceps from a Swiss Army knife are usually not strong enough. If forceps are not available, touching the tick with an extinguished hot match head or covering it with a substance that clogs its breathing pores (sunscreen lotion, camp stove fuel, etc.) may induce it to back out.

During the tick season, outdoor recreationists should inspect each other for ticks nightly. It is important to inspect all hidden and hairy areas carefully, particularly the scalp, armpits, and the perianal and genital areas.

Poisonous Snakes

Of all animals, venomous snakes are the most dangerous to man. Worldwide, there are about 50,000 deaths from snakebite each year. In the United States, between 1,000 and 2,000 poisonous snakebites occur each year, causing about six deaths. Most of these bites occur in the South and Southwest, mainly between the months of April and October. A third of snakebites occur when snakes are purposely handled. The number of bites from exotic poisonous snakes kept as pets is increasing.

There are two general types of poisonous snakes native to the United States: pit vipers and coral snakes (Fig. 24.11). Pit vipers, which include rattlesnakes, copperheads and water moccasins, account for almost all bites by native snakes. They have

Fig. 24.10 *Tick Removal with Forceps*

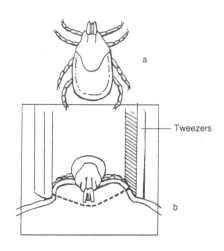

Tweezers

Fig. 24.10

long, slender, hollow fangs that resemble hypodermic needles, which they use to inject their venom deeply into the tissues of their victims (Fig. 24.12a). Coral snakes have solid fangs (Fig. 24.12b); they chew rather than stab.

It is important to distinguish poisonous snakes from harmless ones. All pit vipers have triangular heads and vertical elliptical pupils, while harmless snakes they may resemble have tubular heads and round pupils (Fig. 24.13). Pit vipers have a characteristic depression, or pit, midway between the eye and nostril on each side of the head. They tend to be thicker and heavier for their length than harmless snakes. Rattlesnakes are distinguished by their rattles, which may be missing because of injury. They usually, but not always, will rattle before they strike.

Pit viper bites characteristically leave two fang marks (occasionally three or four marks if older fangs have not been shed), while harmless snakebites leave a horseshoe pattern of small puncture wounds (Fig. 24.13). A pit viper does not jump but can strike up to two-thirds of its length. In striking, the snake opens its mouth widely, erects its fangs so they point forward, lunges, buries its fangs in the victim's flesh with a thrusting motion, and injects a dose of venom. Pit viper venom contains many different enzymes and toxic proteins that damage local tissue, blood vessels, blood components, the heart, and the muscles.

Coral snakes are small, shy snakes related to the cobras. They have brilliant black, yellow, and scarlet bands, which make them resemble the similarly colored but harmless scarlet king snake. The

mnemonic "red on yellow, kill a fellow; red on black, venom lack" helps you to remember the differences in the marking sequences of the two snakes (Fig. 24.14). Their venom acts principally on the nervous system.

The signs and symptoms of snakebite depend on the type, age and size of the snake, and the amount of venom injected. Twenty percent of snakebites do not involve injection of venom (envenomation). Most snakebites occur on the extremities.

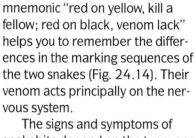

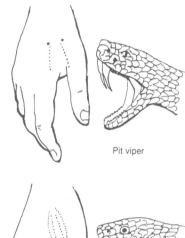

Pit viper

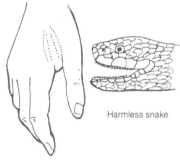

Harmless snake

Fig. 24.11 *Venomous Snakes*

Fig. 24.12 *Fangs of Venomous Snakes*

Fig. 24.13 *Head and Bite Patterns of a Pit Viper and a Harmless Snake*

Fig. 24.14 *Comparison of the Color Patterns of Coral and Scarlet King Snakes*

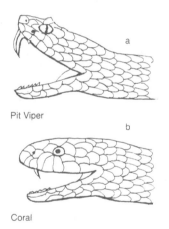

Pit Viper

Coral

Fig. 24.12

Fig. 24.13

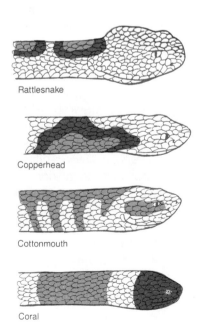

Rattlesnake

Copperhead

Cottonmouth

Coral

Fig. 24.11

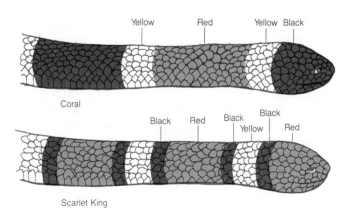

Yellow   Red   Yellow   Black

Coral

Black   Red   Black   Black
                  Yellow   Red

Scarlet King

Fig. 24.14

Signs and Symptoms of Pit Viper Bites

Immediately after pit viper envenomation, the patient develops burning pain at the site. Inspection reveals fang marks 3/16 to 1 1/2 inches (1/2 centimeter to 4 centimeters) apart.

Local swelling occurs within five minutes and slowly progresses proximally to involve the entire extremity. The swelling frequently is accompanied by ecchymosis and blood-filled blisters and blebs. In severe cases, systemic signs and symptoms develop, including nausea, vomiting, sweating, weakness, generalized bleeding, and tingling of the scalp, face, and lips. Damage to blood vessels may cause hypovolemic shock and pulmonary edema.

Emergency Care of Pit Viper Bites

Most patients who are bitten by pit vipers are within a few hours of an urban center where definitive treatment with antivenin is available. The major aims of emergency care therefore are to *do no harm* and to *take the patient to the emergency department as soon as possible.*

If burning pain or swelling do not develop at the bite site within a few minutes of the bite, envenomation probably has not occurred. Bites unaccompanied by envenomation require no care other than wound cleansing and arranging for tetanus prophylaxis, but still should be seen by a physician.

Emergency Care of Bites with Envenomation

1. It is undesirable for the patient to walk or run, because muscular activity may increase venom absorption. Carry the patient by litter from the accident site to the nearest vehicle. However, if help is limited and you are 20 minutes or less from the roadhead, it is permissible for the patient to walk out slowly, stopping frequently to rest on the way. A person who is bitten while alone has no alternative but to walk to help.

2. The patient and bystanders should get out of the snake's striking range (roughly the length of the snake). Killing the snake and bringing its body to the hospital was formerly recommended but is now felt to be too dangerous for general use and usually is unnecessary since hospital treatment of all pit viper bites is the same. *Do not handle* a dead snake or the severed head of a snake since reflex biting can occur for hours after death.

3. Remove all watches, rings, and bracelets from the bitten extremity.

4. Use a commercial negative pressure suction device if available (such as the Sawyer extractor). If used within three minutes of the bite, this device can remove up to 30 percent of the venom. It should be used according to the accompanying instructions and be left on for 30 minutes.

5. Since any motion or muscular activity will speed venom absorption, keep the patient quiet and splint the bitten extremity. Check the splint periodically to detect any danger to circulation caused by swelling of the limb with tightening of the splint.

6. Mark the boundary of swelling with a pen and write the time the mark was made on the patient's skin. Repeat this procedure every 15 minutes until the patient reaches the hospital. It is important for the emergency department physician to know how rapidly swelling is progressing.

7. Take the patient to the emergency department as soon as possible. Call ahead if possible so that antivenin can be ready.

8. Treat shock as indicated (see Chapter 6).

9. Do *not* make incisions, use tourniquets or constricting bands, apply ice or cold water, or give electric shocks. Ice, in particular, has been shown to increase the danger of gangrene.

10. Some authorities, especially in Australia, recommend wrapping the involved extremity with an elastic bandage (Ace, etc.) from the bite site proximally. However, North American pit viper venom differs from Australian elapid snake venom in causing much more local reaction (tissue necrosis, gangrene, blebs, blisters, swelling, etc.). The author and many U.S. authorities feel that local reactions (which theoretically would be aggravated by slowing absorption of the venom from the extremity into the body as a whole) cause more long-term disability and are no less dangerous than generalized (whole-body) reactions. At the present time, use of the elastic wrapping technique cannot be recommended for emergency care of North American pit viper bites.

11. Additional suggestions for emergency care in remote areas where definitive medical care cannot be reached for many hours:
    a. Incising the wound through the fang marks and applying suction has not been

shown to be helpful and cannot be recommended. Incisions performed by excited, inexperienced rescuers may cut important structures or lead to infection or severe bleeding.

b. Some experts recommend the use of a constriction band to slow absorption of the venom in extremity bites. This is a rubber or cloth band tied tightly enough to interrupt lymph flow but not venous or arterial flow. It should be loose enough so that one finger can be inserted easily underneath it. Tie it above the swelling and move it proximally as the swelling moves up the extremity.

c. Commercial negative pressure devices (see 4. above) are useful and should be part of the emergency care kit carried in snake country. They should be used immediately following the bite.

d. Send a party member for help.

e. Clean the bite with soap and water and cover it with a sterile compress.

f. Splint the extremity.

g. Give the patient electrolyte-containing fluids to replace fluid lost from the blood into the bitten area.

h. Set up camp and keep the patient at rest until help arrives. If the group is large enough and a litter can be improvised, carry the patient out.

Signs and Symptoms of Coral Snake Bites

Coral snake bites usually involve much less local burning than pit viper bites. Local swelling, blistering, and ecchymosis usually are minimal. Within an hour or so, the effects of the venom on the nervous system begin to be seen. First, the bitten extremity becomes numb and weak. Later, central nervous system symptoms such as dizziness, paresthesia ("pins and needles all over"), double vision, altered responsiveness, nervousness, involuntary movements, drooling, and increased salivation occur.

These symptoms are followed within several hours by difficulty in talking and swallowing, and occasionally—in untreated cases—death due to respiratory failure and/or cardiac arrest.

Emergency Care of Coral Snake Bites

1. Have the patient lie down and remain as calm as possible.
2. Flush the bite area with several quarts of clean water to remove as much venom as possible.
3. Put a sterile dressing on the wound.
4. Since coral snakes are elapids related to cobras and several types of Australian snakes, some experts recommend treating coral snake bites by wrapping a bitten extremity with an elastic bandage as is done in Australia. This has been shown to delay systemic absorption of venom. It is done by wrapping the extremity from the site of the bite distally to the base of the extremity proximally. The bandage should be loose enough so that your finger can be slid under it, and should not interfere with peripheral pulses.
5. Splint a bitten extremity.
6. Provide basic life support and treat the patient for shock as necessary (see Chapters 4, 6, and Appendix B).
7. Incision and suction or use of a negative pressure device are ineffective and not recommended in coral snake bites, even if there will be a delay in reaching medical care.

8. Transport the patient to a hospital as soon as possible.

Emergency Care of Exotic Snake Bites

Poisonous snakes from other parts of the world are common in zoos and are occasionally kept as pets. Bites from these reptiles should be treated as coral snake bites, with the patient being taken to the emergency department as soon as possible. Specific antivenin is available in some cases.

Advice can be obtained by calling the Poisindex Central Office in Denver (800-332-3037) or the Antivenin Index in Tucson (602-626-6016).

Prevention of Snakebite

In snake country, never put a hand, foot, or other body part in a place that is not in full view. Carry a sturdy walking stick to poke logs and rocks before stepping over them. Use caution when reaching overhead to grasp a rocky ledge or when stepping over a log. Wear sturdy boots that extend to midcalf; special snake-proof boots are available. Avoid hiking at night without a light, and never hike alone.

Gila Monster Bites

The Gila Monster and a close relative, the Mexican beaded lizard, are the only poisonous lizards found in the United States. They are large, ugly, slow-moving reptiles with bead-like scales, large, flat heads, and thick tails (Fig. 24.15). Their colors range from pink to black.

The venom glands are located in the lower jaw, discharging venom at the base of the lower teeth. Envenomation occurs through biting and chewing. The creatures often are difficult to disengage and remove from the patient; teeth may break off in the wound.

Severe, burning pain appears at the bite site within five minutes, followed by local swelling and cyanosis. The patient may feel weak and faint.

Emergency care consists of the following steps:

1. Wash the wound with soap and water, and remove any broken teeth.
2. Splint the extremity.
3. Give basic life support and treatment for shock as needed (see Chapters 4, 6, and Appendix B).
4. Take the patient to the emergency department.

Warm-blooded Animal Bites

Most warm-blooded animals will not attack man unless cornered, teased, or otherwise provoked.

In addition to causing soft-tissue damage, the bites of animals commonly cause infection because their mouths harbor large numbers of bacteria. The greatest danger is contracting **rabies**, a universally fatal disease of the central nervous system. The rabies virus, present in the saliva of infected animals, can be transmitted by biting or licking. Because vaccination of susceptible pets for prevention of rabies is required by law in most states, stray and wild animal bites present the greatest danger to humans.

Emergency Care of Warm-blooded Animal Bites

1. Stop bleeding by direct pressure.
2. Irrigate the wound thoroughly with clean water or sterile saline solution.

Fig. 24.15 *Gila Monster*

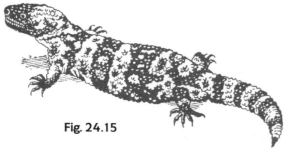

Fig. 24.15

3. Wash the wound thoroughly with soap and water.
4. One-percent povidone iodine, benzalkonium (Zepharin), and Bactine are readily available antiseptic solutions that also have been shown to kill the rabies virus. If one of these preparations is available, soak the wound with it for one minute.
5. Do not close the wound with tape or sutures; leave it open and cover it with a sterile dressing.
6. Splint large wounds on extremities.
7. Take the patient to the emergency department as soon as possible. Tetanus prophylaxis is desirable.

Prevention of Rabies

Do *not* endanger yourself by making attempts to capture a possibly rabid animal.

Domestic Animal Bites (dogs, cats, etc.)

1. It is important to determine the current rabies vaccination status of the animal. When the bite is caused by a pet animal with a current vaccination tag, there is very little danger of rabies, but the animal should still be observed for 10 days.
2. If the animal is not wearing a collar with a vaccination tag, it should be captured or identified. Since attempting to capture an animal can be dangerous, this is best done by properly trained and equipped animal control personnel. Killing or hurting the animal,

especially a pet, should be avoided if at all possible. The animal will be confined and observed by the health department. If it is healthy at the end of 10 days, there is little danger of rabies. If the animal becomes sick or dies within that period, its brain must be examined for rabies.
3. If an animal is inadvertently or intentionally killed, immediately send its head on ice to the state health laboratory for examination.
4. Patients who are bitten by animals confirmed to have rabies should receive rabies vaccine.
5. In the United States, patients who are bitten by unidentified or uncaptured animals should receive rabies vaccine if rabies is known to occur locally in that species. The vaccine need not be given if rabies has not occurred in the region for many years and there is no likelihood that the animal was exposed to rabies.
6. *All* animal bites should be reported to the state health department.

Wild Animal Bites (skunk, bat, fox, coyote, raccoon)

Kill the animal if possible and send its head on ice to the state health laboratory. If the rabies virus is detected in the animal's brain or the animal is uncaptured, the patient should receive rabies vaccine.

Human Bites

The mouth is so bacteriologically "filthy" that a human bite can cause virulent infection. One common method of injury occurs during a fistfight when an assailant strikes an adversary's jaw, and the adversary's tooth cuts the assailant's hand.

Emergency care is the same as for any warm-blooded animal bite except that measures to prevent rabies are unnecessary. Investigation of the HIV and hepatitis status of the participants may be desirable.

Injuries from Marine Animals

This section covers the general principles of emergency care of marine animal injuries likely to occur in North American coastal waters. It is beyond the scope of this text to describe the details of the care of injuries due to every type of hazardous marine animal.

Most injuries are caused by:

1. The bites of vertebrates (sharks, barracuda).
2. The stinging organs of coelenterates (jellyfish, sea anemones, coral, hydras, Portuguese man-of-war).
3. The spines of echinoderms (sea urchins) and vertebrates (stingrays, scorpion fish, stonefish, catfish).

People who live in coastal areas or who practice scuba diving and other salt-water sports should be thoroughly familiar with the animal hazards they may encounter. An excellent reference book is *A Medical Guide to Hazardous Marine Life*, by Paul S. Auerbach, published by C.V. Mosby Co., St. Louis, 1991.

The emergency care of the bites of large fish is similar to the care of other large, open, contaminated wounds. The emergency care of local reactions from the stings of the different coelenterates is similar, and the emergency care of puncture wounds from echinoderms and vertebrates is similar. No specific antidotes are available for the systemic reactions that occasionally occur; the emergency care is for their major manifestations and includes basic life support and care for shock, unresponsiveness, etc., as outlined in Chapters 4, 6, 12, and Appendix B.

Prevention of Injuries from Marine Animals

Stings and puncture wounds can be prevented to some extent by wearing total body suits of thin nylon or Lycra while swimming, and shoes while walking in shallow water and tide pools.

To prevent bites by sharks, barracuda, and other large fish:

1. Avoid waters known to be infested by these fish, especially at night.
2. Avoid solitary swimming.
3. Avoid turbid water, drop-offs, deep channels, and waste-water outlets.
4. Avoid swimming with open wounds. Women should avoid swimming during menstrual periods.
5. Avoid splashing and wearing or carrying fluorescent, bright, or shiny clothing or gear.
6. Do not tease or corner sharks.
7. If a shark or barracuda appears, leave the area with slow, rhythmic movements, keeping the fish in sight.

Emergency Care of Injuries from Marine Animals

Marine Animal Bites

Bites by marine animals such as sharks, barracuda, and other large fish (Fig. 24.16) can cause massive wounds with serious tissue damage and severe blood loss.

The emergency care of such bites includes the following:

1. Remove the patient from the water as soon as possible to avoid exposure to further danger and to expedite emergency care.
2. Control hemorrhage by direct pressure. A tourniquet may rarely be needed to control bleeding from large wounds to the extremities involving major arteries.
3. Give basic life support as necessary (see Chapter 4 and Appendix B).
4. Anticipate and treat shock (see Chapter 6).
5. Irrigate and clean the wound as described above for warm-blooded animal bites. Dress the wound, but do not close it.
6. Splint an involved extremity.
7. Transport the patient rapidly to the emergency department.

Fig. 24.16 *Marine Animals that Bite*

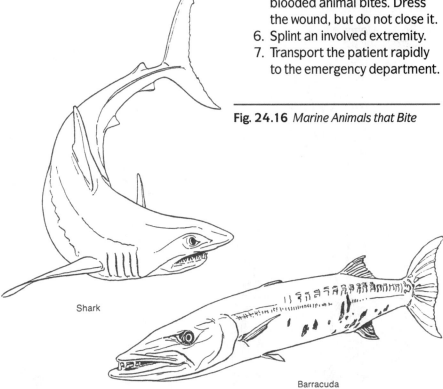

Shark

Barracuda

Fig. 24.16

Marine Animal Stings

Stings from marine animals such as jellyfish, sea anemones, Portugese man-of-war (Fig. 24.17), coral, and hydras can be very painful.

The purpose of emergency care is to inactivate the toxin as follows:

1. Remove the patient from the water.
2. Put on rubber gloves, then wash the affected area well with sea water, *not* fresh water. (Fresh water will cause any remaining stinging organs [nematocysts] to discharge.)
3. Remove any remaining large tentacle fragments with forceps.
4. Next, wash the affected area with one of the following inactivating solutions (listed in order of decreasing preference). Vinegar, (or 5-percent acetic acid solution), rubbing alcohol, household ammonia diluted to one-quarter strength with tap water.

5. Apply shaving cream and gently shave the affected area with a razor or sharp knife.
6. Reapply the inactivating solution for 15 minutes as a soak.
7. Later, apply a soothing non-prescription steroid lotion (Cortaid, etc.) as needed for irritation.
8. On rare occasions, anaphylactic shock may occur. Treat it as described in Chapter 6.

Marine Animal Puncture Wounds

Puncture wounds can be caused by the spines of echinoderms and vertebrates (Fig. 24.18): sea urchins, stingrays, catfish, scorpion fish, and stonefish.

The main purpose of emergency care is to control pain by *inactivating the toxin with hot water*, as follows:

1. Soak the affected part in the hottest non-scalding water the patient can tolerate (up to 113°F [46°C]) for 30 minutes.
2. Remove any visible spines with forceps.

3. Take the patient to a physician for removal of deeply embedded spines. Tetanus prophylaxis may be desirable.
4. In rare instances, anaphylactic shock may occur. Treat it as described in Chapter 6.

Sea Snake Bites

Bites from sea snakes (Fig. 24.19) are treated as described in the section on coral snake bites above.

Food Poisoning

1. **Scombroid.** Eating improperly preserved scombroid fish (tuna, mackerel, etc.) can produce an allergic reaction with itching, hives, nausea, diarrhea, and asthma, due to the production of histamine during decomposition of the fish. Treat these symptoms with an antihistamine such as non-prescription diphenhydramine (Benadryl).
2. **Ciguatera fish poisoning.** This is due to consuming certain fish (barracuda, jack,

Fig. 24.17 *Marine Animals that Sting*

Fig. 24.18 *Marine Animals with Dangerous Spines*

Fig. 24.19 *Sea Snake*

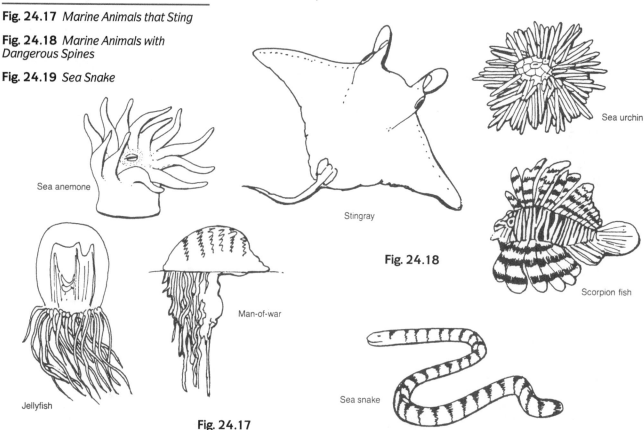

Sea anemone

Stingray

Sea urchin

Fig. 24.18

Man-of-war

Scorpion fish

Jellyfish

Fig. 24.17

Sea snake

Fig. 24.19

grouper, snapper) who have eaten poisonous microorganisms. Signs and symptoms include abdominal pain, nausea, vomiting, diarrhea, weakness, difficulty in walking, and reversal of the perception of hot and cold (hot seems cold and vice versa).

There is no effective field emergency care, and the patient should be taken to the emergency department.

3. **Paralytic shellfish poisoning.** This is caused by consuming shellfish that have eaten poisonous microorganisms. Signs and symptoms include numbness, tingling, lightheadedness, and weakness, followed by drooling, difficulty in swallowing, incoordination, and difficulty in breathing. The patient may progress to complete paralysis.

Emergency care consists of giving basic life support and taking the patient immediately to the emergency department.

Scenario #26 (Fig. 24.20)

The following scenario illustrates the management of a case of poisoning that occurs in the outdoors.

You, your wife Sandy, and the new baby have decided to spend the weekend in an isolated campground in the Granite range, about 20 miles east of Grandstone National Park. You leave right after work on Friday. After turning off the main highway, you drive about 50 miles on a secondary road over a high pass.

The campground is situated where a raging cascade drops through a high mountain valley and empties into the main drainage below. The time is late June; it is too late for good high mountain skiing, and anyway, you want to introduce your 12-month-old son to car camping. You hope that not too many other people have the same idea, but it turns out that the campground is about half full. You pick a site at the back of the campground, not too close to the creek, next to an expensive, three-season dome tent pitched by a four-wheel drive carryall.

It is almost dark when you finish supper and start on the dishes. The baby is in his playpen. There is a commotion at the next campsite, where two couples in their late 20s have just finished eating. One of the men is lying on the ground, groaning. The others seem to be standing around, watching him helplessly, so you decide to see if they need assistance.

You: "Hi, I'm Ben Schussen. Is something wrong?"

Woman: "Yes, there's something wrong with my husband. He says that he has a terrible stomachache and is nauseated. Look at the way he's drooling. I don't know what to do. Are you a doctor?"

You: "No, but I'm on the ski patrol at High Range Ski Area. When did this start?"

Woman: "Just after he finished supper, a few minutes ago."

You: "Was he all right before supper?" (bending down to observe the patient more closely. He is doubled up and in obvious pain but breathing well. His respirations are at least 30 per minute, and his radial pulse is

strong and about 100 beats per minute. His face is pale with beads of sweat on his forehead. There is saliva all over his upper shirt front.)

Woman: "Yes. We went on a hike and he seemed his normal self."

You: (to Sandy) "Please get the first aid kit out of the truck." (To the woman) "What did he have for supper?"

Woman: "We had some venison, fried potatoes, some mixed vegetables, and some cake for dessert."

You: "Has anyone else been feeling sick?"

Woman: "No."

You: "Did he eat anything that the rest of you didn't eat?"

Woman: "Why, yes. He found some yampa by the side of the creek on the way back and dug up some roots. I boiled them for him. None of the rest of us ate any."

You: "What's his name?"

Woman: "Don Eaton."

You: "Don, what did this plant look like that you ate?" (You take a pair of

Fig. 24.20 *Scenario #26*

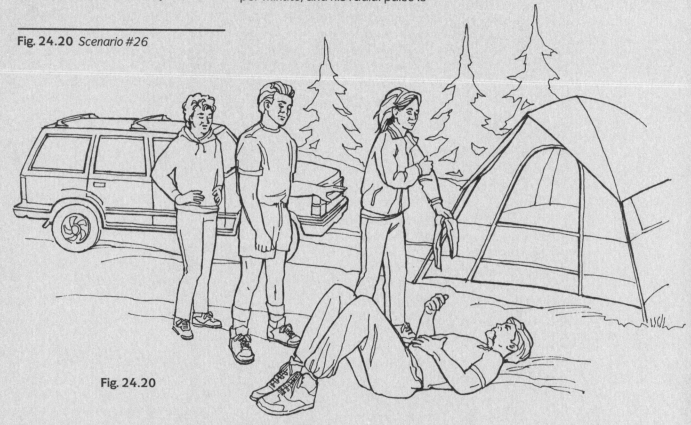

Fig. 24.20

rubber gloves from the first aid kit, put them on, then pull up the patient's shirt and assess his abdomen. There is no distension.)

Patient: "Like a typical yampa." (gasping) "You know, the leaves look like fern leaves, the little cream-colored flowers like Queen Anne's lace." (gasping) "Come to think of it, the root didn't taste quite right."

You: "How much did you eat?"

Patient: "Two, maybe three pieces."

You: "Does this hurt?" (pressing each abdominal quadrant in turn. The patient indicates that the epigastric area is tender.) "Did you save any of it?"

Patient: (moaning) "Yes, there is some there under the tent flap."

You hurry over to the side of the tent and retrieve several roots from under the flap. One of them has a stem with several leaves still attached. It looks like water hemlock to you. He must have mistaken it for yampa. On the way back you take a dishpan, canteen, and cup from the table.

You: "You better get rid of it—I believe it's making you sick. Here, drink this cup of water and I'll help you throw it up."

You help the patient sit up and he is able to drink the water. You take a spoon off the table and gag him with the handle. He vomits a large amount of stomach contents into the dish pan.

You: "Don't throw that away, we need to save it. Whose car is that?" (pointing to the carryall. The other man indicates it is his). "Mrs. Eaton, your husband is quite ill and should be taken to a hospital as soon as possible. I'll send Sandy to the nearest phone to call an ambulance from Sylvan City. Then, we'll load him into the back of the carryall and meet the ambulance on the pass."

You turn back to the patient. He has stopped moaning but does not seem as alert. His respirations seem slower and less deep.

You: (quietly to Sandy) "Take Billy with you and head for the trading post up the road. Call Sylvan City, tell them who we are, and tell them that we have a man with probable water hemlock poisoning and that we'll be bringing him in. We need an ambulance to meet us on the pass and transfer him. Tell them to send a doctor with it if they can, or at least a paramedic. I'll be back as soon as I can." (Sandy zips up the tent and heads for the truck with the baby. You turn to the other man.) "Help me load him into the back of the carryall. We'll need a pad for him to lie on and the pan for him to throw up in. I have a bucket with a lid in the tent that we can carry the vomit in."

In a few minutes everything is ready. You, the patient, and the patient's wife are in the back of the carryall with your first aid kit. You have the plant stem and leaves with you. The driver seems somewhat hesitant and wants to take time to take down the tent and pack up the camp, but after the patient has a grand mal seizure in the back of his vehicle he is more convinced of the urgency of the situation.

You reassess the patient. His airway is open, he is breathing regularly but shallowly at about 16 respirations per minute. His pulse is regular at 120 beats per minute and definitely weaker than it was. You open the first aid kit and take out a set of oropharyngeal airways and your pocket mask. You try to remember the signs and symptoms of water hemlock poisoning. You know that it is probably the most toxic native American plant and that even a single bite can be fatal. It is 60 miles to Sylvan City, the nearest hospital. With luck, you only have 30 miles to go before you meet the ambulance. You ready yourself to start basic life support, which you are fairly sure you will need soon.

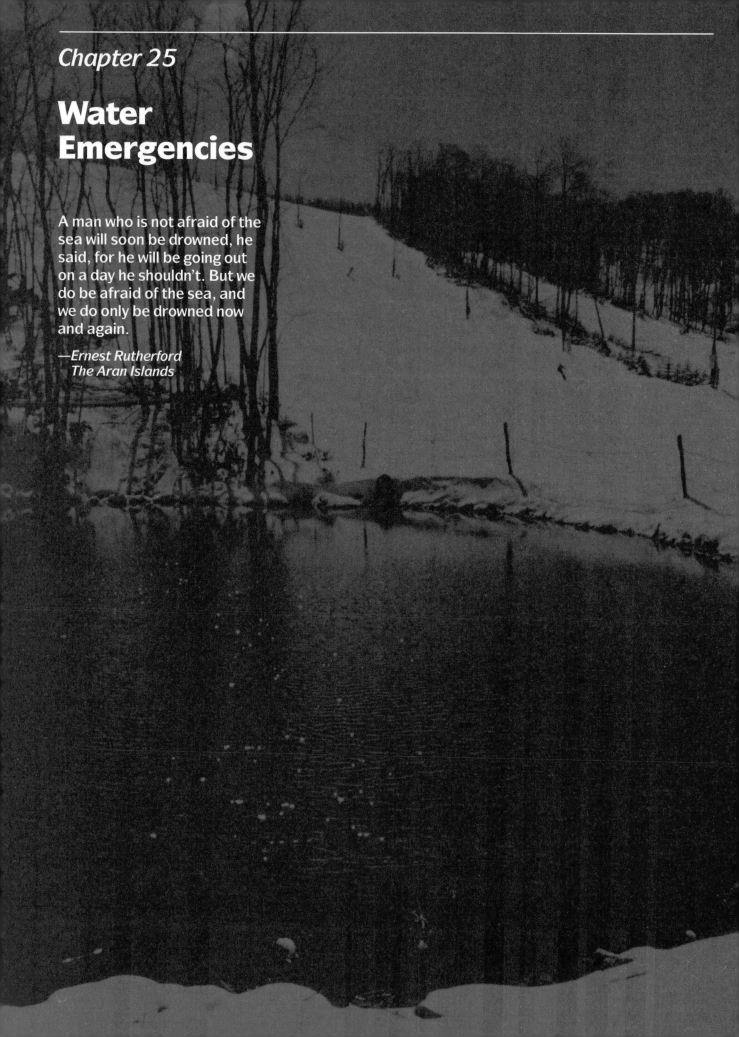

Chapter 25

Water Emergencies

A man who is not afraid of the sea will soon be drowned, he said, for he will be going out on a day he shouldn't. But we do be afraid of the sea, and we do only be drowned now and again.

—*Ernest Rutherford*
  The Aran Islands

Many outdoor injuries are associated with water sports such as swimming, boating, windsurfing, and scuba diving. These injuries are related to the inherent characteristics of bodies of water, water in motion, and the equipment used in water sports. Even cavers can be subjected to hazards from underground bodies of water. Because the number of Americans participating in water sports is growing, more water-related injuries are likely to occur.

The most common cause of death or serious injury in water sports is drowning or near drowning due to **submersion**. Submersion results from such mishaps as exhaustion while swimming, accidental falls into bodies of water, and falls through ice; swimming, water-skiing, and small boat accidents; and entrapments and boat pins during kayaking.

In the United States, there are more than 5,000 drowning deaths and more than 50,000 near-drowning accidents each year. Use of alcohol or other drugs is a factor in at least half of the drowning deaths. One-third or more involve hypothermia caused by cold water. Drowning is the second most common cause of accidental death in children, exceeded only by motor vehicle accidents. About half of all drowning deaths occur during the warm months of June, July, and August. A significant number of drowning victims had never learned to swim; many others lacked basic safety devices such as life jackets.

Although the mechanisms and patterns of injury in water sports may be unique, the care of the specific injuries is generally the same as described in previous sections of this book. Surfers and unsuspecting swimmers who dive into unscouted shallow water can suffer head injuries, cervical spine fractures, and facial injuries; running dives are particularly dangerous. Swimmers can be struck by

power boats and lacerated by propellers. Water skiers can be injured in collisions with floating objects and entangled in tow ropes. Sailboaters can be struck by booms.

Participants in white-water and swift-water sports who capsize their craft or perform poorly executed rollovers can suffer blunt head trauma, contusions, lacerations, broken teeth, chest and abdominal injuries, and fractures. Ankle injuries are common and usually are caused by slipping on wet rocks. Paddle maneuvers that force the arm upwards in abduction and external rotation can dislocate the shoulder. Injuries related to overuse of the thumb, wrist, and shoulders during prolonged paddling, such as sprains and tendonitis, are common. Back injuries can occur from carrying or lifting watercraft.

Environmental injuries include hypothermia; sunburn; ultraviolet conjunctivitis similar to snow blindness; motion sickness; and lightning injury. Swallowing contaminated water can cause gastrointestinal infections. Hazardous plants, land animals, and marine animals can be found, especially in exotic locations.

Skin diving and scuba diving introduce problems related to hypoxia, water pressure, and breathing pressurized gas. These include pressure ("squeeze") injuries of the ears and sinuses, nitrogen narcosis, oxygen toxicity, air embolism, and decompression sickness.

Rescuers should have a strong respect for water, especially cold, deep, or fast-moving water. Only a swimmer well-trained in lifesaving should attempt a direct swimming rescue of a struggling victim. Unless a victim is unable to grasp a floating object, it usually is better to throw or push a lifesaving device to the victim or to use a boat. The maxim to remember is "Throw, tow, or row before you go!" Untrained rescuers—even if they are strong, competent swimmers—are likely to become victims themselves.

When lifting a victim wearing a life jacket into a boat, grasp him or her by the arms or under the armpits. If you lift a victim by the life jacket, you may accidently remove it by pulling it over the victim's head.

Interested persons and those who live in areas where water sports are popular and water accidents are common should take additional training in water safety and water rescue from the American Red Cross, the YMCA, or a similar organization. Persons involved in specific water sports should acquaint themselves with emergency care textbooks written especially for participants in such sports and attend any available special emergency care classes.

Submersion Injury

Submersion injuries are divided into **drowning** and **near drowning**. A drowning victim is dead; a victim of near drowning survives at least temporarily after submersion. Drowning deaths are caused by hypoxia, which if severe and/or prolonged will irreversibly damage the brain and other vital organs.

However, at least in theory, there are two mechanisms that can delay the development of serious hypoxia in *some* submersion victims: the **mammalian diving reflex** and **hypothermia**, both of which are discussed in Chapter 18. Individuals who have been submerged in cold water for up to an hour or more can occasionally be resuscitated with very little residual injury to the brain. The most successful of these resuscitations have involved young children and those submerged in very cold water, but there have been some successes when water temperatures were near 70°F (21°C). These extraordinary survivals appear to be possible because hypothermia slows the body's metabolism and decreases its oxygen requirements. Therefore, submersion victims should be resuscitated vigorously unless they have been submersed for considerably longer than one hour.

Wet and Dry Drowning

After being submersed, the victim first holds his or her breath and may struggle intensely. As hypoxia reduces responsiveness, breath-holding ability and the gag reflex are lost, allowing water to be aspirated into the upper airway. In about 15 percent of victims, this causes the larynx to go into spasm, keeping additional water out of the lungs (dry drowning). In the other 85 percent, the lungs are found to be filled with water at autopsy (wet drowning).

From the standpoint of the patient's response to emergency care, there appears to be no difference between "wet" and "dry" drowning, or between saltwater and freshwater submersion.

Assessment and Emergency Care of a Submersed Patient

1. When a person is found floating face down on the water surface or is brought to the surface by a rescuer, there usually is little question about the cause of unresponsiveness. However, in near drowning in shallow water or in near drowning that is associated with a diving or surfing accident, a head injury may also be present, and *a neck injury should be assumed as well.*

   It is beyond the scope of this book to describe victim assists, tows, and other maneuvers taught in courses in water rescue and lifeguarding. However, it is necessary to bring a submersed victim to the surface to conduct the primary survey and provide emergency care.

   The victim is assumed to be non-breathing, which means that rescue breathing or CPR must be started as soon as possible. Therefore, the patient —if found prone—must be turned immediately to the supine position. This is relatively simple in shallow water where the rescuer can stand on the bottom; it is much more difficult in deep water.

   If two rescuers are available, one can stabilize the victim's head and neck in the neutral, in-line position while the other turns the victim's body, similar to the technique of logrolling the prone patient described in Chapter 13. However, since the patient must be turned as soon as possible and since there usually is only one rescuer available at first, a number of one-rescuer techniques have been developed. The following technique, recommended by the American Red Cross, works well in both shallow and deep water and has the additional advantage of enabling the rescuer to guard the cervical spine (Fig. 25.1).

   a. Swim or walk to the side of the prone victim, facing the head. Grasp the victim's right elbow with your right hand and the left elbow with your left hand. Straighten both of the victim's arms and extend them over the victim's head so that the head is sandwiched between and locked in place by the biceps. Your hands should be at the level of the victim's ears (Fig. 25.1a).

   b. Bring the victim's entire body to the surface by walking or swimming forward a few feet (Fig. 25.1b).

   c. As soon as the body is horizontal at the surface, rotate the victim in the water by pushing down with your right hand and pulling up with your left hand (Fig. 25.1c). This will require you to lower yourself in the water as the victim turns. Continue to splint the victim's head between his or her arms, maintaining the head and neck in-line with the body.

   d. Your right hand will still be on the victim's right arm, but your right arm will be under the victim's neck and shoulders. Rest the victim's head in the bend of your elbow, maintaining the head and neck in-line with the body (Fig. 25.1d).

2. If the victim is found supine instead of prone, splint the victim's head between his or her arms in exactly the same way, except that a 180-degree roll will not be required. Rest the victim's head in the bend of your elbow, maintaining the head and neck in-line with the body.

3. Universal precautions (see Appendix E), while desirable, may be difficult to institute until you are on shore.

4. Conduct the primary survey as with any unresponsive patient. Ask loudly, "Are you okay?" If there is no response, open the airway immediately, using the head-tilt/chin-lift technique. If you suspect a neck injury, use the one-handed jaw-thrust technique. If the patient does not start to breathe, give two rescue breaths as soon as possible. Usually you will not be able to perform rescue breathing until you have reached shallow water where you can stand (Fig. 25.2). In

some cases, you may be able to start rescue breathing in deep water if you are a powerful swimmer, especially if a rescue tube or rescue buoy is available or can be improvised. If there are two rescuers, one can support the patient while the other gives rescue breathing. It is especially important to maintain a water-tight seal over the patient's mouth and nose. A tight-sealing pocket mask with a one-way valve would be ideal, but is rarely available immediately.

Assess the carotid pulse as soon as the first two rescue breaths have been given. If the pulse is absent, CPR will be needed as well; however, because it is almost impossible to perform in deep water, there is no point in wasting time attempting it until the patient is on dry land or some other suitable firm surface.

5. If possible, use a spine board to remove the patient from the water (Fig. 25.3). A rigid collar, if available, should be applied as well. Slide the board underneath the patient, allow it to float up underneath, secure the patient to it, and tow the patient to dry land on the board. If a spine board is unavailable, use the multiple-rescuer direct ground lift and carry (see Chapter 20) to remove the patient from the water once you reach shallow water.

6. After reaching dry land, continue rescue breathing, reassess the carotid pulse, and start full CPR if the pulse is absent. Give oxygen in high concentration and flow rate, using a bag-valve-mask or a pocket mask. Insert an oral airway if the gag reflex is absent. Search for bleeding, lacerations, fractures, and

Fig. 25.1 *Rotating a Submersed Patient*

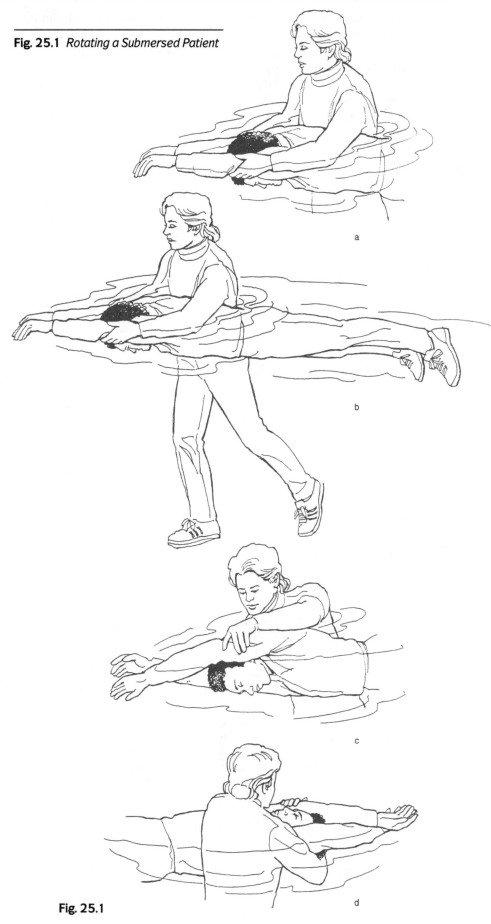

Fig. 25.1

other injuries as time and personnel allow.

7. Following near drowning, the patient's stomach usually is filled with water. Anticipate vomiting, and if it occurs turn the patient to one side to avoid aspiration (see one-rescuer log-roll, Fig. 4.5, Chapter 4). Suction is useful, if available.

The classic Heimlich maneuver (see Chapter 4 and Appendix B) should not be used to remove water from the stomach because of the danger of aspiration. Rarely, there may be so much water in the stomach that the patient's lungs cannot be expanded. In this case, roll the patient onto the side and press on the stomach to expel the water through the mouth (see Fig. B.25, Appendix B). Suction is recommended.

8. Take the patient's rectal temperature, preferably with a low-reading thermometer. Since hypothermia delays the effects of hypoxia in near drowning, time should not be spent correcting it in the field if spontaneous breathing and heart action are absent. *However, prevent further cooling* by providing insulation (see Chapter 18).

9. Take *all* submersion patients to the emergency department as soon as possible, even if they appear normal after they have been revived, since serious delayed complications such as pulmonary edema and pneumonia may occur. On the way, give rescue breathing or CPR if necessary. Monitor and record the vital signs frequently. The emergency department physician will need to know the following information:
   a. The patient's initial rectal temperature and any subsequent readings.
   b. The water temperature.
   c. The patient's age.
   d. The probable length of submersion.
   e. The emergency care that has been given.
   f. Any other important factors such as injuries.

10. A hypothermic victim of near drowning who has spontaneous respirations and heart action can be rewarmed according to the guidelines found in Chapter 18. The techniques appropriate for rewarming depend on the patient's core temperature. However, do not delay transportation of the patient to a hospital in order to warm the patient.

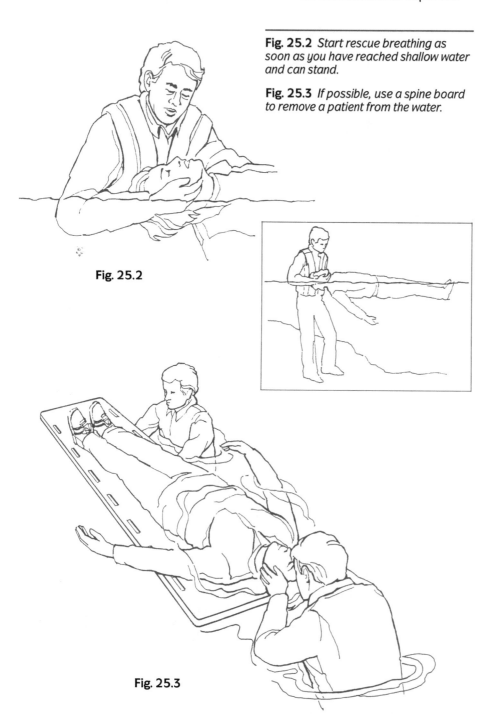

Fig. 25.2 *Start rescue breathing as soon as you have reached shallow water and can stand.*

Fig. 25.3 *If possible, use a spine board to remove a patient from the water.*

Fig. 25.2

Fig. 25.3

Table 25.1

Summary of Emergency Care of a Submersed Patient

1. Turn the patient to the supine position, guarding the neck if indicated.
2. Open and maintain the airway.
3. Institute universal precautions (see Appendix F) if possible.
4. Give rescue breathing.
5. Remove the patient from the water on a long spine board, or use the multiple-rescuer direct lift.
6. Start CPR, if appropriate, as soon as the patient is on dry land or a suitable firm surface.
7. Give oxygen in high concentration and flow rate.
8. Anticipate vomiting.
9. Take the patient's rectal temperature.
10. Transport the patient to a hospital as soon as possible.

Prevention of Drowning

1. *Teach all children to swim.*
2. If possible, fence all swimming pools and other bodies of water in inhabited areas. Keep the water levels of swimming pools close to the pool rim to enable swimmers to climb out easily. Drain rainwater from pool covers.
3. Wear U.S. Coast Guard-approved flotation devices (Fig. 25.4) while aboard small water craft, particularly rafts, sailboats, rowboats, canoes, and kayaks.
4. Wear helmets when kayaking.
5. When swimming, skin diving, or scuba diving, use the "buddy" system. Partners should keep track of each other at all times.
6. Do not leave infants and small children unsupervised near open water.
7. Do not use alcohol, "recreational" drugs, or any other drugs that impair concentration, alertness, or coordination while participating in water sports.
8. If engaged in cold-water sports, wear enough insulation to prevent or delay hypothermia if an unexpected immersion

occurs. The best choice is a dry suit plus a life jacket or an insulated personal flotation device such as a partial or full exposure suit, to provide both flotation and insulation.

9. Obtain competent instruction when learning high-risk water sports such as small boat sailing, kayaking, and canoeing. In white-water sports, be able to recognize and avoid hazards that can cause underwater entrapment, such as hydraulics, strainers, undercut rocks, low head dams, etc. Be familiar with self-rescue techniques such as swimming on your back with your feet downstream if you are thrown into moving water.
10. Do not attempt water rescues beyond your training and ability.
11. Do not participate in water sports alone.
12. Follow U.S. Coast Guard recommendations for safe boating.
13. Swim in guarded areas.

Fig. 25.4 *Flotation Devices*

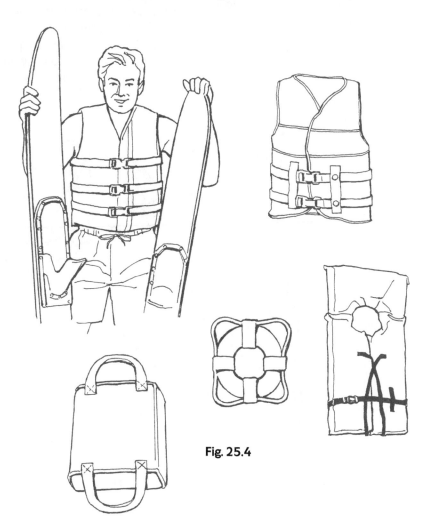

Fig. 25.4

Ice Rescue

The popularity of ice fishing, ice skating, and snowmobiling on frozen lakes increases the likelihood that rescuers may have to aid a person who has broken through the ice. Ice rescue is very hazardous to the rescuer, however. You should have a healthy respect for thin ice and cold water, and you should remember that it is no help to anyone if you fall through the ice to join the victim. The rapidity with which cold water can numb the extremities to the point where swimming and self-extrication are impossible must be experienced to be fully appreciated—it can occur within seconds to minutes.

To allow a victim to reach the shore or a rescuer to reach the victim, an ice rescue must be performed so that the weight of the victim and any rescue equipment is widely distributed over the ice surface. All rescuers should wear personal flotation devices.

An excellent rescue device is a lightweight ladder with a lifeline tied to the shore end. The ladder is shoved out on the ice to the victim, who crawls onto the ladder and edges along it to safety. If the victim is unable to climb onto the ladder, a rescuer may be able to crawl out onto the ladder to help (Fig. 25.5). If the ice breaks under the ladder, the far end will dip and the near end will rise, making it easier to pull the ladder back to safety by the lifeline.

If a ladder is unavailable, one or more wide boards or a stout tree branch can be used instead. Alternatives, especially if the ice is too fragile to support these devices, are to shove canoes, rowboats, or rubber rafts out onto the ice or to throw a spare tire or ring buoy to the victim. A fire hose with the ends capped can be inflated with air to make a semi-rigid, buoyant device that can be shoved out to the victim much like a long pole. Helicopters have been used successfully, especially in multiple-victim disasters. In the past, when no equipment was available, a human chain was sometimes formed by having several rescuers lie on the ice in a line, each grasping the ankles of the person in front. This technique is so dangerous to rescuers that it cannot be recommended.

A person who falls through the ice should attempt self-rescue by extending the arms forward over the ice, kicking the legs up so that the body is in a level position, and working forward onto the ice by kicking and carefully pulling with the forearms, elbows, and hands. A pocketknife can be used to increase traction (Fig. 25.6). This maneuver can be successful even if the ice continues to break ahead of the victim; it should be continued until firm ice is reached. After pulling the entire body onto firmer ice, the victim should carefully roll or edge toward shore, distributing body weight as widely as possible.

All victims of ice breakthroughs are assumed to be hypothermic and are cared for according to the guidelines in Chapter 18.

Fig. 25.5 *Ice Rescue Using a Ladder*

Fig. 25.6 *Ice Self-rescue*

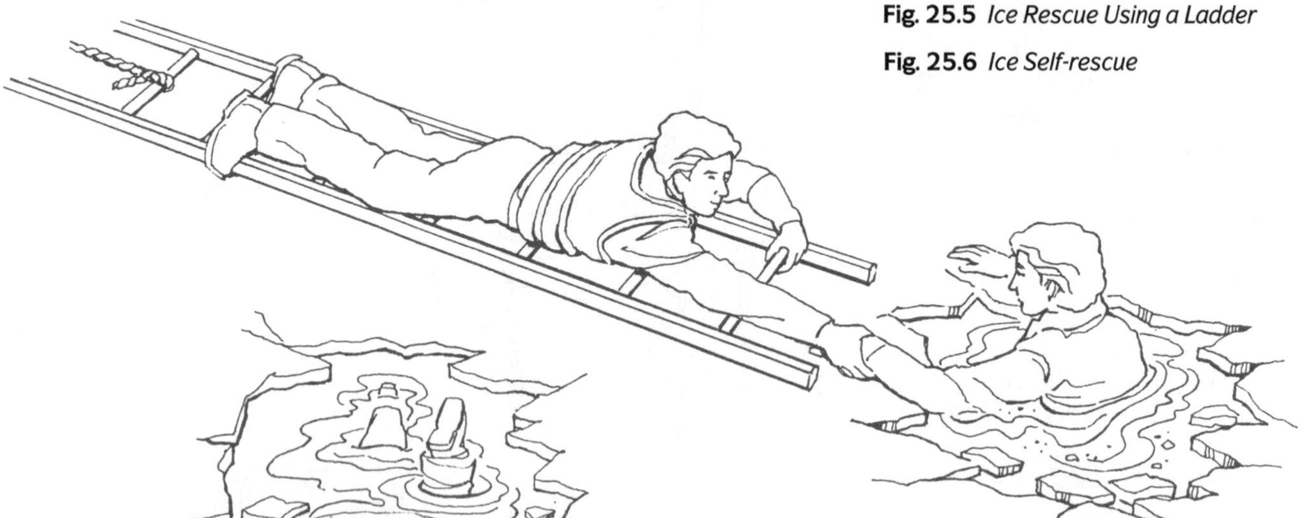

Fig. 25.5

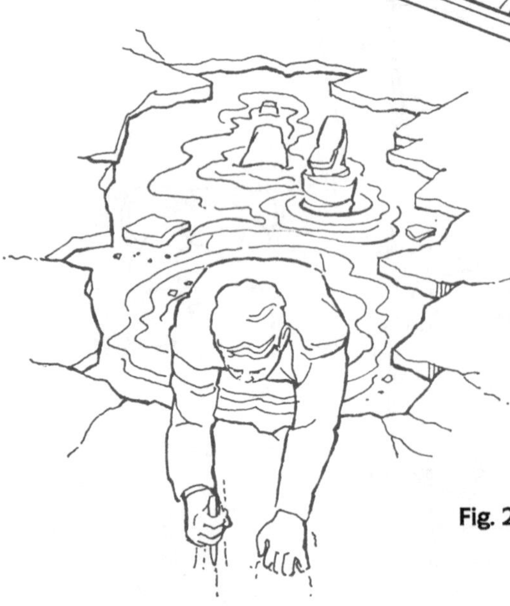

Fig. 25.6

Other Aquatic Problems

Swimmer's Ear

Swimmer's ear is an infection of the outer ear canal, seen in swimmers and divers whose ears are continually wet. Symptoms include pain and tenderness associated with the ear, a white or yellow discharge, and partial deafness.

Patients should see a physician for specific treatment. Swimmer's ear can be prevented by putting several drops of a solution of vinegar diluted to half strength with rubbing alcohol or tap water in both ears after emerging from the water. Commercial preparations containing 2-percent acetic acid in propylene glycol are available (VoSol, etc.).

Breath-holding Blackout

The loss of consciousness that occasionally results when a swimmer hyperventilates before swimming underwater is called breath-holding blackout. Hyperventilation (see Chapter 16) lowers blood levels of carbon dioxide (CO_2) and increases blood levels of oxygen (O_2). Because the breathing control center in the brain uses the amount of CO_2 in the blood as a guide to regulate the rate and depth of breathing, the length of time a swimmer can hold his or her breath underwater is proportional to the amount of CO_2 in the blood. If this is below normal, the breath can be held longer. The danger is that the amount of oxygen in the blood may fall so low during prolonged breath-holding that the swimmer becomes unconscious due to hypoxia before enough CO_2 accumulates to compel surfacing for a breath. Therefore, do *not* hyperventilate before you swim underwater. The emergency care of breath-holding blackout is the same as that described above for near drowning.

Associated Injuries

Kayaking, rafting, canoeing, sailing, windsurfing, motorboating, water skiing, and surfing can all cause injuries. White-water sports are particularly hazardous since the patient may be far from medical help. The additional complication of submersion is always a danger.

The patient must be removed from the water before emergency care can be given effectively. Give basic life support and care for soft-tissue, bone, and joint injuries as outlined in previous chapters. Rigid collars, extremity splints, cylindrical leg splints, and pillow splints can be improvised from life jackets, paddles, kayak float bags, and camping equipment such as pack straps and air mattresses.

The emergency care of injuries caused by hazardous marine life is discussed in Chapter 24.

Scuba Diving Injuries

The increasing popularity of diving with a self-contained underwater breathing apparatus (scuba) has led to increasing numbers of accidents and injuries related to diving techniques, equipment, and the nature of the underwater environment (Fig. 25.7). Many sport dives take place in remote tropical environments where sophisticated medical care may be unobtainable.

The medical problems of diving result from the effects of water pressure and of breathing compressed gas, the natural hazards of the underwater environment, and the human body's lack of gills and consequent dependence on potentially fallible technology to survive underwater. The effects of pressure differences are called **barotrauma**, sometimes known as "squeeze."

Anyone who wants to scuba dive should learn the proper techniques by taking an approved course taught by the YMCA or a similar organiza-tion and becoming a certified diver. *Never* dive alone or with an unqualified partner.

Diving problems can be divided into those that occur upon **descent**, those that occur at the **bottom**, and those that occur upon **ascent**.

Descent Problems

Ear and sinus injuries occur frequently, making them a major problem for the diver. They can involve the ear canal, middle ear, inner ear, or sinuses.

The basic cause is barotrauma due to the difference between the air pressure within these body parts and the water pressure outside. Accessory factors include wax buildup within the ear, failure of the Eustachian tube to open properly, and swelling of the lining of the nose due to allergy or a respiratory infection—all of which can prevent the gradual pressure adjustments that normally occur during a properly conducted dive.

Divers should be thoroughly familiar with methods of equalizing pressure by blowing with the nostrils closed and swallowing, and should not dive if they have an upper respiratory infection or uncontrolled allergy.

Depending on the area involved, symptoms of ear or sinus squeeze can include a feeling of fullness, pain, or ringing in the ear; headache; deafness; and loss of balance. Any diver who experiences these symptoms should halt the dive and return to the surface as soon as possible to reduce the pressure differences. Failure to surface may result in an eardrum rupture or serious injury to the inner ear.

The lungs and upper airway rarely give trouble during descent. However, if a diver holds his or her breath during descent, or the scuba apparatus malfunctions, the diver may suffer lung squeeze with bleeding into the lungs. Air in the gastrointestinal tract usually causes trouble only on ascent. Masks can cause face squeeze unless the pressure differences that develop during descent are equalized by blowing air into the mask through the nose.

Bottom Problems

Bottom problems are uncommon, and those that do occur usually are related to using unsuitable or malfunctioning equipment.

Drowning or near drowning can occur if air is lost from leaking equipment or if the diver runs out of air because of a miscalculation. Malfunctioning air compressors or improper filtering of air when tanks are filled can add small amounts of carbon dioxide or carbon monoxide to scuba tanks; the deleterious effects of these gases are magnified by the increased pressure at depth. Nitrogen narcosis, or "rapture of the deep," is caused by breathing nitrogen at depths below about 90 feet (27 meters), and has an effect similar to alcohol intoxication. Oxygen poisoning with dyspnea, apprehension, changes in hearing and vision, and convulsions can occur if pure oxygen is breathed below 33 feet (10 meters) or if compressed air is breathed below 297 feet (91 meters).

Ascent Problems

Aside from drowning and near drowning, the most serious underwater problems occur on ascent. Ascent problems, including **air embolism** and **decompression sickness**, are related to the effects of decreasing water pressure on the air in the lungs and on the nitrogen dissolved in the body fluids.

Air Embolism

During ascent, the air in the lungs expands as the water pressure decreases. If air expands too quickly or too much, the pressure may rupture the alveoli and force air into the pulmonary capillaries where it forms bubbles. From there, the bubbles are carried by the blood flow into the pulmonary veins, through the left side of the heart, and into the systemic circulation, where they travel until they reach an arteriole or capillary too small to pass through. When they stop, they form a plug, or **embolus**, that prevents blood from flowing through the vessel and reaching the tissues the vessel normally supplies.

Because bubbles can lodge in almost any organ, the signs and symptoms of air embolism are variable. The most common ones are caused by lack of blood to components of the circulatory, respiratory, and ner-

vous systems. They include chest pain, shortness of breath, cough, hemoptysis, and symptoms of pneumothorax (see Chapter 14); signs and symptoms of heart attack (see Chapters 16 and 17); dizziness, confusion, alteration or loss of responsiveness, and seizures (see Chapters 12 and 17); loss of vision, hearing, or speech; and paralysis or loss of sensation. Sudden loss of responsiveness upon reaching the surface is a typical occurrence. Death can occur rapidly if recompression is not available.

Air embolism, a danger during rapid ascent, can be prevented if divers *continually exhale* during ascent to reduce the volume of air in the lungs. *Scuba divers should never hold their breath when under water.* Ascent should be *controlled* at a rate of about 60 feet per minute (1 foot per second). This rate can be estimated by ascending at the same rate as the smallest visible air bubble.

Emergency Care of Air Embolism

1. Remove the patient from the water and place the patient on the left side with the chest *lower* than the feet. This position tends to trap air bubbles in the heart and prevent them from entering important arteries, particularly those supplying the brain.

Fig. 25.7 *The popular sport of scuba diving has led to increasing numbers of accidents.*

Fig. 25.7

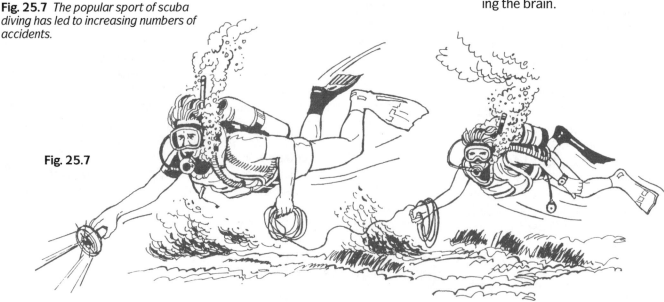

2. Give basic life support (see Chapters 4 and Appendix B) and care for unresponsiveness (see Chapter 12), if necessary.
3. Give oxygen in high concentration and flow rate.
4. Recompression in a pressure chamber (hyperbaric chamber) is the *definitive* treatment for air embolism and should be started as soon as possible. Recompression makes the air bubbles smaller and drives them back into solution. Some diving centers have a hyperbaric chamber as part of their medical facilities. All scuba divers should know the location of the nearest hyperbaric chamber. Usually, there is a chamber within a few hours by air. The aircraft used to transport the patient should fly low or be pressurized at near-sea-level pressure.

Contact the **Diving Accident Network (DAN)** at (919) 684-8111 for assistance in locating hyperbaric chambers and for advice on emergency care. The staff will need to know the following information, which can be obtained from the patient or companions:

1. The age and sex of the patient.
2. The patient's signs and symptoms; the time between surfacing and the onset of illness; and the duration of illness.
3. The depth and the bottom time of the dive or dives.
4. The conditions under which the ascent was made (i.e., the patient was breathing or not breathing), and whether scheduled decompression stops were made.
5. The emergency care that has been given. If a hyperbaric chamber cannot be reached, take the patient to the nearest hospital as rapidly as possible.

Decompression Sickness
("The Bends")

Atmospheric nitrogen is much less soluble than oxygen and carbon dioxide in body fluids. However, during a descent, the increasing water pressure forces a higher proportion of the nitrogen in the lungs into solution in the blood than would occur normally. If ascent is too fast, the rapid decrease in pressure allows the nitrogen to come out of solution even though oxygen and carbon dioxide remain dissolved. The nitrogen forms bubbles in small blood vessels instead of being excreted normally through the lungs. Because these bubbles can form or lodge in any organ, the signs and symptoms of **decompression sickness**, like those of air embolism, are variable and depend on the organs involved.

Common Signs and Symptoms of Decompression Sickness

1. Mottling and/or itching of the skin.
2. Pain in the muscles, joints, or abdomen (the "bends").
3. Weakness, paralysis, and loss of sensation, particularly of the lower extremities.
4. Difficulty in urinating.
5. Chest pain, cough, and shortness of breath.

Table 25.2

Decompression sickness can be prevented by carefully controlling the depth and duration of the dive. Sport divers are advised *not* to dive in a way that requires stops on ascent for decompression.

Tables are available that indicate the safe times at given depths for single and repetitive dives, and the depths and times of decompression stops required on ascent if the safe limits are exceeded. Since the tables are calculated for sea-level dives, they need to be adjusted significantly for mountain-lake diving. Traveling in aircraft for 24 hours before or after any dive using compressed gas may be hazardous.

Emergency care for decompression sickness is the same as for air embolism. The signs and symptoms of air embolism and decompression sickness usually are reversible with treatment in a hyperbaric chamber. Permanent injury may result if recompression is delayed or if the vessels that supply vital organs, such as the heart, brain, and spinal cord, are obstructed. Therefore, treat serious ascent problems as an emergency and arrange for recompression as soon as possible.

Summary of Emergency Care of Air Embolism and Decompression Sickness

1. Remove the patient from the water and place the patient on the left side with the chest lower than the feet.
2. Give basic life support and care for unresponsiveness if necessary.
3. Give oxygen in high concentration and flow rate.
4. Arrange for recompression in a hyperbaric chamber.

Scenario #27 (Fig. 25.8)

The following scenario illustrates the type of complex emergency care problem that can occur with water-related sports

You, your wife Sandy, and the baby are spending a weekend at a friend's cottage at a large nearby lake. The lake shore is ringed with cottages, most of which have boat docks and small sand beaches. By mid-morning, there are many sailboats and small motorboats out in the lake, and a few swimmers are braving the chilly waters. You have your canoe on top of your new 4 x 4 vehicle and are planning to have lunch at a picturesque, uninhabited inlet across the lake.

There seems to be a family reunion going on at the next cabin. Six teenagers in swimwear are playing volleyball on the beach while their parents sit talking under beach umbrellas. They finish their game and race each other to the end of the pier, where they dive head-first into the water, to reappear shortly and stroke awkwardly toward a floating dock 50 yards farther out in the lake.

After they have pulled themselves onto the dock, they seem agitated and keep glancing shoreward, calling someone's name. The parents rise from their chairs and hurry to the shore edge. You cannot make out the details of the exchange of shouts, but there is obviously something wrong.

You: "Sandy, something's going on. I'm going to check it out." (Sandy scoops up the baby and follows you as you trot over to the group of parents.) "What's wrong?" (you ask the nearest parent).

Parent: "George is missing. They all dived off the end of the pier and he didn't come up."

You: "Sandy and I have taken some lifesaving training, we'll see what we can do. Better have someone notify the sheriff and call an ambulance."

You kick off your sandals, peel off your T-shirt, and run to the end of the pier. About 20 feet out you think you see something red in the water. You step down into the water and swim out to where you saw the object, using a strong breaststroke and keeping your eyes on that area. When you reach it, you see that it is a teenaged male wearing a pair of red shorts, floating face down in the water just below the surface near a buried piling.

You: "Sandy, I've found him! Come in and give me a hand."

Sandy hands Billy to one of the women, drops her windbreaker, pulls a mouth shield out of her purse, and runs out to the end of the pier. Meanwhile, you approach the victim's head and lower your feet. The water is about 4 feet deep and you can easily stand on the bottom. You grasp both of his arms, straighten his elbows,

Fig. 25.8 *Scenario #27*

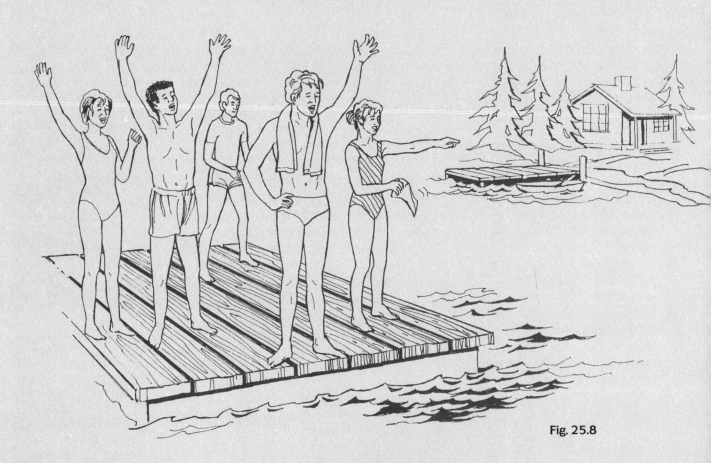

Fig. 25.8

and extend his arms over his head, sandwiching his head between his biceps. You then walk forward a few feet so that his body floats to the surface. You turn his body toward you as a unit until he is face up. At this point Sandy joins you, reaches the victim's side, and opens his airway with the jaw-thrust technique, asking loudly, "George, are you okay?"

There is no answer. She applies the mouth shield and immediately gives two rescue breaths of two seconds each. She listens carefully and watches the victim's chest. It rises with the rescue breaths but he does not start to breathe spontaneously. She feels the carotid pulse; it is fast and regular. She then starts rescue breathing, giving one breath every five seconds. The two of you start walking slowly and carefully toward the shore, keeping his face above water, his head and neck stabilized, and continuing rescue breathing.

By the time you reach a depth of 2 feet, you are about 20 feet from shore. You call several of the parents to enter the water and help you get the victim onto dry land. They get the idea quickly and you are able to change his head and neck stabiliza-tion to the standard type, shift his arms to the side of his body, and raise him out of the water using a direct ground lift. The lift produces no significant spine motion that you can detect. He is carried slowly and carefully a few feet up on the beach and lowered supine onto the sand. Sandy assesses the carotid pulse again. It is strong and regular. She then resumes rescue breathing.

You hear an approaching siren, and in a minute the ambulance arrives and two EMTs join you, carrying a long spine board, oxygen tank, portable suction unit, and trauma kit. By now, the patient is taking an occasional gasping breath on his own. One of the EMTs starts to assist the patient's ventilations, using the bag-valve-mask with added oxygen. The other one pulls out a new eardrum temperature measuring device. When you raise your eyebrows, he remembers that the ear canal is probably full of water and checks a rectal temperature instead; it is 98 °F. The temperature is down one-and-one-half degrees because of the cold lake water, but there is no serious hypothermia.

Sandy tests the patient's ability to move in response to pain, using a painful nail pinch. There is no response in the lower extremities. There is a slight amount of shoulder flexion in the upper extremities.

"Uh-oh," you think. "Probably a fractured neck with some cord injury along with his submersion injury." You are glad you were careful to stabilize his head and neck well. Maybe you spared him a few nerve fibers that he can use later on.

After a few minutes of ventilation and oxygenation, the patient's breathing is deeper and regular. The four of you quickly logroll the patient onto his side and then back onto the spine board. His breathing continues to be assisted with the bag-valve-mask. Just after you finish strapping him securely to the board, he starts to retch. You quickly tip the board on its side while one of the EMTs aspirates his mouth with the portable electric suction unit. He vomits a large amount of lake water mixed with stomach contents onto the sand. You help the EMTs carry the boarded patient to the ambulance and load him onto the gurney. The ambulance drives off with light's flashing and siren screaming, followed by a sedan carrying the patient's parents. You spend a few minutes with the others, discussing the dangers of diving into shallow water.

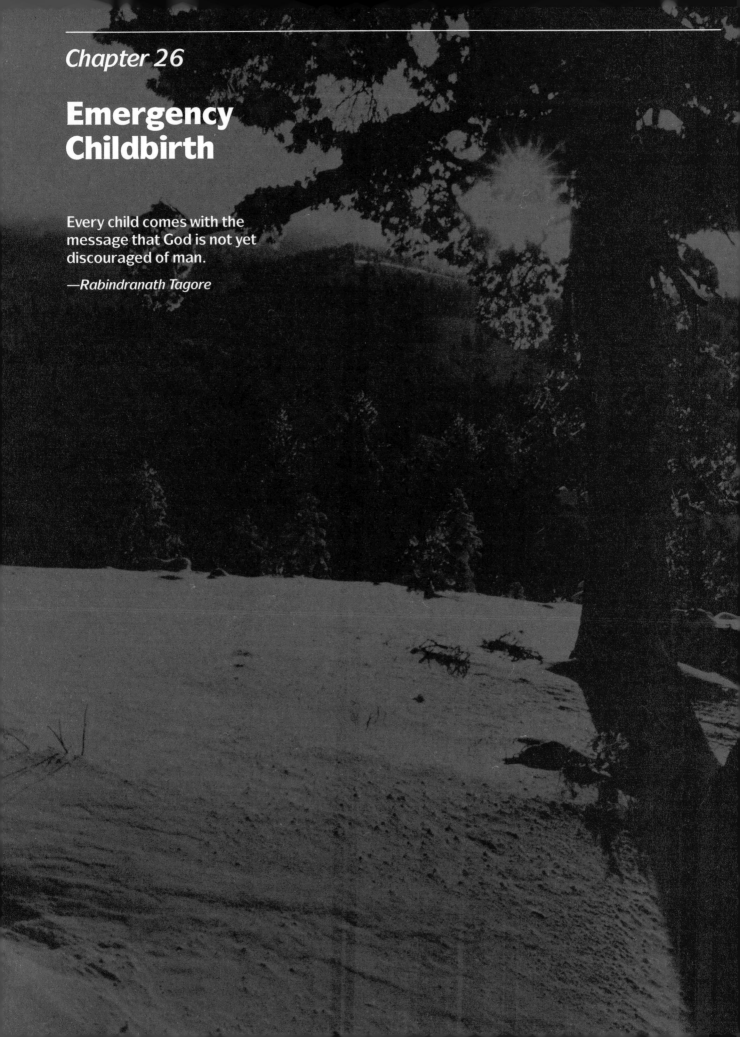

Chapter 26

Emergency Childbirth

Every child comes with the
message that God is not yet
discouraged of man.

—*Rabindranath Tagore*

Even though, in our society, few births occur at home, the fact that the human species has survived on earth for countless years testifies that childbirth is a natural process that can occur in a normal and safe manner outside the hospital. Therefore, "emergency" in the title of this chapter refers more to the rescuer's state of mind than the mother's condition.

Early labor usually begins slowly enough to allow ample time to take the mother to a hospital, but occasionally, because of rapidity of labor, distance, or difficulties with transportation, it may be impossible to reach definitive medical care before the baby arrives.

Although rescuers are not expected to be midwives, they should be familiar with the process of childbirth and be prepared to assist the mother as needed. Afterward, the mother and infant should be taken to a hospital as soon as possible.

Although the overwhelming majority of births are normal, complications are occasionally seen. These are discussed after the normal birth process is described.

Before continuing, please review the anatomy and physiology of the female genitourinary system in Chapter 2.

While in the uterus, the baby is connected to the placenta, or "afterbirth," by the umbilical cord (Fig. 26.1). The placenta is attached to the wall of the uterus. The baby's heart pumps its blood through the umbilical cord to the placenta, where the baby's blood vessels are closely associated with the mother's blood vessels. Then the blood returns to the baby's body through the umbilical cord. This arrangement allows the baby's blood to take up oxygen and nutrients from the mother's blood and to give up carbon dioxide and other wastes.

A crucial time for both baby and mother is when, during birth, first the baby and then its "life support system" —the placenta—are expelled from the uterus, leaving a large, raw area at the former site of placental attachment. Since the baby no longer gets oxygen from its mother, it must start breathing soon after it reaches the outside. Normally, the baby's head comes out before the umbilical cord comes out. In some types of abnormal deliveries, the cord comes out before the head. In this situation, the cord may be compressed by the head as the head comes through the birth canal, cutting off the baby's oxygen supply before the head is out and the baby can breathe. The baby also runs the risk of airway obstruction from mucus and amniotic fluid, which must be cleared from its nose and mouth before it can breathe. In addition, the mother may suffer significant hemorrhage from the raw area where the placenta was attached to the uterus and from any soft-issue injuries to the cervix and vagina that may have occurred during the birth.

The rescuer must know not only how to guide the baby through the birth canal, but also how to support the baby's circulation and breathing, provide ventilation and CPR for the baby if necessary, be able to tell if the mother is losing more than a normal amount of blood during childbirth, and manage abnormal blood loss if it occurs. The rescuer also needs to know when and how to tie and cut the umbilical cord so as much blood as possible remains in the baby's body.

Fig. 26.1 *Anatomical Drawing of a Baby Inside the Uterus*

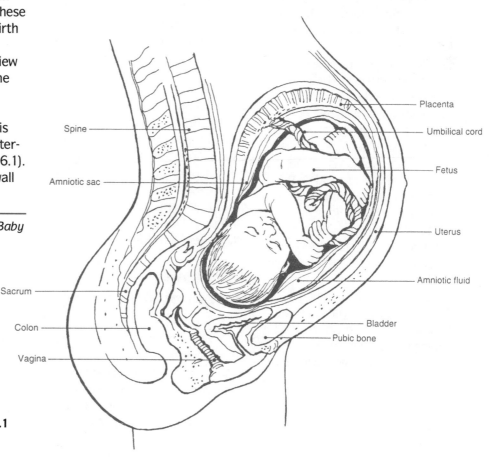

Spine

Amniotic sac

Sacrum

Colon

Vagina

Placenta

Umbilical cord

Fetus

Uterus

Amniotic fluid

Bladder

Pubic bone

Fig. 26.1

The normal length of pregnancy is 280 days: 40 weeks or approximately nine months. At the end of this time, the fetus is fully developed and the pregnancy is said to be "at term." If you are familiar with normal female anatomy, you know that the baby is much larger than the passage it must negotiate to be born. It takes time for the birth process to stretch the elastic tissues of the birth canal—the cervix and vagina—large enough so that the baby can pass through. This is done by repeated contractions of the strong muscles of the wall of the uterus that stretch the canal by slowly pushing the baby through it to the outside, a process called **labor**. The length of labor is variable, tending to be shorter in women who have had previous children.

Labor is divided into three stages:
1. **First stage**. The time from the onset of regular uterine contractions until the lower end of the uterus, the cervix, is completely stretched open.
2. **Second stage**. The time from when the baby starts to leave the uterus until it is completely outside the mother's body.
3. **Third stage**. The time from the delivery of the baby to the delivery of the placenta.

A woman in labor should be encouraged to lie on her *left* side to keep pressure off her inferior vena cava. When the woman is supine, the pressure of the baby's head on the inferior vena cava may interfere with blood returning to the heart, causing dizziness, lightheadedness, and a drop in blood pressure. If she prefers to be supine, place a pillow under her right hip and displace her uterus manually to the left side of the abdomen.

In most cases, the patient's husband or other family members will be expecting the onset of labor, will have been told beforehand how to tell when to take her to the hospital, and will have made the necessary preparations. It is unusual for a rescuer who is not a family member to become involved in these events. However, your help may be requested if labor begins when the patient is far from home, family members or means of transportation are absent, or labor is unusually rapid.

Signs a Pregnant Woman Should Be Taken to a Hospital for Delivery

1. The onset of regular uterine contractions that are five minutes or less apart in a woman at or near term. During a contraction, the woman feels pain in the small of her back as well as in her abdomen. Her uterus, when felt through the abdominal wall, will harden noticeably.
2. A sudden gush of fluid from the vagina (rupture of the membranes or "bag of waters"). This fluid is the amniotic fluid that supports and protects the fetus.
3. Passage of more than a small amount of bloody mucous.

If no private transportation is available, call EMS for an ambulance. If you plan to take the patient to the hospital by private vehicle, she should be assessed to see if there is time to reach the hospital, since *delivery of the infant in the home is much safer and easier than delivery in a vehicle.*

Assessment of a Pregnant Woman

1. Introduce yourself and tell the patient the type and extent of your training.
2. Ask her when the baby is due, whether or not she is carrying more than one baby, how many children she has had before, whether the births were natural or by caesarean section, how frequently the labor pains are coming, how long they are lasting, and whether they are regular. Ask about any complications or problems with past pregnancies and deliveries, any current medical problems, and any expected problems with the current pregnancy or delivery, particularly whether she was advised that she would require a caesarean section. If she has had previous babies, she may be able to tell you if she is about to deliver.
3. Have the patient lie down and undress below the waist. Cover her with a sheet. Place your hand on the patient's lower abdomen so that you can feel her uterus tighten. Time a contraction by measuring from the onset of one contraction to the onset of the next one. Meanwhile, have an assistant start to assemble equipment for home delivery, in case it is needed (see Table 26.1).
4. Wash your hands and put on disposable rubber gloves, preferably sterile. If gloves are not available, wash your hands several times.
5. Inspect the vaginal opening during a contraction to see if the baby's head is visible (Fig. 26.2). If so, you will see an area of wrinkled skin and dark hair. Important considerations in deciding whether there is still time to take the woman to a hospital are the size of the visible area, *how many children* the woman has had previously, and the distance to the hospital.
6. Prepare for home delivery if:
   a. The woman has had one or more children previously and the head is visible during a contraction.

b. The woman is having her first child and the visible part of the head is larger than a 50-cent piece.

c. The woman is bearing down hard with each contraction and feels like she needs to move her bowels.

7. Take the woman to a hospital if:

a. The hospital is no more than 20 minutes away.

b. The head is not visible during a contraction, or in the case of a woman having her first child, is visible but smaller than a 50-cent piece.

c. *The umbilical cord or any part of the infant other than the head* is visible at the vaginal opening. In this case, it will be extremely difficult or impossible for a rescuer untrained in obstetrics to deliver the baby safely. This is an *emergency;* any preparations for home delivery should be stopped and the woman should be taken to the nearest hospital without delay.

d. The woman has been told that she will need a caesarean section.

Fig. 26.2 *Vaginal Opening during a Contraction with the Baby's Head Visible*

Supplies to take along in the car include all the supplies listed in Table 26.1, plus a flashlight, blanket, pillow, and a warm bathrobe for the mother. Tell her not to bear down with contractions, but to take fast, shallow breaths (i.e., pant) with each contraction.

If you are preparing for home delivery, the EMS dispatcher may be able to locate a nearby midwife or other experienced person who can come to the home to assist you. In addition, an emergency department physician may be able to give useful advice by phone.

Home Delivery

1. Arrange for privacy and a place for the woman to lie on a sturdy table, on a bed, or on the floor. A table is more convenient for you because it is higher than a bed. If you use a bed, have the woman lie flat on her back in the middle, knees bent, head on one side of the bed, and feet on the other. Put a small table or chair nearby where you can place your emergency equipment.

2. Lay a piece of waterproof plastic under the woman's buttocks. Lay several layers of newspaper on the plastic and cover them with clean material

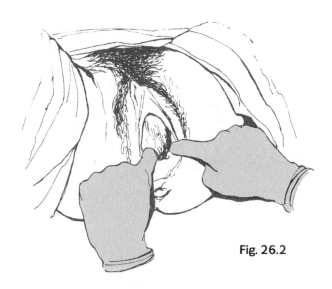

Fig. 26.2

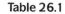

Table 26.1

Equipment for Home Delivery

To protect the mother
Two clean sheets
Several sanitary napkins
Soap and a basin of warm water
At least six sterile compresses
Four clean towels

To protect the infant
Soft rubber bulb syringe, preferably sterilized by boiling
At least one flannel blanket
Several diapers
Several safety pins

To cut and tie the umbilical cord
Two 12-inch pieces of white cloth tape or two white cotton shoelaces, sterilized. (Do not use thin material such as cord or twine, since it may cut through the umbilical cord.)
Scissors or a razor blade
Rubbing alcohol and clean cotton swabs

To protect the delivery room
Newspapers and plastic sheets
A washbasin or large plastic bag for the placenta
Emesis basin or bucket for vomiting

To protect the attendants, mother, and infant
Several pairs of rubber gloves, preferably sterile
A face shield or goggles
Some type of protective clothing such as waterproof or water-resistant parka and pants

A preferable alternative to the above is the "OB kit" carried in all ambulances. All contents are sterile. A typical OB kit should contain: surgical scissors, two cord clamps, two 12-inch lengths of umbilical tape, towels, rubber gloves, a surgical gown, surgical masks, goggles or a face shield, gauze compresses, sanitary napkins, a bulb syringe, a baby blanket, sterile drapes, and two large plastic bags.

such as a sheet or towels. Protect the nearby floor with newspapers or plastic.

3. The woman should be undressed below the waist. Have her lie flat on her back, with both knees bent, feet flat, and thighs spread widely apart. Cover her with a sheet.

4. Station yourself just beyond the woman's buttocks, on her right if you are right-handed or on the left if you are left-handed. Have a basin nearby in case she vomits. Encourage her to rest between contractions. Remember that, since the pelvic outlet is shorter from side to side than from front to back, the baby's body will rotate as it comes out because different body parts of different shapes must accommodate themselves to the shape of the outlet.

5. Delivery of the head:

   a. The baby's head usually will emerge during or after a strong contraction (Fig. 26.3a). The baby usually will be face-down (facing toward the mother's back), but occasionally will be face-up. As the head comes out, feel the baby's neck to see if a loop of the umbilical cord is around it. Hold the head gently, guiding and supporting it with your hand. After the head emerges, allow it to rotate (as the baby's body turns to allow the shoulders to move down and out). Maintain it in its normal position with respect to the body. Do not twist or otherwise manipulate the head.

While the baby's head is emerging, watch the vaginal tissues around the head. Frequently, the head will pop out so fast that these tissues will be torn, especially in a woman who is having her first baby. Sometimes, this can be prevented by supporting these tissues with your other hand while you guide the baby's emerging head through the tightly stretched tissues.

   b. The head may still be covered with the amniotic sac (bag of waters). If the bag does not quickly rupture spontaneously, tear it with your fingers or nick it with a scissor blade and remove it to free the head (Fig. 26.3b).

   c. If the cord is wrapped around the baby's neck,

Fig. 26.3 *Delivery of the Head*

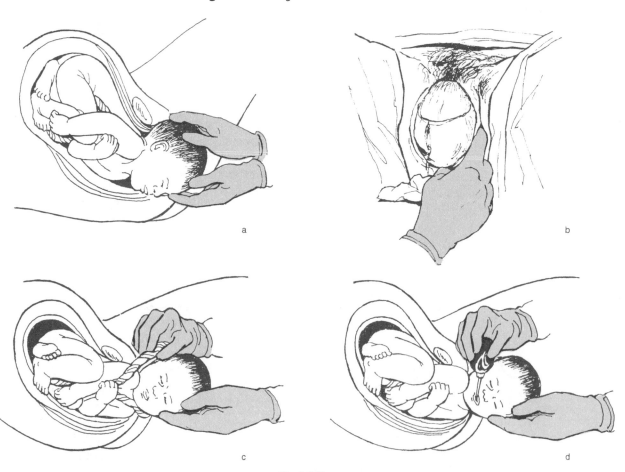

a

b

c

d

Fig. 26.3

unwrap it quickly by passing the loops over the baby's head (Fig. 26.3c). If this cannot be done, quickly tie or clamp and cut the cord as described below in step 9. The ties or clamps must be solid; if they slip off the baby can suffer serious, potentially fatal, bleeding.

d. Usually, there will be a minute or two between the time the baby's head is delivered and the time the shoulders are delivered. During this interval, wipe out the baby's mouth with a clean cloth. If a soft rubber bulb syringe is available, use it instead to gently suction fluid and mucus from both nostrils and the mouth (Fig. 26.3d). Squeeze the air from the bulb, gently insert the tip about 1½ inches into the baby's mouth, and let the bulb inflate. Squirt out any material before reinserting the tip. Suction the mouth and each nostril two or three times. Since babies are nose-breathers and not mouth-breathers, pay special attention to suctioning the nostrils.

6. Delivery of the shoulders: As the body starts to emerge, it will rotate so that the head will face to the side and the shoulders will be vertical (do *not* twist the baby's head).

a. The upper shoulder usually emerges first. Guide the baby's head gently downward without pulling on it to ease delivery of the upper shoulder.

b. After the upper shoulder is out, guide the baby's head gently upward to ease the lower shoulder out. Do not pull or tug on the head or shoulders to get the shoulders out faster, and do not hook your finger in the baby's armpit.

7. Delivery of the trunk: After the shoulders have been delivered, the rest of the body usually will emerge *rapidly*. Be prepared to catch it and hold it securely. Remember that newborn babies are slippery.

8. Care and resuscitation of the baby:

a. To hold the baby properly, grasp the feet with one hand, with the index finger between the ankles and the rest of the fingers and the thumb encircling the feet (Fig. 26.4a). Support the chest and head with the other hand. Set the baby down on a clean sheet between the mother's legs. Have an assistant record the time of delivery. Tell the mother whether it is a boy or a girl.

b. Suction the mouth and nose again with the soft, rubber bulb syringe (Fig. 26.4b).

Fig. 26.4 *Care and Resuscitation of the Baby*

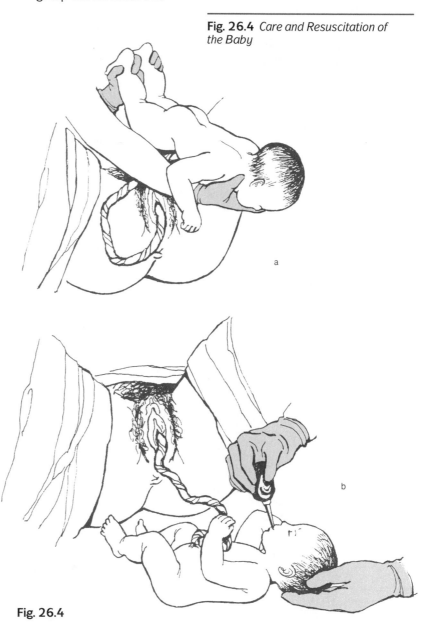

Fig. 26.4

c. If the baby does not start breathing immediately, stimulate it by rubbing its back or sternum gently. Do not hold the baby upside down. If this is ineffective, give rescue breathing or CPR as indicated (see Chapter 4 and Appendix B).

d. As soon as possible, wrap the baby in one or more flannel blankets to keep it warm. Newborn babies lose heat rapidly because of their large surface-to-volume ratio and from evaporation of amniotic fluid on their skin. Thoroughly dry the baby with a clean blanket or a soft towel.

9. The umbilical cord rarely needs to be cut in the field unless it is strangling the baby or there will be a long delay (longer than 20 minutes) in reaching the hospital after delivery. However, the baby should remain at the same level as the birth canal until the cord is cut. If the baby is above this level, blood tends to drain *from* the baby into the placenta.

If you decide to cut the cord, allow it to cease pulsating first if possible, since this allows the maximum amount of blood to flow into the baby from the placenta.

a. To cut the cord, clamp or tie it with a square knot at a 6-inch interval and again at an 8-inch interval from the baby, using a clean, preferably sterile (dipped for a few minutes in boiling water) cotton tape or shoelace (Fig. 26.5a).

b. Cut the cord between the two clamps or ties with scissors or a razor blade sterilized by boiling or wiping with rubbing alcohol (Fig. 26.5b).

c. If you used clamps, be sure to tie off the cord between the clamp and the baby before releasing the clamp on that side.

Fig. 26.5 *Technique of Tying and Cutting the Umbilical Cord*

10. Delivery of the placenta:
    a. After the baby is born, labor pains will return again as the uterus starts contracting to expel the placenta. This usually will take several minutes. Do *not* push on the abdomen or pull on the cord to speed this process. If there are any problems such as the baby not breathing well, the mother bleeding heavily, or the placenta taking more than 20 minutes to deliver, take the mother and baby to the hospital immediately. Remember to keep the baby and placenta at the same level until the cord is cut.

11. Care after delivery:
    a. As soon as the placenta emerges, *gently* massage the top of the uterus through the abdominal wall for a few minutes with one hand to stimulate the uterus to contract strongly and control bleeding. The uterus will feel like a firm, smooth, rounded, grapefruit-sized object in the midline of the lower abdomen just above the pubic bone. This massage is uncomfortable, and you should explain to the mother what you are doing and why.

    b. Continue to massage the uterus gently with a circular motion every 5 minutes for the next hour or until you arrive at the hospital. If the uterus begins to feel soft and there is increased blood flow from the vagina, increase the vigor and frequency of the massage.

    c. If there are any lacerations of the birth canal, stop bleeding with direct pressure and cover the wound with a sterile compress.

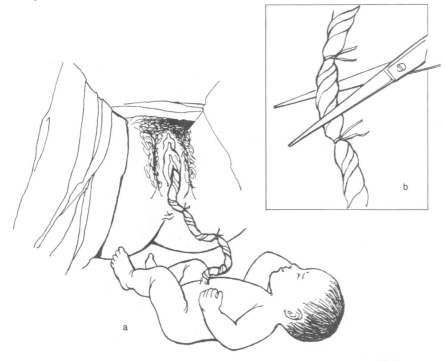

Fig. 26.5

d. Cleanse the mother's genital area by pouring warm, soapy water over it and rinsing it with warm water. Do this while the mother is still lying on her back, so that the water flows from the pubis toward the rectum.

e. Lay a clean sanitary napkin over the vaginal opening (do not place anything in the vagina).

f. Keep the mother and baby warm and check the baby periodically to make sure it is breathing normally. Although you should dry the baby, do not attempt to wash or cleanse it.

g. Once the cord is cut, allow the mother to hold the baby and put it to her breast if she wishes.

h. Take the mother and baby to the hospital. Do not forget to bring the placenta also.

Complications of Childbirth

Nonbreathing Baby

The baby may have died in the uterus days or even weeks before birth. Do not attempt to resuscitate a baby that has a strong, unpleasant odor, large blisters, a very soft head, or obvious deformities incompatible with life. Otherwise, give infant CPR as you have been trained to do in your CPR class (see Appendix B). Do not tie or cut the umbilical cord. Take the mother and baby to the hospital as soon as possible.

Abnormal Presentation or Prolapsed Cord

Occasionally, instead of the head presenting, the baby's "breech" (buttocks or both feet), shoulder, arm, or one foot will present at the vaginal opening. The umbilical cord may come out first ("prolapsed cord"). The only abnormal presentation in which the baby is still "lined up" so that it can move smoothly through the birth canal is the breech presentation. In *all* the others, continuing labor will bring no results and the woman and baby will eventually become exhausted and will die if professional assistance cannot be obtained.

1. **Breech presentation**. The mother should be taken to a hospital without delay. Since labor will continue, however, the rescuer needs to know what to do if the hospital cannot be reached in time.

   The baby will usually be born without any serious problems, but the birth will be more difficult because of the different mechanics involved. The baby's head comes out last. The main danger is compression of the umbilical cord between the baby's head and the tissues of the lower pelvis, cutting off the baby's oxygen before its head has come out and it can start to breathe on its own.

   a. Usually, the baby's body will come out in the prone position. After it has been delivered, let it rest on your forearm with the arms and legs dangling on either side.

   b. If the head does not come out within three minutes, create an airway for the baby by inserting your other (gloved) hand into the vagina, and push the vaginal tissues away from the baby's face. Put a finger gently into the baby's mouth and hold it open, if you can, until the head comes out.

2. **Single foot, arm, shoulder, or umbilical cord**. Have the mother get into the **knee-chest** position (Fig. 26.6), with her buttocks higher than her shoulders. Cover a prolapsed umbilical cord with a clean towel moistened with saline (½ teaspoon of salt in a quart of clean water) to keep it from drying out. Take the mother to the hospital without delay. Give oxygen if available.

   In the case of a prolapsed cord, as the baby's head comes down, there is danger of it compressing the cord and cutting off the baby's blood supply. Put on a sterile glove, insert your hand into the vagina, and push the head away from the cord if you can.

Fig. 26.6 *Knee-chest Position*

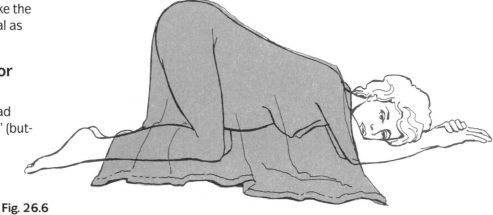

Fig. 26.6

Twins and Other Multiple Births

Twins occur once in 90 births. Usually the mother will know if she is carrying more than one baby. If not, suspect a multiple birth if her abdomen still remains large after the (first) birth.

Delivery is the same as with a single baby, except that a baby may be followed by another baby instead of a placenta. About 10 minutes after the birth of the first baby, labor will start again. Usually, you will have 30 minutes or more before the next baby is born, so use this time to tie and cut the first baby's cord before the second baby comes. In multiple births, the babies usually are smaller than normal and should be handled as premature babies (see below).

Premature Babies

A premature baby is one who is born four weeks or more before it is due, or any baby that looks unusually small, more wrinkled, skinnier, or with a larger head than you would expect. Usually the mother will know when the baby was supposed to have been born.

The premature baby is more delicate and has more trouble breathing, regulating its body temperature, and performing other vital functions. Handle it gently, keep it warm (cover its head but not its face), and watch its airway and breathing. When you call for an ambulance, tell the dispatcher that you have a premature baby so that special equipment will be ready. Give oxygen if you have it, but oxygen should be given into a small "tent" over the baby's face, made of aluminum foil or a blanket.

Abnormal Bleeding

There are two types of abnormal bleeding that are related to childbirth: bleeding before or during the first stage of labor, and bleeding during the second and third stages of labor.

In some cases, the placenta will separate prematurely from the wall of the uterus, usually just before labor begins or during the first stage of labor (abruptio placentae). This is accompanied by dark-colored vaginal bleeding, severe pain in the abdomen and back, and an enlarged, hard, tender uterus. In other cases, the placenta is attached so low in the uterus that it covers the cervix (placenta previa). When labor begins, the placenta will be torn as the cervix stretches, resulting in bright red vaginal bleeding. Abruptio placentae and placenta previa are both dangerous conditions that can cause serious—even fatal—hemorrhage to the mother and death to the fetus.

Any bleeding during late pregnancy and any more than a minimal amount of bloody mucus passed during the first stage of labor is abnormal and should be considered very serious. The patient should be taken to a hospital as soon as possible. Keep the patient on the left side and treat for shock if necessary (see Chapter 6) by elevating her legs and giving oxygen (if available) at high concentration and flow rate. Take soaked pads to the hospital so that hospital personnel can estimate the amount of blood loss.

A mother will lose 1 to 1½ cupfuls (200 to 300 milliliters) of blood normally during the second and third stages of labor. This is enough to soak four or five sanitary napkins from the OB kit. If she loses more than that, or if bleeding does not stop soon after the placenta is delivered, she is in danger of hypovolemic shock and should be taken to the hospital as soon as possible. Meanwhile, treat for shock (see Chapter 6) by elevating her legs, massaging the uterus as described above, and keeping her warm. Give oxygen, if available, at high concentration and flow rate. Tie and cut the umbilical cord and encourage the mother to put the baby to her breast since breast feeding will stimulate the uterus to contract. Do not try to insert any compresses or other material into the vagina. Take the soaked pads to the hospital.

Prolonged Delivery

If you have prepared for a home delivery based on signs that delivery is imminent and, after 20 minutes, there is no progression, the baby may be too big for the vaginal opening or the contractions of the uterine muscle may be too weak. In this case, it is best to stop what you are doing and take the woman immediately to a hospital.

Toxemia

Toxemia of pregnancy is a poorly understood condition characterized by high blood pressure, protein in the urine, blurred vision, headache, and edema, followed in some cases by abdominal pain, convulsions, and/or unresponsiveness. Suspect it if the woman has high blood pressure and swelling of the legs, hands, or around the eyes.

There is no field emergency care other than care of convulsions and unresponsiveness; the mother should be taken to a hospital as soon as possible.

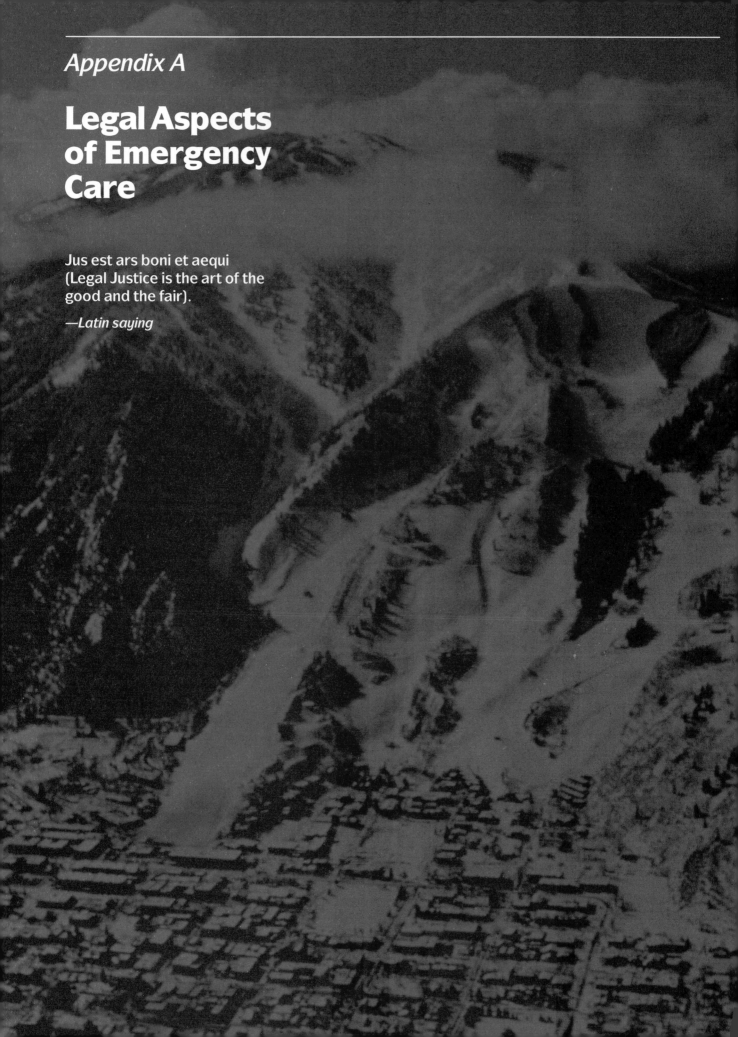

Appendix A

Legal Aspects of Emergency Care

Jus est ars boni et aequi
(Legal Justice is the art of the
good and the fair).

—*Latin saying*

Traditionally in Western society, only physicians have been permitted to diagnose and treat the injured and ill. Preparation for the practice of medicine is long, rigorous, and subject to strict regulation and licensing. Over the years, however, types of medical care that can properly be provided by non-physicians have been identified through experience and general agreement. These have been called by various names: first aid, self-help, and more recently—as sophistication has increased—emergency medical technique, first response, or emergency care.

The following discussion uses the general term "emergency care" to refer to medical care provided by persons who are not physicians, nurses, or physician assistants. Since many physicians have little training in emergency care procedures, these may be performed better by well-trained non-physicians than by physicians.

Emergency care is appropriate under many circumstances, including but not limited to:

1. Medical emergencies when no physician is present and the patient is in danger of death or serious harm unless something is done immediately.
2. Illnesses or injuries in which certain preliminary care is appropriate during the time before the patient is turned over to a physician.
3. Illnesses or injuries that are not serious enough to normally require a physician's care.

Although written material is available for self study, in most cases people who want to learn about emergency care enroll in a specific course taught by a recognized organization such as the American Red Cross or the National Ski Patrol. Upon successful completion of the course, students receive a card specifying that they completed the course and fulfilled its requirements. Such people then are regarded as competent to provide the care that they have been taught. To maintain this competency, they attend refresher courses at regular intervals.

Because of the informal and voluntary way that emergency care has developed in the past, there has been no formal certification or licensing until the past 30 years. With the formation of the EMS system, people trained in emergency care who work in ambulances, helicopters, hospital emergency departments, and similar places have been required to obtain a state certification or license. With the exception of certified or licensed members at the higher levels of the EMS system (such as paramedics or EMT-Intermediates under physician supervision), emergency care providers are not allowed to start intravenous infusions; perform invasive procedures such as needle thoracotomy (use of a needle to drain air or fluid from the chest), cricothyroidotomy (introduction of a tube into the trachea through the cricothyroid membrane) and endotracheal intubation; administer drugs; or perform other advanced life support procedures. To perform these procedures without EMS authority would be "practicing medicine without a license," which is prohibited by the medical practice statutes of every state.

Under common law, emergency care providers, *regardless of their level of training,* are expected to perform as any other reasonable, prudent person *with similar training and experience* would perform under similar circumstances, using their skills as appropriate whether they are in a medical facility or out in the field, and always with due regard for the safety and welfare of both the patient and fellow providers. This is called the **standard of care**.

To adhere to this standard, once you have obtained good training you must practice the learned skills appropriately, correctly, and on a regular basis; have the basic equipment on hand and know how to use it; and keep abreast of advances in emergency care on the level for which you have received training. In case you are called on to demonstrate to the authorities that you have met the standard of care, you should have **documentation** of training, refreshing, and reevaluation of competency in required skills and knowledge.

In addition, you must be able to provide the EMS system (or others who take over care of the patient) with a detailed record of the emergency care given to the patient. This documentation (which also shows that you are adhering to the standard of care) is required by most rescue organizations who provide report forms to be filled out in each case (see Appendix E for examples). Since these report forms may be standardized and brief, in the case of serious or complicated illnesses or injuries it is advisable to attach additional detailed memoranda to the form, including flow sheets used to record vital signs. In certain cases these should include signed statements of witnesses.

Many ski areas have developed incident investigation protocols to be initiated when certain kinds of injuries occur. Typically the protocol requires that someone at the ski area collect the following information:

1. A detailed incident report.
2. Statements from each of the patrollers involved in the incident.
3. Statements from the patient (if possible) and any available witnesses to the incident.
4. Photographs of the incident scene and any applicable signs and markings.

5. Diagrams of the scene.
6. Reports to any regulatory agencies as required by law.

The protocol usually is invoked in the following situations:

1. A death or serious incident with life-threatening injuries or the likelihood of permanent disability.
2. An incident involving a man-made object (chair lift, snow-mobile, etc.) or rental ski equipment.
3. A collision with another skier.
4. An incident occurring in a ski school class or involving ski area personnel or patrollers.
5. Any incident where the injured skier, relative, or friend threatens litigation or makes serious complaints regarding the ski area, the nature of the incident, or the patrol's handling of it.

The patroller should know whether the ski area has an incident investigation protocol and the circumstances in which the area management has directed the protocol be employed. It is imperative that any such investigation be undertaken as soon as the care of the patient permits, and that it be conducted in accordance with the instructions of area management.

If the rescuer makes an inadvertent error when filling out a form, a line should be drawn through it so the error is still legible, and the rescuer should initial the change.

It also is important that the record of care given be consistent with the record of assessment, including the signs and symptoms. In general, if emergency care is *not recorded* in the written report, the presumption is that the emergency care *was not given,* especially if other care was clearly documented. In addition, an incomplete or untidy report implies that the emergency care given also may be incomplete or careless. The rescuer should remember that, in the case of litigation, he or she may be required to testify in court many months or years after the occurrence in question. It is much better to have a complete and accurate written report to refer to than to rely on memory alone.

Despite the ethical and moral obligations people may feel, in most states no *ordinary* citizen has a *legal* obligation to rescue or go to the aid of another individual who is sick, injured, or endangered *unless* he or she has **caused** the sickness, injury, or danger. Some states (Vermont, Minnesota, and Rhode Island at the time of this writing) require that a person who comes upon an emergency either act personally (usually only if it can be done without personal danger) or report the situation to the authorities so that they can act.

However, if the ordinary citizen *does* go to another person's aid, the law obliges him or her not only to act reasonably and prudently but to *continue to care* for the patient, except in the following circumstances:

1. A competent patient refuses care. This should be witnessed and documented in writing and a refusal of care statement should be signed by the patient.
2. The rescuer must go for help.
3. The patient has recovered and no longer requires care.
4. The patient has a minor illness or injury and is placed in the custody of competent friends or family members for transport to definitive care.
5. The safety of the rescuer is endangered.
6. The patient's care is transferred to personnel with an equal or higher level of training, such as another qualified rescuer, EMS team, or definitive care facility staff.
7. The patient is obviously dead (see Chapter 19 for assessment of death).

Otherwise, failure to continue to care for the patient is called **abandonment** and can result in legal constraints or a lawsuit. However, if a citizen has a role or job that presents or implies an obligation to provide rescue or emergency care—such as being a member of a ski patrol or other organized rescue group that has held itself out to the public and to the authorities as an organization of trained, qualified and responsible rescuers—a legal obligation or "duty" *does* exist to search for, rescue, care for, and/or transport the injured and ill within the specific area of operation when requested. Even if the rescuer is an unpaid volunteer, he or she is not an "ordinary" citizen and does not have the option of arbitrarily refusing such a request.

Since state laws differ and impose different responsibilities and types of authority, you should obtain and be familiar with applicable state laws and regulations that pertain to providing emergency medical services, since they impact everything you do. Such laws and regulations may define scope of practice for responders, certification and recertification requirements, relationships with ambulance companies and hospitals, Good Samaritan laws, and immunity from liability laws. Copies may be obtained from the state office of emergency services.

In the eyes of the law, a person's body is inviolate. Interfering with it or even touching it without permission may constitute **battery**, an illegal act in many states. Because any person usually has a right to refuse emergency care, when first approaching a patient the rescuer should identify himself or herself as a trained rescuer and provider of emergency care, and ask "Can I be of help?" The patient may either specifically give consent or may cooperate with your assessment and care in a way that can be taken as actual consent.

If the patient is unconscious, irrational, or a minor, and urgently needs care for a life-threatening or serious illness or injury, consent may be "**implied**." This means that the law presumes that the patient, if able (or the patient's parents or guardian, if present), would consent to the care.

In some cases, a patient who initially refuses necessary or urgent care can be persuaded to accept help by a calm discussion of the risks of not obtaining care. If the patient persists in refusing, it is wise to have responsible witnesses present and have statements from them in writing specifying that care was offered and refused.

Because of the risk that the rescuer may be accused of abandonment, there is one situation in which the rescuer should at least try to provide urgently needed emergency care to a patient, even if the patient initially refuses assistance: when the patient has a life-threatening or very serious condition, the facts and circumstances clearly indicate that the patient is behaving in an irrational manner due to the serious condition (illness or injury), and the patient is not responsible or competent because of irrational behavior.

The risk of being accused of abandonment usually is greater than the risk of being accused of battery. However, this decision remains with the rescuer, who must believe very strongly that any reasonable person would not refuse treatment in this situation or a comparable situation. In addition, it is important that the refusal not be based on a religious belief.

Furthermore, under the legal principle of "choice of evils," a rescuer usually will be protected from liability for battery if he or she preserves the life and health of a seriously ill or injured person who may have refused treatment but who was not in a physical or mental condition to evaluate the situation or to decide about treatment in a rational manner. At this point, law enforcement personnel should be called, if possible, so that they can become involved. This is mandatory when a parent unreasonably refuses urgently needed care for a life-threatening or very serious condition involving a child. These officials generally have strong powers of persuasion and the authority to involuntarily commit a patient (adult or child) for a short period for evaluation, during which necessary medical care can be given. Proper documentation is essential, including a detailed written record, names and addresses of witnesses, and written statements by them. The reader also should refer to the section on **Psychology of Dealing With the Injured or Ill** in Chapter 4.

Despite the best emergency care, unexpected results may occur or the patient may allege that the care or transportation was improper. The result, especially in our current litigious society, may be litigation, which is both costly and time-consuming, even if the rescuer is eventually exonerated. For this reason, every rescuer should be certain that he or she is covered by sufficient insurance to protect against both claims and lawsuits that may arise, whether or not they are supported by the facts. This insurance should cover both awards and the insured's expenses incurred in defending against suits. Each rescuer should *personally* review the level and extent of insurance coverage with his or her insurer and the appropriate officer of any rescue organization before presuming coverage. This is especially true of those certified to practice at basic EMT/ Winter Emergency Care levels and above.

Although a disgruntled patient may allege anything, he or she has the burden of proving four things in court to prevail on a claim of negligence:

1. That the rescuer had a *duty* to the patient.

2. That the rescuer *failed to perform*, or "**breached**," that duty because of an error of commission or omission that *violated the standard of care*.
3. That the patient *actually suffered some injury or loss* that is compensable in money.
4. That the rescuer's failure *caused the patient's injury or loss*.

These four requirements, which place the burden of proof on the plaintiff, are a strong barrier against frivolous or unjustified lawsuits.

Other deterrents are the so-called Good Samaritan laws, whose purpose is to encourage people to help out voluntarily in emergencies. These laws have now been passed by every state but differ significantly from state to state. In some states they apply only to physicians and nurses, in others to other recognized emergency care providers as well, and in still others to *anyone* who renders assistance in an emergency. In some states, organized responders are not covered by the Good Samaritan Law because it has been held that they have a duty to respond.

Although Good Samaritan laws do not prevent suits from being filed, they generally absolve from liability anyone covered by the statute who gives care gratuitously, in good faith, and in accordance with his or her training and expertise in a bona fide emergency, except in the case of **gross or willful negligence**. This means that a physician must perform at the level of a physician, a nurse at the level of a nurse, an EMT at the level of an EMT, and a ski patroller at the level of a Winter Emergency Care (WEC) technician, taking into consideration the facilities and equipment available and the conditions that exist at the time of the emergency. In some states the assistance also must be given "without objection" from the patient.

It is important to remember that physicians, nurses, professional ski patrollers, ambulance personnel and other non-volunteers who are *paid* for their services are not usually covered for emergencies that they care for during their usual duties and in their usual work locations. Every rescuer should be thoroughly familiar with the Good Samaritan laws of all states in which he or she is active.

Negligence can be defined as the breach (failure to perform) of a duty to exercise the degree of care that any reasonable and prudent person would exercise in similar circumstances, resulting in harm to another person.

Gross negligence can be defined as the breach of a duty to exercise the care that even an unreasonable or imprudent person would exercise in similar circumstances, resulting in harm to another person. If bad or malicious intentions are involved, the negligence is referred to as **willful negligence** or willful misconduct.

However, rescuers should realize that the best protection—and also an ethical obligation—is good, up-to-date training, conscientious refreshing of and maintenance of competency in knowledge and skills, and dedicated patient care. Nonetheless, training and refreshing alone are not sufficient unless records are kept that document them, preferably on standardized forms. Detailed notes should be made of dates, names of rescuers attending, and procedures performed. Rescue groups should keep equipment logs that specify the date, type, and duration of equipment use, especially in the case of ropes. All records should be kept indefinitely in a safe place. Equipment should be retired before it becomes unreliable. By following these guidelines, rescuers may well *prevent* incidents in which liability might be incurred.

Table A.1

General Requirements for Good Samaritan Law Coverage

1. Your category of volunteer is covered by the statute.
2. Emergency care is furnished without monetary charge.
3. Emergency care is given in good faith and in accordance with your level of training.
4. A bona fide emergency exists.
5. There is no gross or willful negligence.

General Procedures for Handling Death

Non-highway-related fatalities in the outdoors are uncommon but not rare. The death rate in alpine skiing is around 0.1 per 100,000 skier visits. Collection of data on death rates in such outdoor activities as climbing, backpacking, nordic skiing, ski mountaineering, and wilderness kayaking is difficult because of the informal nature of these activities. In remote areas, a serious illness or injury is more likely to result in death because of the necessary delay in obtaining definitive medical help. Every member of a backcountry rescue group is apt to see at least one fatality during his or her career. Hunters, cavers, kayakers, scuba divers, climbers, and practitioners of similar hazardous sports may see fatalities as well.

Outdoor, off-highway traumatic deaths most often result from head or chest injuries caused by incidents such as falls, snowmobile and all-terrain vehicle accidents, and collisions while boating or skiing. Deaths also may be caused by hypothermia, drowning, avalanche burial, lightning strikes, and medical illnesses such as heart attack, acute mountain sickness, pneumonia, and stroke. Although a legal pronouncement of death can

be made only by a physician or other legally constituted authority, a rescuer can tell from a properly performed patient assessment whether death has likely occurred or is obvious. The signs of death are discussed in Chapter 19.

Because of differences in state and local laws, every rescue group should work with the local coroner and law enforcement authorities to establish procedures for determining that death has occurred and for handling a death, and every group member should be familiar with these procedures. The laws of many states prohibit moving a body or anything associated with the death until authorized by a coroner. This is especially important in the case of death from trauma or when a criminal act is suspected. Failure to obey these laws may be a criminal offense. Backcountry rescue organizations in particular should consult with the coroner beforehand regarding guidelines for handling a body when death occurs in the backcountry and terrain or weather will prevent timely examination of the scene by the authorities.

At a ski area, the area management and local authorities should be involved in the development of procedures for handling a death. These procedures should be posted in a place well known to all patrollers. In general, the following people should be notified:

1. A physician from a ski area clinic or associated with the local patrol, if available. He or she can pronounce the patient dead.
2. The ski area management.
3. The county sheriff, state police, coroner, or other appropriate local law enforcement authority.
4. Any federal, state, or local agency responsible for administration of the land upon which the ski area is located. This includes the local U.S. Forest

Service or National Park Service representative, if the ski area is located on Forest Service or National Park Service land; or the state or local Parks Department, if the area is located on state or local public land.

A person who dies in the first aid room should be covered with a sheet and screened from curious onlookers.

If death occurs in a remote area, rescuers should remember that what they see will never be seen again in the same way. Detailed documentation is necessary both to satisfy the law and for insurance and estate settlement purposes. Also, there is always a potential for learning from the episode to prevent similar happenings in the future. Painstaking records should be kept of all aspects of the death scene; records should include the preparation of written reports, diagrams, maps, and photographs, with dates and times noted. Photographs should be taken of the general area as well as the death scene to orient authorities to the overall picture. Close-up photos should be taken from no nearer than 3 feet and, in daylight, should be taken both with and without flash attachments to record details more accurately. The documented materials along with the photographs are critical in reconstructing the chain of events leading to the fatality.

If the commission of a criminal act is suspected, the sheriff or other appropriate authority should be notified before the death scene is disturbed, if at all possible. Entry into the area where the death occurred should be strictly limited and a record of all persons at the scene should be kept and turned over to the authorities.

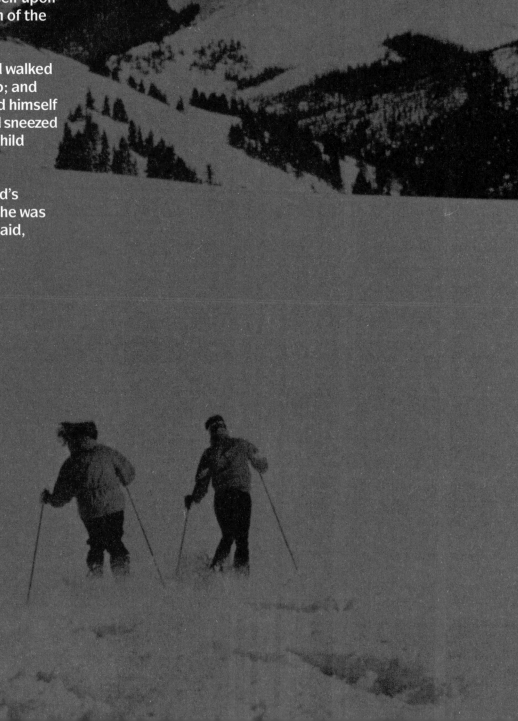

Appendix B

Basic Life Support

And (the prophet Elisha) went up, and lay upon the child, and put his mouth upon his mouth, and his eyes upon his eyes, and his hands upon his hands: and he stretched himself upon the child; and the flesh of the child waxed warm.

Then he returned, and walked in the house to and fro; and went up, and stretched himself upon him: and the child sneezed seven times, and the child opened his eyes.

And he called (the child's mother)....and when she was come in unto him, he said, Take up thy son.

—Holy Bible
  II Kings 4:34-36

When the circulatory and respiratory systems fail to carry out their vital function of delivering oxygen to every body cell, the most frequent cause is heart disease. Heart disease, a major health problem in modern society, usually is secondary to disease of the coronary arteries. More than 6 million Americans are known to have coronary artery disease, which in the United States causes 1.5 million myocardial infarctions and 500,000 deaths a year. About 300,000 of these deaths are sudden deaths due to **cardiac arrest**. About two-thirds of these sudden deaths take place outside the hospital, usually occurring within two hours of the onset of symptoms.

Cardiac arrest is any condition where the blood circulation stops because the heart malfunctions. Either the heart stops beating entirely (asystole) or beats too fast (ventricular tachycardia) or in an uncoordinated manner (ventricular fibrillation). In adults, three-fourths of arrests are caused by potentially treatable abnormal heart rhythms in people whose hearts might otherwise function adequately for many years. In many cases the patient has had no warning of the impending catastrophe. Cardiac arrest from coronary artery disease is the most common serious medical emergency in the United States today. It is a major concern for every emergency care giver and a major topic in every emergency care course.

A technique called **closed chest cardiopulmonary resuscitation** (**CPR**) was developed in the early 1960s to resuscitate victims of cardiac arrest. The rescuer simulates lung action by breathing into the patient's lungs and simulates heart action by rhythmically pressing on the patient's chest. Pressing on the chest raises the pressure inside the chest and squeezes the heart between the sternum and the thoracic spine,

forcing the blood out of the heart into the circulatory system. CPR and techniques for relieving upper-airway obstruction together are called **basic life support** (**BLS**).

CPR provides only 20 to 30 percent of the normal cardiac output of blood, 1 to 5 percent of the normal coronary artery blood flow, and 3 to 15 percent of the normal cerebral blood flow. With each passing minute of delay in starting CPR, the intracranial pressure rises so that by five minutes there is very little cerebral blood flow. Therefore, to be effective, CPR must begin within **four to six minutes** after cardiac arrest.

It is obvious that the only way to save an appreciable number of cardiac arrest victims who collapse outside a medical facility is for *bystanders* to provide CPR. To do this, the technique must be taught to laypersons on a widespread basis. Consequently, the American Heart Association and the American Red Cross have developed courses in basic life support and CPR. More than 50 million people have taken these courses since the early 1970s.

Even so, BLS saves few lives unless it is quickly (within 15 to 20 minutes) followed by advanced cardiac life support (ACLS). In fact, the best results are obtained when BLS is started within four minutes and ACLS within eight minutes of cardiac arrest (see Table C.1, Appendix C). ACLS is performed by paramedics, nurses, or physicians who may reach the patient by ambulance or helicopter. While basic life support requires only the tools that the rescuer carries at all times—the brain, eyes, ears, mouth, and hands—the ACLS team is equipped to do the following:
  1. Restore the patient's normal heartbeat using sophisticated heart monitors and electric defibrillation equipment.
  2. Support the patient with intubation equipment and intravenous drugs.

  3. Administer intravenous substances to dissolve blood clots.

Therefore, an important part of BLS is *contacting the EMS system as soon as possible* so that ACLS can be provided.

Studies have shown that, in a patient with ventricular fibrillation who is receiving BLS, *early defibrillation alone*—even in the absence of full ACLS—will improve survival. This has led to the attempt to make early defibrillation more available by training some EMTs to defibrillate using standard equipment. It has also lead to the development of automatic external defibrillators (AEDs) that can be used by EMTs and other emergency care givers. These are programmed to read the heart rhythm and to automatically deliver a defibrillating shock when a "shockable rhythm" (ventricular fibrillation or ventricular tachycardia) is detected. You may be able to contact EMTs and other individuals trained to use this equipment even if full ACLS is not available. It is estimated that 100,000 to 200,000 lives per year potentially can be saved by prompt basic life support followed rapidly by defibrillation or full advanced cardiac life support. Everyone should memorize the phone number used locally to summon the EMS system, usually 911.

Recognition of the above facts has led experts in CPR to coin the term **chain of survival**. The four components, or links, in the chain are:
  1. **Early activation**, which means recognizing the situation immediately and calling in the EMS system as soon as possible. (Keep in mind that in CPR the **A** in **ABC** should stand for **A**ctivation as well as **A**irway).
  2. **Early CPR**, which means providing ventilation and circulation to keep the heart and brain functioning for as long as possible. This implies immediate CPR from a bystander and re-

Table B.1

Basic Life Support Algorithm

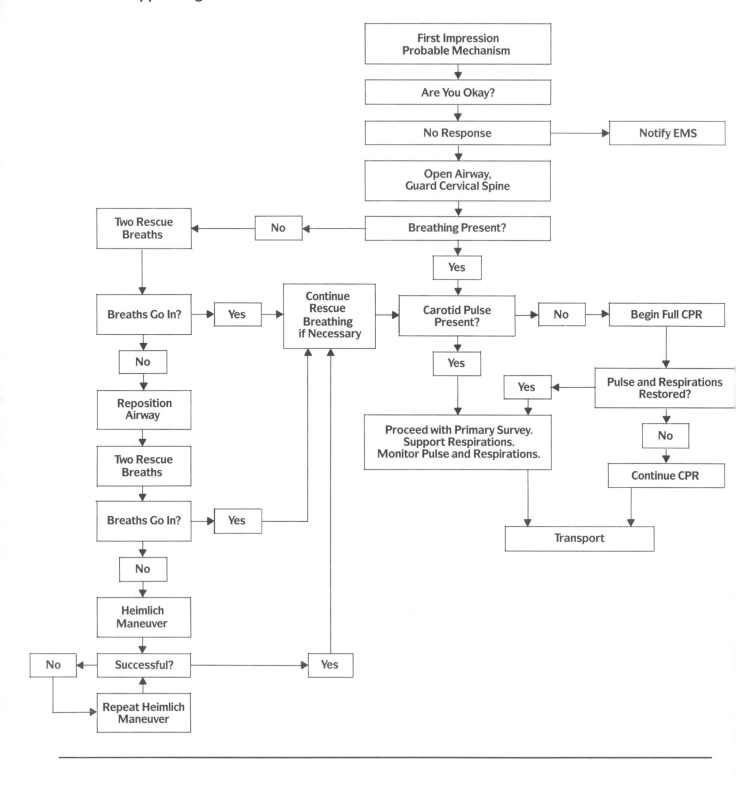

quires widespread training of laypersons in CPR. When there is immediate bystander CPR, the patient is two to three times more likely to survive.

3. **Early defibrillation**, which has been shown to increase survival since it can often restore a spontaneous heartbeat.
4. **Early ACLS**, which stabilizes the patient by securing the airway with intubation and supporting the heartbeat with special drugs.

An even more important public health measure is the *prevention* of coronary artery disease. Some major risk factors such as sex, age, and heredity cannot be changed, but others such as cigarette smoking, high blood pressure, elevated blood cholesterol, and diabetes can be eliminated or treated. Maintaining normal weight and engaging in regular aerobic exercise also appear to help prevent heart disease.

The techniques of basic life support described below follow the recommendations of the 1992 National Conference on Cardiopulmonary Resuscitation (CPR) and Emergency Cardiac Care (ECC) as published in the October 28, 1992, issue of the *Journal of the American Medical Association*. Since instructor's guidelines based on these recommendations have not been published at the time of this writing, I have also made some assumptions based on what I think these guidelines will be. Future conferences may further modify some of the material presented in this chapter. Remember that skills must be *refreshed* regularly if rescuers are to perform effective basic life support.

Basic life support includes techniques for **rescue breathing, closed chest cardiac massage**, and **clearing upper-airway obstruction**. Not everyone who collapses needs these techniques. For example, after an episode of simple fainting (a common

cause of collapse) the patient will recover without any assistance. Therefore, an important part of basic life support is patient assessment to determine which, if any, life support techniques are needed.

The following description is that of basic life support in adults (including children over the age of eight years). In this appendix, the term "child" refers to a child between the ages of one and eight. Because of anatomical and size differences, some modifications are required when the patient is a child or infant. The major modifications will be noted during the description of adult BLS. They are described in detail in the section on **Pediatric Basic Life Support** in this appendix, and are listed in tables B.5 and B.6.

Adult Basic Life Support

Basic life support is more successful and easier when carried out by two rescuers. However, because only one rescuer may be available, at least initially, the technique for one-rescuer adult basic life support is described first.

As soon as you have reached a patient who has collapsed, perform an immediate assessment as follows (also described in Chapter 4), which should only take a few seconds. Follow each step of assessment with the appropriate basic life support measures. Before starting, put on a pair of rubber gloves and have a mouth shield or pocket mask with a one-way valve handy, if possible.

1. **Determine the mechanism of injury or illness**. It is important to distinguish a patient who collapses because of primary cardiac arrest from one who suffers a secondary cardiac arrest as a result of a serious injury. A spine injury must be assumed in any patient who suffers cardiac arrest accompanying significant trauma.
2. **Assess responsiveness** by tapping or gently shaking the patient on the shoulder and shouting "Are you okay?" (In the case of an infant, shake it gently or flick the bottom of its

Fig. B.1 *Shout for help if the patient is unresponsive.*

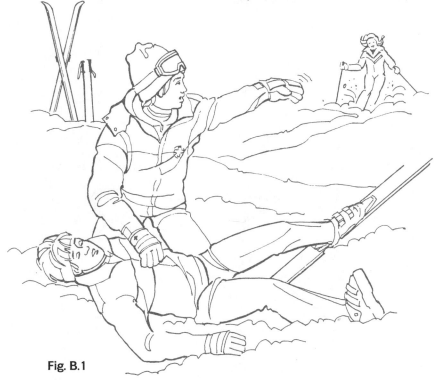

Fig. B.1

foot and call "Baby, baby!") Steady the patient's head with your other hand while you do this. If the patient is truly unresponsive, there will be no reaction. If the patient reacts in any manner, such as by moaning, opening the eyes, or moving, cardiac arrest is not present and you should proceed with the primary survey as described in Chapter 4. Otherwise, immediately shout for help (Fig. B.1). Send someone to telephone the local emergency number (often this is 911) or otherwise notify the EMS system so an ambulance can be summoned. If you are alone and there is a telephone nearby, notify the EMS system yourself.

The EMS dispatcher will need the following information: what happened (i.e., sudden collapse, asphyxiation, drowning, etc.); the location, including street address, directions, and landmarks if

necessary; the telephone number from which the call is being made; the number of patients; the condition of the patient(s); and the type of emergency care being given. The caller should not hang up before the EMS dispatcher hangs up. In the excitement and confusion of the moment, it is easy to forget the essential information you need to give the EMS dispatcher. Regular practice in making this type of telephone call is essential.

3. **Position the patient supine** on a firm, flat surface with the head no lower than the chest. If the patient must be moved or turned, treat the head and body as a unit, if at all possible, so that the back and neck are not twisted or bent (Fig. B.2). Place the patient's arms beside the body. Kneel by the patient's shoulder, facing the patient.

4. **Open the airway.** In the unresponsive patient, the muscles of the upper airway relax,

allowing the tongue to fall back and close the airway by obstructing the pharynx. Because the tongue is attached to the lower jaw, any maneuver that brings the lower jaw *forward* should open the airway. Ideally, such maneuvers should cause minimal bending or twisting of the neck to prevent worsening an undetected neck fracture. However, because the patient will die if the airway is not opened and breathing is not restored, it is acceptable to bend the neck slightly if necessary to open the airway. Neck injuries are unusual in patients who collapse from cardiac arrest.

The preferred method of opening the airway is the **head-tilt/chin-lift technique** (Fig. B.3). Place one hand on the patient's forehead and tilt the patient's head back. At the same time, using your other hand, place several fingertips under the tip of the patient's chin just behind the point of the jawbone and lift to bring the chin forward. Do not use your thumb to lift the chin. The

Fig. B.2 *Positioning a Patient for Basic Life Support*

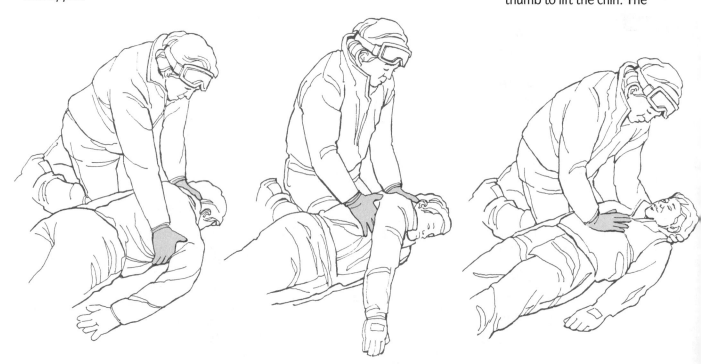

Fig. B.2

patient's mouth should be partly open. If it is necessary to open the patient's mouth, use the **crossed-finger technique** (Fig. B.4a). If the patient is wearing dentures and they are loose, remove them. If they are fixed in place, leave them. Also, remove any visible foreign material with a hooked finger or a piece of cloth (Fig. B.4b).

In the adult or child, if the head-tilt/chin-lift method does not open the airway, or if a neck injury is suspected, use the **jaw-thrust technique** (Fig. B.5). This technique is very effective in opening the airway but is technically difficult and will slow the CPR process if only one rescuer is available. Place the ring and little fingers of each hand behind the angles of the patient's mandible and use them to thrust the jaw forward while stabilizing the patient's head and neck with your thumbs, palms, and remaining fingers. During this maneuver, rest your elbows on the surface on which the patient is lying. Do *not* use the jaw-thrust technique on infants.

5. **Assess breathing** (Fig. B.6). Once the airway is open, determine whether the patient is breathing spontaneously by observing whether the chest rises and falls, listening for the escaping air (place your ear next to the patient's mouth and nose), and feeling for the flow of air. This should only take three to five seconds. If the patient is not breathing, begin rescue breathing (step 6). If the patient is breathing ineffectively (see section on **Respirations** in Chapter 19), assist respirations with rescue breathing. An unresponsive patient in whom trauma is unlikely and who has effective spontaneous respirations should be turned into the semiprone or "recovery" position (Fig. 12.3, Chapter 12).

6. **Rescue breathing** (Fig. B.7). In rescue breathing, air is transferred from the rescuer's respiratory system to the patient's respiratory system. This technique is successful because exhaled air retains sufficient oxygen (16 percent) to maintain life. The AIDS epidemic has caused concerns about contracting AIDS, hepatitis B, and other infections through direct mouth-to-mouth resuscitation. Even though no case of AIDS or hepatitis is known to have been transmitted in this manner to date, the viruses of both diseases have been found in human saliva. It is universally recommended that rescuers carry mouth shields or pocket masks to use when performing rescue breathing or CPR, or use a bag-valve-mask. A mouth shield or pocket mask should be made of clear, soft plastic and have a mouthpiece with a one-way valve (Fig. B.8). Directions for use are found in Chapter 5.

Since much CPR given by laypersons is performed on friends and relatives where the chances of contracting disease are minimal and mouth shields and masks may not be at hand, both mouth-to-mouth and mouth-to-mouthpiece rescue breathing are described. The term "rescue breathing" is used for both mouth-to-mouth and mouth-to-mouthpiece respiratory resuscitation.

Keep the patient's airway open, and if you are not using a mask, pinch the nostrils closed to prevent air from escaping through the nose. If the airway is maintained with the head-tilt/chin-lift technique, use the thumb and index finger of the hand on the patient's forehead to pinch the nostrils closed. If the jaw-thrust technique is used, you may have to press your cheek across the patient's nostrils to close them.

Fig. B.3 *Opening the Airway with the Head-tilt/Chin-lift Technique*

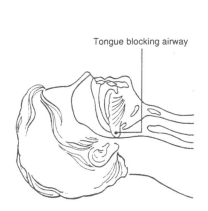
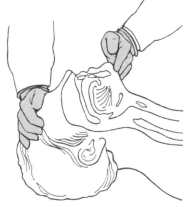
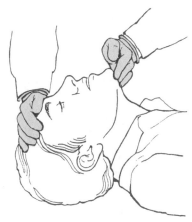

Tongue blocking airway

Fig. B.3

Take a deep breath, and seal your lips around the patient's lips (or in the case of an infant, the mouth and nose) or the mouthpiece of the device. Give two rescue breaths of one-and-one-half to two seconds each. (Counting "one and two" at a normal speaking rate equals approximately one-and-one-half seconds.)

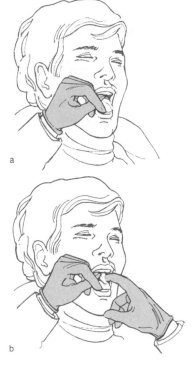

a

b

Fig. B.4

Take a deep breath before each rescue breath. The patient's chest should rise and fall with each breath, and you should hear and feel air escaping during exhalation. Allow the patient to exhale completely between breaths.

If this is unsuccessful, the patient's airway probably is still not open. Reposition the patient's head and chin (or jaw) and repeat rescue breathing. If a second set of breaths is unsuccessful, a foreign body may be blocking the airway. The technique for relieving airway obstruction caused by a foreign body is described below in the section on **Upper-Airway Obstruction**.

Fig. B.4 *Open the patient's mouth with the crossed-finger technique and remove visible foreign material with a hooked finger.*

Fig. B.5 *Opening the Airway with the Jaw-thrust Technique*

Fig. B.6 *Determine if the patient is breathing spontaneously.*

Fig. B.7 *Rescue Breathing*

Fig. B.8 *SealEasy Pocket Mask and Microshield*

After two successful rescue breaths, assess circulation by feeling for the pulse of the carotid artery in the adult or child, or the brachial artery in the infant, for five to 10 seconds (Fig. B.9). The carotid artery lies between the trachea and the sternomastoid muscle, just lateral to the Adam's apple. The brachial artery lies against the humerus at the midpoint of the inner arm. It is important that you do not miss a weak or slow pulse because serious complications can be caused by performing external chest compressions on a patient with a pulse. If there is any question, continue assessing for the pulse for several more seconds. Take up to two minutes in patients with hypothermia, because their pulses may be very slow and weak.

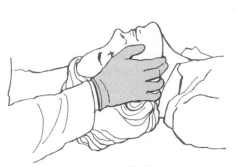

Fig. B.5

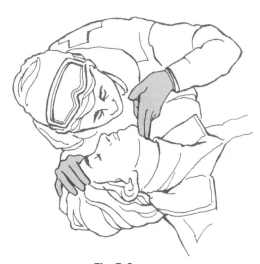

Fig. B.6

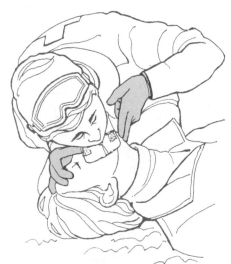

Fig. B.7

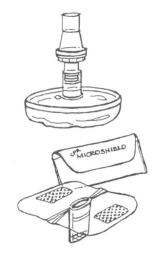

Fig. B.8

If the patient has a pulse but is not breathing spontaneously, continue rescue breathing at a rate of one breath every five seconds for adults (12 breaths per minute), every four seconds for children (15 breaths per minute), and every three seconds for infants (20 breaths per minute). Each breath in the adult should last one-and-one-half to two seconds. Stop rescue breathing every few minutes to see if the patient will start breathing spontaneously. If oxygen is available, attach the oxygen tubing to the intake nipple of the pocket mask or bag-valve-mask. In any unresponsive patient without a gag reflex, an oral airway should be inserted if available.

If you do not have a pocket mask or bag-valve-mask, the **mouth-to-nose technique** (Fig. B.10) may be more effective than mouth-to-mouth in some patients, particularly in the case of facial injury, or when the rescuer cannot open the patient's mouth or achieve a tight seal around the mouth. Maintain an open airway using the head-tilt/chin-lift or jaw-thrust technique, except this time keep the patient's mouth tightly closed. Take a deep breath, seal your lips around the patient's nose, and blow

into the nose. Avoid excessive pressure on injured tissue. Mouth-to-nose rescue breathing is given at the same rate as mouth-to-mouth.

Patients who have had the larynx removed surgically have a permanent opening (stoma) in the front of the neck that connects the trachea directly to the outside. Perform rescue breathing by making an airtight seal around the stoma and blowing until the chest rises, at the same rate as mouth-to-mouth. Other types of patients may have a temporary tube in the trachea (tracheostomy tube). Perform rescue breathing by blowing directly into this tube. To avoid escape of the air through the patient's mouth and nose you may have to seal these with one hand or with a tightly fitting face mask with a one-way valve. Close the valve with your finger.

If there is no pulse, the patient is in cardiac arrest and external chest compressions should be started along with rescue breathing.

Fig. B.9 *Locate the carotid artery lateral to the Adam's apple and check for a pulse.*

Fig. B.10 *Mouth-to-nose Technique of Rescue Breathing*

7. **Start external chest compressions.** Apply pressure over the lower half of the sternum in a regular, rhythmic manner. The cardiac output produced in this way, though only about 20 to 30 percent of normal, is enough to sustain life. Because blood flow to the brain is below normal, the patient's head should not be above the level of the chest. The patient should be lying supine on a firm, flat surface for chest compressions to be effective. If the patient is lying on a soft surface, such as a bed, slide a board under the back or place him or her on the floor.

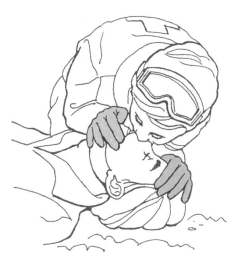

Fig. B.10

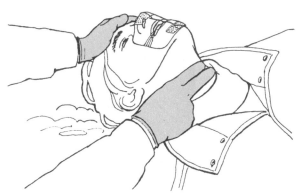

Fig. B.9

The proper hand position is important (Fig. B.11). Continue to kneel facing the patient at shoulder level, and use the middle and index fingers of the hand nearer the patient's feet to locate the costal arch (B.11a). Slide your fingers up the arch until your middle finger is in the notch between the two costal arches (B.11b). Then place your index finger next to your middle finger on the lower end of the sternum. Place the heel of your other hand on the lower half of the sternum, next to your index finger (B.11c). Place the first hand on top of and parallel to the hand on the sternum (B.11d). Your fingers should be pointing across the sternum and should be kept off the patient's chest.

To achieve proper compressions, straighten your arms and lock your elbows. Keep your shoulders above your hands so that the thrust for each compression is directed straight down (Fig. B.12).

Depress the patient's sternum 1½ to 2 inches with each compression. Release pressure on the chest completely between compressions, but do not lift your hands off the chest. Perform compressions at a rate of 80 to 100 per minute. To aid in timing, count briskly "*one*-and-*two*-and-*three*-and," etc. Modifications of the hand positions and compression rates in smaller children and infants are described in the section on **Pediatric Basic Life Support** and are listed in Table B.5.

Fig. B.11 *Locating the Proper Hand Position for Chest Compressions*

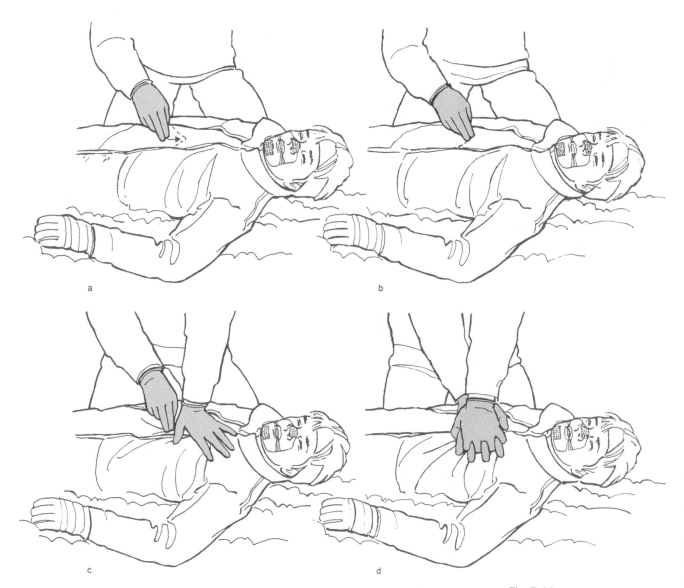

a

b

c

d

Fig. B.11

Table B.2

Information to Give the EMS Dispatcher

1. What happened.
2. Where it happened: Location, street address, map coordinates if appropriate, nearby landmarks or prominent structures, telephone number of phone from which call is being made.
3. Number of patients.
4. Condition of patients.
5. Emergency care being given.

One-Rescuer Adult CPR

In one-rescuer CPR (Fig. B.13), maintain a ratio of two breaths to 15 compressions. After completing 15 chest compressions, move quickly to the patient's head, open the airway, and deliver two rescue breaths of one-and-one-half to two seconds each. Move quickly to the patient's chest, locate the proper hand position, and give another set of 15 chest compressions. Give CPR for one minute (i.e., four complete cycles of 15 chest compressions interspersed with two rescue breaths), and then reassess the patient. Check the carotid pulse for three to five seconds and, if it is absent, resume CPR. The sequence is: 2:15, 2:15, 2:15, 2:15, 2: (pulse check) 15, 2:15, 2:15, etc.

It is obvious that using a pocket mask or employing the jaw-thrust technique of opening the airway may make it more difficult to give the desired number of compressions and ventilations per minute.

If a pulse is present, check breathing for three to five seconds. If breathing is absent, continue rescue breathing at a rate of one breath every five seconds (adult rate), and closely monitor the pulse. If breathing is present, stop CPR and monitor

breathing and pulse. If CPR must be continued, check for the return of a spontaneous pulse and spontaneous breathing every few minutes. Do not interrupt CPR for more than seven seconds except in certain circumstances (see below).

One-rescuer CPR maintains marginally adequate circulation and ventilation. It is less effective and more exhausting for the rescuer than two-rescuer CPR. When a second rescuer

Fig. B.12 *Proper Arm Position for Chest Compressions*

Fig. B.13 *One-rescuer CPR*

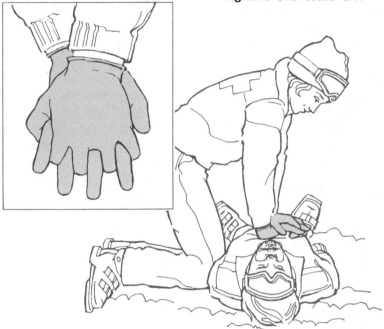

Fig. B.12

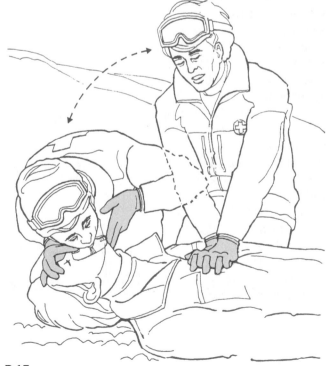

Fig. B.13

arrives, it is preferable to switch to two-rescuer CPR (described below). When changing rescuers in one- or two-rescuer CPR or changing positions in two-rescuer CPR, the change should be done as *quickly and efficiently as possible so that a minimum of interruption occurs.*

A second rescuer who arrives and offers to take over one-rescuer CPR should say, "I'll take over when you've completed the next two breaths and the pulse check," and then move to the patient's chest to locate the hand position. The new rescuer starts chest compressions as soon as the first rescuer says "No pulse."

A suitable sequence is: 2:15, 2:15, 2:15, 2: (pulse check) (new rescuer) 15, 2:15, etc.

Two-Rescuer Adult CPR

If two rescuers are available at the onset, one rescuer goes to the patient's head and determines responsiveness. If the second rescuer will notify the EMS system, the first rescuer initiates one-rescuer CPR. Otherwise, the first rescuer positions the patient, opens the airway, and assesses for breathing. If breathing is absent, the first rescuer says "No breathing" and gives two rescue breaths of one-and-one-half to two seconds each. As in one-rescuer CPR, if the air does not go in, the first rescuer repositions the airway, then gives a second set of two ventilations. If these are also unsuccessful, the first rescuer proceeds with techniques for relieving upper-airway obstruction described below. If the air does go in, the first rescuer then assesses the pulse, and if it is absent, says "No pulse." Simultaneously, the second rescuer, kneeling at the patient's other side, has been locating the proper hand position so that external chest compressions can be started after the first rescuer says "No pulse."

Two-rescuer CPR continues with the rescuer positioned at the patient's side performing external chest compressions and the rescuer on the opposite side at the patient's head maintaining an open airway, providing rescue breathing, and monitoring the carotid pulse for adequacy of chest compressions (Fig. B.14). The ratio of ventilations to compressions is 1:5 rather than 2:15, with a pause of one-and-one-half to two seconds between each set of five compressions to allow for ventilation. Check the pulse during compressions to evaluate their effectiveness. Stop chest compressions for five seconds after one minute (10 cycles of five compressions and one breath) and every few minutes thereafter to see if pulse and breathing have returned.

The sequence is: 1:5, 1:5, 1:5, 1:5...(for 10 cycles), 1: (pulse check) 5, 1:5, 1:5, 1:5, etc.

If the rescuer responsible for compressions becomes fatigued, the two should switch positions. The best time is just after a cycle of five compressions. The rescuer doing the chest compressions calls out "**switch**-and-two-and-three-and-four-and-five-and..." after which he or she moves to the patient's head, takes over the head-tilt/chin-lift position, gives one rescue breath, checks the pulse, and if absent, says "No pulse." Meanwhile, the other rescuer has moved to the chest and located the proper hand position. This rescuer starts chest compressions after the other rescuer says "No pulse."

A suitable sequence is: 1:5, 1:5, 1: "Switch," 2, 3, 4, 5, (rescuers change places) 1: (rescuer who was giving the compressions rechecks pulse) 5, 1:5, 1:5, etc.

If two rescuers arrive to replace a single rescuer giving CPR, the switch is made at a pulse check, in a manner such as the following sequence: 2:15, 2:15, 2:15, 2: (the first rescuer backs off and one of the new rescuers does the pulse check while the other rescuer is locating the hand position on the chest) 5, 1:5, 1:5, 1:5, etc.

If a single rescuer performing CPR is joined by a second rescuer and they change to two-rescuer CPR, the second rescuer locates the hand position on the patient's chest while the first rescuer is giving the two breaths be-

Fig. B.14 *Two-rescuer CPR*

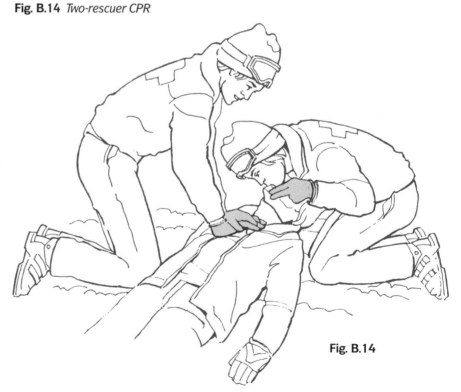

Fig. B.14

fore a pulse check. The second rescuer starts chest compressions when the first rescuer says "No pulse" after the pulse check. A suitable sequence is: 2:15, 2:15, 2:15, 2: (first rescuer rechecks pulse) 5 (second rescuer starts chest compressions), 1:5, 1:5, etc.

Upper-Airway Obstruction

The causes of upper-airway obstruction are listed in Table 1.2, Chapter 1. Upper-airway obstruction may either cause or be the result of unresponsiveness. For example, a patient who is unresponsive due to a head injury or seizure may develop upper-airway obstruction when the tongue, relaxed throat tissues, or vomitus blocks the pharynx. Upper-airway obstruction may lead to unresponsiveness as the brain is deprived of oxygen when the airway is blocked by such things as injured tissue or blood clots in the case of a facial injury or by snow in the case of avalanche burial. Acute airway obstruction caused by food particles can resemble cardiac arrest—the so-called "cafe coronary." Because CPR is ineffective if the airway is obstructed, techniques to relieve upper-airway obstruction are important in basic life support and, if needed, *should be performed before beginning external chest compressions*.

In adults, foreign-body obstruction of the airway most commonly occurs during eating. Meat is a frequent culprit. Important associated factors are drinking alcohol, wearing dentures, and failing to chew food properly. In children, obstruction is most commonly caused by the accidental aspiration of peas, nuts, popcorn, beads, or other small objects.

The following precautions will decrease the incidence of foreign-body obstruction in adults and children:

1. Cut food into small pieces and chew each bite slowly and thoroughly (especially important for those who wear dentures).
2. Avoid laughing or talking while chewing and swallowing.
3. Avoid excessive alcohol intake around mealtime.
4. Prevent children from running or playing with food in their mouths.
5. Prevent children from placing foreign objects in their mouths.
6. Keep small, hard objects such as peanuts, beads, and marbles away from small children.

Upper-Airway Obstruction in Adults

Recognition of Foreign-Body Airway Obstruction

Foreign-body obstruction of the upper airway can cause death quickly yet is treatable if recognized early. Therefore, its prompt recognition is the cornerstone of its successful emergency care. Almost 4,000 deaths occur annually from foreign-body obstruction of the airway.

Airway obstruction must be distinguished from simple fainting, stroke, heart attack, seizure, drug overdose, and other conditions that have similar signs and symptoms but are managed differently. Airway obstruction may be either complete or partial. With partial obstruction, the patient is still able to inhale some air into the lungs. If air exchange is good and the patient can still cough forcefully (although there may be some wheezing between coughs), encourage the patient to cough and attempt to expel the foreign body while being monitored by the rescuer. Either the patient will expel it, the obstruction will persist unchanged, or the condition will progress to poor air exchange or complete obstruction. If the patient does not expel the foreign body rapidly, or if air exchange becomes poor, notify the EMS system. Poor air exchange is indicated by a weak, ineffective cough, increased respiratory distress, and eventual development of cyanosis. Stridor, a high-pitched, crowing noise on *inhalation*, occasionally is present as well.

A *responsive* patient with complete airway obstruction is unable to speak, breathe, or cough, and frequently will clutch the neck (Fig. B.15). This universal distress signal should be taught to the public and to rescuers. Ask, "Are you choking?" If the patient is unable to reply, he or she usually will nod the head. In an *unresponsive* patient with complete airway obstruction, the rescuer will be unable to ventilate the patient even after repositioning the airway.

The Heimlich Maneuver

The Heimlich maneuver is recommended for relieving partial upper-airway obstruction with poor air exchange and complete upper-airway obstruction in adults and children but not in infants. It uses the residual air in the lungs to expel a foreign object blocking the upper airway.

The rescuer, or the patient (Fig. B.19), administers a sudden abdom-

Fig. B.15 *Universal Distress Signal for Choking*

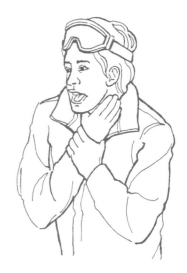

Fig. B.15

inal thrust, which increases intra-abdominal pressure, driving the diaphragm upward and emptying the residual air from the lungs. The force of the expelled air frequently is sufficient to drive the obstructing material out of the airway like a bullet fired from a gun. The maneuver may have to be repeated many times to clear the airway. The rescuer's hands must be properly positioned (Fig. B.16) to obtain maximum effectiveness and to avoid injury to abdominal or thoracic organs. However, despite the best technique the maneuver occasionally causes organ damage or regurgitation of material from the stomach.

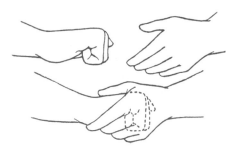

Fig. B.16

Patient Responsive, Standing or Sitting

If the patient is standing (Fig. B.17), stand behind the patient, wrapping your arms around his or her waist. If the patient is sitting, crouch behind the patient's chair and reach around its back and around the patient's waist. The proper hand position (see Fig. B.16) is to place the thumb side of one fist against the midline of the patient's abdominal wall just above the navel and well below the tip of the xiphoid process. With your other hand, grasp the fist and press it into the patient's abdomen, giving repeated, quick, upward thrusts. Relieve the abdominal pressure completely between thrusts.

Patient Lying Down, Usually Unresponsive

If the patient is lying down and is prone, turn the patient to the supine position (see Fig. B.2) and kneel

---

Fig. B.16 *Proper Way to Position the Hands for the Heimlich Maneuver*

Fig. B.17 *Performing the Heimlich Maneuver on a Standing Patient*

Fig. B.18 *Performing the Heimlich Maneuver on a Supine Patient*

astride the patient's thighs, facing the patient's head. Place the heel of one hand on the patient's abdomen just above the navel and well below the tip of the xiphoid, with the second hand on top of the first. Press into the abdomen, giving quick, repeated, upward thrusts at a slow rate (Fig. B.18). When using the Heimlich maneuver, each thrust should always be a separate and distinct movement given with the intent of relieving the obstruction. Relieve the abdominal pressure completely between thrusts.

Use the finger sweep (Fig. B.4) to remove foreign material from the mouth of an unresponsive adult or older child (but not an infant or a seizure patient). Open the patient's mouth, grasp both the tongue and the lower jaw between your thumb and fingers, and lift the mandible. This draws the tongue forward. Insert the index finger of your other hand along the side of the cheek and deeply into the throat at the base of the tongue. Use a hooking motion to bring the foreign body up into the mouth where it can be removed. Be careful not to force the material deeper, and remember that you may be in danger of being bitten.

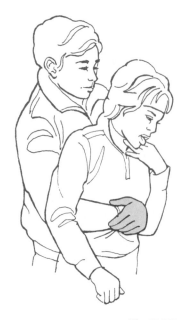

Fig. B.17

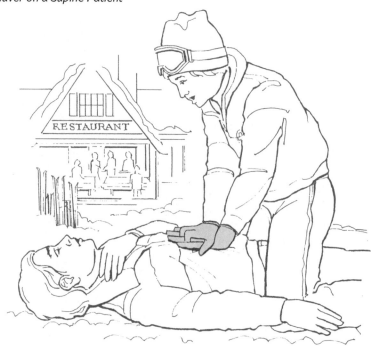

Fig. B.18

Self-Administered Heimlich Maneuver

The self-administered Heimlich maneuver (Fig. B.19) allows you to dislodge a foreign body from your own throat. Position your hands as shown in Figure B.16. If you are unsuccessful after several thrusts, press the upper abdomen quickly and repeatedly against any firm surface, such as the back of a chair, side of a table, or porch railing.

Modifications of the Heimlich Maneuver in Pregnant or Obese Patients

Chest thrusts rather than abdominal thrusts are performed on markedly obese patients or patients in the late stages of pregnancy (Fig. B.20). Stand behind the patient and wrap your arms around the patient's chest under the armpits. Place your fist over the *lower sternum, with the thumb at the middle of the sternum*, avoiding the ribs and the xiphoid process. Grasp your fist with the other hand and press backward, giving quick, repeated thrusts.

The same hand position shown in Figure B.18 is used for the pregnant or obese patient who is lying down, except that it is applied on the *lower half of the sternum* instead of between the navel and the xiphoid. Turn a prone patient to the supine position and kneel close to the patient's body facing the patient's head.

Fig. B.19 *Self-administered Heimlich Maneuver*

Fig. B.20 *Chest Thrusts on an Obese Patient*

Table B.3

Sequence for Responsive Adult with Obstructed Airway

1. When airway obstruction is suspected, ask, "Are you choking?" If the patient cannot speak, use the Heimlich maneuver and have someone notify the EMS system.
2. Repeat the Heimlich maneuver until the foreign body is expelled or the patient becomes unresponsive.
3. If the patient becomes unresponsive, open the patient's mouth and perform the finger sweep.
4. Open the airway and give two rescue breaths.
5. If the breaths fail to go in, perform additional (up to five) subdiaphragmatic abdominal thrusts (or, in the case of the pregnant or obese patient, lower sternal thrusts).
6. Open the mouth and repeat the finger sweep.
7. Position the airway and attempt two rescue breaths.
8. If unsuccessful, repeat the Heimlich maneuver, finger sweep, and attempts at rescue breathing (steps 5, 6 and 7).
9. Continue with these sequences until the airway is clear, you are relieved by another responsible person, you are exhausted, or the patient is pronounced dead by a physician or other qualified person.

Table B.4

Sequence for Unresponsive Adult with Obstructed Airway

1. If you cannot perform rescue breathing although the airway has been opened with the head-tilt/chin-lift or jaw-thrust techniques, reposition the head and chin, or jaw, and repeat two rescue breaths.
2. If unsuccessful, perform up to five subdiaphragmatic thrusts (or, in the case of the pregnant or obese patient, lower sternal thrusts).
3. Perform the finger sweep.
4. Open the airway and repeat two rescue breaths.
5. If unsuccessful, continue to repeat steps 2, 3, and 4 until the airway is clear, you are relieved by another responsible person, you are exhausted, or the patient is pronounced dead.

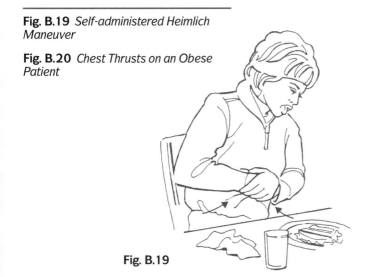

Fig. B.19

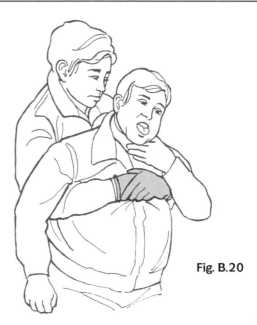

Fig. B.20

Pediatric Basic Life Support

Cardiac arrest in infants and children is more commonly caused by shock or abnormal respiratory system function—particularly respiratory arrest—than by primary heart disease. Both shock and respiratory system abnormalities affect the heart by reducing blood oxygen levels. The long period of hypoxia that usually precedes cardiac arrest in infants and children is one reason for their low survival rate (less than 10 percent) following CPR. Conversely, survival following rescue breathing for respiratory arrest alone is much higher in children (close to 50 percent) than in adults.

Common causes of respiratory and cardiac arrest include head injuries, injuries with shock, suffocation (as from crawling into a plastic bag), aspiration of small objects such as beads or peanuts, smoke inhalation during fires, injuries to the face or neck, respiratory infections, drowning, poisoning, and sudden infant death syndrome (SIDS).

Many of these childhood emergencies are preventable. Do not allow infants and children to play with matches, cigarette lighters, sharp objects, small objects such as beads and marbles, or toys with small, removable parts (Fig. B.21). Keep firearms away from children. Provide smoke detectors for your dwelling. Use car seats and seat belts in moving vehicles. Promote the wearing of helmets when riding bicycles. Teach children swimming and water safety at an early age. Encourage campaigns against drunk driving.

The sequence of CPR for infants and children follows the same principles as that for adults, but the techniques are modified somewhat because of the smaller size, anatomical differences, and higher metabolic rates of these patients. An infant usually is defined as a child under one year of age (i.e., who has not yet begun to walk well and who is small enough to be supported on your forearm or thigh).

Basic life support always is given with the patient in the supine position. If the child is found prone, turn its body as a unit, firmly supporting the head so that the neck is not bent or twisted. The child's air passages are smaller and more easily obstructed by mucus, blood, or vomitus. The head-tilt/chin-lift technique is the preferred method for opening the airway. The jaw-thrust technique is not used in infants. It is used in children only if the head-tilt/chin-lift technique fails or if a neck injury is likely. Avoid overextension of the neck, which may cause or aggravate airway obstruction. In a patient with respiratory arrest, open the airway and give one minute of rescue breathing *before* you activate the EMS system.

In smaller children and infants, perform rescue breathing with the rescuer's mouth over *both* the mouth and nose of the child (Fig. B.22). Rescue breaths should last one to one-and-one-half seconds ("one and" said at a normal speaking rate equals one second) and should make the patient's chest rise. The volume of air needed is less than for an adult. The rescue breathing rate is once every three seconds (20 times a minute) for infants and small children and once every four seconds (15 times a minute) for larger children.

In infants, the brachial artery pulse usually is easier to feel than the carotid pulse, which is used in children. If external chest compressions are required, they are modified as described below:

In a child, compress the chest to a depth of 1 to 1½ inches, using *one* hand rather than two (Fig. B.23a). The hand position is the same as for adults. Chest compressions for infants are performed with only two or three fingers rather than the entire hand (Fig. B.23b). The finger position for chest compressions is as follows: draw an imaginary line between the infant's two nipples, and place the index finger of the hand closest to the infant's feet just under this line where it crosses the sternum. The area of compression lies under the middle and ring fingers. Using these two fingers, compress the sternum to a depth of one-third to one-half of the depth of the chest (usually about ½ to 1 inch).

Fig. B.21 *Keep small objects away from small children.*

Fig. B.22 *Cover both the child's mouth and nose during rescue breathing.*

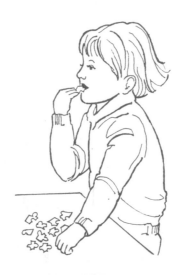

Fig. B.21

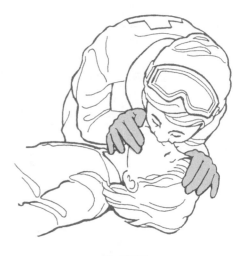

Fig. B.22

For infants and children, maintain a 5:1 ratio of compressions to ventilations. For children, this applies to *both one- and two-rescuer CPR*. The compression rate is 80 to 100 per minute for children and 100 per minute or more for infants.

During one-rescuer CPR in infants, relocating the finger position for chest compression takes so long that the necessary compression rate of 100 or more per minute cannot be maintained. To achieve adequate chest compressions, attempt to maintain an open airway *with the head-tilt only*, so that the finger position on the infant's chest is not lost by using that hand to lift the chin. Watch the infant's chest to make sure it rises and falls with each rescue breath. If the head-tilt alone cannot keep the airway open, the chin-lift will have to be performed before each rescue breath also. In this case, it may be possible to give adequate chest compressions by relocating the finger position *visually* rather than manually. Also consider using a ballpoint pen to mark the finger position location with an X.

In children, usually *both the head-tilt and chin-lift* are needed to maintain an open airway. In one-rescuer CPR, during chest compressions maintain the head-tilt with the hand closest to the patient's head. After every fifth compression, use the hand doing the compressions for the chin-lift and give a rescue breath. Relocate the hand position for chest compressions visually, since finding the landmarks manually requires using both hands and takes so much time that too few chest compressions and rescue breaths will otherwise be given.

Airway Obstruction in Infants and Children

Recognition of Airway Obstruction

A child with airway obstruction is unable to cough, breathe, or speak; may choke; and, as with an adult, may clutch the throat. Ask the child, "Are you choking?" The child may nod. An infant with airway obstruction may choke, turn blue, and is unable to cry, breathe, or cough.

As in the adult, suspect airway obstruction in the unresponsive child or infant if, after positioning the airway twice, rescue breaths still do not go in.

Foreign-body obstruction must be *carefully* distinguished from infections such as croup that cause airway swelling sufficient to obstruct the airway. A foreign body always should be suspected when there are *sudden* signs or symptoms of obstruction in a previously well child, especially when the child has been playing with or eating objects of suitable size.

Airway obstruction caused by croup usually develops slowly and is preceded by a period of hoarseness and the signs and symptoms of an upper-respiratory infection such as runny nose, sore throat, fever, sneezing, and cough. When a child suffers from airway obstruction caused by *infection*, attempts to relieve the obstruction with rescue techniques will be futile. Take the patient to a hospital without delay, assisting ventilations as needed.

Care of Airway Obstruction

Foreign-body airway obstruction in children can be relieved by the Heimlich maneuver; for infants, chest thrusts are used instead because abdominal thrusts are likely to cause damage to the liver or other organs.

Use the Heimlich maneuver for children with complete airway obstruction or partial airway obstruction and poor air exchange in whom aspiration is witnessed or strongly suspected. Also use this maneuver for unconscious, non-breathing children whose airways remain obstructed after the usual maneuvers for opening airways have been attempted. If the child is breathing well and coughing forcefully, do not attempt to relieve the obstruction unless the cough becomes ineffective or the child develops increased difficulty in breathing. This may be accompanied by stridor.

Perform the Heimlich maneuver on children exactly as described above for adults, only do not use blind finger sweeps in small children. In the infant, a modified technique is used to avoid injuring the liver. Lay the infant prone over your forearm so the

Fig. B.23 *Use the heel of one hand for chest compressions on a child, and use two fingers for chest compressions on an infant.*

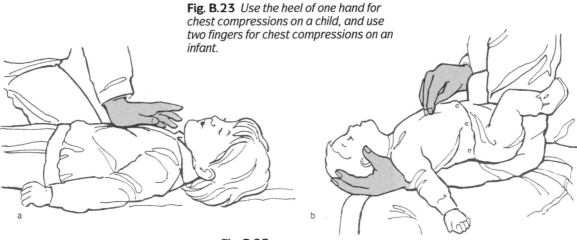

a

b

Fig. B.23

head is lower than the body. Sit with your forearm resting on your thigh. Support the infant's head by grasping the jaw firmly with your fingers. Then, using the heel of your hand, deliver four forceful blows to the infant's back between the shoulder blades (Fig. B.24).

Next, place one hand on the infant's back and turn the infant's body as a unit to the supine position. Place the infant on your thigh or in your lap with the head lower than the body. Deliver four chest thrusts with your fingers at the same location as for CPR external chest compressions but at a slower rate. Open the infant's mouth and perform a visual sweep for a foreign body, removing it with a finger sweep if one is seen. Reposition the airway and attempt to ventilate the infant again. If the breaths do not go in, turn the infant to the prone position on your forearm again and give four more back blows. Continue to alternate back blows and chest thrusts until the airway is clear, you are relieved by another responsible person, are exhausted, or the infant is pronounced dead.

Blind finger sweeps are *not* performed on infants and small children because of the danger of pushing the foreign body further down into the airway.

Tables B.5 and B.6 compare the BLS techniques used in adults, children, and infants.

When to Withhold or Discontinue CPR

In general, CPR should be started on all persons in cardiac arrest, unless it would be futile (i.e., the patient is dead or has a lethal injury); it is not wanted by the patient; or it is not in the patient's best interest (i.e., the patient is in the terminal stages of a fatal disease). Few would insist that CPR be started on a person who is obviously dead or who has sustained a lethal injury such as decapitation, massive open injuries of the head, chest, or abdomen, a severed trunk, or consumption of the body by fire. The signs of death are described in Chapter 19.

CPR also can be withheld when performing it would seriously endanger the rescuer (e.g., one-rescuer CPR with no shelter in very cold, windy weather, or when a valid DNR [Do Not Resuscitate] order is presented to the rescuer).

To ensure that patients whose illnesses are terminal are not inappropriately given CPR, greater emphasis is being given to preparation of living wills and DNR orders that are kept with the patient, with the existence of these documents being made known to caretakers and other household occupants.

Once started, CPR should not be discontinued except in the following situations:

1. Effective spontaneous breathing and circulation are restored.
2. The patient's care is transferred to another trained and responsible person who continues basic life support.
3. The patient's care is transferred to a physician or advanced life support team.
4. The rescuer is unable to continue because of exhaustion.
5. Significant danger to the rescuer(s) develops.
6. An authorized person certifies death. In most states, only physicians are legally authorized to pronounce a person dead.

These rules, while reasonable and proper in an *urban* environment, may be less applicable in a *wilderness* environment. This aspect of CPR is discussed in Appendix C.

Special Situations

A patient in an unsafe location, such as a burning building, should be moved immediately to a safe one before CPR is started. Otherwise, the patient should not be moved until effective CPR has produced a spontaneous pulse or enough help arrives so that CPR can be performed during transport. If a patient must be transported up or down stairs, give CPR for a minute or more before interrupting it, then, at a predetermined signal, move the patient rapidly up or down or to a landing where CPR can be resumed. Special problems at alpine ski areas are discussed in Chapter 17; special problems in the wilderness are discussed in Appendix C.

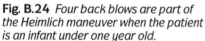

Fig. B.24 *Four back blows are part of the Heimlich maneuver when the patient is an infant under one year old.*

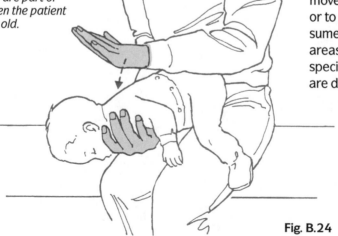

Fig. B.24

Table B.5

CPR Techniques for Patients of Different Ages

	Adult	Child	Infant
Hand position	Middle finger in notch of costal arch, index finger on lower sternum, heel of second hand next to index finger on lower end of sternum. First hand then placed on top of second.	Same as adult	Draw imaginary line between infant's nipples, place index finger of hand closest to infant's feet on sternum, just below this line. Area of compression is at location of middle and ring fingers.
Part of rescuer's hand(s) on chest	Heel of second hand with first hand on top (fingers off chest)	Heel of one hand only	Two or three fingers
Depth of compression of sternum	1½ to 2 inches	1 to 1½ inches	½ to 1 inch
Rate of compressions	80 to 100/min.	80 to 100/min.	>100/min.
Ratio of breaths to compressions *a. One rescuer* *b. Two rescuers*	2:15 1:5	1:5 1:5	1:5 —
Rescue breathing rate: ("one and" equals 1 second)	12/min. (one every 5 seconds)	15/min. (one every 4 seconds)	20/min. (one every 3 seconds)
Rescue breathing duration	1½ to 2 seconds	1 to 1½ seconds	1 to 1½ seconds
Artery monitored for pulse	Carotid	Carotid	Brachial
Recheck carotid pulse for 5 seconds	a. One rescuer: after 1 minute (four cycles), then every few minutes b. Two rescuer: after 1 minute (10 cycles), then every few minutes	a. One rescuer: after 1 minute (10 cycles), then every few minutes b. Two rescuer: Same as adult	Same as child —
Preferred technique of opening airway	Head-tilt/chin-lift or jaw/thrust	Same as adult, avoid over-extension of neck	Head-tilt/chin-lift only, avoid over-extension of neck
Rescue breathing	Mouth (occasionally nose)	Mouth (mouth and nose in small child)	Mouth and nose
Special considerations		One rescuer CPR usually requires both head-tilt and chin-lift, so relocate hand position visually rather than manually to maintain adequate chest compression rate.	To maintain adequate chest compression rate, try to maintain open airway with head-tilt only without losing finger position on chest. If head-tilt and chin-lift both required, relocate hand position on chest visually rather than manually.

Table B.6

Techniques for Relieving Upper Airway Obstruction

	Adult	Pregnant or Obese Adult	Child	Infant
Rescuer's body position	Conscious: Stand or sit behind patient. Lying: Kneel astride patient's thighs.	Conscious: Stand or sit behind patient. Lying: Kneel at patient's side.	Conscious: Same as adult Lying: Same as adult	Conscious: Seated Unconscious: Seated
Hand position	Conscious, standing or sitting: Thumb side of one fist in midline just above navel. Grasp fist with other hand. Lying (unconscious): Heel of hand in midline just above navel with second hand on top of first.	Conscious, standing or sitting: Same as adult, except midsternum instead of abdomen. Lying: Same hand position as standing/sitting but use heel of hand.	Conscious, standing or sitting: Same as adult Lying: Same as adult	Conscious or unconscious: Infant prone on forearm with head lower than body. Support head by grasping jaw with fingers. Give four back blows between scapulae with heel of other hand. Turn infant over on thigh. Give four chest thrusts (same hand position as infant CPR).
Direction of thrust	Upward	Backward	Upward	Backward
Blind finger sweeps?	Yes	Yes	No, visual sweeps only	No, visual sweeps only
Back blows?	No	No	No	Yes
Number of thrusts before repeating rescue breaths	Up to five	Same	Same	Four

Complications of CPR

Gastric Distention

During rescue breathing, air can enter the stomach instead of the lungs, causing the stomach to swell (**gastric distention**). If this swelling is severe, it may interfere with lung expansion by preventing downward motion of the diaphragm. Gastric distention frequently is associated with regurgitation of gastric contents, which may be aspirated into the airway. Although some degree of gastric distention probably occurs in even the most

skillfully performed CPR, it can be minimized by the following steps:

1. Paying attention to proper airway positioning (especially during exhalation).

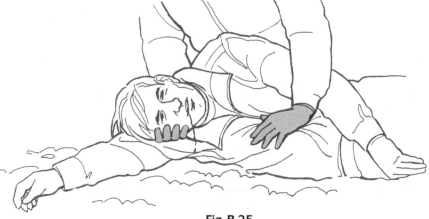

Fig. B.25 *Relieve gastric distention by turning the patient onto one side and pressing on the epigastric area.*

Fig. B.25

2. Providing slow ventilations.
3. Ensuring that the air is going into the lungs and not into the stomach. (See that rescue breaths are making the chest rise rather than the abdomen distend.)
4. Limiting the amount of air blown into the patient's mouth to just enough to make the chest rise.

The latest methods of CPR described in this chapter replace the several rapid breaths used in earlier methods with two slower breaths and are less likely to force air into the stomach. Use of the "Sellick maneuver" also can prevent gastric distension. In this maneuver, one rescuer closes the esophagus by gently pressing backward on the cricoid cartilage each time another rescuer gives a rescue breath.

Massive gastric distention often can be relieved by turning the patient onto one side and pressing on the epigastric area with the hand (Fig. B.25). When this is done, equipment should be available to suction the airway because the patient may regurgitate gastric contents as well as air.

Organ Damage

Rib fractures commonly occur during CPR, especially in older people whose bones are more brittle. While these fractures cannot always be avoided, the rescuer can reduce their frequency by making certain that he or she delivers the compressions to the center rather than the side of the sternum and that compression pressure is not excessive.

Rib fractures usually heal without complications. Damage to the heart, lungs, stomach, and liver occasionally can occur but should be rare in properly performed CPR.

Appendix C

Principles of Wilderness Emergency Care

On the pitiless slabs of the
   Nordwand
Where the bivouac sites are few.
The Ghosts of the hosts of
   Old Masters
Are calling this warning to you:
Live it up, fill your cup, drown
   your sorrow.
And sow your wild oats while
   ye may.
For the toothless old tykes of
   tomorrow
Were the Tigers of Yesterday.

—Tom Patey, M.D.
   "The Last of the Grand
      Old Masters"

The information in this appendix has been included as a guide for wilderness travelers, including members of recreational parties, wilderness search and rescue (SAR) teams, mountain rescue groups, and nordic ski patrols. For these purposes, wilderness means any area where there is no "911" to call; where there are no sophisticated medical facilities and the only emergency care equipment you have is what you have brought along or can improvise; where communications are primitive or nonexistent; where environmental conditions may be so severe you cannot move; and where evacuation to medical care is usually prolonged or delayed.

When most people hear the word "wilderness," they see a mental picture of thick woods or high, snow-covered mountains. Wilderness also can mean arctic ice, subarctic tundra, desert, seashore, tropical savannah or rain forest, the ocean, the underwater world, caverns, and remote, surging rivers.

Exposure to the wilderness may be brief or prolonged. In a sense, an alpine skier caught in a blizzard on a mountaintop is in wilderness, but only briefly unless he or she strays outside the ski area boundary. Nordic skiers or hikers out for a day may be in wilderness for a time, as may cavers in a deep cavern, rafters on an isolated river, scuba divers in the depths, pilots downed in the desert, or mountaineers on the heights. Small-boat sailors, inhabitants of isolated Alaskan villages, and victims of urban disasters whose electricity is cut off and whose medical facilities and communications have been destroyed all can be said to be in wilderness. Wilderness is usually remote but in some cases, areas of true wilderness are so close to inhabited areas that sophisticated rescue teams or helicopters with advanced life support capability can reach a patient within an hour or two after notification.

Successful wilderness existence requires a respect for the forces of nature and at least minimal wilderness-survival training and equipment. Rescuers who operate in nonurban areas also need training in **wilderness emergency care**. The basics of this care have been presented in the previous sections of this textbook and at this point should have been mastered by the reader. In most cases, the emergency care of illnesses and injuries in the wilderness is fundamentally similar to outdoor emergency care anywhere. Most differences arise because the rescuer has to care for the patient over a longer period of time, during which the illness or injury may evolve or be modified by the environment.

The information in this appendix is designed mainly for the reader's personal edification and protection. *Some of this information goes far beyond what rescuers are legally authorized to do at the present time in most states unless they are physicians or physician's assistants. This is particularly true of the sections on the use of prescription drugs and the reduction of dislocations.* Procedures such as inserting Foley catheters, performing cricothyroidotomies, and doing a needle thoracotomy for a tension pneumothorax are reserved for those trained to the paramedic level. They are mentioned here because they are basically simple, easily understandable procedures that require minimal equipment and their risk is outweighed by their value in saving lives or relieving distress. *Even though these procedures may be medically indicated, their inclusion does not imply that the National Ski Patrol endorses procedures or practices that go beyond the usual levels of emergency care described in the body of this text.*

Wilderness emergency care differs from outdoor emergency care in the following specific ways:

1. It is practiced in the wilderness environment, where extreme conditions of heat, cold, altitude, and weather are common and difficulties in obtaining food, water, and shelter are significant. Dangers such as snow avalanches, rockfalls, flash floods, forest fires, and lightning may be present. Hazardous microorganisms, insects, marine animals, land animals, and plants may endanger the health of wilderness travelers, and preexisting medical conditions may recur or flare up at awkward times.

2. Definitive medical care may be many hours or days away because of distance, adverse environmental conditions, interruption of infrastructure components, lack of transportation, or difficulties in communication.

3. Illnesses rarely seen elsewhere, such as acute mountain sickness and deep frostbite, may occur.

4. It may be desirable to train intelligent laypersons to carry out advanced procedures for common injuries and illnesses in which a delay in treatment of more than a few hours or days may cause significant, but otherwise preventable, adverse effects. Simple procedures requiring a minimum of training and equipment but with the potential for saving life or limb are emphasized.

5. There is a need for rescuers to learn extended care (basic nursing care) of an injured or ill person so they can provide for the patient's ordinary day-to-day requirements until medical assistance can be reached.

Wilderness emergency care can be rendered on several levels of complexity and sophistication. The simplest level is self-help first aid for recreational wilderness groups carrying limited emergency equipment and relying on improvisation. The next level is SAR emergency care, in which rescuers trained to the advanced EMT or paramedic level may be available and rescue kits may include more complex and sophisticated equipment. The highest level is expeditionary emergency care and care given by medical workers in isolated villages. In these situations, personnel are highly trained, medical equipment usually is sophisticated, and there is less emphasis on choosing equipment based on its portability.

To apply Otto von Bismarck's comment on politics to the inherent nature of wilderness travel, wilderness emergency care is "the art of the possible." Rescuers cannot carry the equivalent of a hospital emergency room on their backs; instead, they must make do with carefully chosen but limited equipment and rely on thorough training, ingenuity, and their ability to improvise. Patients who are seriously ill or injured may die despite the best care provided in a modern hospital. Thus, rescuers should have a realistic view of their limitations, while at the same time resolving to keep skills sharp and do their best at all times.

Because rescuers who are prepared for potential wilderness hazards can avoid many otherwise inevitable difficulties, prevention is emphasized in previous sections of this text and in this appendix. Enjoyment of the wilderness is enhanced by the knowledge that one has the training to prevent many problems and to deal successfully with those that are unpreventable. Regardless of preparation and training, if a member of a wilderness party is significantly ill or injured, the trip must be aborted and the patient evacuated.

Each member of a wilderness party should start out in good basic health, in good physical condition, and free of acute or chronic infectious disease. If health questions arise, the party leader should require a physician's certificate of physical ability sufficient for the anticipated level of physical stress. Many minor physical abnormalities and illnesses can be controlled sufficiently to allow wilderness travel. These conditions include mild hypertension, minor valvular heart disease, hay fever, asthma, diabetes, and similar ailments.

Other conditions are relative or absolute contraindications to wilderness travel because the condition may flare up under the stress of high altitude or long hours on the trail and/or be difficult to treat in isolated circumstances. These conditions include active peptic ulcers, known kidney, bladder, or gallbladder stones; coronary artery disease; chronic obstructive pulmonary disease; metastatic cancer; a history of severe, recurrent high altitude illness; and disabilities of the musculoskeletal system such as recurrent, severe back pain and severe knee and hip joint disease. Even in its mild form, sickle-cell anemia is a contraindication to high altitude travel and a relative contraindication to severe physical exertion. In borderline or questionable cases, consult a physician familiar with wilderness medical problems.

The party leader should know if any party members have significant health impairments or take any medicines regularly. People who take tranquilizers, antidepressants, beta blockers, and anticholinergics on a regular basis may be more susceptible to wilderness stresses. Beta blockers are mentioned in particular because they are commonly used to treat high blood pressure and can cause chronic fatigue, depression, and deconditioning, poor exercise tolerance, and poor recovery from strenuous exercise.

People who have had anaphylactic reactions to foods, drugs, or arthropod stings should carry emergency kits containing adrenalin and an antihistamine. At least one other party member should know how to use these kits. Those who wear prescription eyeglasses should carry a spare pair, and contact lens wearers should carry a pair of regular glasses as well. Contact lenses can actually freeze to the eyes under severe winter conditions.

Routine immunizations, particularly tetanus, should be up-to-date.

For those wishing to obtain formal instruction in wilderness emergency care, there are a number of organizations that teach Wilderness-EMT and Wilderness First Responder courses. In most cases, prior training to the EMT-basic, Winter Emergency Care, or First Responder level is a prerequisite. A list of currently available courses can be obtained by writing to the Wilderness Medical Society, P.O. Box 2463, Indianapolis, IN 46206, or the National Association for Search and Rescue, P.O. Box 3709, Fairfax, VA 22038.

Patient Assessment in the Wilderness

Patient assessment is the same in the wilderness as in the outdoors in general. Extreme environmental conditions may delay detailed assessment until shelter has been reached. Rescuers should be thoroughly familiar with the assessment of both injured and ill patients, as described in Chapters 4 and 19.

CPR in the Wilderness

Guidelines for starting or stopping CPR are discussed in Chapter 4 and Appendix B. These guidelines, while reasonable and proper in a *traditional* environment, might not be suitable in a remote, outdoor environment.

Eisenberg and his associates studied the rate of survival for patients in cardiac arrest due to ventricular fibrillation, relative to the length of time before basic life support (BLS) and advanced cardiac life support (ACLS) were started. Their findings (Table C.1), reported in the *Journal of the American Medical Association* (241:1905, 1979), showed that the survival rate was only 10 percent if it took more than 16 minutes to start ALS, even if BLS was started within four minutes. If BLS was started after more than eight minutes and ACLS after more than 16 minutes, there was no chance of survival.

Therefore, in a remote area where ALS assistance may be many hours or days away, CPR has little or no chance of success. In addition, administering CPR under wilderness conditions may put group members in serious danger because of physical hazards and exhaustion.

Based on the above data, several suggestions can be made regarding CPR in remote areas. Even though they seem reasonable, they should be viewed as suggestions only. Currently, a rescuer *who begins CPR* is probably obligated to continue unless or until one of the conditions listed in Appendix B is fulfilled. In a remote environment, giving CPR is useless and probably *should not be started* if:

1. The patient is in cardiac arrest caused by trauma.
2. The patient is a drowning victim who has been immersed for over an hour.
3. The patient is in cardiac arrest and advanced life support is more than an hour away, especially if the patient must be carried out.
4. The cardiac arrest was unwitnessed and the time of onset unknown.
5. The patient is hypothermic with an incompressible chest.
6. The patient appears to be dead, based on rigor mortis (stiffening) or livor mortis (discoloration of the body parts next to the ground), lethal injuries, or a body core (rectal) temperature below 60°F (16°C).
7. Giving CPR would be hazardous to rescuers.
8. The patient has a well-defined "do not resuscitate" status.

Moreover, after 30 minutes of CPR with no sign of life, further CPR probably is useless and may reasonably be discontinued. Giving CPR to a patient who is being evacuated by litter or toboggan is very difficult, if not impossible. Unless an ambulance or helicopter can be brought in rapidly, chances of survival are minimal.

Exceptions to the above include the following:

1. Patients with a compressible chest in cardiac arrest caused by hypothermia per se.
2. Patients with another illness or injury complicated by hypothermia (such as avalanche burial and near drowning in cold water).
3. Patients in cardiac or respiratory arrest caused by lightning injury (see Chapter 18).

In all these cases, the outlook is theoretically more favorable and CPR should be given aggressively.

Extended Patient Care (Nursing Care) in the Wilderness

In addition to requiring specific care for illnesses and injuries, patients in the wilderness have certain basic requirements for survival, which for the most part rescuers in the wilderness share.

Basic Survival Requirements for Wilderness Patients

1. Oxygen.
2. Shelter and maintenance of normal body temperature.
3. Water.
4. Food.
5. Psychological support.
6. Assistance with natural processes such as eating, drinking, urination, and defecation.
7. Basic faith and the will to live.

Attention to these requirements will ensure the patient is in the best possible physical and psychological condition during stabilization and transport to definitive medical care.

Table C.1

% Survival Rate

	Time to Advanced Cardiac Life Support		
Time to Basic Life Support		< 8 Min.	8-16 Min.	> 16 Min.
< 4 Min.	43%	19%	10%
4-8 Min.	27%	19%	6%
> 8 Min.	7%	0%	

The initial care of an ill or injured person is no different in the wilderness than anywhere else. While the rescuer performs the primary survey and treats urgent conditions as described in Chapter 4, other party members construct a shelter and prepare to stabilize the patient's body temperature (Fig. C.1).

In cold weather, place insulation beneath and around the patient, cover the patient's head, and replace wet clothing with dry clothing. Also lay out a sleeping bag, start a fire or stove, and erect a tent or prepare a snow shelter. In hot weather, rig a tarp or other shelter as protection against the sun, and in desert conditions prepare a cool surface for the patient to lie on either by scraping away the upper 6 inches of hot earth or by building a platform with backpacks or natural materials. Add or subtract clothing as appropriate to protect the patient against the sun or to prevent a rise in body temperature.

The mechanisms for stabilizing body temperature are always impaired by illness or injury, so that both hypothermia and hyperthermia can develop more easily in an invalid than in a healthy person. The rescue party must look to its own safety, since party members are subject to the same environmental stresses as the patient.

After caring for urgent problems and stabilizing the patient's body temperature, treat less urgent problems and perform the secondary survey so that nothing is missed. In cold weather, expose one small body area at a time for examination.

Normal daily requirements for food and fluid are discussed in Chapter 1. Daily fluid requirements may increase substantially at high altitude, in hot weather, or when the patient has vomiting, diarrhea, extensive burns, or has been perspiring heavily. Give fluids in the form of plain water, soup, bouillon, flavored fruit drinks, or electrolyte-containing sport drinks such as Gatorade or Exceed. Limit the intake of caffeine-containing beverages such as tea, cocoa, and coffee, because caffeine is a diuretic and may increase fluid loss through the kidneys, thereby contributing to dehydration. When a patient is losing large amounts of fluid through vomiting, diarrhea, or extensive burns, measure or estimate the amount of fluid lost and try to replace the lost fluid volume-for-volume with bouillon, sport drinks, or other electrolyte-containing fluids.

The World Health Organization has recommended a standard elec-

Fig. C.1 *Caring for an injured person in the wilderness includes constructing a shelter and stabilizing the patient's body temperature.*

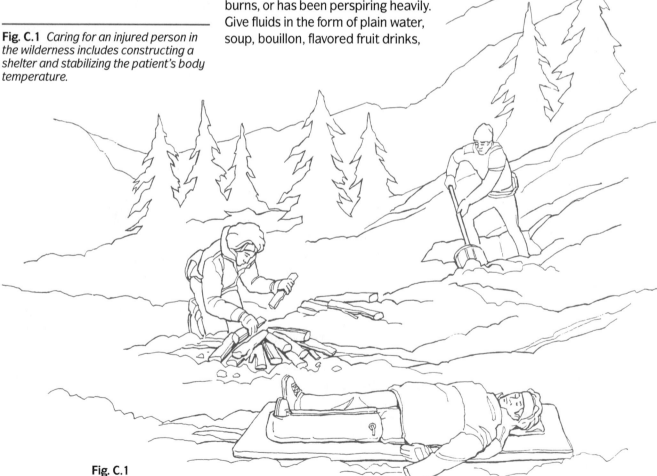

Fig. C.1

trolyte replacement solution for diarrheal illness, designed for use in underdeveloped countries where such illnesses are endemic. This solution for severe diarrheal illness, called Oralyte, contains 90 milliequivalents (mEq) of sodium, 20 mEq of potassium, 80 mEq of chloride, 30 mEq of bicarbonate, and 111 millimoles of glucose per liter. It is prepared by mixing 3.5 grams of table salt, 2.5 grams of sodium bicarbonate (baking soda), 1.5 grams of potassium chloride (available in many pharmacies), and 20 grams of glucose in a liter of water just before use. The solution can be flavored to taste with small amounts of lemon extract or another flavoring agent. Packets containing the right proportions of these compounds can be made up beforehand and carried in first aid kits. Oralyte is better than sport drinks for initial replacement of fluids lost by vomiting and diarrhea because it contains more electrolytes. After the patient improves, sport drinks can be used instead of Oralyte.

In patients with diarrhea, fluid losses sometimes can be reduced by giving drugs that control diarrhea by slowing the motility of the bowel (see **Stomach and Bowel Problems** below). Patients who are vomiting because of an illness that does not interfere greatly with stomach or bowel function, such as acute mountain sickness, headache, or mild gastroenteritis, may be able to eat and drink if vomiting can be controlled with an anti-vomiting suppository such as thiethylperazine (Torecan) or prochlorperazine (Compazine). Side effects of these drugs are similar, and include drowsiness, dizziness, blurred vision, skin rash, and low blood pressure. Muscle spasms, especially of the neck, occur occasionally, particularly with prochlorperazine. They can be relieved by the antihistamine diphen-

hydramine (Benadryl, see Appendix D), available without prescription. Take two 25-milligram (mg) capsules immediately by mouth.

Do not give these drugs or, for that matter, anything by mouth to patients who are vomiting because of a head or abdominal injury, who are unconscious, who have abdominal injuries, or who are expected to have surgery within six to eight hours.

Some SAR groups include members who are trained and licensed to give intravenous fluids, which are very useful in these circumstances. An average daily IV fluid prescription for a patient unable to eat or drink is 2,500 milliliters (ml) of 5-percent glucose in 0.45-percent ("half-normal") physiological saline solution with 20 milliequivalents potassium chloride added per liter. If the patient also is having vomiting or diarrhea, estimate the additional fluid losses and replace this lost fluid volume with equal amounts of the same solution or with lactated Ringer's solution *in addition* to the daily fluid prescription. In most cases, normal kidneys select what the body needs and excrete the remainder.

Collect and measure the volume of all urine excreted by the patient. If urine output is less than 500 ml (17 ounces) per 24 hours, the patient probably is dehydrated and needs more fluid. Urine normally is light yellow when hydration is adequate, but it may be orange-colored in patients with severe illness or injury, cola-colored in patients who have liver disease with jaundice, and bright yellow in people who take vitamin tablets containing riboflavin (Vitamin B2).

Liquids are a more urgent requirement than food, because a previously healthy person can go without eating for many days without permanent damage. Patients who are nauseated and would vomit ordinary amounts of liquid may be able to tolerate frequent sips of small amounts. Those who are able to tolerate solid food

should eat a light, bland diet with no spicy or rich foods. Water, oatmeal, Cream of Wheat, bland soup, broth, Jello, bread, hard candy, and sweet herb tea usually are well tolerated. The invalid should be allowed to eat as desired and not be forced to eat.

Provisions must be made so that the patient can urinate and defecate. A wide-mouth screw-top polyethylene bottle ("pee bottle") of 500- to 1000-ml capacity can be used as a urinal. SAR teams can carry lightweight commercially marketed plastic urinals. Patients can defecate in the supine position if they are placed on an Ensolite pad with a hole cut in it or on carefully arranged clothing, and then positioned over a hole dug in the ground or snow. Always ask patients whether they have to urinate or defecate and allow them to do so *before* they are packaged in a litter or on a spine board.

Unconscious or severely injured patients may be unable to urinate. Members of SAR groups and expeditions should be encouraged to obtain the special training necessary to insert Foley catheters, which should be included in SAR first aid kits. If a catheter is unavailable, nothing can be done except to evacuate the patient with a pee bottle or urinal lying in place to catch urine that may be voided spontaneously. It is important to prevent the patient's clothing from becoming wet with urine, especially in cold weather.

Adequate pain relief is necessary for humanitarian reasons and to prevent shock. Serious wilderness travelers may wish to have their physicians prescribe pain medicines such as acetaminophen with codeine (Tylenol with codeine), meperidine (Demerol), or propoxyphene with acetaminophen (Darvocet-N) so that small amounts of these drugs can be carried for personal use. Side effects of acetaminophen with codeine and meperidine are similar and can include lightheadedness, dizziness, sleepiness, shortness of breath, nausea, vomiting, and constipation. Meperidine can also cause sweating and respiratory depression. Propoxyphene can cause dizziness, sleepiness, nausea, and vomiting.

As with all drugs in first aid kits, the containers should be labeled with the name of the medicine, the rescuer's name, the prescribing doctor's name, and directions for use. Ask your druggist to add the expiration date of the lot as well. Try out pain medications at home first on headaches and other painful conditions to ensure that they are effective in relieving pain and do not cause dizziness, sleepiness, or other undesirable side effects. Leaders of prolonged wilderness trips should consider requiring *each* trip member to carry such drugs since current state and federal regulations do not allow a rescuer to *give* these drugs to patients unless the rescuer is appropriately licensed or under physician supervision. However, a patient may *take* such drugs under his or her *own* responsibility and may be assisted if necessary. No one should take a drug to which he or she is known to be allergic.

For extended wilderness trips and expeditions, injectable pain medication is useful—especially in patients who cannot swallow pills—but must be administered by an individual who is trained and authorized to inject it. Wyeth Laboratories markets codeine, meperidine, and morphine in prefilled, single-dose Tubex containers. These pain drugs should *not* be given to patients with head injuries or high altitude cerebral edema (HACE).

Rescuers must not let reliance on pain medication lead them to neglect traditional pain-reducing emergency care procedures such as aligning and splinting fractures.

Adhere to the usual habits of cleanliness and sanitation as closely as possible in the wilderness. Carry soap, preferably the biodegradable kind, and use it to wash your hands after a bowel movement, before cooking and eating, and before dressing open wounds. Cover food against flies. Carry and put on rubber gloves before handling vomitus, feces, and other secretions of a patient. If soap is unavailable, wash your hands in plain water or snow.

Defecate *downhill* from and as far as possible *away* from camp, drinking water sources, or snow to be melted for water. Bury feces and burn used toilet paper. Do not camp closer than 100 feet from a water source such as a lake, stream, or spring.

Providing the patient with psychological support (see Chapter 4) is extremely important to reinforce faith and the will to live, and to encourage optimism, patience, and cooperation. Discuss plans for emergency care, evacuation, etc., out of the patient's hearing. Attendants should remain calm, unhurried, and deliberate, and should avoid the appearance of indecision, pessimism, fear, or panic. The general situation can be discussed with the patient, adhering to the principle of "emphasizing the donut and not the hole." Warn the patient in advance if any unpleasant or painful procedures are to be performed.

If the illness or injury is so severe that the patient must be evacuated, a decision must be made on whether to attempt an evacuation using the party members and resources alone or to send for help. This will depend on the weather, party size, available equipment, distance and terrain involved, the patient's condition, and the availability of local SAR groups, helicopters, and other assistance. Generally speaking—unless the weather is excellent, the party is strong and well equipped, the route short and easy, and the patient comfortable and stable—the best course of action is to make a comfortable camp and send for help. Send the two strongest party members for help, and perhaps have them take along any other party members who are demoralized or otherwise a liability. If the party is so small that it will be necessary to leave a patient alone in order to reach help, leave an adequate supply of food, fuel, and water within the patient's reach, and reassure him or her that you will return with help.

Stabilize the patient before he or she is moved. "Stabilizing the patient" means that you have controlled bleeding, cleaned and bandaged all wounds, immobilized fractures, and taken care of any urgent physical needs, such as urination and defecation. Pain should be controlled, by medication if appropriate. The patient's body temperature should be stable and the attendants should be fed, rested and ready to go.

The Wilderness Medical Society in its 1989 Position Statements recommends that in any person with one or more of the following conditions, further travel be postponed and/or evacuation be started:

1. Sustained or progressive physiological deterioration, manifested by fainting, abnormally slow or fast heart rate, shortness of breath, altered mental status, progressive weakness, intractable vomiting or diarrhea, or dizziness after arising from the recumbent position.
2. Debilitating pain.
3. Inability to sustain travel at a reasonable pace due to a medical problem.
4. Inability to tolerate oral fluids.
5. Passage of blood by mouth or by rectum, if not from an obviously minor source.
6. Loss of consciousness following a head injury.

7. Signs and symptoms of serious high altitude illness.
8. Infections that progress despite the administration of appropriate treatment.
9. Chest pain that is not clearly musculoskeletal in origin.

Wilderness Injuries

Wilderness injury management follows the same basic principles as management of any injury, except for certain modifications necessary to avoid infection, interference with circulation, or other complications during the time needed for evacuation. Repeatedly monitor circulation of an injured extremity to detect changes caused by swelling and tight splinting, since reduced circulation enhances the danger of gangrene and frostbite. Maintain the injured patient's temperature at a normal level.

Lacerations and Other Open Wounds

In the wilderness, improperly treated open wounds can partially immobilize a patient because of pain, stiffness, swelling, and infection, making self-evacuation difficult. After bleeding is controlled, all open wounds should be cleaned to prevent infection (as outlined in Chapter 7). Disinfect high-risk wounds by pouring a 1-percent solution of povidone-iodine (Betadine, etc.) directly onto the wound. Before doing this, be sure the patient is not allergic to iodine. High-risk wounds are defined as those more likely to become seriously infected, such as animal and human bites; open fractures or dislocations; wounds with exposed tendons; large, ragged wounds; or those containing considerable dirt or devitalized tissue.

The povidone-iodine solution can be prepared on the spot by diluting the standard 10-percent stock solution 10:1 with clean water. Then cover the wound with a sterile dressing moistened with 1-percent povidone-iodine solution, immobilize it, and transport the patient to medical care.

In addition, consider removing impaled objects if they cannot be stabilized effectively or if they interfere with patient packaging or transport, but only if removal is simple and easy.

Small wounds can be closed with butterfly bandages or sterile tape (Steri-Strips), but large wounds should be bandaged open, except in cold weather when they should be taped closed to prevent cold injury. If at all possible, avoid wrapping tape completely around an extremity, since the tape may cause a tourniquet-like effect if the extremity swells. Antibiotics are recommended to prevent infection in high-risk wounds (see **Antibiotics** below). Abrasions heal faster if they can be kept moist. They should be cleaned with mild soap and clean water and covered with plastic wrap or a special dressing such as Opsite.

Dressings can be improvised from clean material such as pillowcases, sheets, towels, underclothing, shirts, and sanitary napkins. Clean toilet paper and tissues (Kleenex, etc.) are quite absorbent and can be used if nothing better is available. Bandages can be improvised from pack straps, belts, strips torn from clothing, cord, or nylon webbing. Kerchiefs and bandannas can be used as cravats and triangular bandages. Rolled T-shirts also can be used as cravats and clean socks as hand or foot bandages. Plastic sandwich or garbage bags can be placed over sterile compresses to make an occlusive dressing.

Depending on immunization status, a patient with an open wound should consider getting a tetanus booster injection as soon as medical help is reached (see Chapter 7 for guidelines).

Fractures

The proper first aid for any fracture is immobilization. Because of weight considerations, few wilderness travelers are able to carry a large variety of pre-made splints. Splints usually must be improvised from natural materials, ski poles, ice axes, ice hammers, and parts of packs such as hip pads and shoulder straps (see Chapter 8 and Fig. 8.11). Wire and malleable metal splints and air splints are lightweight and easy to carry, especially by large parties and SAR groups. Below timberline, tree branches and small trees can be cut and used for improvised splints. A sling can be improvised by pinning the shirt sleeve to the shirt with a large safety pin ("blanket pin"). An all-purpose forearm and hand splint can be improvised from two pairs of socks: one rolled up sock held in the palm of the hand and two to three socks pulled over the hand and wrist like a mitten. Uninjured body parts can act as splints, i.e., a fractured upper arm can be splinted against the chest wall with a sling and swathe, and a fractured hip can be splinted by tying both lower extremities together.

A patient with an open fracture should take antibiotics (see **Antibiotics** below) in addition to receiving the care for a high-risk wound described above and in Chapter 8.

The most marked modification of traditional splinting in the wilderness is that which involves the emergency care of a fractured femur (Fig. C.2). The standard emergency care for a fracture of the middle one-half to three-fifths of the femur is traction splinting, but traction applied to a boot for more than a few hours can cause pressure damage to the ankle tissues. Even when a padded traction harness is used, traction applied to a bare foot or one wearing a sock can injure these tissues if applied for more than a few hours. Therefore, unless evacuation time will be short, avoid pressure on the ankle entirely with the following method:

Remove the patient's boot and socks, roll up the pant leg or open it with a seam ripper, and apply a strip of 2-inch-wide adhesive tape from just below the knee down one side of the leg, under the sole of the foot, and then up the other side of the leg so that a stirrup is formed. Next, wrap the leg from toes to knee with an elastic bandage. Make sure the bandage is firm but not too tight and that the color and temperature of the toes remain normal. Insert a piece of wood into the stirrup as a spreader to keep pressure off the sides of the ankle. After this, apply a traction-type splint (described in Chapter 8), which can be an improvised single ski or ski pole traction splint or a commercial splint such as the Hare, Sager, or Kendrick traction device. Because the stirrup prevents replacing the sock on the foot, keep the foot warm by wrapping it in a spare jacket. Unwrap the jacket at intervals to inspect the toes for color, warmth, sensation, and movement.

Fig. C.2 *Modified Traction Splinting Technique for a Fractured Femur*

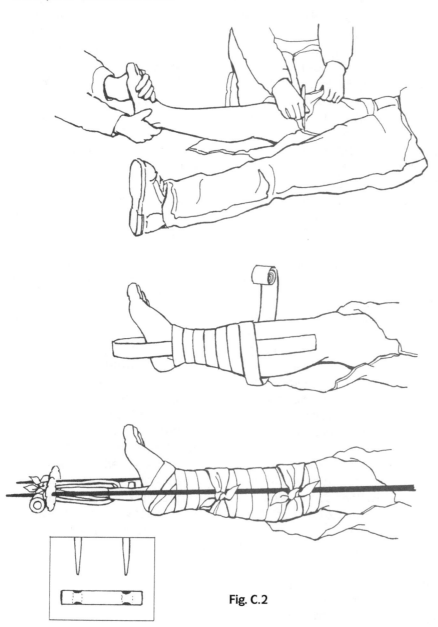

Fig. C.2

Dislocations

In line with traditional emergency care, standard teaching in this text is to treat a dislocation by splinting it in the position found without attempting to straighten or align it unless there is interference with circulation or nerve supply. However, a dislocation usually is more painful than a fracture and causes considerable pressure on joint cartilage and other structures, resulting in additional injury. When a dislocation is splinted in the position found, ligaments, tendons, and nerves are stretched more and circulation is more often impaired than when a fracture is splinted this way. Thus, when medical help is more than a few hours away, there is considerable justification for attempting to align a dislocation so that normal anatomy is restored.

Alignment usually provides marked pain relief, makes it much easier to evacuate the patient, and may prevent a good deal of future disability. This type of alignment is called **relocation** of the dislocation. The process of relocation should be slow and steady, without any quick jerks. Circulation and nerve function should be assessed and documented before and after any attempt at relocation. If one attempt is unsuccessful or causes severe pain, abandon further attempts at relocation and splint the dislocation in the most comfortable position.

Relocation works best if it can be done *immediately* after the dislocation occurs, before the injured part stiffens and muscles go into spasm, and while it is still numb. Otherwise, the patient should take a dose of pain medication and the relocation should be delayed until the medication has had time to work (45 minutes to one hour). For the techniques described below, the author is indebted to Dr. Joseph Serra, whose pioneering work in this area has greatly improved the management of wilderness injuries.

Shoulder Dislocations

In the wilderness, the shoulder is the most commonly dislocated joint; the injury usually is an anterior dislocation (see Chapter 10). The mechanism is a force applied with the shoulder in abduction and external rotation, such as a high brace while kayaking, a slip while the arm is over the head with the hand wedged in a crack, or a fall on an externally rotated, outstretched hand. A dislocation also can occur from a hard fall with a direct blow to the shoulder, but this is more likely to fracture the upper end of the

Fig. C.3 *Technique of Relocating a Dislocated Shoulder Using Gravity*

Fig. C.4 *Technique of Relocating a Dislocated Shoulder Using Two Rescuers*

humerus as well as dislocate it. Circulation and nerve function—especially the function of the axillary nerve (see Chapter 19)—should be checked and documented before and after any attempt at alignment. Several methods are available for relocating a simple shoulder dislocation if there is no associated fracture.

First, the examiner carefully puts several fingers into the patient's armpit. The head of the humerus, which feels like a ball, usually can be palpated. The examiner then moves the extremity slightly. A grating sound or feeling means a fracture also is present. If there is any possibility of a fracture, do *not* attempt to relocate the dislocation; splint it as described in Chapter 10. Fortunately, fracture-dislocations of the shoulder are quite rare in young, healthy persons unless large forces are involved and the dislocation is caused by a direct fall on the shoulder.

An excellent and safe method for relocating a dislocated shoulder is to have the patient lie prone on an elevated platform such as a large, flat rock or log, high enough to allow the injured extremity to hang free. Tie a 10-pound weight to the patient's wrist (Fig. C.3). The gradual pull usu-

ally will relocate the shoulder within one to one-and-one-half hours. If an elevated platform is unavailable or is unsafe due to severe weather conditions, try the following method (Fig. C.4):

The patient sits on the ground with the rescuer kneeling, facing the patient's injured side. An assistant sits behind the patient opposite the rescuer and anchors the patient by wrapping both arms or a sling around the patient's chest. The rescuer ties two cravats together with square knots to make a large loop and slips the loop around his or her waist. The loop should be large enough so that it can be pulled out in front of the waist about 8 to 12 inches. The rescuer then grasps the patient's injured upper extremity in both hands and flexes the patient's elbow to a right angle. The loop around the rescuer's waist is slipped over the patient's hand and worked down to where it is just distal to the bend of the elbow. Keeping the patient's forearm bent with both hands, the rescuer slowly leans backward while the assistant applies countertraction in the opposite direction. The shoulder should slip back into place, frequently with an audible pop. The patient often sighs with relief as the pain disappears.

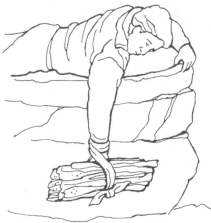

Fig. C.3

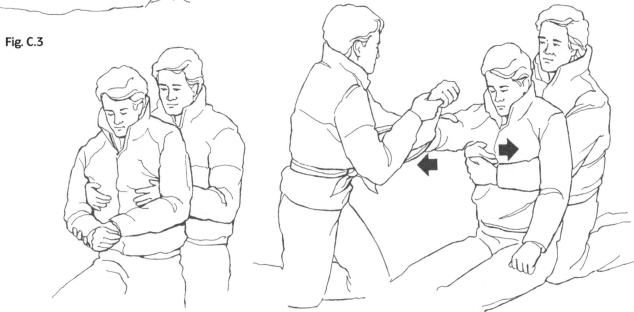

Fig. C.4

When no help is available, self-relocation of a dislocated shoulder may be successful if done immediately. It is easier if the shoulder has been dislocated before. The method is as follows (Fig. C.5):

The injured person sits on the ground with the knees bent, locking both hands together around the knees. The person then slowly leans back and straightens the hips. With luck, the shoulder slips back into place.

After relocation, the injured upper extremity should be immobilized with a sling and swathe until medical help is obtained, or for a minimum of three weeks.

Elbow Dislocations

When an elbow is dislocated, the forearm usually is forced backward on the upper arm, producing a marked deformity with the point of the elbow much farther back than it should be and a large notch above the olecranon process. When seen from the front, the forearm on the involved side appears shorter than the opposite, normal forearm; if not, the patient probably has a fracture above the elbow rather than a dislocated elbow. When seen from the side, the size of the elbow from front to back is greater than normal and there is a bulge in the antecubital space (area in front of the elbow). The circulation and nerve supply of the forearm and hand frequently are compromised. Crepitus should be absent; if present, a fracture is likely.

To relocate a dislocated elbow, the rescuer pulls steadily on the forearm with the elbow partly flexed while an assistant holds the upper arm tightly. The normal shape of the elbow should be restored and the notch above the olecranon process should disappear. The relocated elbow is immobilized as described under the section on **Upper Arm Fractures** in Chapter 10.

Fig. C.5 *Self-relocation of a Dislocated Shoulder*

Fig. C.6 *Technique of Relocating a Dislocated Finger*

Fig. C.7 *Technique of Relocating a Dislocated Hip*

Finger Dislocations

To relocate a dislocated finger, the rescuer uses his or her thumb and forefinger to firmly hold the part of the patient's finger proximal to the dislocation. With the other hand, the rescuer partly flexes the finger distal to the dislocation, while pulling on it and pushing the base of the dislocated part back into position (Fig. C.6). The relocated finger is splinted by an (improvised) all-purpose forearm and hand splint or, if the patient must self-evacuate, by taping the injured finger to an adjacent, uninjured finger.

Hip Dislocations

Attempting to relocate a dislocated hip in the field is justifiable since a prolonged hip dislocation interrupts the blood supply to the head of the femur, eventually causing its death and making a total hip replacement operation likely in the future. The most common type of hip dislocation is a posterior dislocation. The lower extremity is characteristically bent at the hip, rotated inward, and adducted. Attempts to move the hip are very painful. The technique is as follows (Fig. C.7):

An assistant straddles the patient, facing the patient's feet, and places

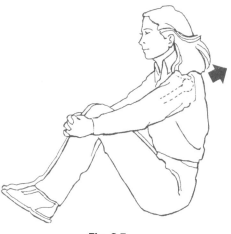

Fig. C.5

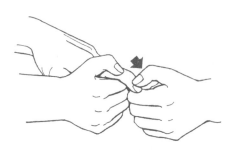

Fig. C.6

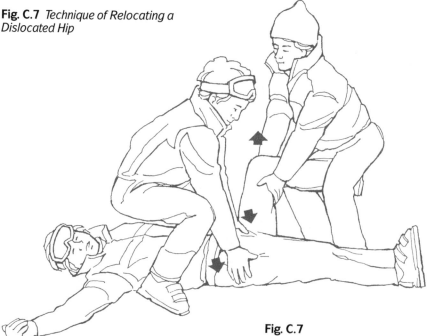

Fig. C.7

one hand on each side of the front of the pelvis to provide countertraction. The rescuer straddles the leg on the patient's injured side, holding it tightly between his or her legs, and gently bends the patient's knee to 90 degrees. The rescuer bends his or her own knees slightly and grasps the back of the patient's leg tightly just below the knee with locked hands. Next, the rescuer exerts steady traction in an upward direction by straightening his or her knees, while the assistant leans hard on the patient's pelvis. After the hip is relocated, put padding between the knees and ankles, tie the lower extremities together, and transport the patient on an (improvised) long spine board.

Patella Dislocations

In the case of a patella dislocation, ask the patient to bend the hip to a right angle, which will relax the quadriceps muscle on the front of the thigh. Then gently straighten the knee while pushing the patella back toward its normal location at the front of the knee joint. The extremity should then be splinted in extension. If the patient cannot be carried out, a "walking splint" can be fashioned with a short Ensolite or Therm-a-Rest pad wrapped around the extremity to keep the knee straight. The patient should use a "cane" (ski pole, ice ax, stick, etc.).

Knee Dislocations

Great force is required to dislocate a knee because of its strong ligamentous and muscular attachments. Most of the major ligaments of the knee must be torn for the joint to dislocate. A dislocated knee usually is unstable, and the circulation and nerve supply usually are impaired. Amputation will likely result if the dislocation cannot be reduced within six to eight hours. Therefore, there is considerable reason to attempt relocation in a wilderness setting.

Relocation consists of simple axial traction to realign the joint so that the leg and foot are in the most normal position possible and the pulses in the foot are the strongest. Afterward, immobilize the extremity in a long-leg type of fixation splint, continuing to monitor and document the circulation and nerve supply at 15-minute intervals. If either becomes compromised, remove the splint and realign the injury in the position that gives the strongest pulses in the foot.

Ankle Dislocations

An ankle dislocation is almost always a fracture-dislocation; impairment of the circulation and nerve supply are a danger. Relocation consists of simple axial traction (Fig. C.8) to return the foot to a normal position with strong pulses, and immobilization of the extremity with a fixation splint. Monitor and document circulation and nerve supply at 15-minute intervals

---

Fig. C.8 *Technique of Relocating a Dislocated Ankle*

Fig. C.9 *An adhesive tape boot can support a sprained ankle.*

after relocation. If either becomes compromised, remove the splint and realign the injury in the position that gives the strongest pulses in the foot.

Sprains

The standard assessment and emergency care for an ankle sprain is discussed in Chapter 11. Under wilderness conditions, a patient with an ankle sprain may have to self-evacuate. A sturdy hiking, mountaineering, or telemark boot alone may provide the necessary support, but an adhesive-tape boot (Fig. C.9) usually is needed to stabilize the sprain enough to allow walking. Consider shaving the lower leg and foot before applying the tape.

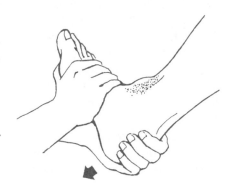

Fig. C.8

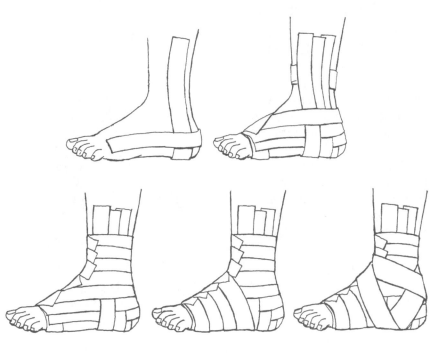

Fig. C.9

Hold the patient's foot at a right angle to the leg and apply overlapping vertical and horizontal strips of tape that are 1-inch wide and 20 to 30 inches long. Run vertical strips from the lower leg on the *uninjured* side across the sole of the foot and up the opposite side of the ankle; run horizontal strips from the top of the foot around the back of the heel to the other side of the top of the foot. Alternate application of these vertical and horizontal strips. Avoid ring-like strips extending all the way around the ankle or foot at the same level since, if swelling occurs, they may function as tourniquets.

Continue taping until most of the ankle, lower leg, and posterior two-thirds of the foot are covered. Conclude with a figure-of-eight wrap around the ankle, heel, and arch to stabilize the arch and provide additional heel stabilization. Then replace the patient's boot on the foot. Usually the patient will need one less sock on the injured foot because of the thickness of the tape. Note: it is less painful to remove the tape if it is peeled off from *top to bottom*.

Injuries to the Head, Spine, Chest, Abdomen, and Pelvis; Multiple Injuries

Rockfall accidents, falls while climbing, and high-speed skiing accidents can cause multiple injuries similar to those seen in motor-vehicle accidents. Serious head, neck, back, chest, abdominal, pelvic, and extremity injuries can occur singly or in various combinations, sorely taxing the emergency care skills of rescuers. The immediate care of these injuries is the same as described in Chapters 4, 7, 8, 19, and 22 and in the chapters on specific injuries. Give the patient oxygen, if available. Keeping the upper airway open may be difficult if there are facial injuries. In the unrespon-

sive patient without a gag reflex, an oropharyngeal airway should be used if possible.

It is useful to have the ability to give intravenous fluids; to intubate or perform a cricothyroidotomy when the upper airway cannot be opened by the usual measures described in Chapter 4; and to insert a needle or tube into the chest for a tension pneumothorax. The techniques for doing a cricothyroidotomy and a needle thoracotomy will be described briefly below; however, these and other similar skills require special training, licensing, and equipment.

Surgical Cricothyroidotomy
(Fig. C.10)

Because of the danger of damage to the cricoid cartilage, this procedure is not performed in children younger than 12 years of age (see **Needle Cricothyroidotomy** below). You will need a scalpel or other sharp knife and a commercially available emergency cricothyroidotomy tube, a small endotracheal tube (about #5), or a large pediatric size tracheotomy tube.

If there is time and you have the equipment, cleanse the skin over the anterior neck with 10-percent povi-

done-iodine solution (Betadine) and put on a pair of sterile rubber gloves. Locate the "Adam's apple" (thyroid cartilage) and run your finger down it until you feel the cricothyroid membrane, a soft area between the lower end of the thyroid cartilage and the cricoid cartilage (refer to Chapter 3 and practice locating this area on yourself and others). With the scalpel, make a horizontal cut about ¾-inch (2 centimeters) long in the skin over the lower half of the membrane (Fig. C.10a). Carefully cut a hole in the membrane, insert the scalpel handle in the hole and rotate it 90 degrees to open the hole (Fig. C.10b). Then take the tube you have chosen and insert the end into the hole so that it points footward and the flange, if any, is up against the skin (Fig. C.10c). Tie it in place and put a piece of sterile gauze between it and the skin.

Needle Cricothyroidotomy

This technique is preferable in children less than 12 years of age. It requires a #12-gauge needle covered with a plastic catheter (Intracath, etc.) and a 20-cc syringe to provide a better grip on the needle. Attach the needle to the end of the syringe. Prepare the skin as described under **Surgical Cricothyroidotomy**, except that

Fig. C.10 *Surgical Cricothyroidotomy*

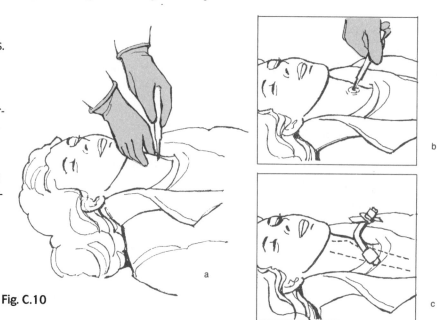

Fig. C.10

instead of making an incision, insert the needle into the cricothyroid membrane so that it points toward the patient's feet, withdraw the needle, and tape the catheter in place. Because of the small size of the catheter, this technique does not provide more than 45 minutes of adequate ventilation.

Needle Thoracotomy (Fig. C.11)

This technique can be life-saving in a patient with a tension pneumothorax (see Chapter 14 for signs and symptoms). A #14-gauge 3- to 6-centimeter Intracath needle and a 20- to 35-cc syringe are needed.

Clean the skin with 10-percent povidone-iodine solution (Betadine) and put on a pair of sterile rubber gloves if you have time. Locate the sternal angle, which is where the second rib attaches to the sternum, and follow this rib out to the midclavicular line (an imaginary line perpendicular to the midpoint of the clavicle). The second intercostal space is *below* the second rib. Since the nerves and blood vessels run along the lower edge of each rib, the needle should be introduced *just over the top* of the third rib to avoid injury to these. The

patient should be sitting up if possible and if there is no cervical spine injury. The site of insertion is in the second intercostal space at the midclavicular line. Attach the needle to the syringe and insert it carefully through the chest wall while maintaining negative pressure in the syringe by pulling back slightly on the plunger. Air will enter the syringe as soon as the needle enters the pleural space. Withdraw the needle, leaving the plastic catheter in place, aspirate as much air as possible, then connect the hub of the catheter to a flutter valve. Tape the catheter to the skin of the chest.

A flutter valve can be improvised by taking a sterile glove, rinsing the talcum powder from its inside by filling it with clean (preferably sterile) water, cutting a finger off the glove, cutting a small hole in the fingertip, and tying the base of the finger around the hub of the catheter. When the patient exhales, air will come out through the needle, fill the glove finger, and exit through the hole in its tip. When the patient inhales, the drop in air pressure as the air tends to move back into the pleural space through the needle will collapse the glove finger and seal the hole in its tip.

Open Abdominal Wound

A loop of bowel protruding through an open abdominal wound can be successfully replaced if discovered and treated *immediately*. Replace the loop as aseptically as possible and tape the wound shut. If much time has elapsed, however, the loop will swell and be impossible to replace. In this case, it should be covered with a clean—preferably sterile—cloth moistened with warm physiological saline or clean water with ½ teaspoon of table salt added per quart, (preferably disinfected or brought to a boil and then cooled (Fig. 15.3, Chapter 15). Keep the dressing moist during evacuation, using repeated applications of one of the above solutions warmed to body temperature.

Spine Injury

Standard emergency care protocols require immobilization of a patient on a long spine board if there is a suspicious mechanism of injury alone (see Chapter 13), even if the patient has *no* signs or symptoms of spine or spinal cord injury. Because of the difficulty of obtaining or improvising a spine board and transporting a boarded patient, many authorities feel that, under wilderness conditions, a patient with a normal mental status and no signs or symptoms of spine or spinal cord injury need not be boarded on the basis of mechanism of injury alone. In this case, the patient must have a full range of spinal motion; no spine pain, tenderness or deformity; and normal motor and sensory function.

Since it is difficult to improvise a serviceable long spine board, safe evacuation of a patient with a neck or back injury is almost impossible if you have to rely on the resources of a small, poorly-equipped party alone. In almost every case, it is preferable to camp on the spot and send for help rather than try to evacuate a seriously injured patient who is partly immobilized with substandard equipment.

Fig. C.11 *Needle Thoracotomy*

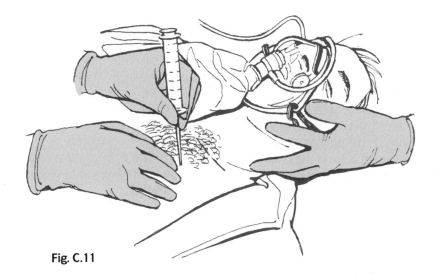

Fig. C.11

If the patient must be moved because of incoming bad weather or a hazardous location, a spine board can be made of several poles or skis tied side by side with crosspieces or several external or internal frame packs tied together in an overlapping fashion and covered with Ensolite or a Therm-a-Rest pad as described in Chapter 20. Backcountry rescue groups usually use the combination of a vest-type device (such as the KED or Oregon spine splint II) and a rigid litter (such as the Ferno-Washington or SKED). At times, a vest-type device can be improvised using the patient's pack frame and adding groin straps.

Shock

In the wilderness, shock is most often caused by one of the following.

1. Loss of whole blood because of:
   a. Severe or uncontrolled external bleeding.
   b. Bleeding from a fractured femur, fractured pelvis, or multiple injuries.
   c. Internal bleeding from a bleeding ulcer, ruptured ectopic pregnancy, etc.
2. Loss of the fluid part of the blood because of:
   a. Severe vomiting or diarrhea.
   b. Extensive burns.
3. Heart attack.
4. Spinal cord injury with neurogenic shock.

There is no good field emergency care for any of these conditions except for controlling bleeding and trying to replace fluids lost by vomiting or diarrhea. The care given is designed to buy time until the patient can reach a hospital. When a patient has a condition commonly known to cause shock, anticipate shock and start to evacuate the patient as soon as possible, *before* shock actually develops.

In the hospital, a patient in shock is treated by re-expanding the blood volume with whole blood, plasma, and/or intravenous fluids, and by correcting the condition that caused the shock. Many rescue groups have members who are trained and licensed to administer intravenous fluids. Although it is rarely possible or practical to transfuse whole blood in the field, rescue groups can carry intravenous fluids. Lactated Ringer's solution is the best standard intravenous preparation to carry for treating shock. In cold weather, intravenous preparations must be protected from freezing. This is frequently done by having rescuers carry the bags of fluid inside clothing against the body. Portable intravenous fluid warmers also are available.

PASGs provide widely distributed direct pressure to the lower half of the body, thereby tending to stop or slow any bleeding in that area. This pressure also collapses shell blood vessels, thereby reducing the vascular volume so that, if the cardiac output remains the same, the blood pressure will rise. PASGs are of some value in the prehospital treatment of hypovolemic shock, but special training and licensing are required to use them. They are most useful in treating neurogenic shock associated with spinal cord injuries and hypovolemic shock due to pelvic fractures, multiple injuries, and intra-abdominal bleeding. However, they are rarely available outside of helicopters and specially equipped rescue groups.

Minor Problems

Blisters

Blisters are annoying injuries produced when an ill-fitting boot or a wrinkled sock rubs repeatedly against the skin. Blisters are most common on the heels, toes, and soles of the feet. The best treatment is prevention. Always wear at least two pairs of socks, preferably a thin inner pair of polypropylene or silk socks next to the skin with one or two outer pairs of heavy wool socks, so that friction tends to occur between sock layers rather than between the sock and your skin. Cut your toenails before a trip and wear properly broken-in boots that are correctly fitted for length so that the toes will not jam against the tip of the boot during downhill walking.

If a sore spot develops, call for a halt, immediately remove the boot and socks, and look for a reddened area of skin. Overlay this area with four layers of 2-inch-wide adhesive tape or a piece of moleskin. Replace the socks, making sure they are not creased or wrinkled, and lace the boot snugly enough to keep the foot, and especially the heel, from moving around inside it.

If a blister has already developed (and you discover it before it has already broken), protect it by overlaying it with several layers of tape. Cut holes slightly larger than the blister in the bottom layers (Fig. C.12). Clean and dress a broken blister as you would any other open wound.

Occasionally, a blister is so painful or awkwardly located that it has to be drained. Wash your hands with soap and water, then wash the skin with an antiseptic solution, sterilize a needle over a flame, insert the needle under the skin about ¼ inch from the edge of the blister, push it up into the blister, and withdraw it while pressing on the blister (Fig. C.13). Then bandage the drained blister.

Subungual Hematoma

Subungual hematoma, or bleeding under the nail, usually is caused by a hard object such as a hammer striking the fingertip with enough force to break blood vessels underneath the nail. The pressure and consequent severe, throbbing pain of a subungual hematoma can be relieved by draining the hematoma.

Wash the fingertip with soap and water, then heat a piece of thin, rigid wire (e.g., a straightened paper clip or the blunt end of a needle from your sewing kit) on a stove or over a candle flame (a match flame is not hot enough) until it is red-hot. Next, press the red-hot end firmly into the nail at the center of the hematoma and allow it to burn through the nail (Fig. C.14). Maintain close control so that the hot object does not penetrate too far. A pop and sudden give means that the object is through the nail. When the object is withdrawn, it usually is followed by a drop of blood, and the pain is relieved. Bandage the nail with a pre-packaged bandage strip such as a Bandaid.

Jewelry Removal

Immediately remove any jewelry from an injured upper extremity. If a ring is not quickly removed and the finger swells, the ring will cause a tourniquet-like effect (Fig. C.15a). Swelling may be so great that cutting it off might seem to be the only way to remove the ring. Fortunately, the following simple technique almost always works.

You will need a small spool of strong thread or dental floss. Work the loose end under the ring in a proximal direction and pull several inches through. Starting just distal to the ring, wind the thread snugly around the finger, working toward the fingertip (Fig. C.15b). Each turn is made next to the previous one so that the finger is wrapped solidly from the ring over the next distal joint down to the midpoint of the next phalanx (Fig. C.15c).

You will note that the pressure of the closely laid thread reduces the swelling to some extent. Cut the thread at the spool end, leaving several inches of loose thread. Then, pull the end that was worked under the ring in the direction of the fingertip (Fig. C.15.d). This will cause the thread to unwind off the finger and pull the ring over the joint and off the finger as it unwinds.

Fishhook Removal

There are two techniques for removing a fishhook embedded in the skin. If a wire cutter or heavy pair of scissors is available, the barbed end of the hook can be pushed up through the skin and cut off, allowing the hook to be backed out of the hole (Fig. C.16).

The second method consists of disengaging the barb of the hook from the tissues so that it can be directly

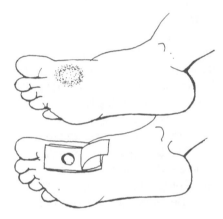

Fig. C.12

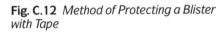

Fig. C.12 *Method of Protecting a Blister with Tape*

Fig. C.13 *Technique of Draining a Blister*

Fig. C.14 *Technique of Draining a Subungual Hematoma*

Fig. C.15 *Technique of Removing a Ring from a Swollen Finger*

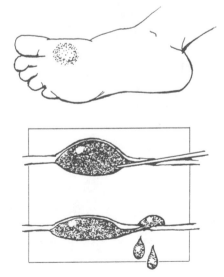

Fig. C.13

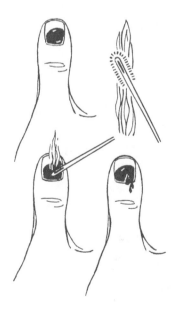

Fig. C.14

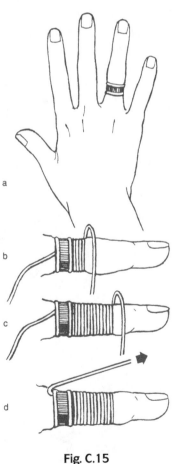

Fig. C.15

backed out of the hole. This technique, recommended by hook manufacturer O. Mustad & Son of Auburn, New York, has the advantage of not damaging a valuable fly (Fig. C.17).

First, loop a long piece of 20- or 30-pound test line or other thin, strong line around the curve of the hook and grip it firmly with one hand (Fig. C.17a). Next, determine the exact location of the hook and the direction of penetration by rocking and rotating the hook gently with your other hand, trying to find the position of least resistance. Then, while holding the hook in this position, apply firm downward pressure with your thumb on the shank of the hook directly over the barb and simultaneously push up on the eye of the hook. This disengages the barb of the hook from the tissues. Guide the barb back along the line of entrance, then, while maintaining pressure on the shank (Fig. C.17b), release the eye and quickly snatch the hook out by

pulling on the looped line horizontally or at a slightly upward angle (Fig. C.17c). If the eye part of the hook has broken off, remove the hook using a pair of pliers instead of a loop of line. Finally, clean the wound with germicidal soap. Afterward, the patient should be considered for a tetanus prophylaxis shot, depending on immune status (see Chapter 7).

This technique is unsuitable when a hook is imbedded in an area of the body where it is difficult to apply strong downward pressure on the shank, e.g., the sides of the neck, earlobes, and around the eyes. A hook cannot be removed by this method when the barb has already come through the skin. If the hook is in the eyeball itself, cut off the line at the base of the hook and take the patient to an ophthalmologist as soon as possible.

Skin Cracks

Small, painful skin cracks are annoyances that mainly affect the fingertips. Common in winter and in dry climates, skin cracks can be prevented to some extent by liberal use of hand cream and by avoiding frequent hand washings.

A thick greasy ointment and protection with a Bandaid will speed healing. In some cases, it is more effective to squeeze the crack shut and apply a small amount of Super Glue to seal the crack. The thin variety of glue works better than the thick variety; it is waterproof and protects the skin while the skin heals underneath, but usually has to be reapplied at least daily. The residual glue will fall off eventually as the surface area of healing skin is shed normally.

Leg Cramps

Because of demands placed on lower extremity muscles by unaccustomed use, many wilderness travelers suffer from leg cramps. At times, excessive perspiration with loss of salt may contribute to this condition (see section on **Heat Illness**, Chapter 18). The cramps occur most often in the evening of the first few days of a trip. Treatment consists of massaging the muscle and stretching it in the direction opposite to the cramp. Nocturnal cramps can be prevented to some extent by taking a 325-mg tablet of quinine sulfate (nonprescription) or two 25-mg tablets of diphenhydramine (Benadryl, also nonprescrip-

---

Fig. C.16 *Technique of Using Wire Cutters to Remove a Ring from a Swollen Finger*

Fig. C.17 *Technique of Using Test Line to Remove a Ring from a Swollen Finger*

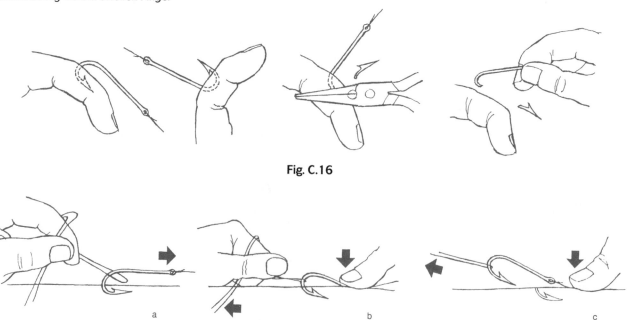

Fig. C.16

a   b   c

Fig. C.17

tion) nightly at bedtime. Side effects of quinine include blurred vision, ringing in the ears, dizziness, headache, nausea, and vomiting. Side effects of diphenhydramine include sleepiness, dizziness, and abdominal pain.

Splinter Removal

Splinters, slivers, and thorns occasionally become imbedded in the skin of the wilderness traveler. First wash the involved area of skin with soap and water, then use a sterile (flamed) sewing needle to free up one end of the splinter so that it can be grasped and pulled out with a small forceps. The forceps from a Swiss Army knife may work, but a special splinter forceps works better (available at most pharmacies).

Use of Prescription Drugs

Federal and state laws prohibit laypersons from prescribing or dispensing prescription drugs. In addition, transporting and even using the prescription drugs described in this appendix may be illegal under various state and/or federal statutes *unless* the drugs in the individual's possession have been prescribed for him or her by a physician and this fact is documented by labels that give the individual's name, the physician's name, and directions for use.

Under certain conditions, the proper drug may prevent or control serious illness or even prevent loss of life. For this reason, wilderness travelers may wish to become familiar with the carefully selected drugs described in this appendix and possibly obtain these drugs by prescription from their physicians for inclusion in first aid kits for personal use. Prescription drugs *should not* be offered to others.

No one should take a drug to which he or she has a known allergy. Common allergic reactions to both pre-

scription and nonprescription drugs include hives and a generalized skin rash. More serious reactions include fever and anaphylactic shock. Anyone who develops skin changes or starts to feel unwell while taking a drug should consider stopping that drug.

The doses of all drugs mentioned in the following sections of this appendix are for adults. Those who wish to obtain such drugs for children's use should consult a pediatrician for the correct doses based on the age and size of the child.

Cold Injuries

The prevention and emergency care of cold injuries are discussed in Chapters 1 and 18. The current recommendation for emergency care of a patient with frostbite is to leave blisters unopened and protect them from damage. However, blister fluid contains prostaglandins and other substances that can injure tissues. Some authorities recommend sterile aspiration of pink (but not purple or bloody) blister fluid with a syringe and needle.

There is evidence that prostaglandin inhibitors such as ibuprofen (Advil, Nuprin, Motrin) may be beneficial in preventing some of the tissue injury associated with frostbite. Ibuprofen can be purchased in 200-mg tablets without prescription. For greatest benefit, immediately begin taking the ibuprofen in a dosage of two tablets four times daily after meals and at bedtime with food if hazardous environmental conditions develop. The major side effects of ibuprofen are epigastric distress, heartburn, nausea, and vomiting.

Acute Mountain Sickness (AMS)

The prevention and care of acute mountain sickness is discussed in chapters 1 and 18.

Oxygen is very useful, if available. It is given by nasal cannula at 4 to 6 liters per minute or by mask at a rate

of 8 to 12 liters per minute. Because oxygen supplies are always finite, simultaneously begin preparations for descent. A new portable hyperbaric chamber, the Gamow bag (see Chapter 18) has been shown to be as effective as medical oxygen and can be carried by large mountaineering groups and expeditions.

A number of drugs have been advocated as having some use in preventing or treating acute mountain sickness. Acetazolamide (Diamox), a carbonic anhydrase inhibitor, has definite value in *preventing* acute mountain sickness but is less useful in *treating* all but mild cases. It is particularly useful for preventing AMS in rescuers who do not have time to ascend slowly. The dose is 250 mg by mouth every 12 hours (or one long-acting 500-mg capsule daily) for three to four days. Start the medication 24 hours before ascent or at the first sign of discomfort, which usually begins at 10,000 to 12,000 feet (3,048 to 3,658 meters). Side effects include tingling of the extremities and intolerance to carbonated beverages.

For early AMS or mild advanced AMS, take aspirin or acetaminophen with codeine for headache, plus 250 mg of acetazolamide every eight hours for two to three days to speed acclimatization. For nausea and vomiting, take 10 mg of prochlorperazine (Compazine) orally every four hours or 25 mg by rectal suppository every 12 hours as needed. Because prochlorperazine also stimulates breathing, it is preferred over other antinausea agents such as thiethylperazine (Torecan).

In treating severe advanced AMS, acetazolamide is of less value. Studies in Europe have shown that nifedipine (Procardia, Adalat) shows promise in treating and preventing high altitude pulmonary edema, probably through its ability to reduce pulmonary artery pressure. The treatment dose is one to two 10-mg capsules chewed and swallowed for fast effect, followed by 30 mg of a long-acting form (Procardia XL 30) every eight hours or 20 mg (Adalat) every six hours. Although the drug is not recommended at the time of this writing for prevention, a dose of 20 mg of the long-acting preparation given at bedtime on the third and second days before ascent, increased to 20 mg every eight hours the day of the ascent, has been suggested and probably would be well tolerated. Mountaineers who intend to carry nifedipine in their first aid kits are advised to try it out at home beforehand to see if it causes significant side effects (dizziness, headache, weakness, low blood pressure).

Dexamethasone, taken in an initial oral or intramuscular dose of 6 mg followed by 4 mg every six hours, is helpful in reducing increased intracranial pressure in patients with high altitude cerebral edema. Side effects of short-term use include epigastric discomfort, heartburn, nausea, vomiting, muscle weakness, and sodium retention with edema.

It cannot be emphasized too strongly that *no* drug or device should be relied upon alone to correct severe acute mountain sickness; the definitive treatment is *rapid descent*.

Use of Antibiotics

Because infectious diseases can occur in the wilderness, it is wise for travelers who expect to be very far from the roadhead for very long to carry antibiotics and have some idea of the indications for their use.

The principal antibiotic-requiring infections likely to be seen are upper and lower respiratory tract infections, dysentery, urinary tract infections, and wound and skin infections. Antibiotics also are used to prevent infection in high-risk wounds.

The principal bacteria to worry about are *streptococci* (including *pneumococci*) and *Hemophilus influenzae,* which cause respiratory infections; *Campylobacter, Shigella, Salmonella,* and toxicogenic *Escherichia coli,* which cause dysentery; *Escherichia coli* and *Proteus,* which cause urinary infections; and *staphylococci,* which cause skin infections.

Under ideal circumstances, the causative microorganism should be identified in each illness and its sensitivity tested so that the correct antibiotic can be chosen. However, the wilderness traveler does not have this luxury and must rely on a small number of carefully selected antibiotics and some general rules of thumb to choose the best drug based on the signs and symptoms of a given illness, the organism(s) most likely responsible, and the known spectrum of activity of each drug. Fortunately, this empiric process is not difficult and is usually successful.

Many different antibiotics are available and are quite safe when used according to directions by people who are *not* allergic to them. If the decision is made to use an antibiotic, it should be given for a minimum of five and preferably for seven to 10 days.

The traveler who will be out a week or more and will be more than two or three days from the roadhead should have antibiotics in the first aid kit. Experts disagree on how many antibiotics should be carried and which ones should be chosen. Choices are dictated to some extent by geographic location and cost. The following recommendations are based on the author's personal experience in North America. Travelers to developing countries, especially in other continents, are advised to consult one of the many excellent travelers' medical guides that are available.

If you wish to carry a *single, inexpensive, multiple-purpose antibiotic,* the best choice is probably trimeth-

oprim/sulfamethoxazole (TMP/SMZ), which has some activity against all the bacteria mentioned above except for *Campylobacter* and perhaps *staphylococci.* Its main brand names are Septra and Bactrim; generic forms also are available. The dose is one double-strength (DS) tablet twice daily. The principal side effects are nausea, vomiting, loss of appetite, and allergic skin rash.

Another good multiple-purpose antibiotic is ciprofloxacin (Cipro), which has some activity against all the bacteria mentioned above. It has less activity against *streptococci* than does TMP/SMZ. Its dose is one 500-mg tablet twice daily. Side effects are uncommon but can include nausea, vomiting, diarrhea, abdominal pain, and headache. Ciprofloxacin is one of the quinolones, a new group of oral antibiotics that also includes norfloxacin (Noroxin), ofloxacin (Floxin), and lomefloxacin (Maxaquin). Although the quinolones look promising, they are quite expensive, and it is uncertain to what extent they will replace older antibiotics in treating wilderness infections.

An alternative is to carry *two separate antibiotics:* a semisynthetic penicillin, a cephalosporin, or erythromycin; and tetracycline or a tetracycline derivative. The frequency of allergy to penicillin makes semisynthetic penicillins less useful for larger party kits than cephalosporins. Together, these two groups of drugs are likely to control most infections that may be contracted in the wilderness in temperate latitudes. Large expeditions, groups traveling to undeveloped countries—especially in the tropics—or rescue groups may wish to include additional antibiotics, including parenteral (injectable) forms for patients who are vomiting or who cannot swallow.

Cephalosporins are active against all the previously mentioned organisms except *Campylobacter, Salmonella, Shigella,* and toxin-producing (toxicogenic) *E. coli.* Therefore, they are a good choice for upper and lower respiratory infections, skin infections, and urinary tract infections. Cephalexin (Keflex), a moderately priced example, is given in a dose of 250 to 500 mg four times daily. Other, probably better but more expensive, choices are cefaclor (Ceclor, dosage 250 mg three times daily), and cefuroxime (Ceftin, dosage 250 to 500 mg twice daily). Side effects are uncommon but include nausea, vomiting, diarrhea, and occasionally an allergic rash.

Amoxicillin, a semisynthetic penicillin, is active against the same bacteria as the cephalosporins. It is taken in a dose of 250 mg every 8 hours. It probably is preferable to choose a brand in which amoxicillin is combined with potassium clavulanate (Augmentin, etc.). Clavulanate is a beta lactamase blocker that increases amoxicillin's action against *staphylococci, Hemophilus, E. coli, Proteus,* and other important pathogens. Unfortunately, the addition of clavulanate also increases the cost. Side effects include nausea, vomiting, diarrhea, allergic skin rash, and hives.

Erythromycin is active against *streptococci,* some *staphylococci,* and some *Hemophilus.* It is also active against mycoplasma (a common cause of bronchitis), amoebae, and *Campylobacter,* but not against other dysentery organisms. The dosage of the ethyl succinate form is 400 mg four times daily. Delayed-release forms are also available (500 mg twice daily). Side effects include occasional nausea, vomiting, diarrhea, and abdominal discomfort.

Tetracycline is active against rickettsial diseases (typhus, Rocky Mountain spotted fever), undulant fever, tularemia, plague, Lyme disease, *mycoplasmal* infections, *E. coli,* amoebae, and to some extent *streptococcus* and *Hemophilus.* The tetracycline derivative doxycycline is also active against some dysentery organisms. Tetracycline is taken in a dosage of 250 mg four times daily, at least one hour before or two hours after eating. Avoid milk and milk products while taking tetracycline. Pregnant women and young children should not take this drug because it stains developing teeth. The dosage of doxycycline is 100 mg twice daily.

Because tetracycline deteriorates, supplies should be replaced yearly (fortunately, it is inexpensive). Patients taking tetracyclines, especially doxycycline, occasionally experience severe sun reactions, which can be prevented to some extent by wearing protective clothing and liberally applying a sunscreen with a high SPF value (see Chapter 18). Other side effects include abdominal discomfort, nausea, vomiting, diarrhea, black tongue, sore mouth, and anal discomfort.

To obtain drugs with the longest shelf life, tell the pharmacist that the drugs are to be used in a first aid kit. Request that the expiration date be typed on each label. Try to protect drugs from temperature extremes.

For empiric treatment, a cephalosporin, amoxicillin/clavulate, or erythromycin should be taken for severe colds, coughs, and sore throats, especially if the patient is producing yellow or green material from the chest or nose, or has white spots on the tonsils, an earache, a high fever, or sore neck glands beneath the mandible. These antibiotics also should be taken for suspected pneumonia or pleurisy, skin and wound infections, abscesses, and to prevent infection in high-risk wounds, open fractures, and open wounds of the chest and abdomen (if the patient is able to swallow). Amoxicillin/clavulanate, a tetracycline, or a cephalosporin should be taken for suspected urinary or prostate infections; and amoxicillin/clavulanate or doxycycline for severe diarrhea (see **Stomach and Bowel Problems** below).

If there is no improvement after 48 hours of treatment with an antibiotic from one group, substitute a member of the other group. Continue taking antibiotics that are producing the desired improvement for a minimum of five days.

Treat abscesses and wound infections with hot packs as well as antibiotics, and cover them with dressings moistened with 1-percent povidone-iodine solution. A wound that becomes swollen, hot, red, tender, and painful is probably infected, especially if there is pus draining out of it. If the wound has been taped closed, remove the tape and allow the wound to drain. Apply hot, wet packs to the wound four times daily for 30 minutes to speed healing.

A hot pack is made by bringing a piece of cloth to a boil in water to make it hot and sterile, then wringing it out, folding it, and placing it against the wound. Test the temperature of the hot pack against your own (cleaned) skin to make sure that it will not burn the patient.

Suspect an abscess in any patient with fever who has a hot, swollen, red, tender area in the skin or muscles. Apply hot packs as described above to speed the formation of pus, which will collect in a tense, shiny, yellow or reddish spot on the surface of the abscess. To allow pus to drain, clean this spot with an antiseptic and nick it with a razor blade or sharp knife sterilized over a flame. Try to introduce a small, sterile gauze wick (cut from a sterile, gauze pad) into the abscess cavity to help it drain and keep it from sealing off prematurely. Continue applying hot packs to promote continued drainage of the pus.

Treat small, infected cuts by applying an antibiotic ointment such as Neosporin topical-ophthalmic or Garamycin ophthalmic ointment three times daily. These ointments also can be used in the eye for conjunctivitis, which is characterized by a red, sore eye that may discharge pus. Unless conjunctivitis clears rapidly, evacuate the patient.

Stomach and Bowel Problems

The type of food usually consumed in the wilderness (freeze-dried food, candy, nuts, lunch meat, dried fruit, cheese) frequently produces an unusual amount of intestinal gas and softer-than-normal stools. Some individuals may experience cramps, usually in the lower abdomen. Gas may accumulate in the left upper abdomen, causing pressure and/or sharp pains in the chest that can be mistaken for more serious illnesses. These symptoms usually disappear when the offending foods are removed from the diet.

Occasionally, patients with altitude sickness, headache, food poisoning, or gastroenteritis may vomit. Vomiting usually can be controlled with medicated rectal suppositories such as thiethylperazine (Torecan) in 10-mg doses inserted every four hours as necessary, or prochlorperazine (Compazine) in 25-mg doses, inserted every 12 hours as necessary.

Mild diarrhea, often caused by food or gastroenteritis, can be controlled by taking one 2.5-mg tablet of diphenoxylate/atropine sulfate (Lomotil) every four hours as needed. Side effects include numbness of the extremities, sleepiness, dizziness, constipation, and inability to urinate. An alternative is to take one 2-mg capsule of nonprescription loperamide (Imodium) every four to six hours.

Side effects include abdominal pain, nausea, vomiting, constipation, sleepiness, fatigue, and dry mouth.

Patients with severe diarrhea and diarrhea accompanied by chills, fever, severe cramps, and blood or pus in the stools should *not* use these drugs, but should start taking an antibiotic and be evacuated, staying hydrated as well as possible. Bismuth subsalicylate (Pepto-Bismol) also is quite useful in treating mild to moderately severe diarrhea, but bulkier to carry, especially the liquid form. It should not be taken by patients who are allergic to aspirin. The dosage is two tablespoonfuls or two tablets four times daily.

A study done in Mexico a few years ago found that trimethoprim/sulfamethoxazole (Septra, Bactrim), when used as empiric treatment for travelers' diarrhea, was effective in 95 percent of cases. Travelers to developing countries are advised to obtain this medication on prescription from their physicians and use it for moderate to severe diarrhea. The dose is one DS (double-strength) tablet (containing 160 mg trimethoprim and 800 mg sulfamethoxazole) twice daily for at least five days. People who are allergic to sulfa should not use this medication. Doxycycline and amoxicillin/clavulanate also have value in treating severe diarrhea. Bismuth subsalicylate should not be taken with doxycycline since it will inactivate the antibiotic. Ciprofloxacin has recently shown considerable value in the empiric treatment of travelers' diarrhea in developing countries and is probably the new treatment of choice.

Giardiasis, caused by the protozoan *Giardia lamblia,* is a hazard for wilderness travelers in temperate as well as tropical climates. Symptoms include gastric distress, mild diarrhea, and foul-smelling flatus. It does not respond to any of the antibiotics mentioned above but can be effectively treated with metronidazole (Flagyl),

a drug mentioned below in **Special Problems of Women**. Fortunately, giardiasis usually develops slowly enough to allow the patient to be evacuated for definitive medical care.

When patients with any kind of stomach or bowel disturbance are able to eat, they should be given a simple-carbohydrate-containing light diet consisting of broth, bland soup, tea, Jello, pudding, and toast. They should avoid milk, spices, rich foods, and fruit juices at first. Dehydration should be corrected as described earlier.

Any patient with persistent or severe abdominal pain should be evacuated promptly (see section on **The Acute Abdomen** in Chapter 16).

Proper sanitation and attention to water and food supplies often will prevent much gastrointestinal misery. Always wash your hands after defecating and before eating. When washing dishes, rinse off soap *thoroughly* since it is a gastrointestinal irritant. Keep food covered in order to protect it from flies. Avoid eating native food in developing countries, unless it can be peeled or has been well cooked shortly after preparation and is still hot. Do not eat raw vegetables, unpeeled fruit, cooked food that has cooled, or food that has been exposed to flies. Avoid iced drinks because the ice may be contaminated. Drink only bottled, boiled, or disinfected water.

Respiratory Problems

People with head colds or sore throats should avoid wilderness trips because the stressful environment may bring on complications such as pneumonia or a sinus infection. Suspect pneumonia or pleurisy in a person who has a cough with fever and chest pain, especially if the cough is producing yellow or green sputum and the pain is located in the side of the chest underneath the armpit or beneath the scapula and is aggravated by deep breathing and coughing. Patients with suspected pneumonia or other severe respiratory infections should take amoxicillin/clavulanate, erythromycin, or a cephalosporin, and be evacuated promptly to medical care.

Urinary Problems

Symptoms of urinary tract infection include painful urination, frequent voiding of small amounts of urine, a feeling that the bladder has not been emptied, chills, fever, and backache in the costovertebral angle.

The patient should drink plenty of fluids and take amoxicillin/clavulanate, a cephalosporin, or tetracycline. The double-strength size of trimethoprim/sulfamethoxazole and the quinolones are also very effective.

Special Problems of Women

Wilderness travel without the customary amenities of civilization may pose special problems for women. Vaginal infections that may occur can be divided into two general types for purposes of treatment.

Yeast infections, characterized by thick, whiteish discharge and severe itching, usually respond promptly to miconazole vaginal suppositories (Monistat 7, available without prescription), inserted once daily at bedtime for seven days. Side effects include burning, itching, and irritation.

Other types of vaginitis commonly involve a thinner, yellowish discharge, sometimes with an objectionable odor. These infections usually are caused by either *Trichomonas vaginalis* or *Gardnerella vaginalis*. They both usually respond to one 250-mg tablet of metronidazole (Flagyl) taken three times daily for seven days. While taking metronidazole, the patient should *not* drink alcohol because the combination produces symptoms similar to those associated with Antabuse (flushing, copious sweating, severe headache, vomiting, dyspnea, and heart irregularities). Other side effects include abdominal pain, nausea, vomiting, diarrhea, and a metallic taste in the mouth.

Women who customarily have menstrual cramps should carry a medication that previously has been found to give relief. Otherwise, 200-mg tablets of ibuprofen (nonprescription Advil, Nuprin, etc.) usually are effective. Prescription pain pills such as acetaminophen with codeine (Tylenol with codeine) and propoxyphene with acetaminophen (Darvocet) also can be used.

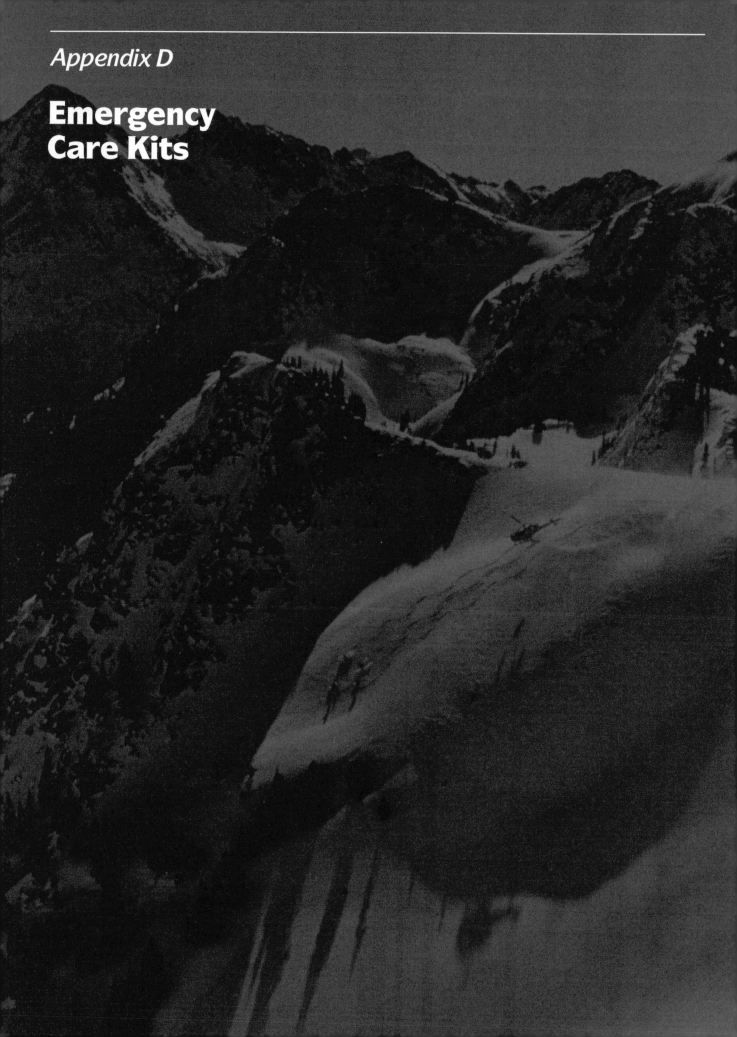

Appendix D

Emergency Care Kits

Recreational Emergency Care Kit

The amount of equipment carried in an emergency care kit depends on the length of the planned trip, the difficulty of obtaining medical help, the number of party members, and the type of transportation. The requirements of a one-day cross-country ski tour obviously are different from those of a four-week Alaskan expedition.

The following lists are suggestions only and can be modified to suit individual needs. Prescription medications are marked with an asterisk (*) and controlled substances are marked with two asterisks (**) except where listed as part of a physician's kit. Controlled substances include narcotics, sleeping pills, tranquilizers, and other drugs with abuse potential. They can be prescribed only by a physician who has registered with the Drug Enforcement Administration (DEA) of the U.S. Department of Justice. The physician is given a DEA number that must be included on every prescription written for a controlled substance.

In each instance, the quantity of each item (dressings, bandages, pills, etc.) recommended is the *minimum* quantity. Determination of the actual quantity to be taken along should be based on the number of persons in the party and the total trip time.

Emphasis is on minimal weight and bulk, low cost, maximum chance of use, favorable cost/bulk/weight-to-benefit ratio, and multiple use.

A **basic kit** is suitable for a day trip or to be carried by each member of a party on a multi-day trip. It can be stored in a small stuff-sack.

Contents of a Basic Kit

Items	Comments
Items	*Comments*
2 cravats	Use for bandage, sling, etc.
1 or 2 rolls of 3-inch or 4-inch self-adhering roller bandage (e.g., Kling)	Bandaging material.
1 roll of 2-inch adhesive tape	Can be torn in half lengthwise to make 1-inch tape. Small strips can be torn off to make butterfly bandages. Also can be used for blister prevention and treatment.
4 sterile gauze compresses, 3-inch x 4-inch or 4-inch x 4-inch (nonadhesive—Telfa or equivalent)	Can be cut up and used with pieces of tape to make small bandages (if you do not wish to carry regular pre-packaged bandage strips).
6 or more pre-packaged bandage strips (Bandaids, Curads)	
20 325-mg aspirin or acetaminophen (Tylenol), and/or 200-mg ibuprofen tablets	For headache and other mild pain, take 1 to 2 every 3 hours as needed. Ibuprofen preferred if frostbite risk (take 2 tablets 4 times daily after meals or with food during hazardous conditions).
Sunscreen or sunblock	See Chapter 18.
Lip salve	Preferably a type that stays relatively soft in cold weather. Use proper SPF number (see Chapter 18).

Items	Comments
Multiple-use knife with scissors and tweezers ("Swiss Army knife")	
Safety pins	Various uses; include large sizes to improvise upper-extremity splint by pinning sleeve to front of jacket.
Plastic sandwich bags	Fill with snow to improvise cold pack, various other uses.
Personal medications, if any	Diabetics include tube of glucose or 2 ampuls of glucagon with syringes and needles (as well as insulin, injection equipment, and blood glucose measuring equipment).
Water purification equipment (Potable Aqua tablets, First Need filter, etc.)	1 set for every 2 people.
Small flashlight or headlamp with spare batteries	Headlamp may be preferred because its use frees both hands.
1 pair of disposable rubber gloves	In 35 mm film can or plastic bag.

Optional

Items	Comments
One sheet of Moleskin	For blister prevention and treatment (some prefer this to 2-inch tape).
Antacid (Digel, Tums, etc.) or antacid/anti-gas preparation (Mylanta, etc.)	Combination of an antacid and an anti-gas preparation may be preferred for increased intestinal gas common at high altitude.
Small, foil-packaged, disposable, moist towelettes	For hand washing if water is unavailable.

Optional For Multi-day Trip

Items	Comments
**Sleeping pills of choice, if desired, with directions for use (consult physician)	Try these out at home to be sure they are effective. Use with caution above 12,000 feet (3,658 meters). Sleeping aids such as ear plugs and eye shields may be sufficient alone.
Pee bottle	Anyone who has had to get out of a warm sleeping bag to make a nocturnal pit stop knows what this is for. Women may wish to add a Sani-Fem funnel.

Contents of a Master Kit

A master kit is designed for multi-day recreational tours. Each party should have one master kit, which can be carried in a nylon stuff-sack, with injectables and other breakables in a separate, hard-sided container.

Items	Comments
Additional cravats to provide at least 6 per party	At least 6 are needed to improvise a Thomas splint from ski poles or to strap a patient to an improvised long spine board.

12 additional sterile, non-adhering gauze compresses

4 ABD pads or Surgipads, 2 medium, 2 large

3-inch wide rubberized bandage (Ace, etc.)

4 extra self-adhering roller bandages, 2 2-inch, 2 3-inch

6 tongue blades — Multiple uses such as improvised finger splints, etc.

30 inches of 1/8- to 1/4-inch diameter nylon cord (or several tongue blades taped together) — Use in setting up pulley traction (or Spanish windlass).

Spreader for ski pole splint — Such as an 8-inch piece of an old ski pole with two holes in it. The ski pole tips go in the holes (see Fig. C.2, Appendix C)

Seam ripper — Use instead of cutting expensive clothing.

Sewing needle — Can be part of a sewing kit and has many uses, including blister care.

Small bottle of antiseptic cleanser (10-percent povidone-iodine [Betadine], Phisohex) — Dilute povidone-iodine 1:10 with clean water for high-risk wound care (see Appendix C).

Thermometer — Rectal type is more versatile. For cold weather trips, low-reading thermometer recommended instead of, or in addition to, standard clinical one.

Single-edge razor blade or packaged sterile #15 scalpel blade — For incising and draining abscesses, etc.

30-cc syringe and #18-gauge needle — For wound irrigation.

Turkey-baster syringe or 60-cc syringe and Foley catheter — For upper airway suction.

2 extra pairs of disposable rubber gloves (consider sterile ones) — Use when dressing open wounds or to avoid contact with body fluids.

Pocket mask with one-way valve, or mouth shield — To increase effectiveness of rescue breathing and avoid contact with patient's saliva.

Notebook and pencil — To record vital signs and other important data.

Oropharyngeal airways (at least 2 sizes such as large and small adult) — To manage airway of unresponsive patient.

Medications

5-gm tube *Neosporin or *Garamycin ophthalmic ointment — Can be used in eyes or on skin for eye infections, infected cuts, etc. Apply 3 times daily.

24 25-mg or 12 *50-mg diphenhydramine hydrochloride (Benadryl) capsules

Alternatives:
*Tripelennamine (Pyribenzamine)
*Dexchlorpheniramine (Polaramine)
*Terfenadine (Seldane), etc.
Consult physician for doses of alternatives.

— For itching, hives, drug reactions, 1 50-mg or 2 25-mg capsules every 4 hours as needed. The 25-mg size is nonprescription.

12 30-mg **acetaminophen with 30-mg codeine (Tylenol #3) tablets

Alternative:
**propoxyphene napsylate 100 mg and acetaminophen (Darvocet N 100), 1 every 3 hours as needed

— For pain, 1 to 2 every 3 hours as needed. Codeine-containing drugs also can be used for diarrhea, 1 every 3 hours, as needed.

Optional

SAM splint — Small, multi-purpose fixation splint; can be used as improvised rigid collar.

Kendrick traction device — Alternative to ski pole traction splint.

12 2.5-mg **diphenoxylate with atropine sulfate (Lomotil) tablets — For diarrhea, 1 to 2 every 3 hours as needed.

Alternative:
2-mg capsules of loperamide (Imodium A-D), 2 with first loose bowel movement then 1 with each subsequent movement (not over 4 in each 24 hour period) — Loperamide is nonprescription.

6 10-mg *thiethylperazine (Torecan) rectal suppositories. — For vomiting. Insert 1 every 3 hours as needed.

Alternative:
25-mg *prochlorperazine (Compazine) suppositories, insert 1 every 12 hours as needed — Prochlorperazine is preferred for high altitude.

Optional for Those With Special Training and Licensing

16-gauge over-needle catheter (Angiocath, etc.) — For relief of tension pneumothorax.

Foley catheter with lubricating jelly — For urinary retention.

Cricothyroidotomy set

Additional Considerations

12 100-mg **meperidine (Demerol) tablets — For severe pain, 1/2 to 1 every 3 hours as needed.

Alternative:
*oxycodone and acetaminophen (Tylox, etc.) capsules — 1 every 3 hours as needed. Meperidine and oxycodone are strong narcotics.

Injectable *epinephrine (Ana-kit, Epi-pen) — For anaphylactic reactions (preferable to have susceptible person carry own kit as well).

For Extended Trips into Remote Country, Add:

Several packets of powdered sport drink (Gatorade, etc.) or Oralyte (see Appendix C)	Electrolyte replacement solution.
20 *trimethoprim/ sulfamethoxazole (Septra DS, Bactrim DS) tablets, or	Good, (inexpensive), multipurpose *single* antibiotic. See Appendix C. 1 twice daily for 5 or more days.
20 *ciprofloxacin 500-mg tablets (Cipro), or	Good, (expensive) multipurpose *single* antibiotic. 1 twice daily for 5 or more days.
1 from each of the following two groups of antibiotics: (see Appendix C)	Broader coverage than with a single antibiotic, but more complicated to use.
1. 20 *Cephalexin (Keflex) capsules, 250 mg, 1 capsule 4 times daily	For upper- and lower-respiratory infections, wound and skin infections, high-risk wounds.
Alternatives: *Cefaclor (Ceclor) 250 mg three times daily; *cefuroxime (Ceftin) 250 mg twice daily; *amoxicillin/clavulanate (Augmentin) 250 mg three times daily; *erythromycin ethyl succinate (EES 400), 400 mg four times daily	
2. 14 *doxycycline 100-mg tablets, 1 tablet twice daily	For urinary tract infections and dysentery.
Alternative: *tetracycline 250-mg tablets, 1 tablet 4 times daily	Do not take tetracycline with milk or dairy products or close to meals. Exaggerated sunburn reaction may occur, especially at high altitude or on snow. Stop drug at first sign of unusual skin redness.

Note: If there is no improvement with a drug in one group after two days, switch to a drug in the other group.

Recommended for High Altitude

12 or more 250-mg *acetazolamide (Diamox) tablets	See Appendix C for details.
30 4-mg *dexamethasone (Decadron or Hexadrol) tablets	See Appendix C.
6 10-mg and 20 long-acting (20 to 30 mg) *nifedipine (Procardia, Adalat)	See Appendix C.

Recommended for Undeveloped Countries

20 *trimethoprim/sulfa-methoxazole (Septra, Bactrim) DS tablets or 20 *ciprofloxacin (Cipro) 500-mg tablets	For dysentery, 1 tablet twice daily for 5 to 10 days. See Appendix C.
Pills for malaria prophylaxis if needed.	Consult physician.

Optional for Women

7 miconazole nitrate (Monistat 7) vaginal suppositories	For yeast vaginitis. Insert 1 at bedtime for 1 week. See Appendix C.
21 250-mg *metronidazole (Flagyl) tablets. 1 tablet 3 times daily for a week.	For all other types of vaginitis. See Appendix C. Do not drink alcohol while taking this drug. Do not take if pregnant.

Recommended for Snake Country

Sawyer extractor	Powerful suction syringe for injected poisons. See Chapters 23 and 24.
Occlusive band	To delay absorption of snake venom.

Wilderness Search and Rescue (SAR) Emergency Care Kit

Dressings, Bandages, and Wound Care

10 3-inch x 4-inch nonadhesive gauze compresses
4 ABD pads or Surgipads, 2 medium, 2 large
4 self-adhering roller bandages, 2 2-inch, 2 3-inch
2 packs of povidone-iodine pledgets or bottle of 10-percent povidone-iodine
1 500-ml bag (with IV tubing) of sterile physiological saline, sterile 30-cc syringe with sterile 18-gauge needle for wound irrigation
2 packets Vaseline gauze
1 roll each, ½-inch, 1-inch, and 2-inch adhesive tape
4 feet of plastic wrap such as Saran, folded or rolled
24 Bandaids
Steristrips, ⅛-inch and ¼-inch
1 3-inch rubberized bandage
1 2-inch rubberized bandage
12 plastic storage bags, 6 small, 6 medium
4 pairs disposable rubber gloves, nonsterile
2 pairs disposable rubber gloves, sterile
2 disposable face shields (see Appendix F)

Splints and Litters

Rigid collars (Stifneck set, medium Stifneck, or improvised from SAM splint)
Sager splint or Kendrick traction device with 55-gallon clear plastic garbage bag
Pneumatic splint for lower extremity, long size
Kendrick extrication device or Oregon spine splint II
8 cravats
2 SAM splints
1 litter (SKED, Ferno-Washington, etc.) Preferably lightweight or break-in-half for backpacking

Cardiorespiratory

6 oropharyngeal airways, 2 each of 3 sizes
Nasopharyngeal airways, 2 each of 3 sizes
Pocket mask with one-way valve and oxygen intake nipple
Suction apparatus (V-Vac, Res-Q-Vac, or portable battery operated)
Bag-valve-mask

Drugs

Same as drugs suggested above in the master kit. Add epinephrine injection kit (*Epipen, *Ana-kit, etc.) for anaphylactic reactions, sublingual nitroglycerine tablets (Nitrostat 0.4 mg), and instant glucose (Glutose, etc.) for hypoglycemia.

Other

Lightweight stethoscope	Penlight
Blood pressure cuff	Razor blade, single-edge
Hypothermia thermometer	Seam ripper
Clinical thermometer	Steel sewing needle
Blood glucose test strips	Lubricant jelly
Bandage scissors	Safety pins
Paramedic shears	Tweezers
Tags	Notebook and pencil
Urinal or pee bottle	Headlamp

Additional Items for Hypothermia

Rewarming equipment such as chemical heating pads, Heat-pac, hydraulic sarong, device for heating inspired air (UVIC Heat Treat, APPLINC Saving Breath, Res-Q-Aire, etc.) See Chapter 18.
Extra sleeping bag or casualty bag
Tent

Optional

PASG
Oxygen backpack (2 tanks, regulator, masks, nasal cannulae, and tubing)

Wilderness SAR Physician/Paramedic Kit

Stethoscope
Blood pressure cuff
Small otoscope/ ophthalmoscope with tongue blades
Cricothyroidotomy set
Endotracheal intubation kit
14-gauge Intracath for needle thoracotomy
Flutter valve (Heimlich or improvised from finger of rubber glove)
Intravenous fluids:
    Liter bags of lactated Ringers/5-percent glucose solution
    Liter bags of 10-percent glucose/half-normal saline solution
IV administration sets
18-gauge Intracath needles
1-inch adhesive tape
½-inch adhesive tape
Alcohol swabs
Tourniquets
Parenteral drugs, general (include sterile syringes and needles for injection):

Meperidine	Diphenhydramine
Thiethylperazine or prochlorperazine	Digoxin
	Furosemide
Morphine	50-percent glucose (requires 50 cc-syringe)
Epinephrine 1:1000	
Naloxone	Dexamethasone
Aminophylline (requires 50-cc syringe)	Diazepam

Optional

Chest tube set and insertion pack
Water seal apparatus and bag of sterile water
Nasogastric tubes
Foley catheter (18 French) with collection bag and clamp
Lubricant
Povidone-iodine swabs
Monitor/defibrillator or automatic external defibrillator
Parenteral drugs, ACLS:
(monitor/defibrillator desirable)

Include additional sterile syringes and needles	Verapamil
	Morphine
Atropine	Procainamide
Lidocaine	Adenosine
Epinephrine 1:10,000	Dopamine
Bretylium	

Ski Patrol Emergency Care Equipment

Recommended Minimum Contents for Alpine Patrol Belt

4 triangular bandages, folded as cravats	Flashlight
2 rolls self-adhering roller bandage: 1 2-inch, 1 3-inch	Release of responsibility form (Appendix E)
6 bandaids	Paramedic shears or bandage scissors
1 roll 2-inch adhesive tape	Several clean tongue blades in plastic bag
9 assorted sterile compresses, 3 each of 3 sizes	Two pairs of disposable rubber gloves in plastic 35-mm film box or plastic bag
Pocket knife such as Swiss army type	
4 large safety pins	Pocket mask (preferable) or disposable mouth shield (either should have one-way valve)
Notebook and "space pen"	
Flow sheet for vital signs (Appendix E)	

Additional considerations:

1 tube instant glucose	Three oropharyngeal airways, 1 each of 3 sizes (adult, child, infant)
Blood glucose test strips (Chemstrip bG)	
Screwdriver, pliers, small wrench, "Leatherman tool"	Map of ski area
	Fire starter
Matches in waterproof container	Plastic storage bags, several sizes
Cigarette lighter	Ankle hitch (EZ-TRAC) with 30 inches of ⅛- to ¼-inch cord for traction
Wire splint or SAM splint	
Avalanche cord	Seam ripper

Note: Avalanche transceiver is preferred, especially at ski areas with high avalanche hazard. It should be worn around the neck on a cord and not be in the patrol belt.

Recommended Minimum Contents for Nordic Patrol Emergency Care Kit

4 or more cravats	Sterile, nonadhesive gauze compresses, assorted sizes
3 rolls self-adhering roller bandage, 1 each of 3 sizes	
	4 ABD pads or Surgipads, 2 large, 2 medium
1 roll, 2-inch adhesive tape	

Bandaids
Betadine pledgets
Vaseline gauze
4 feet of plastic wrap (folded or rolled) or 4 large plastic storage bags
1 3-inch rubberized bandage
2 pairs disposable rubber gloves
SAM splint
Three oropharyngeal airways, 1 each of 3 sizes
Pocket mask with one-way valve and oxygen intake nipple
One tube instant glucose (Glutose)
Tweezers
Bandage scissors or paramedic shears

Single-edge razor blade or #15 scalpel blade in sterile packet
Four large safety pins
Spreader for ski pole splint
Notebook and pencil
Flow sheet for vital signs (see Appendix E)
Flashlight
Seam ripper
Steel sewing needle
Ankle hitch (EZ-TRAC) with 30-inches of nylon cord for pulley traction
Hypothermia thermometer
Matches in waterproof container
Firestarter

Optional

Rewarming device for hypothermic patient (Heatpac, chemical heating pads, hot air inhalation device)
12 25-mg diphenhydramine (Benadryl) capsules
20 aspirin or acetaminophen tablets, 325 mg
12 doses of pain medicine such as **acetaminophen with codeine, 30 mg (Tylenol #3), or **propoxyphene napsylate and acetaminophen, 100 mg (Darvocet N 100)

Additional Considerations

*Sterile saline for irrigating
30-cc syringe and 18-gauge needle for irrigating
Pneumatic splints
*Injectable epinephrine (Ana-kit, Epipen) for anaphylactic reactions
12 2.5-mg **diphenoxylate with atropine sulfate (Lomotil) tablets or 20-mg loperamide (Imodium) tablets
High altitude drugs (see Master Kit above)

Kendrick traction device
Two anti-vomiting suppositories such as:
*thiethylperazine (Torecan) or
*prochlorperazine (Compazine)
12 100-mg **meperidine (Demerol) tablets
*Antibiotics (see Master Kit above)
Urinal or pee bottle
Blood glucose test strips (Chemstrip bG)

Toboggan Pack

Piece of Ensolite to pad bottom of toboggan
Blankets or sleeping bag
Waterproof cover

Quick splint or cardboard splint
Canvas stretcher
Cravats and padding material

Additional Considerations (usually kept at top of hill)

Long and short spine boards
Pneumatic splints
Traction splints
Extra sleeping bags

Portable oxygen with masks, nasal cannulae, and tubing
Extra toboggan packs
Bag-valve-mask
Suction equipment

Patrol First Aid Room

The following are recommended minimum items. Final selection should be based on local needs and consultation with area management, the patrol medical advisor, and WEC instructors.

Basic Equipment

Cots or beds
Bed pans and urinals
Warming mechanism for cold skiers: infrared lamps, electric blanket, hot water bottles, heating pads, etc.
Portable screen or curtains for privacy
First aid cabinet
Oxygen equipment
Suction equipment
Bag-valve-masks
Pocket masks with one-way valve

Sink with running water, soap, towels
Toilet
Waste receptacles
Infectious waste disposal and contaminated clothing containers (see Appendix E)
Telephone and radio
Pipe cutter (for shortening impaled objects)
Large container for rewarming frozen hand or foot in warm water

Contents of Emergency Care Cabinet

Self-adhering roller bandages
Pre-packaged bandage strips (Bandaids, Curads)
Butterfly bandages or Steri-Strips
Standard thermometer
Low-reading thermometer
Cravats
Sterile dressings, assorted sizes including non-adhering types
Tweezers
Plastic bags (add snow to make cold pack)
Adhesive tape, assorted widths
Single-edge razor blades
Povidone-iodine or other skin preparation solution
Sewing kit
Compound Tincture of Benzoin
Safety pins
Bandage scissors

Disposable paper cups
Paramedic shears
Rubbing alcohol
Washpan, large metal or plastic
Emesis basin
Urinal
Laboratory thermometer, to measure water temperature in frostbite rewarming
Stethoscope
Blood pressure cuff
Flashlight
Tongue blades
Sanitary napkins
Blood glucose measuring equipment: (One-Touch II blood glucose meter, Chemstrip bG)
Disposable gowns
Disposable face shields
Disposable rubber gloves, including sterile pairs
Accident and other report forms

Medical Kit for Physician or Paramedic***

The following are suggested items. Final determination should be made through consultation with area management and the patrol medical advisor and members of the Doctors' Patrol, if any.

Intravenous fluids, IV sets, IV needles
Cardiac monitor-defibrillator or automatic external defibrillator
PASG
Endotracheal intubation kit with endotracheal tubes
Drugs (see above under physician/paramedic and SAR kits)
Equipment for needle thoracotomy and cricothyroidotomy
Flutter valve (Heimlich, etc.)
Chest tube set and insertion pack
Small oto-ophthalmoscope set

***Consider commercial self-contained kits, such as the Banyan, available from Banyan International Corp., P.O. Box 1779, Abilene, TX 79604.

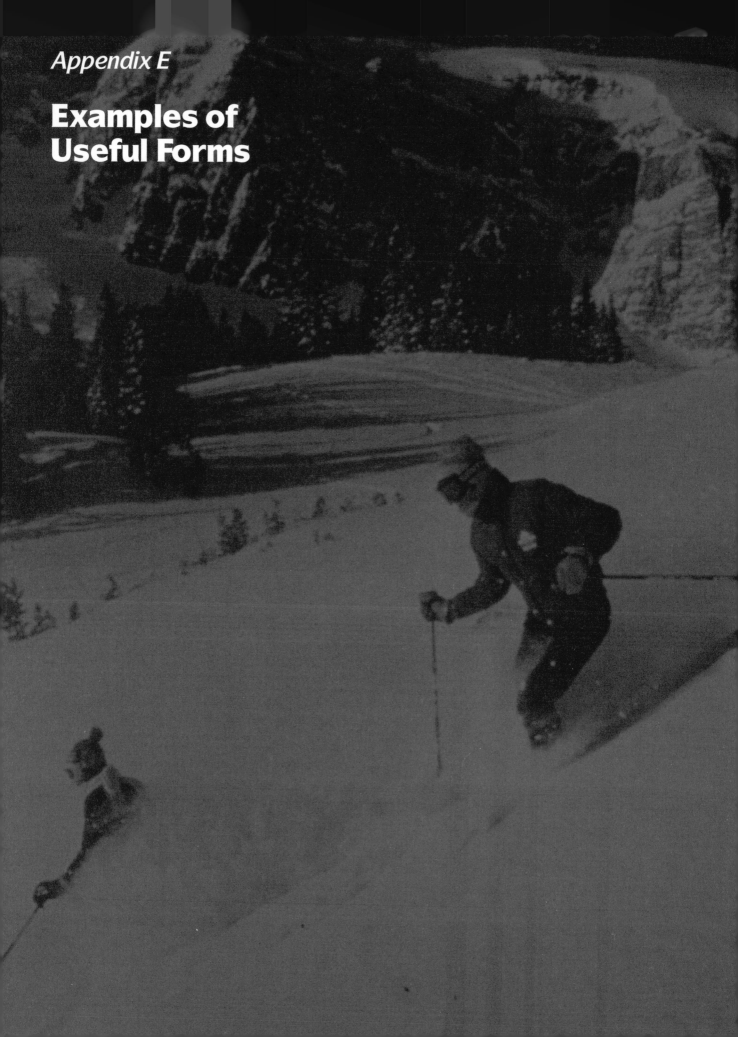

Appendix E

Examples of Useful Forms

This appendix contains samples of four useful forms ski patrollers should carry whenever they may be called on to provide emergency care services for area management. Insurance companies often provide their clients with the appropriate forms for this purpose.

1. Sample Form E.1
   Refusal of Care
2. Sample Form E.2
   Incident Report
3. Sample Form E.3
   Flow Sheet for Seriously Injured Patient
4. Sample Form E.4
   Site of Trauma Figure

Note: Before adopting any of the following forms for ski patrol use at any ski area, the ski patrol director should obtain approval from area management.

REFUSAL OF CARE

Patient Name _____ Incident No._____

I acknowledge that the _____ Ski Patrol has offered me (or the patient) the following assistance:

Check	Initials of Signatory	Type of Assistance
		Emergency Care
		Transportation to a medical facility
		Arrangements to transport to a hospital

    I further acknowledge that the _____ Ski Patrol has explained the nature of my (or the patient's) probable injuries or illness, the possibility that the injuries or illness may be more serious than now known or suspected, the possibility that other injuries or illnesses may be present and undetected, and the potential consequences of refusing the assistance noted above.

    Despite the injuries or illness, and the possible consequences of refusing assistance, I refuse the assistance noted above on behalf of myself (or the patient).

    I agree the _____ Ski Patrol has no further duty to provide assistance to me (or the patient), and I release and discharge the _____ Ski Patrol from any duty of any kind to provide further care or assistance to me (or the patient).

This document is signed and initialed by:

Name _____

Address _____

City _____ State _____ Zip _____

Telephone Number _____ Age _____

Relationship to Patient _____

Date _____ Signature _____

Witness _____ Signature _____
                   Name

If applicable:

Patient / Parent / Spouse / Next of Kin / Other _____
    (circle all that apply)

refused the assistance noted above, and refused to sign this form when requested to do so.

Patroller _____ Signature _____
                Name

Witness _____ Signature _____
               Name

INCIDENT REPORT

Ski Area _____ Date: ___/___/___ Time of Incident _____ ☐ AM ☐ PM Incident No. _____

LOCATION	☐ Trail _____ Skied Trail Before? ☐ Yes ☐ No ☐ Lift # _____ Ridden Lift Before? ☐ Yes ☐ No ☐ Premise: Exact Location _____ ☐ Ski School _____ Instructor _____	**TRAIL RATING** ☐ ○ Easier ☐ ● More Difficult ☐ ◆ Most Difficult ☐ ◆◆ Extremely Difficult

INJURED PERSON	Name _____ Occupation _____ Address _____ City _____ State ___ Zip _____ Phone _____ Parent/Group Leader _____ Medical Insurance: ☐ Yes ☐ No Corrective Lenses: ☐ Yes ☐ No	☐ Male ☐ Female Age _____ Weight _____ Height _____

DESCRIBE INCIDENT IN INJURED PERSON'S OWN WORDS	_____ _____ _____ How could you have prevented incident? _____

WITNESS ☐ INVOLVED IN COLLISION	Name _____ Address/City/State/Zip _____ Phone _____ Name _____ Address/City/State/Zip _____ Phone _____

PROBABLE INJURY	☐ Fracture ☐ Puncture/Laceration ☐ Abrasion ☐ Dislocation ☐ Multiple ☐ Sprain ☐ Bruise/Contusion ☐ Concussion ☐ Frostbite ☐ Other _____

INJURY ZONE	☐ Left ☐ Right ☐ Both	☐ Thigh ☐ Knee ☐ Lower Leg ☐ Ankle ☐ Foot	☐ Hip ☐ Abdomen ☐ Chest ☐ Back ☐ Neck	☐ Shoulder ☐ Arm ☐ Wrist ☐ Hand ☐ Thumb	☐ Head ☐ Face ☐ Eye ☐ Nose ☐ Mouth	☐ Teeth ☐ Other Previous Injury ☐ Yes ☐ No

EMERGENCY CARE RENDERED	On Hill _____ By Whom _____ In Aid Area _____ By Whom _____ Transport: ☐ Toboggan ☐ Self ☐ Snowmobile ☐ Other _____

TRANSPORT & DESTINATION	☐ Walked Out ☐ Auto/Bus ☐ Returned to Skiing ☐ Ambulance Time ___:___ ☐ AM ☐ PM ☐ Lodge/Home ☐ Hospital

EQUIPMENT	☐ Alpine ☐ Owned ☐ Area Rental # _____ ☐ Nordic ☐ Rented ☐ Shop Name _____ ☐ Snowboard ☐ Borrowed ☐ Binding Model _____ ☐ Other ☐ Other ☐ Type Skis _____	**SKIS REMOVED BY** Fall ☐ R ☐ L Injured ☐ R ☐ L Patrol ☐ R ☐ L Other ☐ R ☐ L

SKIING HISTORY	**ABILITY** ☐ Beginner/Novice ☐ Lower Intermediate ☐ Intermediate ☐ Advanced/Expert	**DAYS SKIED THIS SEASON** THIS AREA ANY AREA ☐ 1st Day ☐ 1st Day ☐ 2-9 Days ☐ 2-9 Days ☐ 10 or more ☐ 10 or more days	Falls Today ☐ 1st ☐ 2-9 ☐ 10-more How many years skied this season? ___ ☐ Season Pass Holder # _____

SIGNATURE	Injured Person THE ABOVE INFORMATION IS CORRECT. (X) _____ Parent or Guardian I REFUSE EMERGENCY CARE. (X) _____

SNOW AND WEATHER CONDITIONS	**CONDITIONS** ☐ Powder ☐ Soft ☐ Deep ☐ Packed Powder ☐ Corn ☐ Icy ☐ Hard ☐ Heavy ☐ Variable	**WEATHER** ☐ Fair ☐ Snowing ☐ Overcast ☐ Raining ☐ Fog	**TEMPERATURE** ☐ Below 0 °F ☐ 0-32°F ☐ Above 32°F

PATROLLER COMMENTS	_____ _____ _____ Use Separate Sheet if Necessary

PATROLLER COMPLETING REPORT	Photos Taken ☐ Yes ☐ No By Whom _____ Date _____ Time _____ Name _____ Signature _____ Patrol Number _____

FLOW SHEET FOR SERIOUSLY INJURED

_____ Ski Patrol

Incident No. _____

| Patient's Name | Age | Sex | Date |

Patroller's First Impression/Mechanism of Injury   Time of Arrival on Scene

_____

_____

PRIMARY SURVEY

AIRWAY
- ☐ Open
- ☐ Partial Obstruction
- ☐ Total Obstruction

BREATHING
- ☐ Normal
- ☐ Shallow
- ☐ Labored
- ☐ Absent

BLEEDING
- ☐ Severe
- ☐ Minor
- ☐ None

CIRCULATION
- ☐ Normal Pulse
- ☐ Weak Pulse
- ☐ Strong Pulse
- ☐ Irregular Pulse
- ☐ Absent Pulse

LEVEL OF RESPONSIVENESS
- ☐ Alert ☐ Oriented to:
- ☐ Person ☐ Place ☐ Time ☐ Event
- ☐ Lethargic ☐ Confused
- ☐ Anxious ☐ Violent
- ☐ Uncooperative
- ☐ Responds to verbal
- ☐ Responds to pain
- ☐ Unresponsive

CERVICAL SPINE PROBLEM
- ☐ Mechanism ☐ Pain
- ☐ Tenderness ☐ Numbness
- ☐ Weakness ☐ Paralysis
- ☐ Not Applicable

PUPILS
- ☐ Equal
- ☐ Unequal
- ☐ Fixed
- ☐ Dilated
- ☐ Pinpoint Size
  (see pupil gauge)

PUPIL GAUGE (MM)
2   3   4
5   6   7
____ R   ____ L

VITAL SIGNS

TIME	P	R	BP	AVPU	R Pupils L	Comments

PROCEDURES

TIME	PROCEDURES
	Toboggan Arrival Time
	Extrication
	CPR
	Bandaging
	Oxygen
	Suction
	Oral Airway
	Bag-Valve-Mask
	Rigid Collar
	Spine Board
	Splint Upper R L Other
	Lower R L
	Traction R L
	PASG
	Leave for Base
	Arrive Base

SECONDARY SURVEY

SKIN TEMPERATURE/MOISTURE
- ☐ Normal ☐ Dry
- ☐ Warm ☐ Moist
- ☐ Cool ☐ Sweaty
- ☐ Hot ☐ Cold

SKIN COLOR
- ☐ Normal ☐ Pale
- ☐ Flushed ☐ Cyanotic

CAPILLARY REFILL
EXTREMITY:	NL	ABNL
RU		
LU		
RL		
LL		

PAIN
- ☐ None ☐ Minimal
- ☐ Moderate ☐ Severe

PATIENT'S CHIEF COMPLAINT OR DESCRIPTION OF ACCIDENT

PRE-EXISTING ILLNESS

MEDICATIONS

ALLERGIES

HEAD ☐ Normal ☐ Raccoon Sign
Drainage: ☐ Ears   R   L
           ☐ Nose
☐ Vision Grossly Intact
Other _____

NECK ☐ Normal ☐ Trachea Deviated
Other _____

CHEST ☐ Normal ☐ Symmetrical ☐ Subcutaneous Emphysema
☐ No Expansion ☐ Breath Sounds R ___ L ___
☐ Heart Sounds Muffled   Other _____

ABDOMEN ☐ Normal ☐ Distended
☐ Tender: ☐ RUQ ☐ LUQ ☐ RLQ ☐ LLQ
☐ Absent Bowel Sounds   Other _____

PELVIS ☐ Normal ☐ Unstable ☐ Bleeding
☐ Urethra ☐ Rectum ☐ Vagina
Other _____

EXTREMITIES ☐ Normal
☐ Abnormal Pulses: ☐ RU ☐ RL ☐ LU ☐ LL
☐ Abnormal Sensations: ☐ RU ☐ RL ☐ LU ☐ LL
☐ Abnormal Motor: ☐ RU ☐ RL ☐ LU ☐ LL
Other _____

BACK ☐ Normal ☐ Pain ☐ Deformity
Other _____

Signature of Person Completing This Form

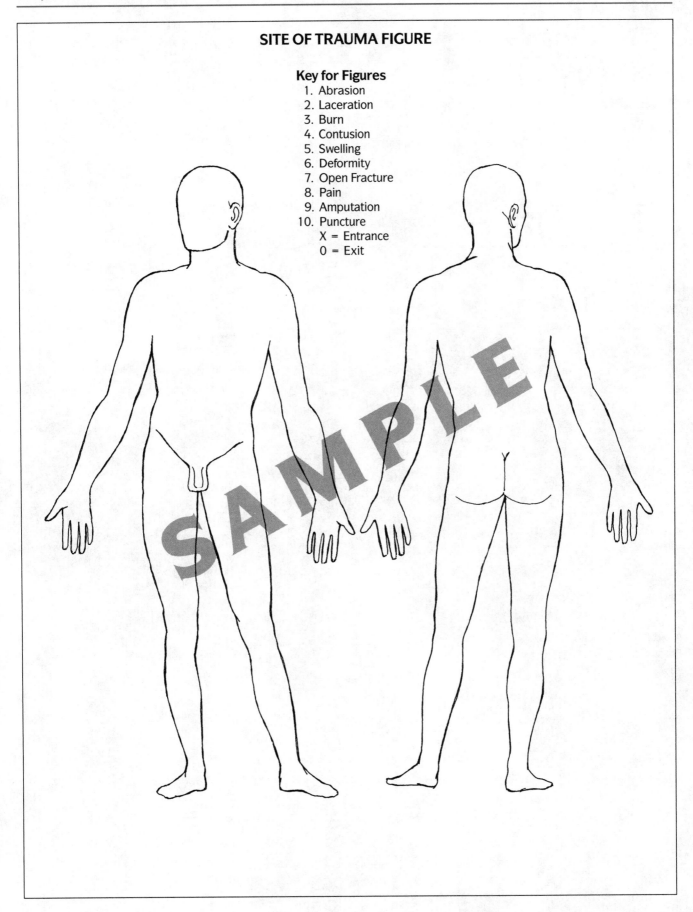

SITE OF TRAUMA FIGURE

Key for Figures
1. Abrasion
2. Laceration
3. Burn
4. Contusion
5. Swelling
6. Deformity
7. Open Fracture
8. Pain
9. Amputation
10. Puncture
    X = Entrance
    0 = Exit

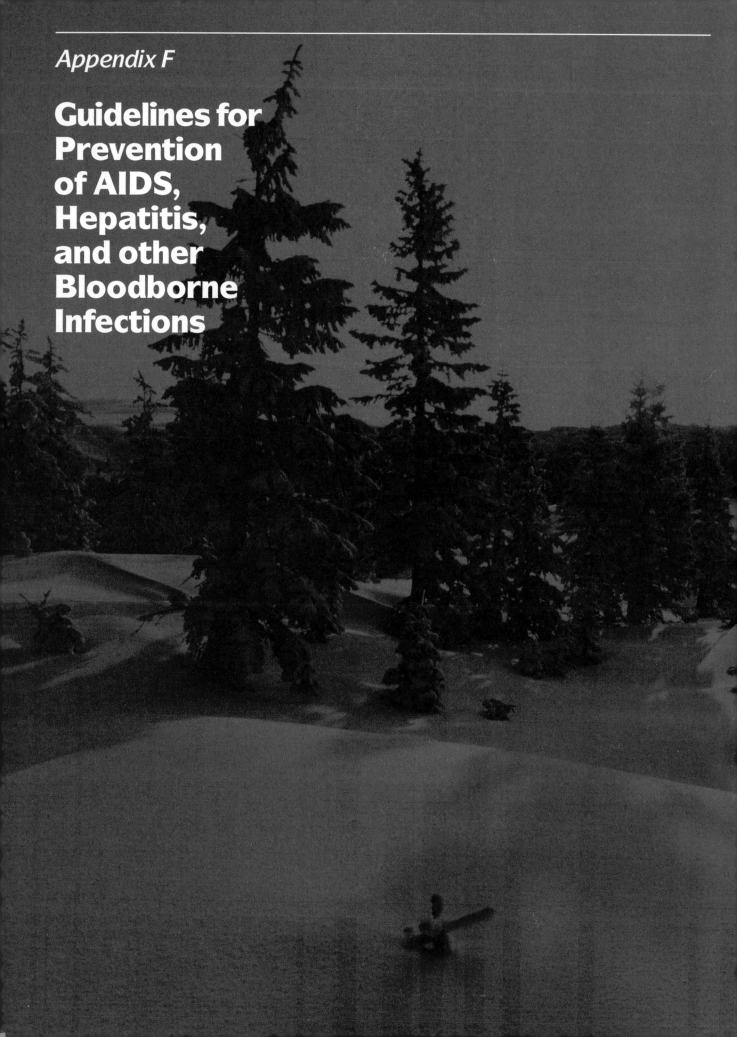

Appendix F

Guidelines for Prevention of AIDS, Hepatitis, and other Bloodborne Infections

This appendix has been prepared with the aid of "Guidelines for Prevention of Transmission of Human Immunodeficiency Virus and Hepatitis B Virus to Health-Care and Public-Safety Workers," published by the Centers for Disease Control of the U.S. Public Health Service, February 1989; and the guidelines issued by the Occupational Safety and Health Administration (OSHA) in December 1991 (Part II, Department of Labor, Title 29, Code of Federal Regulations, Part 1910.1030: Bloodborne Pathogens).

Before 1981, the risk of contact with human body fluids was unappreciated and unemphasized. Rubber gloves and gowns worn by health care workers were for the *patient's* protection rather than the worker's protection. This unsophisticated concept of risk evaporated rapidly after the first cases of acquired immunodeficiency syndrome (AIDS) were identified in 1981, the significance and magnitude of the AIDS epidemic became apparent, and the route of spread was identified. In some cases there was over-reaction, leading to hysterical rather than rational protective measures. One purpose of this appendix is to discuss the actual risks of contact with body fluids and to list reasonable and effective measures to counteract them. No one of us needs to refuse to give care or to resign from his or her emergency care activities because of the fear of contracting AIDS or any other contagious disease.

AIDS is caused by the human immunodeficiency virus (HIV), a retrovirus that attacks human T lymphocytes, causing a progressive depletion of the CD4 helper-inducer subset with resulting destruction of the body's ability to fight off certain infections and resist certain cancers. Although tests for HIV infection may

be positive as early as one to three months after exposure to the virus, there usually is a period of a few to many (even 10 or more) years of asymptomatic HIV infection before the patient develops signs and symptoms of AIDS. Although the patient may feel perfectly healthy during this asymptomatic period, he or she is capable of passing the infection to others.

AIDS is regarded as 100-percent fatal. As of this writing, well over 300,000 cases of AIDS have been reported from 156 countries. Approximately 200,000 of these cases have been reported from the United States; over 130,000 of these patients have died. In the United States, about 1.5 million persons are currently infected with HIV, almost all of whom either have AIDS or will eventually develop it. It is estimated that by the end of 1993 —12 years after the report of the first case—between 390,000 and 480,000 cases of AIDS will have been diagnosed in the United States and at least 250,000 persons will have died.

Although HIV has been found in blood, semen, vaginal fluid, breast milk, saliva, and tears, most infections are acquired through transmission by blood, semen, or vaginal fluid; rarely through breast milk. There have been no reported incidents of transmission through saliva or tears. HIV infection usually is acquired by having unprotected homosexual or heterosexual intercourse with an infected person, by sharing needles with an infected person (intravenous drug addicts), by receiving infected blood or blood products through transfusion, by the fetus through an infected mother during pregnancy, or (rarely) by the infant through breast feeding.

The concept of AIDS as a disease of homosexuals and intravenous drug abusers is changing as more and more cases are seen in heterosexuals. Heterosexual teenage girls form the fastest growing group of new AIDS patients.

A few cases of HIV infection in health care workers have been caused by contaminated material introduced through intact skin by needle sticks or accidental cuts. In rare instances, infected material splashed onto mucous membranes (eyes or mouth) or non-intact skin (i.e., dry winter skin, chapped, cracked, or inflamed skin) has caused HIV infection. When the patient is HIV positive, the emergency care worker's risk of becoming positive through a cut or needle stick is about 0.3 percent; from a splash onto mucous membranes or non-intact skin considerably less than that, and from a splash onto intact skin probably zero. As of 1988, *no* emergency care worker below the paramedic level had acquired HIV infection from emergency care activities.

A more important problem for the emergency care worker is hepatitis, because of its higher infectivity and greater prevalence (one to three per 1,000 persons in the general population are carriers). The types of hepatitis of concern are hepatitis B, C, and D, caused by the hepatitis B, C, and D viruses respectively. By far the most prevalent type is the hepatitis B virus (HBV). In 1990, 250 health care workers died of job-related hepatitis while none died of job-related AIDS. In some parts of the world, 5 to 15 percent of all people are positive for HBV. Patients in institutions, intravenous drug users, homosexual males, and household contacts of carriers all have high rates of infection. The mode of transmission of the hepatitis viruses is similar to that of HIV.

Household contacts of infected patients can acquire hepatitis by sexual contact, close personal contact such as kissing, and through sharing toothbrushes, razor blades, nail clippers, and other items where blood may be exchanged. Because of the high concentration of virus in the blood of infected individuals, the risk from an accidental needle stick or splash on non-intact skin is considerably higher than with HIV, i.e., 15 to 40 percent. About 12,000 health care workers become infected with hepatitis B each year, of which 250 die of fulminating hepatitis. Since a potent hepatitis B vaccine is available, *all* health care workers are strongly advised (many are required by law) to be vaccinated against HBV.

Volunteer emergency care providers who do not give injections or start IVs (such as basic EMTs or ski patrollers) are at minimal risk for HIV or hepatitis infection. What risk there is results from getting an infected patient's blood or other high-risk substances on non-intact skin or splashed into an eye, mouth or nose; or from accidentally being cut while working on such a patient.

Feces, nasal secretions, sputum, sweat, tears, urine and vomitus, if uncontaminated with blood, have not been shown to be dangerous. However, since *any* body fluid can contain blood and under emergency conditions you cannot easily tell what type of fluid you are dealing with, *avoid* contact with *all* body fluids. Although surgeons in the operating room frequently end up with blood anywhere from the top of the head to the shoes, studies have shown that most blood contamination during surgery is on the hands, forearms, and abdomen. This is probably also true of emergency care providers working on patients with severe hemorrhage or multiple open injuries.

The following **universal blood and body fluid precautions** are based on recommendations from the U.S. Centers for Disease Control, modified to some extent for the outdoor environment. They apply to high-risk substances and are designed to protect you from *all* blood-borne infectious agents and to *give a wide margin of safety*. They are especially important if you are *pregnant*.

High-risk substances include the following:

1. Blood (including menstrual blood) and any other body fluid visibly contaminated with blood.
2. Certain other body fluids such as semen; vaginal secretions; amniotic fluid (from childbirth or miscarriage); cerebrospinal fluid (from an open head injury); joint fluid; pleural, peritoneal, or pericardial fluid; breast milk; and saliva.
3. Clothing, bedding, and other absorbent materials soiled with blood or the other body fluids listed above. HBV can survive on the surface of clothing at room temperature for a week and thus can be spread by contact with dirty laundry.

However, *the most important source of infection is blood*. Most of the following recommendations are concerned with avoiding exposure to blood.

Although health care workers are at more risk in areas with a high incidence of AIDS and hepatitis than those in areas of a low incidence, since you rarely know the HIV and hepatitis status of a patient you should assume that *all patients are infectious for HIV and other blood-borne pathogens*.

1. Wear rubber (latex) gloves when handling high-risk substances. Have extra pairs available, and when you are caring for more than one patient, change gloves between patients to prevent transmission from one patient to another. If a prolonged period of care is anticipated, put on two pairs of gloves. Inspect the gloves before and after you put them on. About 1.5 percent of gloves are defective to begin with; 20 percent fail after being used two hours. If a glove breaks while you are working on a patient, wash your hands before putting on a new pair of gloves. Remove gloves contaminated with high-risk substances as soon as possible, taking care to avoid skin contact with the contaminated surface of the gloves. Dispose of the gloves according to the local protocol for infectious waste.
2. If you have non-intact skin or skin that is broken by a rash, skin crack, open cut, or sore, do not handle high-risk substances even while wearing rubber gloves. If handling is absolutely necessary, wear two pairs of gloves. In the classic emergency situation where direct pressure is required immediately to stop serious bleeding, try to get the patient to apply the direct pressure.
3. Unbroken skin provides good protection. However, if you cannot avoid handling high-risk substances *without* gloves or if other body parts are exposed to contamination or contaminated clothing, wash yourself immediately afterward, preferably with soap and water, or if these are not available, with waterless antiseptic hand cleanser. If no soap or hand cleanser is available, use water alone; if there is no liquid water, use snow if feasible. Afterward, wash thoroughly with soap and water as soon as you reach a facility where it is available.
4. Be careful to avoid cutting or sticking yourself with sharp objects while working on a patient.

5. Wear protective clothing when there is a chance of being splashed by blood or other high-risk fluids, i.e., as in a patient with massive arterial bleeding. Protect your face with goggles plus a face mask, or a disposable face protector (face shield). Protect your body with a surgical gown, preferably a reinforced, fluid-resistant, disposable one. The type of clothing usually worn by ski patrollers and other nonurban rescuers—goggles and water-resistant parka and pants—offers good protection. Zip your parka, put on your goggles, and put on latex gloves as you approach an accident where a patient has obvious bleeding.

6. Wash your hands with soap and water as soon as possible after removing gloves and other protective clothing. Pull the gloves off so they are inside-out and the contaminated side is not exposed. Wear gloves while handling contaminated clothing and other materials; store these contaminated items in a plastic bag while awaiting cleaning or disposal. Do not eat, drink, or smoke while wearing gloves. Clean up all spills of blood and blood-containing fluids promptly, wearing rubber utility (household) gloves. Remove visible material with disposable towels, wash the area with soap and water, then scrub it thoroughly with a 1:10 solution of sodium hypochlorite (household bleach).

7. When giving rescue breathing or CPR, protect yourself from the patient's saliva with a mouth shield or a pocket mask that has a mouthpiece with a one-way valve, or use a bag-valve-mask if available.

8. Wear gloves when inserting an oropharyngeal airway, using a bag-valve-mask, giving CPR, or using suction. The use of goggles and a face shield also is recommended.

9. Wear gloves, goggles or a face shield, and fluid-resistant clothing when attending an emergency childbirth.

10. Wear rubber utility (household) gloves while cleaning instruments and other medical equipment contaminated with blood or other body fluids. Contaminated goggles and eyeglasses can be washed with soap and water. Disinfect reusable household gloves and equipment with one of the following substances, which have been shown to effectively inactivate HIV and the hepatitis viruses: 0.3-percent hydrogen peroxide, 25-percent ethyl alcohol, 35-percent isopropyl alcohol, 0.5-percent Lysol, 0.25-percent povidone-iodine, and 1:10 to 1:100 dilution of sodium hypochlorite (household bleach). Blood can be removed from clothing with hydrogen peroxide and the clothing cleaned in an automatic washer (hot water cycle) or dry cleaned.

11. Disposable gloves and a pocket mask or mouth shield should be in every first aid kit or ski patrol first aid belt so they are easily available no matter how urgent the situation. A pair of ski goggles or a disposable face shield also are highly recommended.

12. Splinting open fractures involves the risk of contaminating splints and splint straps with blood. This can be prevented by covering the bandaged extremity with a clear plastic bag before applying the splint. A 55-gallon clear plastic garbage can liner is suitable for a lower extremity; a smaller size for an upper extremity. The top of the bag can be rolled down and after the hand or foot is inserted can be rolled back up the extremity like a long sock. All straps including traction hitches are put in place over the bag. (This procedure is suggested by Jim Gale, Briggs Allen, and John Chandler, M.D., of the Beech Mountain Ski Patrol, North Carolina.)

13. Disposable rubber gloves, disposable face shields, and disposable, reinforced, fluid-resistant gowns should be available in every ski patrol first aid room.

14. Consult local regulations regarding disposal of infectious waste. Your local hospital is a good source of information.

15. *Immunization with hepatitis B vaccine is highly recommended* for all health care workers with more than minimal exposure to blood or other body fluids.

16. If significant exposure occurs (i.e., unprotected exposure or exposure despite protective clothing), it is advisable to contact your physician promptly. Testing of the patient's blood for HIV and hepatitis may be indicated. (Local laws regarding consent for testing and confidentiality must be observed.) Measures to prevent the establishment of infection in yourself may be indicated and follow-up testing of your blood to see if you have become infected may be advisable. Counseling should be provided.

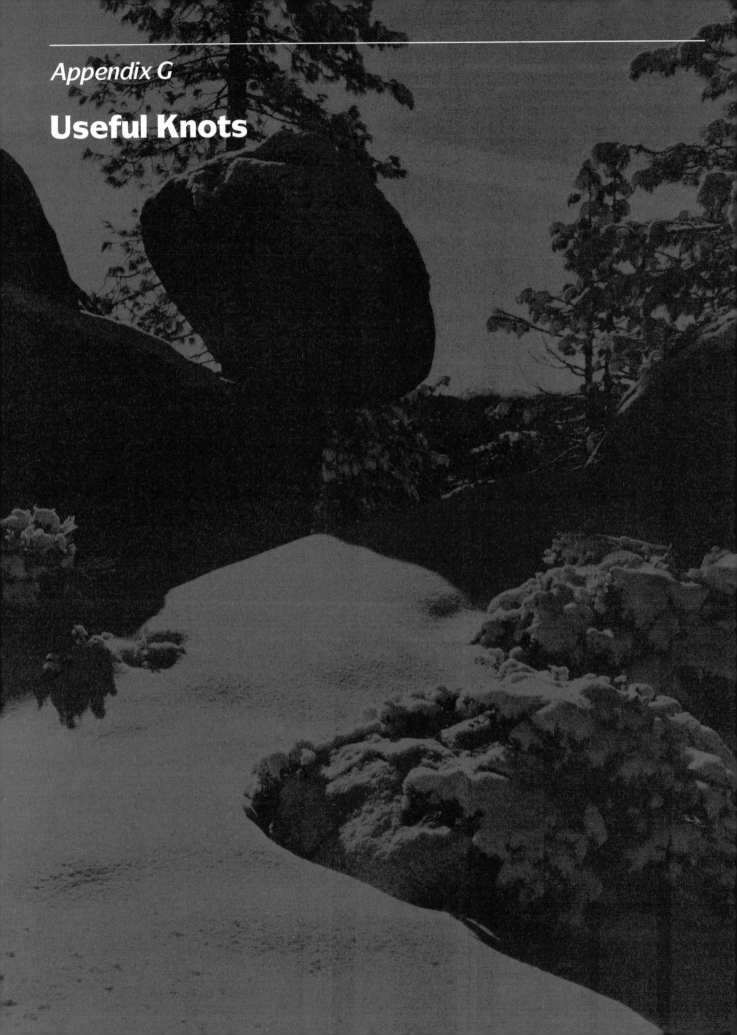

Appendix G

Useful Knots

This appendix contains illustrations of the following eight knots that are used frequently in emergency care and outdoor activities in general.

1. Figure G.1
   Square Knot
2. Figure G.2
   Figure-of-eight Knot
3. FigureG.3
   Figure-of-eight Follow-through Knot
4. Figure G.4
   Double-overhand Knot
5. Figure G.5
   Girth Hitch
6. Figure G.6
   Clove Hitch
7 Figure G.7
   Prusik Knot
8. Figure G.8
   Two Half-hitch Knots

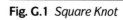

Fig. G.1 *Square Knot*

Fig. G.2 *Figure-of-eight Knot*

Fig. G.3 *Figure-of-eight Follow-through Knot*

Fig. G.4 *Double-overhand Knot*

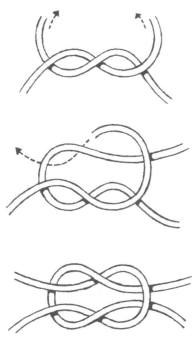
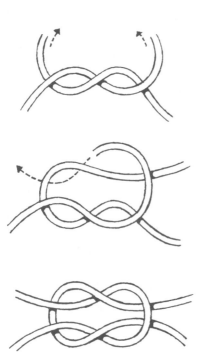

Fig. G.1

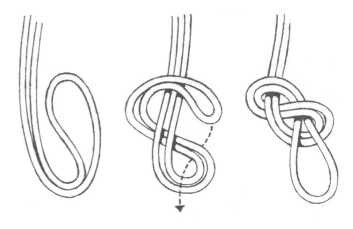

Fig. G.2

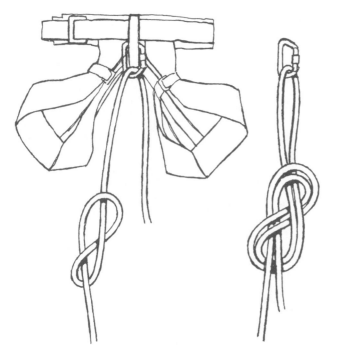

Fig. G.3

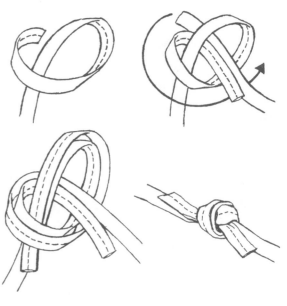

Fig. G.4

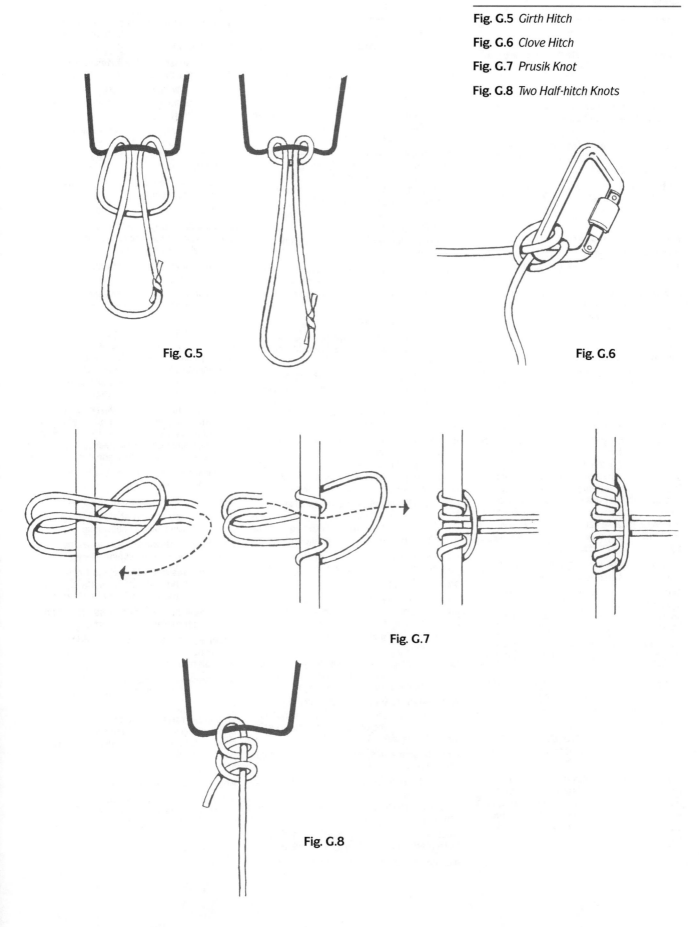

Fig. G.5 *Girth Hitch*

Fig. G.6 *Clove Hitch*

Fig. G.7 *Prusik Knot*

Fig. G.8 *Two Half-hitch Knots*

Fig. G.5

Fig. G.6

Fig. G.7

Fig. G.8

Glossary

A

abandonment—failure to continue care until the patient is transferred to the care of another qualified person.

ABCDE—a mnemonic aid to remember components of the primary and secondary surveys (**A**irway, **B**reathing, **C**irculation, **D**isability, and **E**xposure).

abdomen—the part of the body that lies between the chest and the pelvis and contains the abdominal cavity.

abdominal cavity—the cavity in the lower part of the trunk that contains parts of the digestive and urinary tracts and associated organs.

abduct—to pull away from the midline.

abrasion—a superficial injury caused by moving contact between the skin and a parallel rough surface.

abruptio placentae—a premature separation of the placenta from the uterus wall, usually just before labor begins or during the first stage of labor.

absence—brief loss of responsiveness without muscle movements.

absorption—the transfer of digested substances through the intestinal wall into the blood.

acceleration—to increase the speed; the rate of change of velocity with respect to time.

accident investigation protocol—a protocol that requires the appropriate ski area representative to collect a detailed incident report, statements from each of the rescuers involved in the incident, statements from the patient (if possible) and any available witnesses to the incident, photographs of the incident scene, and any applicable signs and markings, diagrams of the scene, and reports to any regulatory agencies as required by law.

acclimatization—the process by which the body adjusts to a new environment.

acetabulum—a cup-shaped depression at the point where the three pelvic bones are joined laterally. The acetabulum forms a socket of the hip joint into which the head of the femur fits.

acetazolamide (Diamox)—a prescription drug that improves acclimatization in people going to high altitude.

Achilles tendon—the tendon that joins the calf muscles to the heel of the foot.

acid—a substance that forms hydrogen ions in solution.

acidosis—an abnormal condition due to accumulation of acids or loss of bases from the body.

acquired immunodeficiency syndrome (AIDS)—a universally fatal infection with the human immunodeficiency virus (HIV) that attacks the body's immune system and reduces the body's resistance to certain infections and malignant tumors.

acromioclavicular (AC) joint—the joint between the clavicle and the acromion of the scapula at the point of the shoulder.

acromion—the lateral extension of the spine of the scapula, which forms the highest point of the shoulder.

acute—sharp, severe. Having rapid onset, severe symptoms and a short course; not chronic.

acute abdomen—medical jargon for an acute abdominal condition that usually requires surgery within a few hours.

acute mountain sickness (AMS)—a condition that can occur at altitudes above 7,500 feet caused by lack of oxygen, which injures body cells both directly, through interference with oxygen-requiring chemical reactions, and indirectly, through changes in the circulatory, respiratory, and nervous systems.

Adam's apple—a projection at the front of the neck formed by larynx cartilage.

addiction—a behavioral state of compulsive drug use that includes tolerance, physical dependence, and physiological dependence on a drug.

adduct—to draw toward the midline.

adult onset diabetes—type II, or non-insulin-dependent diabetes mellitus (NIDDM) that affects adults.

advanced assessment—an elaboration on the techniques of basic assessment for students who are familiar with these techniques; emphasizes the many things that may be found on assessment and what they may mean.

advanced cardiac life support (ACLS)—techniques used by paramedics, nurses, or physicians using technical equipment and intravenous drugs to treat patients with cardiac arrest or other serious heart problems.

advanced life support (ALS)—the use of cardiac monitoring, defibrillation, intravenous fluids and drugs, and other sophisticated equipment in the treatment of life-threatening illness.

agitation—restlessness and increased activity accompanied by fear or anxiety.

aerobic—oxygen requiring.

aerobic exercise—rhythmic, nonstop, endurance-building exercise that requires a constant supply of oxygen and relies little on anaerobic mechanisms such as lactate production.

aerobic fitness—the capacity for performing endurance exercise. Implies ability to extract oxygen efficiently from the inhaled air.

AIDS-related complex (ARC)—illness in a patient with antibodies to the human immunodeficiency virus who does not fulfill the criteria for diagnosis of AIDS.

air embolism—an illness caused by blockage of small blood vessels by air bubbles.

airway obstruction—complete or partial blockage of the airway by a foreign body, vomitus, blood clots, the tongue, or by swollen or relaxed soft tissues of the throat.

alcohol—an intoxicating liquid obtained by fermentation of carbohydrates with yeast.

alcoholism—addiction to alcohol.

algorithm—a step-by-step formula for solving a problem.

alignment—the process of bringing a deformed (fractured or dislocated) limb into correct anatomical position.

alkali—a substance that forms hydroxyl ions in solution; a base.

alkalinity (alkalosis)—an abnormal condition due to accumulation of bases or loss of acids from the body.

allergy—a state of hypersensitivity to a specific substance so that reexposure causes reactions in the skin, respiratory tract, and/or gastrointestinal tract.

alpha-methyl-fentanyl—designer street drug called "China white."

alveoli—the smallest air sacs of the lungs.

amino acids—organic acids containing carbon, oxygen, and nitrogen that form the chief structural units of proteins.

amniotic fluid—the amniotic sac fluid that supports and protects the fetus.

amniotic sac—the fluid-filled sac ("bag of waters") within which the fetus grows and develops.

amphetamines—highly addictive stimulant drugs once used in medicine as mood elevators and appetite suppressants. Side effects of amphetamine use include rapid pulse, elevated blood pressure, excitement, agitation, insomnia, irritability, and inability to concentrate.

AMPLE—a mnemonic to help remember the sequences of questioning a patient about his or her history. (**A**llergies; **M**edicines or drugs, both legal and illegal; **P**ast medical history; **L**ast meal; **E**vents prior to the incident in question.)

amputation—the complete tearing away of a body part from the body.

AMS—see **acute mountain sickness**.

analgesic—an agent that alleviates pain without causing loss of consciousness.

anaphylactic shock—shock caused by an immediate and overwhelming allergic reaction.

anatomic position—the position in which the patient is standing erect, facing the examiner with arms at the side and palms facing forward.

anatomy—the science of the structure of the body and the relation of its parts.

anemia—a condition characterized by too few red blood cells or a decrease in the amount of hemoglobin in the red cells.

aneurysm—a bulging weak spot on a blood vessel that can rupture and cause internal bleeding.

angina pectoris—a pain of characteristic type and location in patients with coronary artery disease. It occurs when the heart muscle temporarily does not receive enough blood for its needs.

Angle of Louis—see **sternal angle**.

ankle joint—a hinge joint formed by the lower ends of the tibia and fibula proximally and the talus bone of the foot distally.

anterior—nearer the front surface of the body.

antibiotics—chemical substances produced by microorganisms that have the capacity to kill other microorganisms. Some antibiotics are used in the control of infectious diseases.

anticholinergic drug—a drug that blocks the passage of impulses through parasympathetic nerves.

antidepressant—a drug that prevents or relieves depression.

antidote—a remedy for counteracting a poison.

antihistamine—a drug that counteracts the action of histamine and relieves allergic symptoms.

anus—the terminal opening of the alimentary canal.

aorta—the major artery of the body into which blood is pumped from the left ventricle of the heart.

apex—the top or highest point.

appendicitis—inflammation or infection of the appendix.

appendicular skeleton—the bones of the upper and lower limbs and the pelvis (see **axial skeleton**).

appendix—a worm-sized organ with no obvious useful purpose that is attached to the beginning of the large bowel.

aqueous humor—the watery fluid contained in the anterior compartment of the eyeball.

arachnoid—the middle of the three layers of membranes (meninges) that cover the brain and spinal cord.

ARC—see **AIDS-related complex**.

arch—the portion of the foot made up of the calcaneus, talus, and tarsal bones.

arterial blood—oxygenated blood flowing through the arteries to the tissues.

arterial pressure points—points where the pressure of a hand can easily occlude an artery to stop or reduce blood flow to a wound.

arteriole—the smallest size of artery.

arteriosclerosis—a disease characterized by the thickening and loss of elasticity of arterial walls because of fatty deposits and scar tissue, leading to stiffening and narrowing of the arteries.

artery—a tubular vessel that carries blood away from the heart.

arthropoda—phylum of invertebrate animals with jointed bodies and limbs, including insects, spiders, and ticks.

artificial kidney—a mechanical device used in patients with kidney failure to remove wastes from the blood that are ordinarily excreted in the urine.

articular process—a projection of a bone that forms part of a joint.

aspiration—the act of sucking in. Aspiration usually refers to sucking foreign matter into the airway.

assessment—examination of a patient in emergency care.

asthma—a condition in which periodic episodes of bronchial narrowing occur, causing attacks of coughing, wheezing, and shortness of breath.

asymmetry—lack of symmetry or balance, as when one side of the body does not correspond to the other side (see **bilateral symmetry**).

asystole—complete cessation of heart contractions.

ataxia—loss of muscle coordination leading to difficulty in maintaining balance.

atrium—either of the two smaller chambers of the heart.

aura—a peculiar sensation, which can be a sound, sight or smell, that signals the onset of a generalized (grand mal) epileptic seizure.

auscultation—listening for sounds within the body.

automatic external defibrillator (AED)—an electronic device that, when attached to a patient, interprets the patient's heart rhythm and automatically initiates or advises defibrillation as needed.

autonomic nervous system—the system that is composed of the sympathetic and parasympathetic nervous systems and controls the activity of the cardiac muscle, smooth muscle and glands, and other automatic functions of the body.

AVPU Scale—an acronym the rescuer uses to grade the patient's responsiveness for normalcy to complete unresponsiveness. (**A**) Is **A**wake and **A**lert; (**V**) Responds to **V**oice; (**P**) Responds only to **P**ain; and (**U**) Is **U**nresponsive.

avulsion—a body part torn loose from underlying tissues and left hanging by a flap.

axial skeleton—the skull, spine, ribs, and sternum (see **appendicular skeleton**).

axial traction—a pull parallel to the long axis of a body part.

axilla—the armpit.

axon—the long process of a neuron.

B

back carry—an emergency one-rescuer technique for moving a conscious patient short distances over very rough terrain or for belaying both the patient and rescuer over a short, vertical distance. The technique involves fashioning a seat from a sling or climbing rope so the patient can be carried on the rescuer's back.

bag-valve-mask (BVM)—a mechanical device consisting of a mask, an oxygen reservoir, a squeezable rubber bag, and a unidirectional valve that is used to deliver oxygen-enriched air to a nonbreathing patient.

"bag of waters"—the amniotic sac containing the amniotic fluid that supports and protects the fetus in the uterus.

ball-and-socket joint—a joint that allows rotation as well as flexion and extension.

bandage—the material used to hold a dressing or compress in place.

bandaging—the process of applying a dressing (or compress) and bandage to a wound.

barbiturates—a class of sedative drugs that depress the nervous system. Usually used as sleeping pills or tranquilizers. Examples are phenobarbital and decobarbital.

barotrauma—injury due to pressure differences.

basal heat production—heat produced by constant internal metabolic processes (50 kilocalories per square meter of body surface per hour in an average adult male).

basic assessment—in a patient with an illness or injury, a protocol consisting of a linked series of actions performed in a certain order for detection and treatment of urgent medical problems.

basic life support (BLS)—techniques of rescue breathing, cardiopulmonary resuscitation, and clearing upper airway obstructions without the aid of mechanical devices to reestablish the proper function of the respiratory and circulatory systems.

battery—interfering with a person's body or even touching it without permission; an illegal act in many states.

Battle's sign—ecchymosis at the tip of the mastoid process behind the ear, a sign of internal bleeding from a skull fracture.

benign—nonmalignant.

Betadine—the brand name of a povidone-iodine antiseptic solution used for sterilizing instruments and cleaning wounds.

biceps muscle—the major muscle of the anterior upper arm, which flexes the elbow.

bilateral symmetry—the state of each body half being a mirror image of the opposite half.

bile—a substance produced by the liver and stored in the gallbladder which contains an emulsifying agent that prepares fat for digestion.

bilirubin—a yellow compound that is a byproduct of the normal breakdown of red blood cells. It is removed by the liver and excreted through the bile into the intestines.

bladder—a hollow organ with muscular walls that stores urine before it is passed out of the body through the urethra. The bladder lies in the pelvic cavity.

bleb—a small, blister-like swelling.

blink reflex—an instantaneous blink caused by sudden eye irritation, as by a foreign body in the eye.

blood—thick fluid made up of plasma; red cells, which carry oxygen; white cells, which fight infection; and platelets, which aid in blood clotting. The blood carries oxygen and nutrients to the cells of the body and removes carbon dioxide and waste materials.

blood pressure—the pressure transmitted to the walls of the arteries by the blood as it is propelled by the rhythmic contractions of the heart.

blood pressure cuff—the part of a sphygmomanometer that goes around a patient's arm.

blood volume—the quantity of blood in the circulatory system.

blunt trauma—compression trauma.

body—any mass of matter that is distinct from other masses of matter.

boot-top fracture—a fracture of the tibia and/or fibula at the level of the top of the ski boot.

Bourdon gauge flowmeter—a pressure gauge calibrated to record flow rate when attached to a tank of compressed gas.

brachial artery pulse—a pulse that can be felt beating against the humerus on the inside of the upper arm, midway between the shoulder and elbow.

brachial plexus—a network of nerve trunks that gives rise to the major nerves of the upper extremity. The brachial plexus lies in the neck above and behind the clavicle.

brain—the portion of the central nervous system contained within the cranium.

brain contusion—bruising of brain tissue.

brain stem—the most inferior portion of the brain, attached directly to the spinal cord. Centers in the brain stem help regulate breathing, heart function, and blood pressure. Long nerve fibers from upper parts of the brain pass through the brain stem to the spinal cord.

breach—failure to perform a duty.

breathlessness—shortness of breath. Breathlessness also can refer to absent breathing.

breech presentation—a delivery in which the baby's buttocks or one or both feet, instead of the head, present at the vaginal opening.

bronchi—the tubular air passages of the lungs.

bronchioles—the smallest bronchi.

bronchitis—an infection or inflammation of the bronchi.

burn—a type of wound caused by excessive thermal, electrical, or radiant energy, or a similar injury caused by certain chemicals.

bursa—a fluid-filled sac that is located between moving body parts and acts to decrease friction.

bursitis—inflammation or infection of a bursa.

C

Caladium—a common household plant that is poisonous.

Calamine—the brand name of a soothing non-prescription lotion used for symptomatic relief of insect bites.

calcaneus—the heel bone.

callus—the calcified tissue formed during the process of bone healing.

calorie content—the capacity of food to produce heat and energy in the body.

Campylobacter—a bacterium that causes dysentery.

Cannabis sativa—Indian hemp plant, source of marijuana.

cancer—a malignant tumor that tends to become progressively worse and can cause death because of invasion or spreading.

cantharidin—an irritating substance excreted by blister beetles.

capillary—a tiny blood vessel that connects an arteriole to a venule and has thin walls that allow the interchange of substances between the blood and tissue cells.

capillary refill—the ability of the circulatory system to refill small vessels after blood has been squeezed out of them.

carbohydrate—organic compounds composed of carbon, hydrogen, and oxygen present in food mainly as sugars and starches. When oxidized in the body, they produce energy, heat, carbon dioxide, and water.

carbon monoxide—a colorless, odorless, poisonous gas that causes asphyxiation by combining irreversibly with the blood hemoglobin, thus blocking the transport and use of oxygen.

cardboard splint—an effective, disposable, easy-to-apply, fixation splint often used to replace a quick splint before the patient leaves the first aid room.

cardiac arrest—any condition where blood circulation stops because the heart malfunctions.

cardiac monitor—an electronic device that records and displays on a screen the electrocardiogram, pulse rate, blood pressure, and other important data related to the state of the heart.

cardiac output—the quantity of blood pumped by the heart.

cardiac tamponade—a condition in which the sac around the heart fills with blood or fluid, causing interference with heart contractions.

cardioaccelerating center—an area in the brain that receives signals from pressure monitors in the circulatory system and responds by increasing heart rate and blood vessel tone to counteract a fall in blood pressure.

cardiogenic shock—a form of shock due to failure of the pumping function of the heart.

cardioinhibitory center—an area in the brain that tends to slow the heart rate in response to elevated blood pressure.

cardiopulmonary resuscitation (CPR)—a technique of resuscitating victims of cardiac arrest by using rescue breathing to restore ventilation and external chest compressions to maintain blood circulation.

cardiovascular exercise—aerobic (oxygen-requiring) exercise that develops the heart and circulatory system to meet the body's changing needs for blood.

carotenemia—yellowing of the skin caused by eating large quantities of foods, such as tomatoes and carrots, that contain high levels of the vitamin A precursor carotene.

carotid arteries—the two arteries that supply blood to the head and neck. The pulses can be felt between the sternomastoid muscles and the larynx.

carpal bones—the wrist bones.

cartilage—a specialized fibrous connective tissue that covers opposing bony surfaces (riding surfaces) of joints and forms the anterior portions of the ribs and parts of the nose and ears.

cauda equina—(Latin for "horse's tail") a fan-like arrangement of peripheral nerves at the lower end of the spinal cord.

cecum—the pouch-like first part of the large intestine.

cell—the basic unit of all living matter.

central nervous system—the brain and spinal cord.

cerebellum—the portion of the brain that lies below and to the rear of the cerebrum and regulates posture, balance, muscle tone, and body movement.

cerebral hemispheres—the largest part of the brain, responsible for conscious functions including voluntary movement and the sensations transmitted by the sensory organs for sight, hearing, touch, taste, and smell.

cerebrospinal fluid—a watery, colorless fluid that bathes the brain and the spinal cord. This fluid fills the space between the arachnid and pia mater membranes.

cerebrovascular accident (CVA)—stroke, caused by interference with the blood supply to a part of the brain, usually because an artery either clots or it ruptures with hemorrhage into the brain substance.

cerebrum—the portion of the brain that is composed of the outer right and left cerebral hemispheres and the inner thalamus and hypothalamus.

cervical collar—see **rigid collar**.

cervical spine—the uppermost portion of the spine formed by the seven cervical vertebrae in the neck.

cheekbone—the bony ridge of the maxilla below the orbit and above the soft part of the cheek.

chest cavity—a hollow, cage-like structure whose semirigid wall surrounds and encloses a large cavity (see **thoracic cavity**).

Cheyne-Stokes respirations—waxing and waning of the depth of breathing interspersed with regular periods when breathing stops.

child—in basic life support, a person between the ages of one and eight.

choke—to interrupt respiration by obstruction or compression of the airway.

cholecystitis—inflammation or infection of the gallbladder.

cholera—a specific bacterial bowel infection that involves profuse diarrhea, dehydration, and shock, and is caused by the organism *Vibrio cholerae*.

cholesterol—a type of fat implicated as a cause of arteriosclerosis.

chondromalacia of the patella—roughening and deterioration of the cartilage of the posterior surface of the patella caused by excessive physical activity with the knee in the partly flexed position.

chronic—of long duration.

chronic obstructive pulmonary disease (COPD)—a lung disease in which the alveoli become larger due to expansion or breakdown of some of the walls between them. COPD is caused by chronic inhalation of irritants such as tobacco smoke and polluted air (see **emphysema**).

cirrhosis—a chronic liver disease characterized by destruction of liver cells and an increase in liver fibrous tissue.

clavicle—the collarbone, which is attached medially to the sternum and laterally to the acromion of the scapula.

closed fracture—a fracture where the overlying skin is intact.

closed injury—damage to the skin and deeper tissues that does not involve a break in the skin.

coastal alpine zone—refers to mountain ranges near the east or west coast of the United States, where temperatures are moderate and rain is common, even in winter.

CO₂—carbon dioxide.

cocaine—a widely used illegal drug produced from the coca plant. Cocaine induces marked euphoria.

coccyx—the vestigial tail-like structure that is formed by the fusion of the lower four vertebrae and hangs below the sacrum.

"coffee grounds" matter—refers to the appearance of partly digested blood vomited from the stomach.

colic—an intermittent, severe, abdominal pain caused by obstruction of a hollow, muscular organ such as the bowel or ureter.

colitis—colon inflammation.

collateral ligaments—the medial and lateral ligaments of the knee.

Colles' fracture—a fracture of the distal radius that produces a characteristic "silver fork deformity" resembling an upside-down dinner fork.

colon—the portion of the large intestine extending from the cecum to the rectum.

comminuted fracture—a fracture in which there are two or more fracture lines with three or more fragments.

comminuted—broken or crushed into multiple small fragments.

compress—(see **dressing**).

compound fracture—usually called an "open fracture," a compound fracture is any fracture involving a wound of the overlying skin.

compression trauma—trauma caused by an impact between a body part and a blunt object.

concussion—a temporary loss of consciousness or other brain dysfunction following a blow to the head.

conduction—the transmission of heat, sound waves, nerve impulses, or electricity.

conductor—a substance or body that conducts.

condyle—a projection on the end of a bone, usually part of a joint.

conjunctiva—the delicate transparent membrane that lines the interior of the eyelid and covers the visible part of the sclera of the eye.

conjunctivitis—inflammation or infection of the conjunctiva.

consciousness, level of—(see **responsiveness**).

consolidation of the lung—stiffening of the lung in a pneumonia patient, caused by the filling of alveoli with fluid and inflammatory cells.

constipation—the passage of hard, dry stools at less than normal intervals.

constrict—to narrow or decrease in size.

contrecoup injury—an injury to parts on the side opposite the primary injury, such as when the brain is forced against one side of the skull by a blow to the opposite side.

contusion—a closed soft-tissue bruise caused by an impact between the body and a blunt object.

convection—transmission of heat by a moving gas or liquid.

convulsion—an involuntary contraction or series of contractions of the skeletal muscles.

core—the central nervous system, heart, lungs, liver, and other important internal organs of the body (see **shell**).

core temperature—the temperature of the body core (central nervous system, heart, lungs, liver and other important internal organs), usually measured with a rectal thermometer.

cornea—transparent anterior surface of the eyeball.

coronary arteries—the arteries that supply blood to the heart.

coronary artery disease—arteriosclerosis of the coronary arteries.

coronary veins—the veins that carry blood away from the heart.

costal arch—the arch formed by the cartilage that connects the sixth through tenth ribs to each other and to the base of the sternum.

costovertebral angle (CVA)—the triangular space on each side of the back between the lowest rib and the spine.

cough—a sudden, noisy expulsion of air from the lungs.

CPR—see **cardiopulmonary resuscitation**.

CRAMS Scale—a triage device useful in assigning patients to a high mortality group (score of 6 or less) or a low mortality group (score of 7 or more). **C**irculation, **R**espiratory, **A**bdomen, **M**otor, **S**peech.

cranial nerves—the nerves that arise directly from the brain, including nerves responsible for sight, hearing, taste, and smell, and nerves that supply sensory and motor fibers to the head.

cranium—the part of the skull that encloses the brain.

cravat—a long bandage, several inches wide, made by folding a triangular bandage lengthwise.

crepitus—a grating sensation caused by broken bone ends grinding together.

cricoid cartilage—a ring-like cartilage that forms the lowest part of the larynx.

cricothyroid membrane—a ligament that connects the thyroid and cricoid cartilages and can be felt as a soft spot between the thyroid and cricoid cartilages at the front of the neck.

cricothyroidotomy—surgical opening of the cricothyroid membrane between the thyroid and cricoid cartilages to provide an airway.

Critical Incident Stress Debriefing (CISD)—group support that is provided to rescuers involved in extremely distressing events.

crossed-finger technique—a technique for opening the patient's mouth that is used when necessary to open the airway for rescue breathing.

crown—the topmost part of the tooth that is covered with enamel.

cruciate ligaments—the anterior and posterior ligaments of the knee that originate in the groove between the femoral condyles, cross each other, and insert in the middle of the tibial plateau. Along with the medial and lateral ligaments (collateral ligaments), the cruciate ligaments make up the four important ligaments of the knee.

crushing injury—an injury caused by compression that involves both direct tissue injury and injury secondary to circulatory disturbance caused by pressure on the blood vessels.

cumulonimbus clouds—huge, billowing vertical clouds with anvil-shaped tops that may tower to 60,000 feet or more (thunderheads).

cutaneous system—the system made up of the skin and subcutaneous tissues that protects the internal body parts, controls body temperature, and contains special organs responsible for sensations of pain, touch, and temperature. The cutaneous system protects the body from dehydration and infection, and regulates body temperature by producing perspiration and adjusting surface blood flow.

cyanosis—a bluish discoloration of the skin, fingernails, and mucous membranes that occurs because the blood is not adequately oxygenated.

cyst—a closed cavity or sac containing liquid or semisolid material that develops in the skin, a body cavity, or other body part.

cytoplasm—the fluid material within the cell that is outside the nucleus.

D

deceleration trauma—trauma from dissipation of kinetic energy caused by rapid slowing of the body, such as when a skier collides with a tree.

decompression sickness—an illness caused when too rapid ascent from a deep dive allows nitrogen to come out of solution in body fluids and form bubbles in small blood vessels. The symptoms are due to obstruction of blood flow to various tissues. This condition also is called "the bends."

decongestant—a substance that reduces enlargement or swelling.

deep frostbite—a full- or partial-thickness freezing of a body part, most commonly the hands or feet.

defibrillator—an electronic device used to treat abnormal heart rhythms by applying a brief electrical shock to the heart.

definitive medical care—care given in a hospital or physician's office (see also **first aid** and **emergency medical care**).

deformity—malformation, distortion, or disfigurement of the body or its parts.

dehydration—the condition that results from excessive loss of body water.

deltoid muscle—a muscle in the upper extremity that forms the rounded part of the shoulder and is the main muscle that lifts the upper extremity upward and outward.

dendrites—the short processes of a neuron.

dermis—the inner layer of the skin that contains hair follicles, oil glands, sweat glands, blood vessels, nerves, and the sensory organs that perceive pain, touch, and temperature.

designer drug—a substance intended for recreational use that has been modified from an existing, legitimate drug just enough to avoid current legal restrictions.

deviation—a turning away from the regular standard or course.

diabetes mellitus—a metabolic disorder in which the ability to use glucose as fuel is lost because of an absolute or relative insufficiency of insulin.

diabetic coma—unconsciousness caused by loss of fluid and increased acidity that occurs in people with previously undiagnosed diabetes mellitus and in known diabetics who have taken insufficient insulin. Signs and symptoms include confusion, stupor, or coma; rapid, deep respirations; flushed, dry, warm skin; weakness; and fatigue. The patient's breath has a fruity odor and there may be signs of shock.

diabetic ketoacidosis—a serious condition occurring in patients with severe, uncontrolled diabetes. The condition is caused by a lack of insulin, which results in the inability to metabolize glucose and the accumulation of acidic breakdown products of fat in the blood and other body tissues.

diagnosis—identification of a disease or injury based on the results of examination.

diaphragm—the muscular partition separating the abdominal and thoracic cavities.

diarrhea—the passage of soft or liquid stools with abnormally high frequency.

diastolic blood pressure—the lowest point of the blood pressure curve.

Dieffenbachia—common poisonous household plant.

digestion—the breakdown of food into simpler substances that can be more easily absorbed into the bloodstream.

digestive system—the system that consists of the digestive tract—a tube that conducts food through the body from mouth to anus—and associated organs that produce substances to aid digestion. This system ingests, digests, and absorbs food and fluid, and eliminates wastes.

dilate—to enlarge.

direct ground lift—a technique by which three or more rescuers lift and move a patient.

direct pressure—a technique to reduce external bleeding by applying manual pressure over a compress placed directly on a wound.

disc, intervertebral—the donut-shaped ring of fibrous cartilage with a pulpy center that separates one vertebra from another.

discharge—an excretion of material from a body orifice.

disease—any deviation from or interruption of the normal structure or function of the body as manifested by a characteristic set of symptoms and signs.

disinfection—the removal of disease-causing organisms by means of chemical treatment.

dislocation—a disruption of a joint that occurs when the joint is forced to move beyond its normal range.

disorientation—a state of mental confusion regarding time, location, or identity.

displaced fracture—a fracture in which the bone ends are moved out of their normal in-line position.

dissipation—the dispersal of the energy from a moving object through deformation of body tissues. The amount of injury is roughly proportional to the amount of energy that has to be dissipated.

distal—closer to the tips of the extremities.

distention—the state of being swollen or enlarged.

distraction trauma—trauma caused by stretching.

diuretic—an agent that promotes the excretion of urine.

diverticulitis—inflammation of a small, finger-like pouch (diverticulum) on the side of the colon.

Diving Accident Network (DAN)—an organization that provides assistance in locating hyperbaric chambers and advice on emergency care of scuba-related medical problems. Telephone number: (919) 684-8111.

dorsalis pedis pulse—the pulse felt on the top of the foot between the first and second metatarsals.

dorsiflex—to flex the foot upward, or dorsally.

dressing—a sterile material placed directly on a wound.

drop attack—sudden loss of muscle tone.

drowning—death by suffocation after being submerged in water or another liquid.

drug—any substance that alters mental or physical function when introduced into the body.

drug dependence—a behavioral state of psychological dependence in which the abuser becomes obsessed with taking the drug and continues to take it despite obvious physical, mental, or social harm.

duodenum—the first part of the small intestine, which connects the stomach to the jejunum. Duodenum is from the Latin term "duodeni" (12 each), because it is the length of 12 fingers laid side by side.

dura mater—the outermost of the three layers of meninges that cover the brain and spinal cord.

dysentery—a severe bowel infection causing profuse diarrhea, chills, fever, and prostration. Blood and pus typically are present in the stools.

dysphagia—difficulty in swallowing.

dyspnea—difficult or labored breathing.

dysuria—painful urination.

E

ear—the organ of hearing and equilibrium.

ear canal—the portion of the ear whose external opening is surrounded by the pinna (external ear) and which leads to the middle and inner ear.

ecchymosis—a blue or purplish spot in the skin or mucous membranes caused by bleeding; a bruise.

ectopic pregnancy—a pregnancy in which the fetus develops outside of the uterus, usually in the fallopian tube.

edema—the escape of fluid from vascular or lymphatic spaces into tissues, causing local or generalized swelling.

egg—the female germ cell.

ejaculation—sudden, forceful expulsion.

E^k—kinetic energy.

elbow joint—the joint that connects the humerus proximally with the radius and ulna distally.

electrocardiogram (EKG)—the graphic recording of the heart's electrical activity.

electrocution—death caused by a high-voltage electrical current passing through the body.

electrolytes—ionic components of inorganic salts found in cells and body fluids.

elimination—the expulsion of indigestible residues of food from the body.

embolus—a clot or other plug brought by the blood from a larger vessel to a smaller one where it obstructs the circulation.

embryo—the developing unborn offspring in the first eight weeks of pregnancy, which is the period of most rapid growth.

emergency medical care—prehospital medical care in an emergency, usually delivered by emergency medical technicians and similarly trained individuals rather than doctors or nurses. Emergency medical care is more sophisticated than first aid. (See also **definitive medical care** and **first aid**.)

Emergency Medical Services (EMS) system—an interconnected network of hospitals, emergency departments, and emergency vehicles manned by physicians, nurses, and emergency medical technicians and designed to provide immediate services to patients with sudden or unexpected illness or injury.

emergency medical technician (EMT)—an individual who has passed a basic or advanced EMT course sanctioned by a state and the United States Department of Transportation. EMTs work in the Emergency Medical Services (EMS) system and are trained to reach patients rapidly, provide emergency care, and transport them to a hospital.

emphysema—a chronic, progressive, obstructive pulmonary disease, often caused by cigarette smoking, that involves the loss of some alveoli in the lungs, enlargement of other alveoli, and narrowing of the bronchi. Patients have a barrel-chested appearance, their breath sounds are quieter than normal, and exhalations are prolonged.

emphysema, subcutaneous—air in the subcutaneous tissues due to injury to air-containing parts of the respiratory tract in the neck or chest. Typically accompanied by a unique, crackling sensation described as "Rice Krispies under the skin."

endogenous—developing or originating within the body.

endotracheal intubation—opening and maintaining an airway by inserting a special tube through the nose or mouth into the trachea.

endotracheal tube—a breathing tube inserted through the mouth or nose into the trachea.

energy—the capacity for doing work. Energy can be either potential, which is derived from the position of a body in a gravity field, or kinetic, which is created by motion.

engorgement—excessive fullness of an organ, vessel, or tissue because of the accumulation of blood or other fluids.

envenomation—the process of being poisoned by the bite or sting of an animal.

environmental illness—a term usually applied to illness caused by physical components of the environment as opposed to mechanical, toxic, or infectious components. Examples are hypothermia, hyperthermia, sunburn, snow blindness, and lightning injury. The term frequently is expanded to include injuries due to wilderness and marine animals and plants.

enzyme—a substance produced by the body that catalyzes a specific chemical reaction.

epicondyle—a bony projection located above a condyle.

epidermis—the outer layer of skin composed of many layers of flat, closely adhering cells, the innermost layer of which is the germinal layer that constantly multiplies to renew the outer layers.

epigastrium—the area of the abdomen below the xiphoid process and between the costal arches.

epiglottis—a thin, lid-like cartilaginous flap overhanging the entrance to the larynx. Its action allows air but not food or liquid to enter the larynx and trachea.

epiglottitis—inflammation or infection of the epiglottis, which occasionally causes swelling sufficient to obstruct the upper respiratory tract.

epilepsy—recurrent episodes of seizures caused by an abnormal focus of electrical activity within the brain that may be manifested as impaired consciousness, abnormal movements, or psychic, sensory, or autonomic disturbances.

epinephrine (adrenalin)—a hormone produced by the adrenal gland that stimulates the sympathetic nervous system and heart muscle, raises the blood pressure, increases the heart rate, and relaxes bronchial smooth muscle.

erection—enlargement and hardening of tissue due to filling with blood.

esophageal varices—large, dilated veins in the upper stomach and lower esophagus in patients with chronic liver disease. Rupture of these vessels can cause severe hemorrhage.

esophagus—the tubular organ that connects the oropharynx with the stomach.

eustachian tube—the channel that connects the tympanic cavity of the ear with the nasopharynx and serves to equalize the pressure of the air in the cavity to the pressure of the outside air.

evaporation—conversion of a liquid into a vapor.

exhalation—breathing air out of the lungs.

exposure—(see **hypothermia** and **frostbite**.)

expressive aphasia—a characteristic speech impairment marked by the ability to understand what is said but the inability to choose the right words to reply.

extend—to straighten a joint.

extremities—the arms and legs.

extremity, lower—the thigh, leg, and foot.

extremity, upper—the shoulder, arm (upper arm), forearm, wrist, and hand.

extremity lift—a method of moving a patient with a splinted lower extremity from the first aid room to a nearby vehicle.

extrication—the process of freeing or removing a patient from an awkward, confined, or poorly accessible situation or position.

extrication collar—(see **rigid collar**.)

eye—the organ of vision.

eyeball—a hollow globe about 1 inch in diameter that lies in the eye socket of the skull and is connected with the brain by the optic nerve that passes through the back of the socket.

eyes-front position—when the head is in the anatomical position with the body, with the eyes looking straight ahead and the head at right angles to the shoulders.

F

fallopian tube—the tubular structure that conducts the ovum from the ovary to the uterus.

false motion—limb motion where there is no joint (a sign of bone fracture).

fascia—tough, fibrous tissue that forms a cover for muscles and other body organs.

fast-twitch fibers (type I)—muscle fibers that are capable of rapid contraction, tend to rely on anaerobic metabolism, and readily form lactic acid (see also **slow-twitch fiber**).

fat—organic substance containing carbon, oxygen, and hydrogen that is usually a compound of one or more fatty acids with glycerol.

fat, polyunsaturated—fat containing fewer hydrogen atoms than normal that is found in fish oil and vegetable products.

fat, saturated—fat that contains normal numbers of hydrogen atoms and usually is of animal origin.

fatigue—a state of discomfort and decreased efficiency resulting from prolonged or excessive exertion or lack of rest.

fatigue fracture (stress fracture)—a bone fracture caused by the strain of repeated stresses such as prolonged walking or exercise.

febrile illness—an illness with fever.

feces—the residue remaining in the bowel after digestible material has been removed.

femoral artery pulse—the pulse that can be felt just below the midpoint of the inguinal ligament, which lies between the anterior superior iliac spine and the pubis.

femoral condyles—the two rounded projections of the distal end of the femur.

femoral nerve—a major nerve of the lower extremity that enters the front of the thigh lateral to the femoral artery and provides sensation to part of the front of the thigh and the inner leg, as well as supplying the muscles that flex the hip and extend the knee.

femoral shaft fracture—a fracture of the middle one-half to three-fifths of the femur.

femur—the thigh bone.

fetus—the developing unborn offspring between the eighth week of pregnancy and birth.

fever—an increase in body temperature of more than 1°F (0.5°C) above normal.

fibrillation—rapid, uncoordinated wormlike movement.

fibrin—an insoluble protein that forms the essential part of a blood clot.

fibula—the lateral of the two bones of the lower leg.

filtration—a method of purifying water using substances that contain microscopic pores through which most microorganisms cannot pass.

finger sweep—the technique of using a hooked finger to clear a foreign body lodged in the mouth of an unconscious adult or older child.

fireman's carry—an emergency technique that allows a single rescuer to carry a patient while crawling on the hands and knees.

fireman's drag—an emergency technique that allows a single rescuer to drag a patient while crawling on the hands and knees.

first aid—simple emergency care techniques that require little equipment and rely on speedy coordination with the Emergency Medical Services (EMS) system (see also **definitive medical care** and **emergency care**).

first impression—the earliest effect, image, or feeling that is registered during an experience.

first-degree frostbite—mild, superficial damage to tissue caused by environmental temperatures below freezing. On thawing, the affected part is warm, swollen, and tender. Blisters are either absent or are few and small.

fissure—a crack or small ulcer.

fixation splint—a splint that prevents motion at the site of a fracture or other injury when applied firmly above, below, and across the injury site.

flail ankle—an injured ankle that is abnormally mobile.

flail chest—a loose section of the chest caused by multiple adjacent rib fractures.

flank—the part of the side of the body below the ribs and above the ilium of the pelvis.

flashback—unintentional recall.

flat bones—bones found in the skull and pelvis, as opposed to long bones, found in the limbs, and irregular bones, such as the vertebrae.

flatus—gas expelled through the anus.

flex—to bend a joint.

flotation device—an device that keeps a person from sinking in water.

floating ribs—the eleventh and twelfth pairs of ribs, which lack a connection at the front of the chest.

"floor burn"—a type of abrasion commonly seen in gymnasts.

flowmeter—a flow measuring gauge attached to a regulator used with an oxygen tank.

food poisoning—an illness caused by a toxic substance or a microorganism. This illness is characterized by abdominal pain, vomiting, and/or diarrhea.

foot drop—inability to dorsiflex the foot because of paralysis of the anterior leg muscles.

foramen magnum—a hole at the base of the skull through which the spinal cord passes from the base of the brain to the spinal canal.

foramen—a small opening in a bone.

force—any action that changes the state of rest or motion of a body to which that force is applied.

fore-and-aft carry—an emergency two-rescuer technique for moving an unconscious patient with no serious injuries.

forearm bones—the radius and the ulna.

forehead—the area of the face above the eyes.

foreskin—a covering of folded skin over the glans of the penis.

fourth-degree frostbite—serious, full-thickness damage to tissue caused by subfreezing environmental temperatures. On thawing, there are no blisters or swelling. The part remains numb, cold, and bloodless. It is gray or white initially but soon turns dark purple and becomes gangrenous within a few days.

fracture—any break in the continuity of a bone.

fracture-dislocation—an injury that includes both a break in bone continuity and a disruption of joint continuity.

frequency—in urology, abnormally frequent urination.

front cradle—an emergency one-rescuer technique for carrying a small patient.

frostbite—damage to tissue caused by subfreezing temperatures. Before thawing, frostbite is categorized as superficial or deep; following thawing, it can be categorized as first-degree, second-degree, third-degree, or fourth-degree based on the extent of blistering, swelling, and skin color.

fulcrum point—the hinge-like point about which a lever turns.

G

gallbladder—a sac-like reservoir for bile storage located on the undersurface of the liver.

"gamekeeper's thumb"—see **"skier's thumb."**

Gamow bag—a portable hyperbaric chamber used to treat patients with advanced acute mountain sickness.

ganglia—small clusters of autonomic nervous system neurons that lie outside the spinal cord.

gangrene—tissue death followed by bacterial invasion and putrification, usually caused by loss of blood supply.

gastric distention—enlargement of the stomach and intestines caused by such things as infection, overuse of alcohol, food poisoning, irritating drugs, or emotion.

gastric juice—the liquid secretion of the stomach glands, containing hydrochloric acid and an enzyme that digests protein.

gastroenteritis—inflammation of the stomach and intestines caused by such things as infection, overuse of alcohol, food poisoning, irritating drugs, or emotion.

gastrointestinal system—the organs of the stomach and intestines that are involved in the digestion of food and excretion of the solid waste products of digestion.

Gatorade—the brand name of an electrolyte preparation.

genitalia—the male and female reproductive organs, usually referring to the external ones.

genitourinary system—the organs of reproduction together with the organs for the production and excretion of urine.

Giardia lamblia—an organism that is present in the feces of infected animals, often contaminates outdoor water sources, and causes a diarrheal illness.

Glasgow Coma Scale—a standardized approach to evaluation of neurologic function, utilizing eye opening, response to verbal stimulation, and motor ability.

glottis—the part of the larynx that produces speech, i.e., the vocal cords and the opening between them.

glucose—a simple sugar containing six carbon atoms that is the chief source of energy for most living organisms; also known as dextrose.

gluteus muscle—one of the large muscles that form the buttocks and allow extension and abduction of the hips.

glycogen—a complex carbohydrate that is the chief storage form of carbohydrate in animals. It is found in the muscles and liver and is readily broken down into glucose.

goiter—an enlarged thyroid gland.

"golden hour"—the average time before a patient with multiple injuries starts to deteriorate rapidly; for every half hour following the first hour, the patient's chances of survival are cut in half.

Good Samaritan laws—statutes that protect an individual who gives emergency care against lawsuits. The care must be given gratuitously, in good faith, in accordance with the rescuer's training and expertise, in a bona fide emergency, and without gross or willful negligence.

grade I sprain—a sprain in which the ligaments are stretched but not torn.

grade II sprain—a sprain in which the ligaments are badly stretched or partly torn.

grade III sprain—a sprain in which the ligaments are completely torn.

grand mal seizure—a severe generalized seizure involving abnormal muscle movements.

gray matter—groups of nerve cells in the brain and spinal cord that derive their name from their color.

greater trochanter of the femur—the prominent knob on the outside of the upper end of the femur.

greenstick fracture—an angulated fracture that passes partway through the shaft of a bone.

groin—the region where the abdomen joins the thigh.

gross negligence—injury to another person caused by failure to provide even the degree of care that an unreasonable or imprudent person would exercise in similar circumstances (see also **negligence** and **willful negligence**).

guarding—tightening of abdominal muscles overlying a tender area.

gurney—an adjustable, wheeled stretcher developed for ambulance use.

H

hallucination—a perception by the brain of a sight, sound, smell, touch, or taste that has no origin in an external stimulus.

hallucinogen—a drug such as LSD, psilocybin, mescaline, and peyote that alters perceptions of the environment, sometimes producing hallucinations or delusions.

hamstring muscles—the major muscles of the posterior thigh, which flex the knee.

hamstring tendons—the tendons of the muscles that flex the knee joint and can be felt on either side of the popliteal fossa behind the knee.

Hare splint—a commercially available modification of the Thomas type of traction splint that replaces cradle hitches with Velcro straps and uses a mechanical ratchet device to provide traction.

hay fever—an allergic condition of the upper respiratory tract that causes symptoms similar to those of a head cold.

head-tilt/chin-lift—a method of opening the airway by tilting the head back and lifting the chin with the fingers.

heart—the hollow, muscular organ that maintains the circulation of the blood by functioning as a pump.

heart attack—a term commonly used for any sudden episode caused by malfunction of the heart (see also **myocardial infarction**).

heart disease—any organic, mechanical, or functional abnormality of the heart.

heart failure, chronic—a clinical syndrome that is caused by the inability of the heart to pump an adequate amount of blood, and characterized by shortness of breath, weakness, and swelling of the abdomen and legs.

heartburn—a type of indigestion characterized by a burning sensation in the epigastric area or beneath the sternum, often accompanied by increased saliva production.

heat cramps—cramping in active muscles that results from excessive loss of fluid and electrolytes because of perspiring in the heat.

heat exhaustion—a form of hypovolemic shock caused by either excessive sweating or the inadequate replacement of water and electrolytes lost by sweating.

heat syncope—a mild form of hypovolemic shock that resembles simple fainting. Heat syncope can result from sitting or standing for long periods in the direct sun or in hot weather.

Heatpac—the brand name of a lightweight stove fueled by a charcoal cartridge.

heatstroke—an illness characterized by prolonged elevation of the body core temperature above 104 to 105°F (40 to 40.6°C).

Heimlich maneuver—a technique for relieving upper-airway obstruction in adults and children (but not infants) that uses a sudden push on the abdomen or chest to expel residual air in the lungs and remove a foreign object blocking the upper airway.

hematoma—a localized tumor-like collection of blood within an organ or tissue.

hematuria—blood in the urine.

hemiplegia—paralysis of the arm and the leg on the same side.

hemopneumothorax—air and blood in the pleural space.

hemoptysis—blood coughed up from the lungs.

hemorrhage—profuse bleeding.

hemorrhagic shock—hypovolemic shock due to blood loss.

hemorrhoid—an enlarged vein in the anal area.

hemothorax—blood in the pleural space.

hepatitis—an inflammatory or infectious disease of the liver, usually caused by a virus.

hepatitis A—hepatitis caused by the hepatitis A virus (HAV) that is transmitted by direct contact with an infected individual or through contaminated food or water.

hepatitis B—hepatitis caused by the hepatitis B virus (HBV) that is spread by contact with blood and body fluids.

hernia—the abnormal protrusion of an organ or tissue through an opening.

high altitude cerebral edema (HACE)—a type of acute mountain sickness characterized by swelling of the brain.

high altitude pulmonary edema (HAPE)—a type of acute mountain sickness characterized by filling of the lungs with edema fluid.

high alpine zone—the Rocky Mountains and other inland ranges. The high alpine zone is colder and drier than the coastal alpine zone.

hip fracture—a fracture of the upper end of the femur.

hip joint—a ball-and-socket joint formed by the acetabulum proximally and the head of the femur distally.

histology—the branch of anatomy that deals with the minute structure, composition, and function of the tissues.

Hg—chemical symbol for mercury.

Homan's sign—pain produced in the calf when the foot is bent upward at the ankle, usually indicating the presence of a blood clot in the veins of the calf.

hoarseness—a rough, low-pitched quality of the voice.

homeotherm—a human or other warm-blooded animal that maintains a relatively constant body temperature despite changes in environmental temperature.

hooked-finger technique—a method of clearing solid debris from the oral cavity.

hormones—organic compounds that are produced by glands and regulate the activity of other organs.

human immunodeficiency virus (HIV)—a retrovirus that attacks human T lymphocytes, causing a progressive depletion of the CD4 helper-inducer subset with resulting destruction of the body's ability to fight off certain infections and resist certain cancers.

humerus—the upper arm bone.

hydraulic sarong—an apparatus for rewarming a hypothermic patient that uses a backpacking stove to heat a pot of water and a bilge pump to circulate the water through plastic tubes sewn into a blanket that can be wrapped around the patient's trunk.

hyperbaric chamber—a pressure chamber used for recompression of patients suffering from air embolism and decompression sickness.

hypercarbia—excess carbon dioxide.

hyperextension—extreme or abnormal extension.

hyperflexion—extreme or abnormal flexion.

hyperpigmentation—abnormally increased pigmentation.

hyperpnea—an increase in breathing depth.

hyperthermia—unusually high body temperature (above 104 to 105°F [40 to 40.6°C]). See **heatstroke**.

hyperventilation—deep, rapid breathing. The term hyperventilation usually refers to a common, benign form of respiratory distress that starts with an increase in the rate and depth of breathing, which produces an excessive loss of carbon dioxide, making the blood more alkaline.

hypervitaminosis—a toxic condition caused by excess intake of vitamins.

hypoglycemia—low blood sugar.

hypothalamus—the portion of the cerebrum of the brain that controls automatic functions such as the regulation of the heart, circulation, digestion, and blood pressure, as well as water balance, sexual function, sleep, appetite, and body temperature.

hypothermia—a fall in the body core temperature to below 95°F (35°C).

hypovolemic shock—shock caused by a decrease in circulating blood volume resulting from a loss of whole blood or a decrease in the fluid portion of the blood due to vomiting, diarrhea, or severe burns.

hypoxia—low oxygen content.

hysteria—a type of psychoneurosis characterized by lack of control over acts and emotions, by morbid self-consciousness, by anxiety, and by simulation of the signs and symptoms of various diseases.

I

ileum—the distal portion of the small intestine, extending from the jejunum and connecting to the large intestine at the cecum.

iliac arteries—the arteries that supply blood to the lower extremities.

iliac crest—the long curving portion of the ilium.

iliac veins—the veins that carry blood away from the lower extremities.

iliopsoas muscle—one of the two muscles that lie at the back of the abdominal and pelvic cavities on either side of the spine and flex the hip joints.

ilium—the most lateral of the three fused bones making up the pelvis.

illness—a condition marked by deviation from the normal healthy state; sickness.

immersion hypothermia—low body temperature caused by immersion in cold water.

impaled object—an object that is left protruding from a wound after an injury.

implied consent—the legal presumption that a patient (or the parent or guardian if present) would consent to accepting care if able to do so in situations where care is urgently needed for life-threatening or serious illness or injury and the patient is unconscious, irrational, or a minor.

immunization—the process by which resistance to an infectious disease is produced.

incident command system—a management plan designed for controlling, directing, and coordinating emergency response resources.

incision—a type of laceration caused by a knife or other sharp object.

incontinence—the uncontrolled passage of urine or feces.

indigestion—disturbance of the normal function of the stomach, producing symptoms such as heartburn, pain, nausea, and vomiting.

infarct—an area of tissue death due to interruption of its blood supply.

infection—the invasion and multiplication of microorganisms (e.g., viruses, bacteria, or parasites) in body tissues, and the reaction of the tissues to their presence and to the toxins they produce.

infectious disease (communicable disease)—a disease that is caused by bacteria, viruses, and other microorganisms and can be transmitted from person to person by transfer of the causative microorganism.

inferior—nearer to the soles of the feet.

inflammation—a tissue condition caused by injury or infection and marked by swelling, pain, heat, redness, and loss of function.

influenza (flu)—a moderate to severe type of respiratory infection caused by a virus. The symptoms are the same as those of the common cold, plus a high fever, generalized aching, sore throat, and severe cough.

infrared radiation—invisible heat waves beyond the red end of the visible spectrum.

ingestion—to take into the body.

inguinal hernia—protrusion of a loop of bowel through a weak spot in the abdominal wall at the groin.

inhalant—in toxicology, a substance taken into the body by breathing, such as the fumes of gasoline, organic solvents, and glue, inhaled for their central nervous system effects.

inhalation—breathing air into the lungs.

injury—damage to the body, usually inflicted by an external source.

insidious—of gradual and subtle development.

insomnia—the inability to sleep.

insulators—materials that resist transmission of electricity, heat, or sound.

insulin—a hormone that is produced by the pancreas and is essential for use of glucose as fuel by the cells. Insulin quantities are deficient in patients with diabetes.

insulin shock—a state caused by an abnormally low blood glucose level in a patient with diabetes mellitus, usually caused by too much insulin or insufficient food. The hallmark of insulin shock is alteration of the mental state, progressing from personality changes and confusion to stupor or coma.

intensive care unit—a hospital unit using special equipment and skilled personnel to care for seriously ill patients who require immediate and continuous attention.

intercostal muscles—the muscles between the ribs.

intercostal spaces—the spaces between the ribs.

interspaces—see **intercostal spaces**.

intervertebral disc—see **disc, intervertebral**.

intestine (bowel)—the part of the digestive tract that extends from the distal opening of the stomach to the anus. The small intestine is the proximal portion of the bowel, while the large intestine is the distal portion.

intracranial pressure (ICP)—the pressure inside the cranium.

involuntary muscle—muscle whose contractions are not under conscious control.

ion—a particle carrying an electric charge.

iris—the muscle-containing ring of tissue that surrounds the pupil, forming the colored part of the eye.

irregular bones—bones of irregular shape, such as the vertebrae.

irreversible shock—prolonged shock marked by the production of toxic substances from injured organs, which prevent reestablishment of the circulation despite treatment.

ischial tuberosity—the large, bony knob that can be felt deep in each lower buttock.

ischium—the most posterior of the three fused bones making up the pelvis.

-itis—suffix denoting infection or inflammation, e.g., appendicitis or bronchitis.

IV—intravenous, within a vein. IV usually refers to a drug or solution injected into a vein.

J

jaundice—yellowing of the skin and whites of the eyes caused by the accumulation of bilirubin in patients with liver disease and certain types of anemia.

jaw ramus—a process projecting superiorly from the posterior part of either side of the mandible.

jaw-thrust—a method of opening the airway by thrusting the lower jaw forward with the fingers.

jejunum—the portion of the small intestine, extending from the duodenum to the ileum.

joint—the junction between two or more bones.

joint capsule—a sac of fibrous tissue enclosing movable joints.

Joule— one Kg/m²/second².

juvenile diabetes—type I, unstable, insulin-dependent diabetes mellitus (IDDM) usually affecting children and adolescents.

K

Kendrick extrication device (KED)—a lightweight, collapsible, vestlike, short backboard made of nylon strengthened with vertical wooden slats.

Kendrick traction device—a traction splint similar to the Sager splint.

ketoacidosis—acidosis characterized by accumulation of ketones in the body.

ketone—a compound containing the carbonyl group C = O. Formed by incomplete fat metabolism in uncontrolled diabetes.

kidney—one of a pair of organs that lie on either side of the spine against the upper part of the posterior abdominal wall. The kidneys filter the waste products of cellular metabolism from the blood and regulate the body's content of water and essential minerals by adjusting salt retention and urine excretion.

kidney stone—a stone formed by precipitation of mineral salts in the kidney. A kidney stone can cause excruciating pain if it travels from the kidney to the bladder through the ureter.

kinetic energy—energy created by motion.

knee joint—the joint between the tibia distally, the femur proximally, and the patella anteriorly.

L

labor—in obstetrics, the process by which the baby is pushed by the contractions of the uterine muscles from the uterus through the vagina into the outside world.

laceration—a tear in the skin.

lactic acid—an intermediate product of carbohydrate metabolism that accumulates in the blood during exercise and normally is metabolized to carbon dioxide and water if sufficient oxygen is available.

ladder splint—a fixation splint made of heavy, rigid wire.

large intestine—see **colon**.

laryngitis—infection or inflammation of the larynx.

larynx—the organ that connects the pharynx with the trachea and contains the vocal cords responsible for production of the voice.

lateral—farther from the midline of the body.

lateral malleolus—the outer portion of the ankle joint formed by the distal end of the fibula.

lateralized extremity weakness—weakness of both extremities on one side or the other.

latissimus dorsi muscle—the muscle that extends like a wing from each shoulder girdle to the spine and adducts the upper arm. The muscle can be felt as it extends downward from the armpit to the side of the chest; it is attached to the humerus laterally and the spinous processes of the thoracic vertebrae medially.

Law of Conservation of Energy—energy can be neither created nor destroyed but may be changed from any form to any other form.

lens—the transparent biconvex body that forms part of the optics of the eye. The lens is located behind the cornea and separates the anterior compartment of the eye from the posterior compartment.

leprosy—a chronic, communicable disease caused by *Mycobacterium leprae* that affects the skin and peripheral nerves.

level of responsiveness (LOR)—(also known as level of consciousness [LOC]). The degree to which a patient responds to stimuli such as the human voice or pain.

ligament—a band of thick, strong, fibrous tissue that connects bones or cartilages. A ligament may be a localized thickening of the joint capsule.

lightheadedness—a feeling of "floating," slight unsteadiness, or faintness that is most commonly caused by chronic anxiety.

liver—a large gland essential to life that is located in the upper right quadrant of the abdomen. The liver has many functions, including storage and filtration of blood, secretion of bile, excretion of bilirubin and other substances formed elsewhere in the body, and numerous metabolic functions including assistance in fat metabolism, detoxification of drugs and other substances, conversion of sugars to glycogen, and storage of glycogen.

LLQ—left lower quadrant.

"lockjaw"—see **tetanus**.

logroll—a technique used to roll a patient 180 degrees or to the side so that a spine board can be slipped underneath without causing bending or twisting of the spine.

long bones—one of the three major types of bones (the others are flat bones and irregular bones), long bones are found in the limbs.

lower airway obstruction—blockage in the larynx, the trachea, the major bronchi, or the other air passages within the lung.

LPM—liters per minute.

LSD—lysergic acid diethylamide, a commonly used hallucinogenic drug.

lumbar spine—the five lumbar vertebrae.

LUQ—left upper quadrant.

Lyme disease—a tick-borne infectious disease caused by a spirochete. Manifestations include a characteristic skin rash, neurologic and cardiac abnormalities, and arthritis.

M

M—scientific abbreviation for "mass" when used in an equation.

"magic" mushroom—(*Psilocybe mexicana*). The source of psilocybin, a commonly used hallucinogenic drug.

malaria—mosquito-borne tropical disease caused by protozoa of the genus Plasmodium. The organism is a parasite of red blood cells. Symptoms include cyclic fever, chills, and fatigue.

malignant—cancerous.

malleable metal splint—a fixation splint made of soft sheet metal padded with thin sheets of foam.

mammalian diving reflex—slowing of the heart rate, cessation of breathing, and diversion of blood flow from the shell to the body core in response to immersion of the face in cold water. The reflex acts to conserve vital oxygen for the most important tissues.

mandible—the lower jaw, containing the lower teeth.

manual stabilization—using the rescuer's hands to stabilize the head and neck of a patient with a possible neck or back injury.

manual traction—traction using the hands alone.

marijuana—a product of the Indian hemp plant *Cannabis sativa*, marijuana causes mild euphoria, relaxation, and drowsiness when ingested or smoked.

mass-casualty incident (MCI)—a disaster that initially overwhelms the resources of the community and requires triage to ensure that the greatest good is done for the greatest number (see **multiple-casualty incident**).

masseter muscle—one of the two large, powerful muscles that close the jaws (see **temporalis muscle**).

mastoid process—the sharp tip of the mastoid part of the temporal bone that can be felt just behind the ear.

maxilla—the upper jaw, containing the upper teeth.

mechanism of injury—the mechanical forces involved in producing an injury. Identifying this helps the rescuer predict and recognize the type and extent of injury.

medial—nearer to the midline of the body.

medial malleolus—the distal end of the tibia that forms the inside part of the ankle joint.

median nerve—a major nerve of the upper extremity that supplies sensation to the lateral side of the ring finger, most of the thumb, and the first two fingers; and supplies the muscles that flex the wrist and enable the hand to form a grip.

median plane—an imaginary plane separating the body into right and left sides.

mediastinum—the space in the chest that separates the two thoracic cavities and contains the heart, the roots of the great vessels, and other important structures.

medical history—information about a patient's past health problems that may affect the current illness or injury. The rescuer obtains this information during the secondary survey.

medical-alert tag—a bracelet, necklace, or card stating the patient's medical problems.

meninges—the three layers of protective membranes that cover the brain and spinal cord.

meningitis—inflammation of the meninges.

meniscus—a crescent-shaped cushion of cartilage found in some movable joints, e.g., the medial and lateral menisci atop the tibial plateau that cushion the knee joint.

menstrual period—the normal, cyclic discharge consisting of blood and mucosal tissue from the lining of the uterus, which normally occurs every 28 days in a nonpregnant woman of reproductive age.

mescal cactus—(*Lophophora williamsii*). The source of mescaline and peyote, two commonly used hallucinogenic drugs.

mesenteric adenitis—painful inflammation of intra-abdominal lymph nodes in a patient with a respiratory infection.

mesenteric arteries—the arteries that supply blood to the digestive tract.

mesenteric veins—the veins that carry blood away from the digestive tract.

mesentery—a thin sheet of connective tissue that attaches the organs of the abdominal cavity to the body wall.

metabolism—the oxygen-requiring chemical reactions by which the body produces or uses energy.

metacarpal bones—the five bones found in the palm of the hand that form a base for the fingers and thumb and connect with the eight carpal bones that form the wrist.

metatarsal bones—the five long slender bones that form the arch of the foot and are located between the tarsals proximally and the digits distally.

micron—a unit of measurement equalling 0.000039 inches or 0.001 millimeter.

midclavicular line—an imaginary line running perpendicular to the midpoint of the clavicle.

midline—the intersection of the median plane with the body surface in front and in back.

migraine—a recurrent, throbbing, one-sided headache accompanied by nausea and preceded by abnormal visual phenomena such as blurred vision or bright, moving lights.

minerals—inorganic elements and compounds that are found in the earth's crust. Many minerals are necessary for normal metabolic body functioning.

miscarriage—the spontaneous expelling of the fetus from the pregnant uterus before the fetus is capable of life outside the uterus.

modified hinge joint (knee)—a joint in which motion is mainly in the single plane of flexion-extension. Some degree of rotation of the tibia on the femur can occur during full flexion and full extension.

monitor—to check constantly or repeatedly on a condition or phenomenon, i.e., the vital signs of a patient.

motor area—the part of the cerebral cortex of the brain that controls the movement of the voluntary muscles.

motor fibers—fibers composed of the axons of nerve cells that regulate muscle motion.

motor fitness—the development of strength, power, balance, agility, flexibility, and, to some extent, endurance.

motor nerves—nerves that transmit impulses to the skeletal muscles.

mouth-to-mouth breathing—see **rescue breathing**.

mouth-to-nose breathing—a rescue breathing technique used in infants, small children, patients with facial injuries or mouths that cannot be opened, or when it is difficult to achieve a tight seal around the patient's mouth.

mucoid—mucus-like.

mucous membrane—a thin, moist mucous-producing tissue that lines the mouth, nasal cavity, and other body cavities.

mucus—the slimy material that is found on the mucous membranes and lubricates body openings; the secretions of the mucous glands.

multiple-casualty incident (MCI)—an emergency in which there are more patients than rescuers (see **mass-casualty incident**).

muscle—a special tissue composed of cells that can shorten, or contract, and lengthen, or relax.

muscle tension headache—a headache caused by chronic contraction of the muscles of the head and/or neck.

musculoskeletal system—all the bones, joints, muscles, and tendons of the body, collectively.

muscular system—the muscles of the body. The muscular system acts together with the skeletal system to permit body movement.

myelin—a fatty substance that encloses the axons of the neurons and acts like the insulation that prevents short circuits in electric wires.

myocardial contusion—a bruise of the heart.

myocardial infarction—death of the heart muscle caused by lack of oxygen, usually because of a blood clot or sudden narrowing of an artery in a patient with coronary artery disease.

myocardium—the heart muscle.

myoclonic seizures—seizures characterized by muscle jerks without loss of responsiveness.

N

narcotic—a pain-relieving drug that suppresses the central nervous system, producing stupor, insensibility, or deep sleep. Narcotics are derived from the opium poppy or are manufactured synthetically, e.g., heroin, codeine, methadone, meperidine, and Dilaudid.

nasal cannulae—a low-flow oxygen delivery system consisting of a thin tube with two small tubular prongs that slip into the nose, capable of delivering 24 to 40 percent oxygen when operated at a maximum of 6 L/min.

nasal cavity—the interior cavity of the nose, separated into two halves by the nasal septum.

nasal septum—the thin partition that divides the nasal cavity into two nostrils and is composed of membrane, cartilage, and bone.

nasopharyngeal airway—a soft rubber tube that is inserted into the nose so that its tip lies in the nasopharynx. It does not prevent the tongue from obstructing the airway.

National Association for Search and Rescue (NASAR)—a national association consisting of volunteer and professional rescuers; covers all aspects of search and rescue.

NATO position—the semiprone or stable side position recommended for all unconscious or semiconscious patients without neck or back injuries.

nausea—an unpleasant sensation in the epigastrium that often leads to vomiting.

navel—the umbilicus; a depression in the abdominal wall marking the site of attachment of the umbilical cord in the fetus.

near drowning—survival, at least temporarily, after submersion in water.

negligence—injury to another person caused by failure to provide the degree of care that any reasonable and prudent person would provide in similar circumstances (see also **willful negligence** and **gross negligence**).

neoplasm—new growth; a benign or malignant tumor.

nervous system—the system of nerve cells and their supporting structures that collects and processes stimuli from the environment and coordinates the activities of the other major organ systems.

neurogenic shock—shock due to dilation of blood vessels, caused by paralysis of the nerves that control them; usually due to spinal cord injury.

neurons—special cells that react to stimuli and are able to conduct impulses rapidly through their cytoplasm. The primary cells of the nervous system.

neurosurgical—relating to surgery of the nervous system.

Newton's First Law of Motion—a body at rest will tend to remain at rest, and a body in motion will tend to remain in motion unless acted upon by an outside force.

nicotine—a poisonous alkaloid in tobacco that accounts for the addictive nature of cigarette smoking.

nipple—the pigmented projection on the anterior surface of the breast.

nitrogen narcosis—("Rapture of the deep"). An effect similar to alcohol intoxication that is caused by breathing nitrogen-containing gas (i.e., air) at depths below about 90 feet (27 meters).

nitroglycerin—a medication dispensed as a small white tablet that is placed under the tongue to treat patients with angina pectoris. Nitroglycerin relaxes vascular smooth muscle and increases blood flow and oxygen supply to the heart muscle.

non-rebreather mask—a transparent mask fitted with a plastic reservoir bag and one-way valve that allows the patient to inhale oxygen from the bag but prevents exhalation into the bag.

normothermic—characterized by normal body temperature.

nostrils—the external openings of the nasal cavity; the nares.

numbness—a lack of or decrease in sensation in a part.

O

O$_2$—oxygen.

occiput—the back of the head.

occlusive dressing—airtight dressing, consisting of a universal dressing or several layers of sterile, moist compresses, covered with Vaseline gauze, foil, plastic wrap, or a plastic bag. Occlusive dressing is used to keep organs from drying out or to prevent air from entering the pleural space.

olecranon of the ulna—the bony projection of the ulna at the elbow, to which the triceps muscle tendon is attached.

olfactory organ—the part of the nose that contains the end organs for smell.

open fracture—any fracture that involves a wound of the overlying skin.

open injury—any injury that involves a break in the skin as well as damage to the tissues beneath it.

ophthalmologist—a physician specializing in the treatment of eye disease and injury.

optic nerve—one of the paired cranial nerves that transmits nerve impulses from the light-sensitive retina cells to the brain.

oral airway—a curved device designed to keep the tongue of an unconscious patient from falling back and occluding the upper airway. Oral airways have an opening down the center or along either side to transmit air and allow suctioning.

orbit—the bony socket that contains and protects the eye.

Oregon spine splint—the brand name of a portable, vest-like short backboard similar to the Kendrick extrication device.

oropharyngeal (oral) airway—see oral airway.

oropharynx—the portion of the pharynx between the soft palate and the upper edge of the epiglottis.

orthopedics—the branch of surgery concerned with the preservation and restoration of the function of the skeletal system, its articulations, and associated structures.

osmotic pressure—pressure exerted by a solution in direct proportion to the number of particles dissolved in it.

ovary—the sexual gland in the female that produces sex hormones and eggs.

ovum—an egg.

oxygen (O$_2$)—a gas that makes up 21 percent of air and is necessary for normal metabolism.

oxygen debt—a buildup of lactic acid in the blood and muscle tissues during exercise because of a relative lack of oxygen.

oxygen poisoning—convulsions caused by breathing pure oxygen below 33 feet (10 meters) or breathing compressed air below 297 feet (90 meters).

P

PABA—para-aminobenzoic acid; used in sun-protective products.

packaging—the process of securing a patient to a device such as a spine board, litter, or toboggan, and otherwise preparing the patient for transport after initial emergency care has been given.

palpation—feeling; examining by touch.

pancreas—the organ that produces digestive enzymes and makes hormone insulin.

pancreatic juice—a fluid produced by the pancreas that contains enzymes that aid in the digestion of fat, starch, and protein.

pancreatitis—inflammation or infection of the pancreas.

pantothenic acid—a water-soluble vitamin.

pant-leg pinch lift—a technique used to lift a patient's lower extremity onto a quick splint by grasping the clothing rather than the extremity itself.

paradoxical motion of the chest wall—a condition in which a flail section of the chest wall moves in instead of out with inhalation and out instead of in with exhalation.

paralysis—inability to move a part due to interruption of its nerve supply.

paranoia—a psychiatric disorder marked by delusions of grandeur or persecution.

paraplegia—paralysis of both legs.

parasympathetic nervous system—one of the two parts of the autonomic nervous system, the parasympathetic nervous system has many functions, including constriction of the pupils, slowing of the heart rate, and relaxation of body sphincters.

paravertebral muscles—the generic name given to a number of different muscles lying on either side of the spine.

parietal bones—bones that form the superior and lateral surfaces of the cranium.

partial pressure of oxygen (PO$_2$)—the percentage of total atmospheric pressure accounted for by oxygen. At sea level, oxygen partial pressure is 160 mm Hg (21 percent of 760 mm Hg of the total atmospheric pressure).

PASG (pneumatic antishock garment)—a large, pant-shaped air splint for the abdomen and lower extremities. Used to stabilize pelvic, hip, and femoral fractures, and combat hypovolemic shock.

patella—the kneecap.

patellar ligament—the continuation of the quadriceps muscle tendon that extends from the patella to the tibial tuberosity.

patient—an ill or injured person who requires emergency care.

pectoralis muscle—one of the two muscles beneath the breasts that help adduct the upper extremities.

pelvic cavity—the cavity located in the lowest part of the trunk that is continuous with the abdominal cavity. It contains the bladder, rectum, and female reproductive organs.

pelvis—a cone-shaped, bony ring made up of the right and left pelvic bones joined in front at the pubis and in back to the sacrum at the sacroiliac joints. Each pelvic bone is made up of three fused bones—the ilium, ischium, and pubis. The pelvis contains the bladder, rectum, and female reproductive organs.

penetration trauma—trauma caused by a sharp object moving at a moderate to high speed that penetrates the skin, or by a moving body striking a narrow, pointed object.

penis—the male organ of sexual intercourse.

Pepto-Bismol—the brand name of a non-prescription bismuth preparation useful in controlling diarrhea.

pericardial tamponade—the failure of heart action because of blood or other fluid accumulation in the pericardium that leads to increased pressure, which interferes with the heart's ability to relax between contractions and refill with blood.

pericardium—the fibrous sac that surrounds the heart and the roots of the great vessels.

perineum—the area between the pubis anteriorly and the coccyx posteriorly.

periodic breathing—see **Cheyne-Stokes respirations**.

peripheral nervous system—the part of the nervous system that includes the nerves and their branches and the special sensory organs lying outside the brain and spinal cord.

peristalsis—the wave-like movement by which the alimentary canal propels and mixes its contents.

peristaltic activity—the contraction of the muscles in the walls of the small and large intestines that mixes and propels their contents forward.

peritoneal cavity—the body cavity enclosed by the peritoneum; includes the abdominal and pelvic cavities. The term is frequently used to mean the same as "abdominal cavity."

peritoneal dialysis—dialysis using the peritoneum as a dialyzing membrane, with the dialyzing solution being introduced and removed from the peritoneal cavity.

peritoneum—a thin membrane that lines the abdominal cavity and is continuous with the outer coverings of the organs within the cavity, forming a closed sac similar to the pleural cavity. A continuation of the peritoneum lines the pelvic cavity.

peritonitis—inflammation or infection of the peritoneum.

peroneal nerve—one of the branches of the sciatic nerve, the peroneal nerve winds around the head of the fibula before entering the lower leg where it divides into superficial and deep branches. It supplies sensation to the top of the foot and helps move the ankle.

perspiration—the liquid excreted by the sweat glands.

phalanges—the small bones that make up each finger and toe.

pharynx—the cavity that is continuous with the nasal cavities and mouth in front and the larynx and the esophagus below.

phenol—an organic acid containing a single benzene ring and a single hydroxyl (OH) group.

phenothiazines—a group of tranquilizing drugs.

phrenic nerves—nerves that originate in the cervical part of the spinal cord and pass down through the chest to supply the diaphragm.

physical dependence—physiological changes in response to a drug, so that suddenly stopping its use causes well-defined symptoms of withdrawal.

physiological saline solution—(also called "normal saline"). A 0.9-percent solution of sodium chloride in water with the same osmotic pressure as human plasma; used to irrigate an open wound, keep tissue moist, and for intravenous injection.

physiology—the branch of biology dealing with the function of the living organism and its parts.

pia mater—the innermost of the three layers of meninges that cover the brain and spinal cord.

pinna—the external ear, which is made of cartilage covered by skin and surrounds the ear canal.

"pitting edema"—a type of swelling characterized by a depression or pit that remains after a finger is pressed into a swollen area.

pituitary gland—a gland at the base of the brain that controls the male and female reproductive systems, thyroid, adrenal cortex, body growth, and other body functions.

placenta (afterbirth)—an organ that attaches to the lining of the uterus and contains special tissues through which the blood of the mother and fetus are brought in close proximity so that oxygen, nutrients, waste products, and other substances can be exchanged. It is attached to the fetus by the umbilical cord.

plantarflex—to bend the foot downward, in the direction of the sole of the foot.

plasma—the fluid component of blood. Plasma transports the blood cells and contains a large variety of dissolved minerals and inorganic and organic compounds. The compounds include nutrients, waste products, and components involved in immunity and blood clotting.

platelets—disc-shaped bodies in the blood that aid in blood clotting.

pleura—a thin membrane that lines the inner wall of each thoracic cavity and covers the outer surface of each lung.

pleural space—a potential rather than actual space between the pleura lining the rib cage and the pleura covering the outside of the lung; the pleural space is normally filled with a thin film of fluid.

pleurisy—inflammation of the pleura.

pneumatic antishock garment (PASG)—a pant-like garment originally designed to combat hypovolemic shock. The PASG consists of three separate inflatable chambers, one for each leg and one for the abdomen. Each chamber is folded around its respective body part and fastened with Velcro straps.

pneumatic counterpressure device—a term used for inflatable devices used as splints and for control of bleeding. Includes PASGs and air splints.

pneumonia—an infection or inflammation of the lungs that causes consolidation (stiffening) due to filling of the alveoli with fluid and inflammatory cells.

pneumothorax—air in the pleural space caused by an abnormal passage that connects the pleural space with the outside air, either through the chest wall or within the lung. Accompanied by full or partial collapse of the lung.

poikilotherms—cold-blooded creatures.

poison—any substance that impairs the functioning of the body through chemical action that interferes with normal metabolic processes.

poison control center—information telephone center staffed by trained personnel who provide information on nontoxic and toxic exposures.

polycythemia—an increase in the numbers of red blood cells that can occur in association with certain diseases and as an adaptive response to living at high altitude.

poly-drug abuse—abuse involving more than one drug.

polyunsaturated fats—see **fat, polyunsaturated**.

popliteal fossa—the area behind the knee bordered by the hamstring tendons.

position of function—the position in which an immobilized body part functions best.

posterior—nearer to the back surface of the body.

posterior tibial artery pulse—a pulse that can be felt just below and behind the medial malleolus.

potentiator—an agent that enhances the action of another agent.

predisposition—a latent susceptibility.

pregnancy—the condition of carrying a developing offspring inside the body.

pressure irrigation—squirting a cleansing liquid into a wound under pressure.

pressure point—a point where a major artery lies close to the skin and over a bone. Pressure at this point is sometimes used as an aid to control severe bleeding.

priapism—a long-lasting, painful erection of the penis.

primary survey—a rapid and systematic evaluation of the level of responsiveness (LOR) and the function of the respiratory and circulatory systems.

primary organ systems—the circulatory and respiratory systems.

progressive—advancing, increasing in strength or severity.

process—a projection of bone or tissue.

prone—lying face down.

prostate gland—a small gland that lies at the base of the bladder and surrounds the male urethra. It produces part of the seminal fluid.

protein—an organic compound composed of chains of amino acids made up of nitrogen, sulfur, and phosphorus in addition to carbon, hydrogen, and oxygen.

proximal—closer to the trunk of the body.

PSI—abbreviation for pounds per square inch.

psilocybin—a hallucinogenic substance made from the mushroom *Psilocybe mexicana,* or "magic mushroom."

psychological dependence—a state in which a drug user becomes obsessed with taking a drug and continues to take it despite obvious physical, mental, or social harm.

psychosomatic illness—an illness with bodily symptoms but an emotional or mental cause.

pubic bone—see **pubis**.

pubis—the most anterior of the three bones that make up the pelvic bone.

pulmonary artery—the major artery leading from the right ventricle of the heart to the lungs.

pulmonary circuit—the closed circuit of the circulatory system that includes the lungs. The blood is pumped from the right side of the heart through the lungs and back to the left side of the heart.

pulmonary contusion—a bruise of the lung.

pulmonary edema—the abnormal accumulation of fluid in the tissues and air spaces of the lung.

pulmonary embolus—a blood clot that has broken loose and traveled to the lung.

pulmonary emphysema—see **emphysema**.

pulmonary fibrosis—a condition that leads to thickening of the walls of the alveoli in the lungs because of increased fibrous tissue in their walls.

pulse—the rhythmic, expanding tap felt when the fingers are placed over an artery lying close to the body surface. The pulse represents the pressure wave produced each time the heart beats.

pulselessness—absence of a heartbeat.

puncture—a deep wound with a small entrance caused by a sharp, narrow object or by a high-velocity blunt object.

pupil of the eye—the opening in the center of the iris of the eye through which light enters.

pupils, reaction of—ability of the pupils of the eyes to respond to light and other stimulants by enlarging or decreasing in size.

pus—a thick, yellowish or greenish liquid made up of white cells and fluid, produced in response to inflammation.

Q

quadriceps—the major muscle of the anterior thigh, which allows extension of the knee.

quadriplegia—paralysis of both arms and both legs.

quality assurance—methods for ensuring a high level of patient care.

quick splint—a temporary splint made of plywood padded with foam, designed for rapid application.

R

rabies—a universally fatal disease of the central nervous system, caused by a virus present in the saliva of infected animals that is transmitted through biting or licking.

"raccoon eyes"—ecchymosis in the skin around the eyes, a sign of internal bleeding from a skull fracture.

radial artery pulse—a pulse felt anterior to the radial styloid process proximal to the base of the thumb.

radial nerve—a nerve that winds around the humerus at its midpoint, carrying sensations to the back of the hand and controlling extension of the hand at the wrist.

radiating—characterized by divergence from a common center.

radiation—the process of emitting energy in the form of waves or particles.

radius—the lateral of the two forearm bones when the palms are held facing forward.

reclining—lying down.

rectum—the distal portion of the large intestine ending at the anal canal.

rectus muscle—one of the two strap-like muscles covering the front of the abdomen that provide support for the abdomen and allow flexion of the lumbar spine.

recumbent—lying down.

red cell sludging—clumping together of red cells within blood vessels.

reduce—to restore the normal relationship of parts, e.g., to reduce a fractured bone.

reflex arcs—short connections between motor and sensory nerve fibers within the spinal cord that bypass the brain and provide an immediate reaction to noxious stimuli, i.e., pulling a hand away from a hot stove.

regulator—the name given to the device that contains a pressure-reducing valve, pressure gauge and flowmeter, and is attached to the outlet of a gas cylinder.

regurgitation—backward flowing, e.g., the casting up of undigested food.

renal arteries—the arteries that supply blood to the kidneys.

renal pelvis—the funnel-shaped upper portion of each ureter.

renal veins—the veins that carry blood away from the kidneys.

reproductive system—the system of organs that provides the means of producing successive generations of offspring.

reproductive system, female—the ovaries, fallopian tubes, uterus, vagina, and associated glands.

reproductive system, male—the testicles, vasa deferentia, seminal vesicles, prostate gland, and penis.

rescue breathing—a mouth-to-mouth or mouth-to-mouthpiece technique for ventilating a nonbreathing patient.

rescuer—a ski patroller, search and rescue group member, or any other person who provides rescue and prehospital care in an emergency.

respiration—breathing.

respiration (heat loss)—heat loss as inhaled air is warmed to body temperature before being exhaled.

respiratory center—the brain center that controls the depth, rate, and rhythm of breathing.

respiratory distress—abnormal breathing that includes dyspnea (difficult or labored breathing), tachypnea (increase in breathing rate), hyperpnea (increase in breathing depth), and occasionally shallow breathing. The patient is usually aware of the need for extra efforts necessary to obtain enough air.

responsiveness, level of—the patient's ability to respond to stimuli such as a voice or pain. If the level is normal, then the patient is oriented, talks coherently, and can answer correctly when questioned about name, address, location, day, and date.

retina—the lining of the inner surface of the sclera of the eye, which contains light-sensitive cells.

rewarm—to raise the body temperature of a patient with hypothermia, or to raise the temperature of a part affected with frostbite.

rhonchi—coarse sounds produced by air moving through larger air passages partly blocked by sputum or other secretions (see also **wheezes** and **stridor**).

rib—one of 24 paired, curved bones that form and support the chest wall.

rigid collar—a device that limits head and neck motion when applied to the neck of a patient with an actual or suspected neck injury (also called a cervical collar, C-collar, or extrication collar).

rigid splints—splints made from firm material and applied to the sides, front, and/or back of an injured extremity to prevent motion at the injury site.

rigor mortis—the stiffening of a dead body.

RLQ—right lower quadrant.

"road burn"—a type of abrasion commonly seen in cyclists.

Rocky Mountain spotted fever—a severe, acute, febrile illness characterized by muscle and joint pain and a rash. It is caused by a rickettsia transmitted by a wood tick.

rule of nines—a way of estimating the size of a burned area.

RUQ—right upper quadrant.

S

sacroiliac joint—the joint between the sacrum medially and the ilium laterally.

sacrum—a flat, triangular bone formed from the five sacral vertebrae fused together to form a single bone that can be felt below the lumbar vertebrae and above the sharp coccyx.

Sager splint—the brand name of a lower extremity splint that uses a single, adjustable pole.

salicylate—a compound such as aspirin that is a salt of salicylic acid.

saliva—the liquid secretion of the glands of the mouth that serves to moisten and soften food and initiate the digestion of starch.

salmonella—the bacterium that causes a type of dysentery.

SAM splint—the brand name of a malleable metal splint padded with thin sheets of foam.

saturated fat—see **fat, saturated**.

Sawyer extractor—the brand name of a small, powerful suction pump for removing injected poisons.

scalp—the part of the skin of the head that is normally covered by hair.

scapula—the shoulder blade; a large, flat, triangular bone lying against the posterior chest wall.

SCBA—self-contained breathing apparatus.

sciatic nerve—the largest nerve in the body; the sciatic nerve provides sensation to the lateral leg and foot, and supplies the muscles that extend the hip, flex the knee, and move the ankle and foot. In the back of the thigh, the sciatic nerve branches into the tibial and peroneal nerves.

sclera—the dense tissue that forms the posterior five-sixths of the globe of the eye. The visible part of the sclera is called the white of the eye.

scoop stretcher—a lightweight aluminum frame that breaks apart lengthwise. Each side is inserted beneath a patient until the two sides meet in the middle.

scrotum—the sac that contains the testicles and their accessory organs.

search and rescue (SAR)—the process of searching for, locating, obtaining access to, extricating, transferring, giving emergency care to, packaging, and transporting a patient. The patient's initial location is frequently unknown or uncertain.

seated carries—emergency two-rescuer techniques for moving conscious patients without spinal injuries by carrying them in the seated position.

second-degree burn—a burn in which the epidermis and a varying extent of the dermis are damaged; characterized by blister formation.

second-degree frostbite—a type of deep frostbite characterized, after thawing, by large blisters filled with clear or pinkish fluid that form within minutes to hours and enlarge over several days.

secondary survey—the part of patient assessment that involves assessing the vital and other important signs, taking a brief history, and doing a head-to-toe body assessment.

seizure—a sudden, transient alteration of normal brain function.

semen—the fluid that contains sperm and the secretions of the prostate and seminal vesicles that is discharged at ejaculation.

seminal fluid—see **semen**.

seminal vesicle—outpouching of the vasa deferentia that store the sperm.

semiprone—lying face down but on one side, usually with the opposite knee drawn up.

sensory fibers—fibers that are composed of the nerve cell axons that carry sensation to the brain from the organs of touch, pain, and temperature in the skin and muscles.

septum—a bony plate that divides the two sides of the nasal cavity.

sesamoid—a bone that forms within a muscle tendon.

sexually-transmitted infection—an infectious disease transmitted by sexual contact.

shaft (of a bone)—the long, slender part of a long bone between its wider ends.

shell—the skin, muscles, and extremities of the body (see also **core**).

shivering—a method of heat production that involves involuntary trembling or quivering of the body caused by rapid contractions or twitches of muscles.

shock—a form of acute failure of the blood circulation.

shockable rhythm—a heart rhythm (ventricular fibrillation or ventricular tachycardia) that can be returned to normal by an electric shock applied to the heart.

short spine board—a short board used to evacuate patients with spine injuries from wrecked automobiles and other confined spaces.

shoulder girdle—the clavicle, scapula, humerus, sternoclavicular joint, acromioclavicular (AC) joint, and shoulder joint.

shoulder joint—a ball-and-socket joint in the shoulder girdle where the humerus connects distally with a socket in the outer angle of the scapula proximally.

side crutch support—an emergency technique for assisting a conscious patient to walk to safety with the support of one or two rescuers.

sign—an important characteristic of an illness or injury that the observer notes by looking, feeling, listening, or smelling (see also **symptom** and **vital signs**).

silent—producing no detectable signs or symptoms.

silver fork deformity—(see **Colles' fracture**).

simple fracture—a fracture with only one fracture line.

skeletal system—made up of 206 bones and their associated ligaments, the skeletal system provides a rigid framework to protect and support the soft tissues, gives form to the body, and, together with the muscular system, allows body movement.

"skier's thumb"—("gamekeeper's thumb"). A sprain or fracture of the structures at the base of the thumb caused when the skier tries to break a fall with an outstretched hand while holding a ski pole, which bends the thumb backward on impact.

skin—the outer covering of the body, made up of the epidermis and the dermis.

skin perfusion—the flow of blood through the small skin vessels.

skull—the bones of the head, including the eight bones of the cranium, the facial bones, and the mandible.

sling—a triangular bandage tied around the neck to support the weight of the upper extremity (see **swathe**).

slow-twitch (type I) fibers—muscle fibers designed for sustained, slow contractions that rely mainly on aerobic metabolic processes (see also **fast-twitch fibers**).

slipped disc—herniation of the nucleus of the intravertebral disc.

small intestine—the segment of bowel between the stomach and the large intestine, from which most digested food is absorbed before the undigested residue is passed to the large intestine.

smallpox—an acute, viral disease characterized by a severe pustular rash, high fever, prostration, and severe aching.

snowblindness—sunburn of the conjunctiva of the eye.

socket—a hollow or depression into which a corresponding part fits, e.g., the socket of a tooth or joint.

soft fixation splint—a splint made of soft material, i.e., an air splint, splints improvised from folded parkas, blankets or pillows, and the sling and swathe.

soft tissues—skin, subcutaneous tissues, and muscles.

somatic nervous system—the system that controls voluntary activities such as eating, walking, and talking.

sore throat—a painful infection or inflammation of the tonsils and upper oropharynx.

Spanish windlass—a device that provides traction through tightening a twisted cravat.

sperm—the male germ cell.

sphygmomanometer—an instrument used to measure blood pressure.

spinal canal—the tunnel, formed by the successive vertebral arches, in which the spinal cord lies.

spinal cord—the part of the central nervous system that lies in the spinal canal. The spinal cord is connected to the brain above at the foramen magnum of the skull.

spinal nerves—the 31 pairs of nerves that branch off from the spinal cord and exit through notches between the vertebrae.

spine—the bony column, composed of 33 vertebrae, that forms the main support for the body and protects the spinal cord.

spine board—a long, rigid board designed to immobilize the body of a patient with a neck or back injury.

spinous processes—the posterior processes of the vertebrae that form the attachment points for ligaments and tendons.

spiral fracture—a fracture in which the fracture line spirals around the shaft of the bone. A spiral fracture usually is caused by a twisting force.

spleen—a vascular organ, located in the left upper part of the abdominal cavity, that destroys worn-out blood cells, stores blood, produces antibodies, and forms lymphocytes.

splint—a device designed to prevent or reduce motion at the site of a fracture or other injury.

splinting—the application of a splint.

spontaneous pneumothorax—air in the pleural space caused by spontaneous rupture of a bleb or cyst of the lung.

sprain—the stretching or tearing of a ligament or tendon.

sputum—mucoid material from the lower respiratory tract (trachea, bronchi, and lungs), usually produced by coughing.

"squeeze" injuries—injuries to certain body areas caused by failure to equalize pressure between the area and the outside water. The middle and inner ears, sinuses, and lungs are most often affected (see **barotrauma**).

standard of care—the common law requirement that care providers perform as any other reasonable, prudent person with similar training and experience would perform under similar circumstances, with due regard for the safety and welfare of both the patient and fellow care providers.

START—Simple Triage and Rapid Treatment, a four-step technique for managing mass-casualty incidents developed by Hoag Memorial Hospital Presbyterian, Newport Beach, California.

staphylococci ("staph")—a gram positive, spherical bacterium that causes skin and severe internal infections; grows easily in bland, creamy foods left at room temperature for a few hours.

step-off deformity—a step-like deformity of the back due to partial dislocation of a vertebra.

sterile—free from living microorganisms.

sterilize—to make sterile or free from contamination by bacteria or other microorganisms.

sternal angle (Angle of Louis)—a prominent bony ridge at the junction of the upper one-fourth with the lower three-fourths of the sternum.

sternal notch—the notch at the top of the sternum.

sternoclavicular joint—the joint that joins the sternum to the clavicle.

sternomastoid muscle—one of the two strap-like muscles on either side of the front of the neck that are attached above to the mastoid processes and below to the sternoclavicular joints. The sternomastoid muscles help turn the head and flex the neck.

sternum—breastbone.

stethoscope—an instrument used to transmit sounds from the body to the examiner's ears.

stimulant—an agent that excites to greater activity. In toxicology, a stimulant is a drug that excites the mind, increases the heart rate, raises the blood pressure and breathing rate, and provides a sense of euphoria or well-being. Stimulants include caffeine, nicotine, decongestants, and asthma drugs as well as cocaine and amphetamines.

Stokes litter—a basket stretcher shaped like an oblong shell, used for removing patients from heights or over difficult terrain.

stomach—the sac-like organ between the esophagus and the duodenum where food is mixed with gastric juice to form a semifluid substance that is passed on to the intestine for further digestion.

stomach ulcer—a defect in the inner lining of the stomach caused by destruction from infection, inflammation, or self-digestion.

straddle injury—an injury to the groin or perineum caused by a fall when the patient lands with the legs straddling an object such as a fence.

strain—the stretching or tearing of a muscle because of overstretching or overexertion.

streptococcus—a gram positive, spherical bacterium present in short chains that causes severe sore throats, scarlet fever, pneumonia, and other serious infections.

stress fracture—a hairline fracture caused by repeated small traumas to a bone.

stridor—harsh, high-pitched sounds on inhalation produced by air moving through a narrowed larynx (see also **wheezes** and **rhonchi**).

stroke—a sudden lessening or loss of responsiveness, sensation, and/or movement caused by a rupture or obstruction of an artery in the brain.

styloid process—a long, pointed process of a bone.

subclavian arteries—the arteries that supply blood to the upper extremities.

subclavian veins—the veins that carry blood away from the upper extremities.

subcutaneous emphysema—see **emphysema, subcutaneous**.

submersion—to plunge under water.

submersion hypothermia—acute hypothermia combined with hypoxia caused by submersion in cold water (near drowning in cold water).

subnormal temperature—temperature below the normal range.

substance abuse—use of mind-altering chemicals without a legal medical purpose.

substernal pain—pain beneath the sternum.

subtrochanteric fracture—a fracture of the upper part of the femur below the trochanters.

subungual hematoma—bleeding under the nail.

sucking chest wound—an open hole in the chest wall that establishes a connection between the pleural space and the outside air. The lung is collapsed, and when the patient breathes, air moves in and out of the hole in the chest rather than in and out of the lung through the normal airway, making a sucking noise.

suction apparatus—a mechanical device for removing liquid and semi-solid foreign matter from the mouth, nose, and throat by suction.

suffocation—stoppage of respiration; deprivation of oxygen.

sun protection factor (SPF)—a number that refers to how many times longer skin protected by a sunscreen can be exposed to the sun before becoming red compared to unprotected skin.

sunburn—a first- or second-degree skin burn caused by ultraviolet light in the medium-wave range (UVB) with a wavelength of 290 to 320 nanometers.

sunscreen—a preparation that protects the skin from the harmful effects of sunlight. Physical sunscreens block sunlight; chemical sunscreens selectively filter out harmful rays.

superficial frostbite—an injury caused by subfreezing environmental temperatures that causes a mild tingling or pain followed by numbness. Inspection reveals a gray or yellowish patch of skin, usually on the nose, ear, cheek, finger, or toe.

superior—nearer to the top of the head.

superior vena cava—one of the two largest veins in the body; carries blood from the upper extremities, head, neck, and upper chest back to the heart.

supine—lying face up.

supracondylar fracture—a fracture of the lower end of the femur just above the condyles.

swathe—a cravat that is tied around the chest and used with a sling to immobilize the upper extremity to the chest.

swelling—an enlargement of a body part or area.

swimmer's ear—an infection of the ear canal that occurs in swimmers and divers whose ears are continually wet.

sympathetic nervous system—one of the two parts of the autonomic nervous system, the sympathetic nervous system prepares the body for action in response to stress by causing the pupils of the eyes to dilate, hairs to stand on end, the heart rate to increase, sphincters to tighten, and other reactions.

symptom—an important characteristic of an illness or injury that the patient notes and describes to the observer.

synapse—the site at which neurons connect, allowing nerve impulses to be transmitted from one to another.

syncope—see **fainting, simple**.

synovial membrane—the inner lining of the joint capsule which produces the fluid that lubricates and nourishes joint tissue.

syphilis—a contagious venereal disease caused by the spirochete *Treponema pallidum*. It can involve the central nervous system, skin, heart, aorta, and many other organs.

systemic circuit—the closed circuit of the circulatory system where the blood is pumped through all the body except for the lungs.

systolic blood pressure—the highest point of the blood pressure curve.

T

tachycardia—rapid heartbeat.

tachypnea—an abnormal increase in the breathing rate.

talus—a bone of the foot that forms the distal portion of the ankle joint.

tarry stools—tar-colored (reddish black) stools due to partial digestion of blood as it passes through the bowel.

tarsals—the five small bones of the midfoot located between the calcaneus proximally and the metatarsals distally.

taste buds—the bud-like sensory end organs for taste, located mainly on the tongue.

tear ducts—the tube that conducts tears from the eye to the nasal cavity; has two entrances, one located at the inner end of each eyelid.

tear gland—the gland, located above the outer part of the eye, that produce tears.

tears—fluid that is produced by tear glands and keeps the conjunctiva and cornea moist.

temporal pulse—the pulse of the temporal artery that can be felt just in front of and above the opening of the ear canal.

temporalis muscle—one of the two large, powerful muscles that close the jaws (see **masseter muscle**).

temporomandibular (TM) joint—the joint that connects the mandible, or jawbone, to the base of the skull just in front of the ear on either side.

tenderness—abnormal sensitivity to touch or pressure.

tendon—a tough fibrous cord that attaches a muscle to a bone.

tension pneumothorax—a serious complication of pneumothorax that occurs when a defect simulating a one-way valve develops at an injury site and allows air to enter but not escape the pleural space. The pressure in the pleural space increases with each breath until it compresses the lung and interferes with the function of the heart and the opposite, normal lung.

terminal velocity—a final speed of fall reached when the air resistance equals the pull of gravity.

testicle—the male gonad, one of a pair of egg-shaped glands normally located in the scrotum that contain specialized cells that produce hormones and sperm.

testis—see **testicle**.

tetanus—a disease caused by a soil bacterium that grows in open soft-tissue wounds and produces a toxin that provokes serious muscle spasms and interferes with breathing.

tetanus prophylaxis—immunization to prevent tetanus.

thalamus—a part of the cerebrum that contains centers for pain, temperature, touch, and emotion.

thermometer—an instrument for recording body temperature.

third-degree frostbite—a type of deep frostbite that is, after thawing, characterized by proximally located small to medium blisters containing dark reddish-blue to purplish fluid.

Thomas splint—a traction splint for immobilizing a fracture femur; was developed during World War I by Sir Hugh Owen Thomas.

thoracic cage—the hollow cage-like structure formed by the ribs, sternum, and vertebral column that encloses the pleural cavities and mediastinum.

thoracic cavities—the two cavities in the chest that contain the right and left lungs and are separated by the mediastinum.

thoracic spine—the 12 thoracic vertebrae.

thorax—the chest.

thyroid cartilage—("Adam's apple"). The shield-shaped cartilage of the larynx at the front of the neck.

thyroid gland—an endocrine gland consisting of two lobes joined by a isthmus, one lobe lying on each side of the lower larynx and upper trachea. It produces iodine-containing hormones that control the body's metabolic rate.

tibia—the weight-bearing bone that is the medial of the two bones of the lower leg.

tibial plateau—the concave riding surface of the knee on which the femoral condyles sit.

tolerance—a state in which the body adjusts to the presence of a drug so that increasing amounts are required to produce the desired effect.

"tonsil" tip—see **Yankauer tip**.

tourniquet (TK)—a device used to control hemorrhage by exerting circumferential pressure around a limb proximal to the bleeding site.

toxemia of pregnancy—an illness in pregnant women characterized by high blood pressure, protein in the urine, blurred vision, headache, and edema, followed in some cases by abdominal pain, convulsions, and/or unresponsiveness.

toxic—poisonous; manifesting the symptoms of severe infection.

toxin—a poison. The term frequently is used to refer to highly poisonous substances produced by some plants, animals, or bacteria.

trachea—the tube that is attached to the larynx above and that branches below to form the two main bronchi.

tracheostomy—an incision made through the neck into the trachea to allow insertion of a tube to relieve upper airway obstruction and aid ventilation.

"tracks"—multiple, linear, pigmented scars overlying veins; characteristic of intravenous drug abuse.

traction—the action of drawing or pulling on an object.

traction splint—a splint that stabilizes a fracture by means of a steady pull on the limb.

tranquilizer—a drug used to reduce agitation, anxiety, and tension in humans and animals.

transient ischemic attacks (TIAs)— minor transient strokes (cerebrovascular accidents) that occur when blood flow through a narrowed brain artery is temporarily inadequate to support the function of the brain area supplied.

transverse fracture—a fracture in which the fracture line is at or close to a right angle to the long axis of the bone.

trapezius muscle—one of the two muscles that form the web of the neck and are attached to the scapula laterally and to the spinous processes of the cervical and upper thoracic vertebrae and the base of the skull medially. These muscles strengthen the shoulder girdles and lift the shoulders.

trauma—the end effect of a force applied to the body, often used interchangeably with injury; a physical or psychological wound or injury.

tremor—the involuntary shaking of a body part.

triage—the technique of sorting and allocating treatment of patients during a disaster when limited resources and personnel do not allow everything possible to be done for every patient. Designed to maximize the number of survivors.

triceps muscle—the major muscle of the posterior upper arm, which extends the elbow.

tuberculosis (TB)—a chronic infectious disease caused by *Mycobacteria*, characterized by the formation of granulomas (nodular accumulations of inflammatory cells) in many organs, particularly the lungs.

turgor, skin—the degree of elasticity, resistance to deformation, and amount of moisture in the skin.

U

ulna—the medial of the two forearm bones when the palm is held facing forward.

ulnar nerve—one of the five major nerves of the upper extremity, it arises from the brachial plexus. The ulnar nerve controls most of the fine movements of the hand and supplies sensation to the little finger and medial side of the ring finger.

umbilical cord—the cord-like structure that connects the fetus with the placenta.

umbilicus—see **navel**.

unconscious—incapable of responding to sensory stimuli.

universal precautions—an approach to infection control; a consistent set of procedures and use of appropriate precautions to assist in protection from blood and body fluids of all patients.

unresponsive—unaware, incapable of responding to sensory stimuli.

upper airway obstruction—blockage of air flow through the nose, nasal cavity, mouth, pharynx, and/or epiglottis.

upper respiratory tract infection (URI)—infection of the nose, sinuses, tonsils, throat, and/or epiglottis.

uremia—a toxic condition in kidney failure caused by the accumulation in the blood of substances normally eliminated in the urine.

ureter—a muscular tube that drains urine from the kidneys into the bladder. The ureters lie behind the abdominal and pelvic cavities against the back muscle.

urethra—the tube that passes urine from the bladder out of the body. In males, the urethra passes through the penis; in females the urethra opens above the entrance to the vagina.

urinary system—the system that consists of the two kidneys; the two ureters, which drain the urine from the kidneys; the bladder, which stores urine; and the urethra, which drains urine from the body. The urinary system removes waste products of cellular metabolism from the bloodstream and excretes them in the urine.

urinary tract infection (UTI)—an infection of the bladder, prostate (in men), or a kidney.

urine—a fluid excreted by the kidneys that contains water, minerals, and waste products of cellular metabolism.

uterus—the muscular organ within which the fetus develops.

V

V—in an equation, the symbol for velocity.

vaccine—a preparation of living, attenuated, or killed organisms that is administered to produce or increase immunity to a particular disease.

vacuum splint—an airtight plastic or rubber splint filled with small plastic pellets. After being fitted to the body part, it becomes rigid after air is evacuated with a pump.

vacuum spine board—a spine board based on the same principles as the vacuum splint.

vagina—the canal in the female that connects the uterus with the external female genitalia; it receives the penis during sexual intercourse.

vagus nerves—nerves that originate in the brain and pass through the neck into the chest and abdomen. They help regulate the heart rate and digestive tract function.

vapor barrier garment—a waterproof garment worn either next to the skin or over a thin garment of polypropylene or similar material. This traps a warm film of moisture next to the skin, theoretically decreases water requirements by reducing perspiration, and maintains the insulating properties of outer garments by keeping sweat out of them.

vaporization—conversion of water or another volatile liquid into vapor.

vas deferens—one of the two ducts that conduct sperm from the testicles to the urethra.

Vaseline—a brand name for petrolatum or petroleum jelly.

Vaseline gauze—gauze saturated with petrolatum (petroleum jelly).

vasogenic shock—shock due to dilation and relaxation of blood vessel walls caused by failure of the mechanisms that normally control vessel tone.

veins—tubular vessels that carry blood from the tissues back to the heart.

vena cava, inferior—the large vein that drains blood from the lower chest, abdomen, pelvis, and lower extremities.

vena cava, superior—the large vein that drains blood from the head, neck, upper extremities, and upper chest.

venae cavae—the two large veins that carry blood to the right atrium of the heart.

venous blood—deoxygenated blood that flows back from the tissues through the veins.

ventilation—the process of moving air in and out of the lungs.

ventricle—either of the two larger chambers of the heart.

ventricular fibrillation—a sudden, rapid, irregular, worm-like twitching of the ventricular muscle.

ventricular tachycardia—a very fast heartbeat caused by an abnormal electrical focus in the ventricle; may or may not produce a detectable pulse.

vertebra—one of the 33 bones making up the spine.

vertebral arches—the portion of the vertebrae forming the tunnel that contains the spinal canal.

vertebral column—the spine.

vertigo—dizziness; a sensation of whirling.

vital signs—important indicators of body functions necessary to life: pulse, respiration, temperature, blood pressure, and level of consciousness (see also **sign** and **symptom**).

vitamins—organic substances, present in many foods in small amounts, that are necessary for the metabolic functioning of the body.

vitreous humor—a jelly-like fluid that fills the posterior compartment of the eyeball behind the lens.

void—to cast out as waste matter.

vomitus—vomited matter.

voluntary muscles—muscles that are under conscious control and can be contracted or relaxed at will.

vulva—the external female genital organs.

W

"walking wounded"—individuals involved in a mass-casualty incident whose injuries do not present a risk to life and who usually are ambulatory and can wait several hours before being transported to a hospital.

wheezes—high-pitched whistling sounds produced by exhaled air traveling through small air passages narrowed by swelling or spasm (see also **rhonchi** and **stridor**).

whiplash—a type of neck sprain suffered by an occupant of a vehicle struck by another vehicle, usually from the rear.

white matter—groups of myelin-covered axons that derive their name from their yellowish-white color.

white of the eye—the visible part of the sclera covered by the transparent conjunctiva.

willful negligence—negligence involving malicious intentions (see also **negligence** and **gross negligence**).

windburn—irritation of the skin that is caused by exposure to wind and resembles first-degree sunburn.

windchill effect—the cooling effect of wind added to low environmental temperature.

wire splint—a fixation splint made of wire mesh.

wrist drop—weakness in the wrist or fingers produced by injury of the radial nerve.

wrist joint—the joint between the radius and ulna proximally and the carpal bones distally.

X

X-rays—electromagnetic radiations of very short wavelength that can penetrate most substances and can produce an image on film.

xiphoid process—a cartilaginous process attached to the lower end of the sternum.

Y

Yankauer tip ("tonsil" tip)—a rigid, plastic pharyngeal suction tip attached to the rubber tubing of a mechanical suction device.

Z

Zepharin—the brand name of an antiseptic solution containing benzalkonium chloride.

zygoma—the cheekbone; connects the maxilla with the frontal and temporal bones.

Index

A

Abandonment   450
ABCDE mnemonic   84
   steps in caring for a patient   400
Abdomen
   surface anatomy   67
Abdominal injury   257, 487
   advanced assessment of   343
   assessment of   100, 258, 335, 398
   cavity   49
   emergency care of   260, 486
   pain   335
   caused by ski injury   384
Abduct   48, 187, 197
Above-knee femur fracture
   emergency care of   203
   signs and symptoms of   203
Abrasions   137
AC separations
   emergency care of   188
Acceleration   182
Accident scene inspection   184
Accident prevention   387
Acclimatization   11, 12
   high altitudes   11
   hot weather   23
   altitude sickness   315
Acidosis   25, 293
ACLS
   advanced cardiac life support   456
Acromioclavicular (AC) joint   383
Acrylic   15, 21
Activated charcoal   409
Activity
   muscular   13, 15, 18
   physical   15, 27
   to increase heat production   10
   to increase skin circulation   10
Acute abdomen   276
   assessment of   276
   emergency care of   278
   signs and symptoms of   276
Acute mountain sickness (AMS)   317, 491
Adaptation
   to cold weather   10, 15
   to hot weather   22, 23
Addiction   298
Adduct   48, 187
Adult basic life support   457
Advanced AMS   318
   emergency care of   319, 320
   signs and symptoms of   318
Advanced assessment   329
   in medical illness   336
   of responsive patient   329
   of unresponsive patient   329
Advanced cardiac life support (ACLS)   456, 477
AED
   see Automatic external defibrillator
Aerobic
   fitness   29
Agitation
   sign of heat stroke   316
AIDS   89, 267, 297, 509
   guidelines for prevention of   509
Air
   components of   10

Air embolism   434
   emergency care of   434
Air splints   161
Airway   39
   first consideration in injured patient   393
   opening during triage   394
   in unresponsive patient   88
Airway obstruction   90, 211-213
   in adults   91
   emergency care of   469
   in children   91
   in infants   91
   in infants and children   469
   lower   270
   in obese adults   91
   caused by a foreign body   90
   in pregnant persons   91
   recognition of   469
   relief techniques   91
   signs and symptoms of   270
   upper   270
Alcohol   18, 298
   abuse, cause of nausea   274
   advanced assessment of   340
   signs and symptoms of   298
Alcoholism   297
Alignment   157
Alkalis   409
Allergen   132
Allergic reactions   130
Alpine patrol belt   500
Altered mental status   57, 338
Altitude
   effects of   317
   emergency care kit   499
   increased risk of hypothermia   309
Altruism   356
Ambulance rendezvous   372
American Red Cross (ARC)
   advanced first aid   3
American Society for Testing and Materials
   (ASTM)   5
Amino acids
   essential   25
Amphetamines   299
AMPLE mnemonic   105
Amputations   138
Anaerobic metabolism   29
Analgesics
   signs and symptoms of   299
Anaphylactic shock   132
Anatomical positions   357
Anatomy
   human   33
   vocabulary   35
Aneurysm   216, 276
Angina pectoris   272
   emergency care of   287
   symptoms of   288
Animal bites
   emergency care of   420
   warm-blooded   420
Animals
   hazardous   414
Ankle dislocation   206, 485
   emergency care of   206
   signs and symptoms of   206
Ankle fracture
   emergency care of   204
   signs and symptoms of   204
Ankle sprain   201
   emergency care of   201
   signs and symptoms of   201

Anterior   36
Anterior cruciate ligament injury   383
Anterior dislocation   191
Antibiotics   492
Antifriction devices   386
Anxiety
   cause of constipation   275
   cause of respiratory distress   267
Appendicitis   276
Appetite
   loss at high altitude   317
Approach
   to an injured skier   389
Aquatic problems   433
   associated injury   433
Aqueous humor   217
Arachnids   410
   dangerous   415
Arsenic   407
Arteries   36
Arteriosclerosis   25, 288
Arthropods
   stings and bites   414
Artificial ventilation   399
Aspiration
   of vomitus   120
Assessment   65
   of abdomen   100
   of abdominal injury   258
   of acute mountain sickness   319
   advanced   329
   in approaching the patient   86
   of back   101
   basic   83
   of breathing   89
   of chest   99
   of chest injury   230, 249
   of chest pain   273
   of child   85
   of circulation   91
   of electrical injury   322
   examination procedures   97
   of extremities   100, 101
   of face injury   219
   first impression   84
   of gastrointestinal complaint   276
   global   86
   of head   97
   of heat illness   315
   of hypothermia   311
   of ill diabetic   294
   of musculoskeletal injury   155, 157
   of neck   99
   of neck or back injury   229
   objectives   83
   of open wound   138
   of pelvic injury   258
   of pelvis   100
   permission to provide care   85
   of poisoning   408
   of pregnant person   440
   primary survey   84
   psychology of   84
   of respiratory complaint   271
   of responsive patient   102
   of severe, generalized seizure   296
   of shock   130
   standard   397
   of stroke patient   292
   of submersed patient   428
   of suspected substance abuse   300
   systematic   84

of thermal burns   141
of throat injury   219
of trauma   83
triage   397
of unresponsive patient   87
in the wilderness   476
Asthma   267, 270
drugs for   299
ASTM
see American Society for Testing and
Materials
Asystole   289
Ataxia   318
Aura   295
Auscultation
blood pressure   76
Automatic external defibrillators (AED)   455
shockable rhythm   455
Automobile accidents   181
Avalanche   355
Avalanche injury   323
AVPU Scale   77, 96, 104, 212, 400
Avulsions   138

B

Baby
nonbreathing   445
Back
advanced assessment of   346
assessment of   229
emergency care of   231, 239
injury to   227, 360
injury classification of   227
pain   280
signs and symptoms of   229
surface anatomy of   71
Back carries   361
Backcountry skiing   9, 387
Backpack   362, 369
Backpacking
menu   27
"bad trips"
serious effect of hallucinogen use   300
Bag-valve-mask   89, 121, 399
Bandages   143, 499
commonly used   144
improvisation of   145
special types of   143
Barbiturates   299
Barotrauma   433
Basic assessment   103
Basic life support   5, 84, 455, 456, 477
algorithm   456
Basic survival requirements
wilderness patients   477
Battery   450
Battle's sign   216
Behavior
automatic, psychic symptoms   296
inappropriate, in suspected substance
abuse   298
Bending trauma   181
Bile duct colic   275
Bilirubin   276
Bindings
mechanics of   387
mountaineering   387
release of   383
research   385
step-in   383
three-pin   387

Bismuth preparations, effect on stool   275
Black widow spider   415
Bladder
injury, signs and symptoms of   257
obstruction of   278
Blanket lift and carry   366
Blanket stretcher   369
Bleeding
aneurysm   216
assessment of   93
control of   394
emergency care of   216
external   125
internal   127
management in triage   395
sign of heat stroke   316
vaginal   279
Blindness   318
from electrical injury   321
Blink reflex   217
Blisters   488
sign of frostbite   308
Blood   38
arteries   125
capillary   125
cells   38
circulatory system   33
clots   308
in the stools   275
in the urine   278
oxygen-carrying capacity   11
plasma   38
pooling   317
venous   125
vomiting of   277
Blood pressure   126, 129, 316
advanced assessment of   337
cuff   127
vital signs   75
Blood sugar, in hypothermia   310
Blood-borne pathogens
guidelines for prevention of   86, 509
BLS
see Basic life support
Body
motion   180
Body cavities   49, 50
Body heat
avoiding excess of   23
production of   13
Body survey   97
advanced assessment   341
Body temperature
regulation of   12
Body-to-body heat
for rewarming   314
Boot-top fractures   383
Bourdon gauge flowmeter   115
Bowel
disease   273
habits   273
Bowel infarction   276
Bowel problems   494
Brain   56
causes of unresponsiveness   213
control of breathing   11
contusion   216
effects of environmental injury   317
emergency care of   216
organ   14
Brain damage
in unresponsive patient   295
injury   211
Breach of duty   451

Breath-holding blackout   433
Breathing
advanced assessment of   335
assessment of   89
in injured patient   395
rate, caused by environmental
variations   309
rescue   89
Breech presentation   445
Bronchi   39
Bronchitis   269
Brown recluse spider   416
Bulb syringes   120
Burns
chemical   142
electrical   142, 321
first-degree thermal   140
rule of nines   141
second-degree thermal   140
thermal   140
third-degree thermal   140
Bursitis   54
Butterfly bandages   139
Bystanders   456

C

C-collars
see Rigid collars
Caffeine   299
California mussels   407
Calories
diet   27
Cancer
of the skin caused by sun exposure   320
Cannabis compounds   300
Cants   388
Canvas stretcher lift   366
Capillary
advanced assessment of   337
circulatory system   33, 36
Capillary refill time   72, 78
Carbohydrate
diet   27
food sources of   24
Carbon monoxide poisoning   297, 410
emergency care of   297
Cardboard splints   160
Cardiac arrest   289, 455
because of avalanche injury   323
because of electricity   321
because of hypothermia   313
Cardiogenic shock   128, 129, 289
Cardiopulmonary resuscitation
1992 national conference   6
emergency care kit   499
Cardiovascular
disease   29
fitness   29
Cascade litter   367
Cell
functions of   33
Central nervous system
depression   301
injury, signs and symptoms of   299
stimulants   301
Cerebral edema, high altitude   317
Cerebral hemispheres   56
Cerebrovascular accident (CVA)
stroke   291

Cervical collars
    see Rigid collars
Chain of survival   455
Chemical burns   142
    to the eye   218
Chest
    advanced assessment of   342
    assessment of   99, 249, 273, 355
    back injury   248
    cavity   39
    closed   246
    compressions   461
    emergency care of   250, 273
    environmental injury   312
    injury   245, 486
    integrity   11
    open   246
    pain   272
    penetrating injury   247
    signs and symptoms of   245
    surface anatomy   66
    thorax   46
Cheyne-Stokes respirations   12, 318
Child
    definition of   457
childbirth
    abnormal bleeding   446
    abnormal presentation   445
    complications of   445
    delivery care   444
    multiple births   446
    premature birth   446
    prolonged delivery   446
    twins   446
Cholesterol   25
Chondromalacia of the patella   200
Cilia   34
Circulation system   11, 33, 36
    assessment of   91, 398
    important assessment with fractures   203
    normal functions of   245
    signs of loss   157
Cirrhosis, liver disease   299
CISD
    see Critical incident stress debriefing
Clavicle   46
Clavicle fracture   189
    emergency care of   189
Climbing ropes stretcher   370
Closed chest wound   245
Closed soft-tissue injury
    contusions   138
    emergency care of   138
    strains   138
Clothing
    cold weather   19
    protecting patient   371
    protective   511
Clove hitch   515
Clumsiness, in hypothermia   309
Coastal alpine zone   19
Cocaine   299
Coffee grounds, sign of bleeding   275
Cold weather
    clothing   19
    injury   491
    upper respiratory tract infection   268
    survival kit   19
Colic   275
    emergency care of   278
    ureteral   275

Collars
    rigid   173
Collateral ligaments   199
Colles' fracture   191
Collisions, secondary   182
Color   77
Coma
    in heat stroke   316
    in high altitude cerebral edema   318
    in hypothermia   309
    signs and symptoms of   293
Comminuted
    fracture   153, 154
Common cold   268
Compress   143
Compression
    massive injury   248
    trauma   180
Concussion   215
    emergency care of   216
Conduction   13
Conductors   322
Confusion
    sign of heat exhaustion   316
    sign of high altitude cerebral edema   309
Conjunctivitis   217
Consciousness
    see Responsiveness
Constipation   275
    care of   278
Contact lens removal technique   99, 217
Contact poisons
    emergency care of   410
Contagious diseases   89
Contaminated food or water
    cause of diarrhea   275
Contrecoup injury   183
Contusions   138
Convection   14
Convulsions   295
    in heatstroke   316
    sign of high altitude cerebral
        edema   318
Cooling   310
    exposure   309
    to treat heatstroke   316
Coral snake bites   417
    emergency care of   419
    signs and symptoms of   419
Core
    body   13
    central nervous system   13
    heart   13
    liver   13
    lungs   13
Core temperature, in hypothermia   309
Cornea   217
Coronary artery disease   272, 288
    advanced assessment of   340
    risk factors of   288
    symptoms of   288
Cotton   15
Cough   245, 267
    symptom of advanced AMS   318
CPR   455
    in adults   92-94
    in children   94
    closed chest cardiopulmonary
        resuscitation   455
    complications of   472
    for electrical injury   322
    for heart attack   290
    in the wilderness   477

    indications for submersion
        hypothermia   313
    in infants   94
    management in triage   397
    one-rescuer   92
    special situations   470
    techniques of   94
    two-rescuer   93
    when to discontinue   470
"Crack" (cocaine)   299
CRAMS Scale
    significance of   398
    triage device   397
Cranial nerves   57
Cravat ankle bandage   201
Crepitus   100, 101, 154
Cricothyroidotomy
    needle   486
    surgical   486
Crime
    illegal drug use   297
Critical incident stress debriefing
    (CISD)   6
Crossed-finger technique   88, 459
Crowds
    need to control   372
Cruciate ligaments   199
Crushing injury   181
Cumulonimbus clouds   321
Curriculum
    DOT   3
    EMS   3
    WEC   3
Cutaneous system   34
    skin   60
Cyanosis   246, 338
    symptom of acute mountain sickness   319
    symptom of high altitude pulmonary
        edema   318

D

Dacron   20
Death
    advanced assessment of   347
    classifying, in triage   394
    danger of, with hypothermia   309
    determination of   347
    legal procedures   452
    from ski injury   385
    risk with high altitude cerebral
        edema   318
    tissue damage with frostbite   308
Deceleration   181
Decompression sickness   434
    "the bends"   435
    emergency care of   435
    signs and symptoms of   435
Defibrillation
    early   455
Dehydration
    emergency care of   278
Delayed examination
    management of triage   393
Delirium
    sign of heatstroke   316
Deltoids   54
Delusions, effect of hallucinogens   300
Dental injury
    see Oral-dental injury

Dependence
    physical   297
    psychological   297
Depressant
    use, signs and symptoms of   299
Depression
    medical history, advanced
        assessment   340
Dermis   60
Desert survival kit   24
Designer drug   298
Diabetes   293
    diabetes mellitus   293
    adult onset   293
    advanced assessment of   340
    assessment of   294
    comparison   294
    complications of   295
    emergency care of   294
    juvenile   293
Diabetic coma   293
Diabetic ketoacidosis   293
Diaper bandage   258
Diaphragm   39
Diarrhea   275
    advanced assessment of   335
    chronic, mild   275
    emergency care of   278
    severe   275
    symptom of heat stroke   316
Diastolic pressure   75
Diet
    bulk-poor   275
    components of   27
    daily servings   27
Difficulty breathing
    advanced assessment of   335
Difficulty in swallowing   276
Digestion   18
Digestive system   33, 40
    organs   50
Direct ground lift   234
    carry   363
    four-person   171
    multiple-person   234
Direct pressure   126, 125
Disability   400
    serious   333
Discharge
    urethral   279
    vaginal   279
Dislocations   482, 484
    ankle   206
    elbow   192
    finger   192
    hip   205
    knee   205
    patella   206
    relocation   482
    shoulder   191, 483
    wrist   192
Distal   36
Distension
    assessment of   100
Distraction trauma   182
Diverticulitis   276
Diving Accident Network (DAN)   435
Diving reflex   310
Documentation
    legal   449

DOT
    see United States Department of
        Transportation
Double-overhand knot   514
Down   15
Dressings   143, 499
    commonly used   144
    improvisation of   145
    occlusive   260
    special types of   143
Drowning   427
    dry   428
    near   427
    prevention of   431
    wet   428
Drug dependence   298
Drugs
    emergency care kit   500
Dry lime   411
Duodenum   41
Dysphagia   276
Dyspnea   245, 267
Dysuria   278

E

Ear diseases   279
Earache   268
Early defibrillation   455
Ectopic pregnancy   276
Elastic (rubberized) bandages   144
Elbow dislocation   192, 484
    emergency care of   192
Elbow joint   47
Elbow sprains   188
    emergency care of   188
Elderly
    subject to constipation   276
    subject to vertigo   279
Electrical injury
    assessment of   322
    burns   142
    causes of   321
    emergency care of   322
    prevention of   322
Elemental phosphorus   411
Elemental sodium   411
Elevation   126
Emergency cardiac care (ECC)   457
Emergency care
    of abdominal injury   260
    of above-knee femur fracture   203
    of AC separation   188
    of acute abdomen   278
    of advanced AMS   319, 320
    of air embolism   434
    of angina pectoris   287
    of ankle dislocation   206
    of ankle fracture   204
    of ankle sprain   201
    of bites with envenomation   418
    of bleeding inside the skull   216
    of brain contusion   216
    of burns   142
    of carbon monoxide poisoning   297
    of chest injury   250, 252
    of chest pain   273
    of clavicle fracture   189
    of closed soft-tissue injury   138
    of colic   278
    competency in   449
    of concussion   216
    of constipation   278

    of contact poison   410
    of coral snake bite   419
    of decompression sickness   435
    definition of   4, 449
    of dehydration   278
    of diarrhea   278
    of elbow dislocation   192
    of elbow sprain   188
    of electrical injury   322
    of exotic snake bite   419
    of eye burn   218
    of eye contusion   218
    of eye injury   217, 218
    of eye laceration   218
    of face injury   219
    of facial fracture   220
    of femoral shaft fracture   202
    of finger dislocation   192
    of finger sprain   189
    of foot fracture   205
    of forearm fracture   191
    of gastrointestinal complaint   277
    of gila monster bite   420
    of hand fracture   191
    of hand sprain   189
    of heart attack   289
    of heatstroke   316
    of hip dislocation   205
    of hip fracture   202
    of hypothermic patient   311
    of ill diabetic   294
    of indigestion   278
    of ingested poison   409
    of inhaled poison   410
    of injected poison   410
    of internal bleeding   128
    of knee dislocation   206
    of knee sprain   201
    of lower-leg fracture   204
    of marine animal bite   421
    of marine animal injury   421
    of marine animal puncture wound   422
    of marine animal sting   422
    of musculoskeletal injury   157
    of neck or back injury   231
    of open soft-tissue injury   139
    of open wound   138
    of oral-dental injury   220
    of patella dislocation   206
    of pelvic fracture   202
    of pelvic injury   260
    of pit viper bite   418
    of plant poisoning   414
    of poisoning   408
    of respiratory complaint   271
    of scalp laceration   215
    of scapula fracture   189
    of severe, generalized seizure   296
    of shock   130
    of shoulder dislocation   192
    of shoulder sprain   188
    of skull fracture   216
    of stroke patient   292
    of submersed patient   428
    of substance abuse patient   301
    of thermal burn   141
    of throat injury   221
    of unresponsive patient   213
    of upper arm fracture   189

of vomiting   278
warm-blooded animal bite   420
in wilderness   476
of wrist dislocation   192
of wrist fracture   191
of wrist sprain   188
Emergency care cabinet
patrol first aid room   501
Emergency care equipment
ski patrol   500
Emergency care kit
basic contents   497
for extended trips into remote
country   499
for high altitude   499
for snake country   499
for undeveloped countries   499
master kit contents   497
minimum contents for nordic patrol   500
multi-day trip   497
optional items for women   499
options with special licensing   498
options with special training   498
physician/paramedic   500
recreational   497
wilderness search and rescue   499
Emergency care provider
legal   450
Emergency childbirth   439
delivery signs   440
Emergency medical services (EMS)   3
dispatch information   463
EMS system   379
Emergency medical technician (EMT)   4
Emergency move   356, 360
Emotions of patients   398
Emphysema   267, 269
oxygen flow rate for   115
subcutaneous   249
EMS
see Emergency medical services
EMT
see Emergency medical technician
Endotracheal tube   399
Energy
cell   34
kinetic   180
potential   180
Envenomation
bites, emergency care of   418
Environmental emergencies
adapting to the outdoors   9
frostbite   308
heat cramps   316
heat exhaustion   316
heat illness   314
heat syncope   317
hypothermia   309
injury   428
Enzymes
cell   34
Epidermis   60
Epiglottis
infection of   268
Epilepsy   295
advanced assessment of   340
frequency of   295
medication for   295
Epinephrine   132
Esophagus   38
cause of vomiting blood   274

Evacuation
environmental emergency concerns   309
Evaporation   14
Examination
assessment procedure   97
Exposure   309
External bleeding   125
External rotation   197
Extremities
assessment of   100, 101
lower   100
upper   101
Extremity lift   365
Extrication
collars, see Rigid collars
difficult positions   236
equipment   356
principles of   355, 357
Eye injury
anatomy and physiology   217
changes with head injury   218
emergency care of   217, 218
evaluation technique   217
foreign bodies   217
laceration   218
retinal hemorrhage   319
Eyelids   215, 217

F

Face injury   219
assessment of   219
emergency care of   219
Face shield   511
Facial fracture, emergency care of   220
Fainting   131
similarity to heat syncope   317
Fallopian tube
infection of   276
Family members
interview of   338
Fat
diet   27
food source   25
Fatigue   387
factor in ski injury   204, 387
Feel, in advanced assessment   340
Female genitalia
injury to   258
Femoral shaft fracture   202
emergency care of   202
signs and symptoms of   202
Fern leaf burn
characteristic of lightning injury   322
Fever
advanced assessment of   340
Fibers
motor   58
sensory   58
Fibula   48, 197
Figure-of-eight
follow-through knot   514
Figure-of-eight bandage   145, 147
for ankle sprains   201
Finger dislocation
emergency care of   192, 484
Finger sprains   188
emergency care of   189
Fireman's carry   361
Fireman's drag   360
First aid
definition of   4
room   501

First impression   86
advanced assessment of   332
assessment of   84
in triage   399
Fishhook removal   489
Fitness program   30
Flail chest   246
Flashbacks   300
Flowmeters, for oxygen   114
Flying insects   410
Foam   16
Food   27
nutrition   24
poisoning   422
Foot fracture
emergency care of   205
signs and symptoms of   204
Force   180
necessary to cause fracture   383
Fore-and-aft carry   363
Forearm fracture   191
emergency care of   191
Foreign bodies
in the eye   217
Foreign-body airway obstruction   465
Foreskin of the penis
injury to   258
Forms   503
Flow Sheet for Seriously Injured
Patient   506
Incident Report   505
Refusal of Care   504
Site of Trauma Figure   507
Fracture   481
above-knee femur   203
ankle   204
clavicle   189
closed   153
comminuted   154
displaced   154
femoral shaft   202
foot   204
forearm   191
general principles of   153
greenstick   154
hand   191
hip   202
lower leg   204
non-displaced   154
open   153, 158
pelvic   201
rib   246
scapula   189
signs and symptoms of   154
simple   154
spiral   154
stress   154, 204
subtrochanteric   203
supracondylar   203
transverse   154
upper arm   189
wrist   191
Front cradle   361
Frostbite   308
categories of   308
deep   308
first-degree   308
fourth-degree   308
second-degree   308
superficial   308
thawed   308
third-degree   308
Fulcrum point   183

G

Gallbladder   40, 41
  inflammation of   276
Gallstone
  cause of jaundice   276
Gamekeeper's thumb
  see Skier's thumb
Ganglia   59
Gangrene
  complication of frostbite   308
Garments
  insulating   15
  materials   15
Gastric distention
  complications of   472
Gastrointestinal complaint
  acute abdomen   276
  assessment of   276
  blood in the stools   275
  cause of vomiting   274, 335
  colic   275
  constipation   275
  diarrhea   275
  difficulty in swallowing   276
  emergency care of   277
  indigestion   274
  nausea and vomiting   274
Gatorade   316
Genitalia
  female   258
  injury to   258
  male   258
  signs and symptoms of   258
Genitourinary complaints
  abnormal menstrual flow   279
  blood in the urine   278
  inability to urinate   279
  incontinence   278
  injury   257
  painful urination   278
  urethral discharge   279
  vaginal discharge   279
  vertigo   279
Giardia lamblia   28, 275, 335, 494
Gila monster
  bite   419
  emergency care for bite   420
Girth hitch   515
Glasgow Coma Scale   77, 212, 400
Gloves   511
  disposable   511
  rubber (latex)   510
Glucose   293, 294
  carbohydrates   25
Gluteus muscles   54
Glycogen   34
Goggles   321, 388, 511
Golden hour   398
Good Samaritan Law
  coverage   452
Gore-Tex   18
Grand mal seizure   295
Great vessels
  injury to   249
Greenstick fracture   154
Ground currents   322
Gurney   366, 367, 369

H

Hallucinogens   300
Hamstring tendons   201
Hand fracture   191
  emergency care of   191
Hand sprain   188
  emergency care of   189
Handwashing   511
Hard hats   356, 388
Hay fever   268
Hazards
  to patients and rescuers   331
  in difficult extrications   356
Head
  advanced assessment of   341
  assessment of   97
  surface anatomy of   65
Head downhill
  positioning guidelines   390
Head injury   486
  causes of unresponsiveness   213
  secondary injury   211
Head splint technique   6
Head tilt/chin-lift technique   88, 458
Head uphill
  positioning guidelines   390
Headache   280
  advanced assessment of   334, 340
  benign, causes of   280
  cause of nausea   274
  medication for   280
  migraine   280
Headband, for securing dressing   147
Heart
  atriums   36
  blood circulation   37
  circulatory system   36
  valves   37
Heart attack   288
  complications of   289
  emergency care of   289
  signs and symptoms of   288, 289
Heart disease
  arteriosclerosis   288
  coronary artery disease   288
Heart rate
  in stimulant users   300
  with angina   287
Heartburn   274
Heat
  minimize gain   23
  physical mechanisms   13
Heat cramps   316
Heat exhaustion   316
Heat gain
  hot weather   23
Heat illness
  assessment of   315
  environmental emergency   314
  heat cramps   316
  heat exhaustion   315
  heat stroke   315
  heat syncope   315
Heat loss
  body   14
Heat production
  basal   13
Heat stroke   315
  classic   315
  emergency care of   316
  exertional   315
  signs and symptoms of   315

Heat syncope   317
Heatpac   312
Heimlich maneuver   40, 456, 465
  for airway obstruction   90
  modifications of   467
  in obese patient   467
  in pregnant patient   467
  self-administered   467
Helicopter rendezvous   372
Helmets   233
Hematoma
  subungual   488
Hematuria   278
Hemiplegia   227
Hemoptysis   245
Hemorrhage   125
  assessment of   93
  classes of   128
  emergency care of   93
Hemothorax   246, 249, 267
Hepatitis   89
  cause of jaundice   276
  danger in intravenous drug use   297
  guidelines for prevention of   509
Hepatitis B vaccine   511
Heroin   299
High alpine zone   20
High altitude cerebral edema (HACE)   317
  signs and symptoms of   318
High altitude illness   267
High altitude pulmonary edema (HAPE)   317
  signs and symptoms of   318
High blood pressure
  advanced assessment of   340
  cause of headache   280
Hip dislocation   205, 484
  emergency care of   205
  signs and symptoms of   205
Hip fracture   202
  emergency care of   202
  signs and symptoms of   202
Hollofil II   16
Homan's sign   270
Home delivery
  childbirth   442
  equipment   441
Homeotherms   12
Horse collar   172
Hot tubs, to treat hypothermia   311
Hot weather
  acclimatization   22
Human bites   420
Human crutch   361
Human immunodeficiency virus (HIV)   509
Humerus   46
Humidifying device, for oxygen   116
Hydration
  in hot weather   22
Hydraulic sarong   311
Hyperextension   182, 187
Hyperflexion   181
Hyperpnea   245
Hyperthermic temperature   74
Hyperventilation   11, 271
  in altitude sickness   318
Hypervitaminosis   26
Hypoglycemia   293
  signs and symptoms of   293

Hypothermia 309, 427
    assessment of 311
    CPR 313
    emergency care of 311
    emergency care kit 500
    field 310
    immersion 310
    mild 312
    profound 312
    severity 310
    submersion 310, 313
    types of 309
    urban 310
Hypothermic temperature 74
Hypovolemic shock 129
    in spinal cord injured patients 230
Hypoxia 12, 116, 394
Hysterical patient 397

I

Ice rescue 432
Igloos, danger of carbon monoxide
    poisoning 297
Iliopsoas muscles 53
Immobilization 126
    spine devices 160, 169
Immunization 511
    routine 476
Impaled object 138
Impedance, removing from the patient 356
Implied consent 451
Incident command system 355
Incident investigation protocols 449
Incident report 505
Incisions 137
Incontinence
    genitourinary complaint 278
Indigestion 274
    care of 278
Industrial gases 410
Infarct 270
Infection
    causes of unresponsiveness 213
    symptoms of 334
Inferior 36, 191
Inferior dislocation 191
Influenza 268
Ingested poisons
    emergency care of 409
Inhaled poisons
    emergency care of 410
Injected poisons
    emergency care of 410
Injured skier
    approach to 389
Injuries
    abdominal 257
    back of the chest 248
    bladder 257
    closed 257
    genitalia 258
    great vessels 249
    kidney 257
    massive compression 248
    mechanism of 180
    multiple, serious 185
    open 257
    penetrating 247

Insects
    dangerous 414
    symptoms of stings or bites 414
Insulators 322
Insulin 293
Insulin-dependent diabetes mellitus
    (IDDM) 293
Intercostal muscles 53
Internal bleeding 127
    emergency care of 128
    examples of 127
    signs and symptoms of 127
Internal injury 183
Interview
    of witnesses 338
    of family members 338
Intestinal obstruction 276
Intoxication 293, 298
Intracranial pressure (ICP) 211
Intravenous drugs 288
Intravenous fluids
    for profound hypothermia 313
Iris 217
Iron
    effects on stool 275

J

Jakes litter 367
Jams-and-pretzels extrication 6
Jaundice 276, 298
    gastrointestinal complaints 276
Jaw fracture 220
Jaw-thrust technique 88, 231, 233, 395, 459
Jewelry removal 489
Joints
    ankle 49
    ball and socket 44
    carpometacarpal 47
    hinge 43
    immovable 43
    metacarpophalangeal 59
    movable 43
    slightly movable 43
Juvenile diabetes

K

Kendrick extrication device (KED) 173, 367
Kendrick traction device 167
Ketoacidosis, diabetic 293
Kidney
    infection of 276
    injury to 257
    signs and symptoms of 257
Kinetic energy 180
Knee
    anatomy and physiology of 198
    dislocation 205, 485
    emergency care of 201, 206
    injury, signs and symptoms of 200, 206
    sprain 198, 383
Knots 513

L

Labile
    juvenile diabetes 293
Labor 440
Lacerations 137
Ladder splints 160
Laerdal suction device 119
Laryngitis
    larynx infection 268

Larynx 39, 219
Lateral 36
Law of conservation of energy 179
Laws of motion 180
Layering 16, 20
    first layer 20
    fourth layer 21
    hot weather 22
    other considerations 22
    principles of 15
    rain gear 22
    second layer 20
    system 19
    third layer 21
    vapor barrier garments 22
Leader
    in rescue and in lifting 358
Leg cramps 490
Legal aspects 449
Legal principle
    "choice of evils" 451
Legs
    elevation of, to treat shock 395
Lens of the eye 217
Level of responsiveness 57, 76, 297, 299
    advanced assessment of 338
Level of training 450
Life-threatening disturbances 329
Lifting
    carries 360
    patient 358
    proper procedures 360
    straps 359
Ligaments
    damaged 198
    knee joint 199
    medial and lateral 199
    skeletal system 43
Lightheadedness 279
Lightning injury
    causes 321
Listen, in advanced assessment 340
Litters and stretchers 366, 499
    adjustable, wheeled cot-stretchers 369
    improvised 369
    rigid and semirigid 367
Liver 40
    cause of jaundice 276
    deterioration 298
Logroll 231, 234
    four-person 171
Long-axis drag 362
Look, in advanced assessment 340
Lower extremity 48
    advanced assessment of 344
    injury to 197
    nerves 59
    surface anatomy of 69
Lower respiratory infection
    advanced assessment of 335
    symptoms of 335
    tract infections 268
Lower-leg fracture 204
    emergency care of 204
    signs and symptoms of 204
Lung 267
    advanced assessment of 340
    cancer 267
    compression of 267
    consolidation of 269
    function of 11
Lye 409, 411

M

Macula 319
Male genitalia 258
Malignant disease 270
Malleable metal splints 160
Malleolus
    lateral 49
    medial 48
Mammalian diving reflex 427
Mandible (jawbone) 89
Marijuana
    cannabis compound 300
Marine animal 410
    bites, emergency care of 421
    injury, emergency care of 421
    injury, prevention of 421
    puncture wounds, emergency care of 422
    stings, emergency care of 422
MCI
    see Multiple-casualty incident
Mechanism of injury 5
    anticipating complications of 179
    fractures 154
    inspection of 184
    mental reconstruction of 184
    neck and back injury 228
    predicting from observation 179
Median 36
Mediastinum 39, 49
Medical
    advanced assessment 336
    assessment 267
    common complaints 267
    definitive care 4
    emergencies 287
    history, elements of 105
    illness 288
    secondary survey 336
    kit, physician/paramedic 501
Medical-alert tag 293
Medications 498
Meningitis
    cause of headache 280
Menisci 199
Menstrual flow 61, 279
Mental function
    assess in triage 395
Mesenteric adenitis 276
Metabolic abnormalities
    cause of unresponsiveness 213
Metabolism 18, 34
Metacarpophalangeal joint 384
Midline 36
Migraine headache 280
Minerals
    food sources 26
Miscarriage 279
Modified hinge joint 198
Mono-skier 389
Motion sickness
    cause of nausea 274
Motor
    assessment of 398
    fitness 29
Mouth shield 118
    disposable 511
Mouth-to-mouth technique 89
Mouth-to-nose technique 91, 461

Move
    ability to 79
    multiple rescuers 363
Moving joints
    bandaging techniques 145
Multiple injuries 238, 486
    from trauma 185
Multiple-casualty incident (MCI) 394
Muscle fibers
    fast twitch 29
    slow twitch 29
Muscle tension headaches 280
Muscular system 34
    cardiac 51
    skeletal 51
Musculoskeletal injury
    assessment of 155, 157
    emergency care of 157, 158
Myocardial
    contusion 249
    infarction 272, 288

N

Narcotics
    use, signs and symptoms of 299
Nasal cannula 115
Nasal cavity
    respiratory system 38
NASAR
    see National Association of Search and Rescue
Nasopharynx 38
National Association of Search and Rescue (NASAR) 6
National Research Council 3
NATO position 390
Nausea and vomiting 274
    advanced assessment of 335
    in altitude sickness 319
    in high altitude cerebral edema 318
Navel, pain 275
Neck
    advanced assessment of 335, 342
    assessment of 99
    surface anatomy of 66
Neck injury 227
    assessment of 229
    classification of 227
    emergency care of 231, 239
    signs and symptoms of 229
Needle cricothyroidotomy 486
Needle thoracotomy 487
Negligence
    gross, willful 451
Nerve supply
    monitor with fractures 203
    signs of loss 158
Nervous stomach
    cause of chest pain 273
    cause of nausea 274
Nervous system 33
    autonomic 59
    brain 55
    central 55
    nerves 55
    neurons 55
    parasympathetic 59
    peripheral 55, 58
    spinal cord 55
Neurogenic shock 130, 229, 230
Neurosurgical emergency 80, 336

Nicotine 18, 300
Nitroglycerin 287
Non-insulin-dependent diabetes mellitus (NIDDM) 293
Non-narcotic central nervous system depressants
    use, signs and symptoms of 299
Non-rebreather reservoir mask 115
Non-supine position 231
Nonbarbiturates 299
Nonemergency move 356, 360
Nonrotational fall 384
Nonsalvageable patients
    in triage 394
Nonurban
    illnesses and injuries 5
Nordic 390
    types of ski injury 387
    emergency care kit 500
Normothermic
    temperature 74
Nose injury 219
Nosebleed
    emergency care of 219
Nutrients
    carbohydrates 24
    fats 24
    food 24
    proteins 24
    vitamins 24
    water 24

O

Obstacles, to patient access 356
Obstructed airway
    emergency care sequence 467
Occlusive dressing 143, 260
Ohmeda suction device 119
One-rescuer adult CPR 463
One-rescuer techniques 360
Open soft-tissue injury
    abrasions 137
    amputations 138
    avulsions 138
    emergency care of 139
    lacerations 137
    punctures 138
Open wounds 481
    assessment of 138
    emergency care of 138
Oral (oropharyngeal) airways 119
Oral-dental injury 220
    emergency care of 220
Oregon spine splint II 173, 367
Organ
    damage 473
Organ systems
    function of 33
    hollow 50, 257
    primary 33
    secondary 33
    solid 50, 257
    supportive 33
Orlon 15
Oropharyngeal airway 89
Outlet valves, for oxygen cylinders 115
Ovary infection 276

Oversnow rescue
  equipment 390
  techniques 390
Oxygen 10, 35, 113, 402
  administration of 118
  in environmental injury 312
  to head-injured patient 212
  to injured patient 399
  debt 35
  indications for use 116
  inhaled air content 113
  lack of 57
  lung extract content 113
  medical 10
  precautions 117
  procedures for giving 116
  supply 11
  zone 320
Oxygen equipment 114
  content of cylinders, estimating 114
  flowmeter 114
  guidelines on assembly 114
  pressure gauge 114
  pressure-reducing valve 114

P

Pack frames stretcher 370
Packaging patient 355
Pain 158
  advanced assessment of 334
  in chest 272
  in lower back 280
  reaction to 79
  in respiratory tract 268
Palpation
  blood pressure 76
Pancreas 40
Pancreatitis 276
Paralysis 318, 321
Paramedic emergency care kit
  for wilderness search and rescue 500
Paraplegia 227
Paravertebral muscles 53
Parka stretcher 369
Patella dislocation 206, 485
  emergency care of 206
  signs and symptoms of 206
Patient
  positioning in toboggan 390
  in triage 398
  with an illness 334
  with multiple injuries 398
Patient care
  extended in the wilderness 477
Patrol belt
  minimum contents for alpine 500
Patrol first aid room 501
Pectoralis muscles 53
Pediatric basic life support 457, 468
Pelvis
  advanced assessment of 343
  assessment of 100, 258
  cavity 48, 50
  fracture 201
  injury 257, 486
  injury, emergency care of 202, 260
  signs and symptoms of 202
  surface anatomy of 67

Penetrating injury 247
  trauma 180
Penis 62
  amputation of 258
Peptic ulcer
  advanced assessment of 340
  rupture of 276
Pepto-Bismol
  effect on stools 275
Pericardial tamponade 249
Periodic breathing
  see Cheyne-Stokes respirations
Peritoneal dialysis, to treat hypothermia 312
Peritoneum 50
Peritonitis 257
  signs and symptoms of 258, 276
Phalanges 47
Pharynx 38
PHTLS
  see Prehospital trauma life support
Physical conditioning fitness 29
Physical dependence 298
Physician emergency care kit
  for wilderness search and rescue 500
Physiology 33
Pit viper 416
  bites 417
  emergency care of 418
  signs and symptoms of 418
Placenta 440
Pleural effusion 267
Pleurisy 269
Pneumatic antishock garment (PASG) 161,
  202, 260, 313, 399
Pneumatic counterpressure device 126, 127
Pneumonia 268
Pneumothorax 246, 248, 267
  tension 248
Pocket mask 89, 399
  disposable 511
  with an oxygen inlet 118
Poikilotherms 13
Poison control center 408, 409, 411
Poison ivy 410
Poisoning
  assessment of 408
  by plants 414
  emergency care of 408
  food 422
  signs and symptoms of 408
Poisonous plants
  common reactions 414
  emergency care of 414
Poisons 407
  contact with 410
  identification of 408
  ingested 409
  inhaled 410
  injected 410
Poly-drug abuse 298
Polyester 15
Polyprophylene 19
Positioning
  anatomical positions 357
  guidelines 390
  position of function 188
Posterior 36
Posterior dislocation 191
  hip 205
Potential energy 180
Powder cords 388
Pregnancy 61
  assessment of 440
  ectopic 279
  toxemia 446

Prehospital Trauma Life Support (PHTLS) 5
Premature labor 279
Prescription drugs
  use of 491
Pressure
  dressings 143
  gauge, for oxygen 114
  on a major artery 126
  pressure points 125
Primary survey 87
  advanced assessment of 332, 339
  assessment of 84, 360
  of responsive patient 333
  of unresponsive patient 86
Problem surfaces
  special bandaging techniques for 145
Prolapsed cord 445
Prone 87, 231
Protein
  diet 27
  food sources of 25
Proximal 36
Prusik knot 515
Psychogenic shock 131
Psychology
  dealing with the ill or injured 84
Psychosomatic illness
  cause of nausea 274
Pulmonary edema 269, 289
  high altitude 317
Pulmonary embolism 267, 270
Pulse 97
  advanced assessment of 337
  changes in 73
  in environmental injury 309
  in triage 395
  irregular 73
  normal 73
  strong, fast 73
  strong, slow 73
  vital sign 72
  weak, fast 73
  weak, slow 73
Pump
  bilge, for rewarming patients 311
Puncture wounds 138
  marine animals 422
Pupils
  in hypothermia 309
  reaction of 79
  state of 212, 211, 212

Q

Quadriceps femoris 199
Quadriplegia 227
Quallofil 16
Quick splints 160

R

Rabies 420
  prevention of 420
Raccoon eyes 216
Radiation 14
  infrared 17
Radio
  maintain contact 372
Rappeling
  for patient access 356
Reactions
  slowed in hypothermia 309

Red cell sludging   308
Refreezing
    protecting against   308
Refusal of care   85
    form   504
Regulator
    for oxygen cylinder   114
Reproductive system   34, 61
Rescue
    in difficult position   371
    oversnow techniques   390
    overview of process   356
    in remote location   371
Rescue breathing   89, 459
Respiration   14
    advanced assessment of   337
    agonal   338
    assessment of   398
    vital sign   73
    in triage classification   395
    ineffective   338
Respiratory complaint   267, 294
    assessment of   271
    emergency care of   271
Respiratory distress   267, 393
    causes of   268
    chest injury   245
    illnesses   267
Respiratory infections
    medical cause of   268
Respiratory rate
    decreased   338
    increased   337
Respiratory system   33
    lower airway   38
    normal functions   245
    upper airway   38
    system support   113
Responsibility
    order of   356
Responsive patient   57, 101, 329
    advanced assessment of   329
    assessment of   102
    patient   465
    patient lying down   466
    patient standing or sitting   466
    primary survey of   333
    secondary survey of   104
Responsiveness
    altered   80
    assessment of   457
    level of   76
Resuscitation
    of baby   443
Retina   217
Rewarming methods   311
Rhonchi   268
Rib
    chest injury   246
    chest wall   39
    fracture   246
Rigid collar   6, 173, 233
Rigor mortis   309
Risks
    in difficult extrications   356
Roller bandage   139
Rotational   384
    externally   187
    fall   384
    trauma   182
Route, safest   356
Rule of nines   141

S

Safety straps   383
Sager splint   168, 372
Salicylates   315
Salivary glands   40
SAM splint   174
SAR
    see Search and rescue
Sawyer extractor   410
Scalp lacerations   215
    emergency care of   215
Scapula   46
Scapula fracture   189
    emergency care of   189
Scenario
    #1   106
    #2   107
    #3   108
    #4   109
    #5   110
    #6   133
    #7   149
    #8   175
    #9   193
    #10   207
    #11   222
    #12   240
    #13   253
    #14   262
    #15   282
    #16   283
    #17   303
    #18   324
    #19   348
    #20   350
    #21   373
    #22   375
    #23   377
    #24   401
    #25   402
    #26   424
    #27   436
Scene survey   86
Sclera   217
Scoop stretcher   170
Scorpion sting
    emergency care of   416
Scuba diving
    ascent problems   434
    bottom problems   434
    descent problems   433
    injury   433
Sea snake bite   422
Search and rescue (SAR)   355
Seated carries   362
Secondary collision   182
Secondary survey   65, 371
    advanced assessment of   332, 336
    of responsive patient   104
    of unresponsive patient   96, 97
Seizure
    assessment of   296
    cause of unresponsiveness   213
    disorders   295
    emergency care of   296
    sign of heatstroke   316
Self-adhering roller bandages   144
Self-splinting
    of injured upper extremity   187
Semiprone (coma or NATO) position   87,
    120, 231
    positioning guidelines   390
    unresponsive patient   213

Separation, of acromioclavicular joint   188
Sequencing of care
    for multiple-injury patient   398
Shell
    extremities   13
    muscles   13
    skin   13
Shelter
    emergency   19
Shivering
    in hypothermia   308
Shock   128, 488
    anaphylactic   132
    assessment of   130
    cardiogenic   128, 288, 289
    cause of unresponsiveness   213
    complication of substance abuse   302
    early   337
    electric   290
    emergency care of   130
    hypoglycemia   293
    hypovolemic   128
    insulin   293
    irreversible   128
    psychogenic   131
    reversible   128
    signs and symptoms of   130
    special types of   131
    treatment, in triage   394
    vascular   238
    vasogenic   128
Short spine board   356
Shortness of breath   267
Shoulder dislocation   191, 483
    emergency care of   192
Shoulder sprains   188
    emergency care of   188
Signs and symptoms
    of above-knee femur fracture   203
    of advanced AMS   318
    of airway obstruction   270
    of alcohol use   298
    of ankle dislocation   206
    of ankle fracture   204
    of ankle sprain   201
    of bladder injury   257
    of coral snake bite   419
    of decompression sickness   435
    of diabetic coma   293
    of foot fracture   204
    of fracture   154
    of femoral shaft fracture   202
    of genitalia injury   258
    of HACE   319
    of HAPE   319
    of heart attack   288, 289
    of hip dislocation   205
    of hip fracture   202
    of hypoglycemia   293
    of internal bleeding   127
    of kidney injury   257
    of knee dislocation   206
    of knee sprain   200
    of lower-leg fracture   204
    of narcotics use   299
    of neck and back injury   229
    of patella dislocation   206
    of pelvic fracture   202
    of peritonitis   258
    of pit viper bite   418

of poisoning 408
of shock 130
sign, definition 72
of spinal cord injury 229
of spine injury 229
of sprain 155
of stroke 291
symptom, definition 72
Silver fork deformity 191
Single-ski technique
traction 168
Site of Trauma Figure 507
SKED
vest-type device 173
stretcher 356
Skeletal system 34
bones 43
ligaments 43
Ski accidents, types 384
Ski bindings
alpine 383
mono-ski 389
see Bindings
Ski brakes 383, 386
Ski injury
knee sprain 383
likelihood of injury 385
rate of 383
relative frequency of 383
soft-tissue 383
Ski mountaineers 390
Ski patrol
emergency care equipment 500
Ski pole
injury from 384
length 388
use in improvised emergency care
equipment 391
Skier's Responsibility Code 388
Skier's thumb 188
gamekeeper's thumb 384
Skiing
body characteristics 384
equipment 384
Skin
blue 78
cracks 490
pale, dry, cool 78
pale, moist, cool 78
perfusion 337
red, dry, warm 78
red, moist 78
temperature 77
types of 320
wrinkling 320
yellow 78
Skull fracture 44
emergency care of 216
Sleeping bag 366
Sling and swathe 161
for upper extremity injury 188
Slings 369
Smell, in advanced assessment 341
Snake bites 410, 411
emergency care of 419
poisonous 416
prevention of 419
Snow caves
danger of carbon monoxide
poisoning 297

Snowblindness 321
Snowboarding 388
types of ski injuries 388
Soft-tissue injury 383
general principles of 137
Solar radiation 317
Solar stills
water source 28
Sore throat 268
Spanish windlass
traction 165
Speech
assessment of 398
SPF
see Sun protection factor
Spiders
black widow 415
brown recluse 415
Spinal cord 58, 228
cervical 237
high thoracic 237
injury, signs and symptoms of 229
injury to 228
Spinal plane
anatomical position 357
Spine 44, 228
immobilization devices 160, 169
injury to 486
signs and symptoms of 229, 48
Spine board
application technique 171
dimensions 170
immobilization technique 236
short 172
vest-type 172
Spiral fracture 154
Splinter removal 491
Splinting
general principles of 160
purposes of 157
Splints 157, 355, 499
air 161
cardboard 160
fixation 160
improvised 161
improvised traction 168
ladder 160
malleable metal 160
quick 160
rigid fixation 160
soft fixation 161
Sager 168
Thomas 164
traction 160, 163
vacuum 161
wire 160
Sprains 155, 485
AC separation 188
ankle 201
elbow 188
finger 188
hand 188
knee 198
shoulder 188
signs and symptoms of 155
wrist 188
Sputum 269
in high altitude pulmonary edema 318
Square knot 514
Stabilizing dressings 143
START technique 394
Steristrips 139
Sternomastoid muscles 53
Sternum 39, 46

Stiff neck
advanced assessment of 340
Stimulants
signs and symptoms of 299
Stokes litter 366
Stoma 461
Stomach
problems 494
Stools
blood in 275
Straddle injury 258
Strains 138
Streptococcus 268
Stress 270, 272, 274, 275
management of 346
Stress fracture 154
Stretcher-to-bed transfer 366
Stridor 268
Stroke
assessment of 292
causes of unresponsiveness 213
cerebrovascular accident 291
emergency care of 292
signs and symptoms of 291
Stupor
sign of heat stroke 316
sign of high altitude cerebral edema 318
Subcutaneous emphysema 99, 221, 246, 249
Submersed patient 427
assessment of 428
drowning 427
emergency care of 428
Substance abuse 297
assessment of patient suspected of 300
emergency care of 301
Substernal pain 273
Subtrochanteric fracture 203
Subungual hematoma 488
Sucking chest wound 247
Suction devices 119
Sudden death 288
Suicide 297, 300
Sun protection factor (SPF) 320
Sunburn 320
Sunscreen, application of 320
Superior 36
Supine position 87, 231, 233
Supracondylar fracture 203
Surface anatomy
abdomen 67
back 71
chest 66
head 65
lower extremity 69
neck 66
pelvis 67
upper extremity 70
Surgical cricothyroidotomy 486
Survey
body 97
Survival
basic 9
cold weather 9
cold-weather kit 19
desert kit 24
emergency equipment 19
rate 477
requirements 10
triage scan 397
Swallowing, difficulty of 276
Swimmer's ear 433
Symptoms 72
Systolic pressure 75

T

Tachypnea 245
Tactel 18
Tapering cylinders
    bandaging techniques 146
Tear ducts 217
Tear glands 217
Tearing
    symptom of snowblindness 321
Technical rescue equipment 371
Tooth injury 219
Telemark skiing 387
Temperature
    advanced assessment of 338
    body 308
    heat production 15
    involuntary 14
    stabilization of 15
    vital sign 74
    voluntary 14
Temporalis muscles 53
Tension pneumothorax 248
Terminal velocity 179
Terrain 356
Testicle 61
    contusion of 258
Tetanus 138
Thermal burn 140
    assessment of 141
    classification of 141
    emergency care of 141
    to the eye 218
Thermal conductivity
    hot weather 23
Thermax 16
Thermolite 16
Thermoloft 16
Thermometer
    low reading 308
Thinsulate 16
Thintech 18
Thirst
    symptom of heat exhaustion 316
Thomas splint 164
Thoracotomy
    needle 487
Thorax
    chest 46
Threat to life
    advanced assessment of 333
Threat to limb
    advanced assessment of 333
Throat injury 219, 221
    assessment of 219
    emergency care of 221
Thunderheads 321
TIA (transient ischemic attack) 291
Tibia 48, 198, 199
Tibial tubercle 199
Ticks 416
Tobacco 300
Toboggan 356
    commercially-made backcountry 391
    improvised backcountry 391
    pack 501
    positioning the patient 390
Tonsil tip 120
Touch, reaction to 79
Tourniquet 126
    application of 125, 126

Toxemia 446
Trachea
    deviation of 246
Traction 163
    single-ski technique 168
    splinting 202
    two-ski-pole technique 169
Traction splints 163
Transient ischemic attack (TIA) 291
    advanced assessment of 340
Transportation 355
    in triage 394
    to definitive care 356
Transverse
    fracture 154
Trapezius muscles 53
Trauma 180
    deaths from 267
    types of 180
Triage 393
    algorithm 396
    assessment of 397
    technique 394
Triage categories
    black 394
    green 394
    red 394
    yellow 393
Triangular bandages 144
Triceps 54
Tumor
    cause of blood in urine 278
    cause of colic 275
    cause of jaundice 276
    of the brain 279
    of the stomach 274
Two half-hitch knots 515
Two-rescuer adult CPR 464
Two-rescuer moves 362
Two-ski-pole technique
    traction 169

U

Ulcer
    cause of indigestion 274
    cause of vomiting blood 274
Ulna 47
Ultraviolet light 320
Umbilical cord 441
Unconsciousness
    general care of 215
    treatment for 294
    see Unresponsiveness
United States Department of Transportation (DOT) 3
Universal precautions 5, 86, 125, 139, 215, 260
    AIDS 459
    blood and body fluid 510
    hepatitis B 459
    recommendations 510
    regulations 511
Unresponsive patient 57, 156, 237, 329, 465
    airway of 88
    assessment of 5, 87, 212
    causes of 213
    general care of 213
    in triage 399
    not requiring rescue breathing 95
    secondary survey of 97
    serious hemorrhage in 95

Upper arm fracture
    emergency care of 189
Upper extremity 46
    advanced assessment of 345
    nerves 59
    surface anatomy of 70
Upper respiratory infection
    advanced assessment of 334
    symptoms 334
Upper respiratory tract infection
    URI 268
Upper-airway obstruction 465
Upper-extremity injury
    occurring outdoors 187
Urethral discharge 279
Urinary system 33
    bladder 41
    kidneys 41
    problems 495
    ureter 41
    urethra 41
Urinary tract infection (UTI) 278
    symptoms of 335
Urinate
    allow before long transport 372
    inability to 279
    painful 278
Uterus 61

V

Vacuum splints 161
Valve, pressure reducing, for oxygen 114
Vapex 18
Vascular headache 280
Vaseline gauze 143
Vasogenic shock 129
Vehicle
    extrication from 355
    positioning a vehicle in 365
Veins
    circulatory system 36
Ventricular fibrillation 289, 309, 455
Ventricular tachycardia 289, 455
Vertigo 279
    symptom of high altitude cerebral edema 279
Viral infection 268, 274, 275
Vital signs 6, 65, 71, 313, 316, 319, 322
    blood pressure 75
    pulse 72
    respiration 73
    temperature 74
Vitamin-mineral supplements
    effect on stools 275
    food sources 26
Vitreous humor 217
Vocabulary
    anatomy 35
Voiding difficulty
    advanced assessment of 336
Volunteer
    emergency care providers 510
Vomiting 274
    emergency care of 278

W

Walking wounded   395
Wallet cards   295
Water   24, 28
    balance   28
    solar stills   28
Water emergencies   427
Weakness
    complaint of   316
    advanced assessment of   336
Wheezes   268
Wilderness   475
    basic survival requirements of   477
    CPR in   477
    emergency care in   476
    extended patient care in   477
    injury in   481
    patient assessment in   476
    travel postponed   480
Wilderness Medical Associates   357
Wilderness Search and Rescue (SAR)
    emergency care kit   499
Windburn   321
Windchill   15, 17
Wire splints   160
Witnesses
    interview   338
Women, special problems   494, 495
Wool   15
Wound
    emergency care of   499
    chest   245
    closed   245
Wrist dislocation
    emergency care of   192
Wrist drop   59
Wrist fracture
    emergency care of   191
Wrist sprain   188
    emergency care of   188

Y

Yankauer tip   120
Yoke-style regulator   115
Young Adult Male Immortality Complex
    (YAMIC)   385

Z

Zippers   17